D1362349

LONG-TERM
CARE
Perspectives from
Research and Demonstrations

Ronald J. Vogel, Ph.D.
The University of Arizona

Hans C. Palmer
Pomona College

Editors

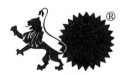

AN ASPEN PUBLICATION®
Aspen Publishers, Inc.
Rockville, Maryland
Royal Tunbridge Wells
1985

Library of Congress Cataloging in Publication Data

Main entry under title:
Long-term care.

"An Aspen publication."
Includes index.
1. Long-term care of the sick—United States. 2. Long-term
care facilities—United States. 3. Community health
services—United States. 4. Nursing homes—United States.
I. Vogel, Ronald J. II. Palmer, Hans C. [DNLM: 1. Long
Term Care—in old age. 2. Home Care Services—United
States. 3. Day Care—in old age. 4. Nursing Homes—
United States. WT 30 L8485]
RA644.6.L664   1985   362.1′6   84-18468
ISBN: 0-89443-572-8

Aspen Publishers, Inc., 1600 Research Boulevard,
Rockville, Maryland 20850.

ISBN: 0-89443-572-8
Library of Congress Catalog Card Number: 84-18468

Printed in the United States of America

3   4   5

Contents

Part 3: The Nursing Home

Preface

Between 1970 and 1980, expenditures on the long-term care population increased at an average annual rate of 27 percent. This rate of increase was greater than that of any other expenditure category in the health care sector. Moreover, the elderly population grew at a more rapid rate than the population as a whole and will continue to do so in the foreseeable future. This combination of financial and demographic realities has generated considerable concern in the Congress, in State legislatures, and in local governments across the country.

Because of this concern, many Federal agencies, such as the Social Security Administration, the National Center for Health Services Research, the Administration on Aging, and the Health Care Financing Administation, funded numerous research and demonstration projects on the multifaceted subject of long-term care during the 1970s. Although some of these studies were done on an intramural basis, the majority were funded extramurally. Consequently, this large accumulated body of knowledge has never been systematically synthesized into a coherent whole, nor has much of this knowledge been pushed to the limits to which it seemed capable.

In the beginning of 1980, certain circumstances made it possible to create such a synthesis. There was a growing recognition throughout the Department of Health and Human Services that long-term care was a pressing issue, and would become even more so, because of its growing financial and demographic magnitude. Task forces had been formed to look into various aspects of the looming problem; the subject of long-term care seemed to be discussed by everyone, both inside and outside DHHS, with much more frequency than in the past. At the same time, a group of individuals had assembled in the Division of Economic Analysis of the Office of Research, HCFA, who were intensely interested in long-term care and all of the problems that it posed, and who had done previous research in the area or in areas related to it.

This project was begun in February 1980 by that group. Its stated purposes were to provide a general synthesis of the research on long-term care that had been done, to push that research forward as much as possible, and to highlight areas of research that might be fruitfully pursued in the future, both inside and outside of HCFA. It is our hope that this volume has achieved those stated purposes, and,

i

consequently, that its contents will provide useful information for policymakers and researchers, stimulate further research, and ultimately benefit those in need of long-term care.

Judith R. Lave, Ph.D.
Director
Office of Research

Acknowledgments

Many people gave us help, advice, and comments during the long course of this study. Judith Lave, Director, Office of Research, HCFA, facilitated the work by providing many scarce resources. The entire manuscript was reviewed by the University Health Policy Consortium, whose Center for Health Policy Analysis and Research is located at the Florence Heller Graduate School, Brandeis University. Stanley Wallack, the Director of the Center, with James Callahan, a Deputy Director, and Christine Bishop, a Senior Research Associate, coordinated and participated in the review. Besides Wallack, Callahan, and Bishop, members of the Consortium who gave critical comments on the various chapters were Leonard Gruenberg, Edward Locke, Marcia Mabee, Thomas McGuire, Mead Over, Alonzo Plough, Alan Sager, Margaret Stassen, Sanford Weiner, Judith Williams, and Paul Youket. The manuscript was also reviewed in its entirety by Judith Feder, John Holahan, and William Scanlon of the Urban Institute.

In addition, the following people gave us advice on various technical points and many times kept us from going astray: Elaine Brody, Philadelphia Geriatric Center; Stanley Brody, School of Medicine, University of Pennsylvania; John Grana, Office of the Assistant Secretary for Planning and Evaluation, DHHS; Sidney Katz, School of Medicine, Michigan State University; Kenneth McCaffree, Emeritus, University of Washington and Batelle Human Affairs Research Centers; Mark Meiners, National Center for Health Services Research; Robert Seidman, formerly at the Office of Research, HCFA and now at San Diego State University; William Weissert, formerly at the National Center for Health Services Research and now at the University of North Carolina; and Thomas Willemain, formerly at Harvard University and the University Health Policy Consortium.

Donna Levin Siegel gave us invaluable editing input throughout the many reviews and revisions of this manuscript, especially in its latter stages in 1981–82. Without her constant attention to detail and her persistence in scheduling, there is doubt that this book would have appeared in such a timely and polished fashion. We especially wish to acknowledge her contribution as editor.

Pat Hough, Annette Johns, Vernice Neal and Melissa Sterling conscientiously typed most of the many drafts necessary for final completion.

While any credit must be shared with all of these people, the authors of the various chapters, as well as the editors, assume full responsibility for what follows. Likewise, the statements and data contained in this monograph are solely those of the authors and do not express any official opinion of or endorsement by the Health Care Financing Administration, nor by the U.S. Department of Health and Human Services.

Introduction and Summary

by Ronald J. Vogel and Hans C. Palmer

Purpose and Framework

Long-term care (LTC) is medical care, nursing care, health care, mental health care, and social services, provided in the context of adequate income, however defined. Its purpose is to relieve the effects of illness and to maintain or enhance functional capacities to maximize personal independence. It may well be the major health and social issue of the next four decades, polarizing society ove₁ the next 20 to 40 years.

Stanford economist Michael Boskin's warning about social security could apply equally to long-term care:

> If we wait until the baby-boom generation retires before we begin to deal with the tremendous long-term deficit in Social Security, we will see the greatest tax revolt and age warfare in the history of the United States.[1]

The financial and resource needs of LTC may compete fiercely with those of defense, education, energy, and welfare, creating much political controversy.

The dimensions of the LTC problem are rooted in the basic demographics of American society. Anne Somers provides a useful catalogue of these developments in an article in the November 1980, issue of *Inquiry:*

- Life expectancy at age 65 rose by nearly 1.5 years between 1965 and 1975. A 65 year old in 1980 could expect to live to age 81, an 85 year old to age 91. In 1975, a 65 year old white female could expect to live to age 83, a black female to 82. Males at 65 could expect to live only to 79 or so, leaving many dependent widows.
- The number of Americans 65 and older has grown from about four million in 1900 to 24 million in 1979, and will continue to rise at least until the year 2035. By 2030, there may be 55 million people over 65.
- Depending on fertility projections, the ratio of retirement-age elderly to the younger working-age groups (18 to 64 year olds) may range from 1:2.4 to 1:4. The resource-absorbing implica-

---

[1] *Newsweek,* June, 1981, p. 25

tions of this burden of dependence and of the associated burdens of LTC and income maintenance are awesome.

- Among the group over 65, the proportion of those over 75 (the "old old") will grow, as will that of the group over 85. By the year 2000, those over 75 will amount to 45 percent of the over 65 group (up from 38 percent in 1980) and by 2040 will account for more than 50 percent, more than the total number of those over 65 today. Most ominous in terms of LTC dependency is the proportion of those over 85, the most LTC-dependent group in the society. They will amount to 12 percent of the over 65 group by the year 2000.
- There will be more single women in the group over 65, a fact suggested by male-female differences in life expectancies. The ratio is now 1.5 women over 65 to every male, and it is not expected to change dramatically. A portent of future need, however, is the expected 2.5 women over 85 for every man over 85 by the year 2000.
- There will be more elderly members of minority groups. The minority elderly population is expected to rise by 60 percent, versus 30 percent for the overall elderly between 1980 and 2000. Blacks will account for 9.5 percent of the elderly by the latter year. This minority increase may result in the growth of an LTC-dependent group which is poorer than earlier elderly groups and which may have aggravated health problems.

Since LTC dependency is very much a function of advancing age, the demographic reality just outlined presents the United States with an extraordinary task in terms of both money and providing services over the next 40 years at least. We have, of course, been dealing with this task to some degree for much of our history, but its real dimensions have only recently been recognized, in light of the introduction of Medicare and Medicaid in 1966 and the growth of the nursing home industry.

An emergent awareness of the scope of the LTC burden and of its implications for the development of a services system raises some important policy and analytical issues:

- Where will and should this LTC be provided? Will we continue the pattern of institutional development so characteristic of the years since 1966? Will we attempt to develop more community-focused systems of services and modes of care to provide the necessary levels of care in a more personally satisfying and/or cost-effective setting?
- If we decide on a more community-oriented care system, will the community supports be available to provide care and other support? Will community-based care serve as a substitute for,

or an add-on to, institutionalized care? Will we find that we still need to develop more institutions as the number of those over 85 continues to grow?

- How much care should we provide? How do we pay for this care and provide the resources it requires? What portion of it should be financed through the government? How will LTC compete for resources as the costs rise for defense, energy, and services to younger people?
- What financial mechanisms most efficiently evoke needed responses from LTC suppliers, and what financial provisions will ensure care for the needy without raising the use of services to unacceptably high levels? How will inflation affect these resource requirements and financial mechanisms?
- How will changes in the family affect members' ability to provide care in the home? How will the need to provide care to a growing group of vulnerable older people affect the family? What will be the result of more women in the labor force?

The Health Care Financing Administration (HCFA) is uniquely well suited to examine past and current research on LTC and to project the future resource needs for LTC in American society. HCFA's two major programs, Medicare and Medicaid, have been important financing sources for LTC in recent years and have undoubtedly influenced, if not determined, the existing structure of LTC provision in the United States.

HCFA, other parts of the Department of Health and Human Services (DHHS), other agencies, private researchers, and private interest groups have all studied various aspects of LTC. Few comprehensive assessments, however, have brought together in a general framework the many user, provider, financing, and regulatory aspects of LTC. For example, one very rich, though relatively unknown and unintegrated, component of the research has focused on demonstrations which test the feasibility, practicability, and outcomes of home care. Many of these were undertaken by States or local governments with HCFA support.

This collection of analytical essays brings together significant aspects of LTC research and relates them to critical policy issues. The perspective is that of the social sciences, although contributions from the medical and biological sciences are also included. No final answers are forthcoming from this effort, which is largely aimed at identifying problems, summarizing the research on those problems, and indicating directions for future research. We hope that this book will help in the common search for solutions to the problems of long-term care in which the Congress, the Department of Health and Human Services, other government agencies, the States, and various private groups are all cooperating.

The book is divided into three parts. Part 1 defines long-term care and places it in its personal and systemic setting. Next, we identify goals and objectives, especially policy goals for LTC. Part 2 analyzes the various forms of community care available for the long-term care population. Finally, Part 3 considers the nursing home as a source of long-term care provision.

Although our pattern is often that of the economist's model of supply and demand, we do not seek determinate solutions or definable demand and supply functions. That is a task for future research. Rather, we have surveyed existing efforts and tried to identify key causes of LTC usage and provision, the latter in part through an institutional analysis of important types of LTC providers. We have also tried to provide some suggestions for future research by highlighting those analytical, historical, and institutional issues about which we need to learn more.

Part 1: Population and System Characteristics

Chapter I

In the first chapter of this section, Palmer examines long-term care within a systems context. A coherent system of long-term care requires a clearly defined set of goals, with trade-offs among conflicting goals explicitly stated. Public goals for long-term care are (1) *access* to care for those who need it, (2) the delivery of *quality* care, and (3) *cost-effectiveness* in the delivery of care. Actual public goals, however, may reflect administrative and bureaucratic imperatives and the political influence of prospective LTC client groups, as much as the publicly stated objectives. Furthermore, the definitions of quality and access have not been clarified, nor do analysts and policymakers all agree on their meanings. Individual goals include restoration of health and/or physical functioning, maintenance of independence, and even death with dignity. Contradictions between public and private goals must be identified, since trade-offs may be required. It must also be recognized that individual goals may be altered by the changes in incentives as public programs pursue their goals to accommodate specific individual requirements. Having identified these goals, we need an economically efficient method for achieving them.

Long-term care is characterized by myriad requirements, multiple services, the central role of the family and other community institutions, and the presence of the government in various forms—provider, paymaster, etc. Because of the multiplicity of services and because of complex supportive relationships, LTC must be considered from a systems perspective, both analytically and organizationally.

Perspectives on the need for LTC and the resulting policy must incorporate interactions between individual needs and perceptions of needs, the role of the family, and the roles of professionals as individual providers and as interdisciplinary team members giving care and guiding the use of care-providing resources. We must also recognize the need for a systemic and systematic approach interpreting and organizing the institutions of LTC—nursing homes, hospitals, home health agencies, adult day care centers, domiciliary care facilities, etc.—so that care and support are cost-effective and enhance the lives of recipients as well as answering the need of society in general. Similarly, we need to devise organizational systems to finance and channel LTC to maximize its effectiveness and minimize duplication and waste. Palmer uses recent analyses of these systemic imperatives to outline the nature of an ideal LTC system and to suggest the organizational and structural dimensions of such a system.

Chapter II

In Chapter II, Horen sets out the beginnings of an operations research (OR) approach to the long-term care problem. Although little operations research work in the United States has been directed specifically to long-term care, OR has been successfully applied in areas of service delivery, such as hospitals, in Great Britain. On the macro level, OR models can explicitly incorporate objectives for the total system of health care or for subsystems such as the various modalities of long-term care. The most important result of these macro models is that they efficiently solve system problems, once the goals and the problems have been clearly defined. Another important outcome of these models is that their construction and solution force policymakers to consider all of the factors that enter into the achievement of stated objectives (that is, their "objective function").

On the micro level, models used for other fields of health care can be adapted for long-term care in the OR context. For example, the efficiency of individual institutions can be studied to determine the amount of benefits achieved in relation to resources used. There are already OR methodologies to measure the efficiency of institutions, such as schools and public transportation, which produce more than one output. There is no reason why similar methodologies cannot be used for the long-term care system. Horen gives heuristic examples of both macro and micro applications to long-term care problems and shows how an operations research approach to long-term care can yield fruitful insights for researchers and policymakers.

Chapter III

In this chapter, Liu, Manton, and Alliston analyze the demographic and epidemiologic determinants of long-term care expenditures. They first contend that prior efforts to estimate public expenditures for long-term care are imprecise because the many determinants have not been thoroughly examined. These influences include population composition, mortality, morbidity, and disability, and their dynamic interrelationships. The authors analyze the relationship between population dynamics and disease and disability and treat the conceptual and operational issues concerning morbidity and mortality. They next examine conventional approaches toward estimating the magnitude of need for long-term care in the U.S. population and discuss bioactuarial models as an alternative strategy to the usual approaches. They conclude that there is a need for further research on the individual roles and interrelationships of the underlying components of long-term care expenditures.

Chapter IV

Quality of care includes a wide range of concepts associated with professionally recognized standards of care. In Chapter IV, Kurowski and Shaughnessy show that the results of long-term care research generally support the conclusion that the relationships between structural measures of quality and the process of care, and between the process of care and its outcomes, are not well established. Nevertheless, a reasonable amount is known about certain aspects of such relationships and, therefore, about specific issues related to measuring the quality of long-term care. Structural criteria are least likely to reflect process and outcome quality in areas such as patient activities, social services, and rehabilitative services. Such criteria do not indicate whether the organization actually has a functioning program and whether it actually provides services to patients who need them. Process criteria generally represent a useful and common tool for evaluating the quality of care. However, the relationship between structural or process measures and patient outcome has not yet been consistently demonstrated. Although patient outcome represents the final validation of the care process, it is difficult to specify appropriate outcomes of care and to relate individual outcomes to the process of care. Moreover, assessment of the outcome of long-term care must consider the initial characteristics and overall potential of the individual patients. Finally, in addition to validated measures and accurate data, other necessary conditions for determining the true relationships between the three types of measures of the quality of care are adequate sample sizes, financial resources, and time.

Research priorities on outcomes and quality include (1) refined measures of the quality of care, (2) the relationship between process and outcome measures of quality, (3) the development of optimal outcomes of care, (4) refinement of case-mix measures, (5) evaluation of incentives to change provider behavior, and (6) study of the relationship between quality and the cost of care.

Chapter V

Chapter V provides the basic LTC data on utilization and provision used in the analytic chapters in Parts 2 and 3. Lloyd and Greenspan examine the major public sources for providing long-term care (Medicare, Medicaid, Title XX, and OAA Title III) with the latest and most extensive data available from HCFA and DHHS. This is the first time that all of these data (on nursing homes, home health and homemaker services, and adult day care) have been compiled in this fashion. The authors review these sources of long-term care provision from the perspective of costs, utilization, and supply. These data yield some interesting overviews of long-term care activity and give some insight into future problems in long-term care.

Chapter VI

In general, the social sciences have achieved some success in broadly predicting responses of individuals and institutions to various incentive systems. However, modern-day governmental programs are often complex and offer myriad incentives. Thus, they reflect the society from which these programs originate and in which they progress and interact with one another. In short, *a priori* knowledge and theory will not always yield precise enough answers to questions about the financial and human consequences of proposed policy enactments, innovations, or changes. For that reason, the Health Care Financing Administration supports a relatively large demonstration program that has two primary purposes: feasibility testing of new models of care and finance and formal experimentation and/or evaluation of existing programs. As an example of the former, HCFA has recently undertaken demonstrations on the human and economic aspects of terminal care hospices. In addition, the Agency has experimented with many aspects of the existing Medicare program (for example, expansions of adult day care) and has encouraged the States to experiment with their Medicaid programs (such as changes in certification procedures for nursing homes) by granting waivers of the Social Security Act, Title XVIII (Medicare), and Title XIX (Medicaid) provisions and/or regulations, and by awarding special Federal research funds to the States. In Chapter VI and its Appendix, Hamm, Kickham, and Cutler describe HCFA's current demonstrations in some detail and report the results and findings of these demonstrations to date.

Part 2: Community Care

Chapter VII

Dissatisfaction with the nursing home as a vehicle for offering appropriate, high-quality care at reasonable cost has stimulated a focus on alternatives to nursing homes. As a prelude to analyzing specific alternatives in the following chapters, in Chapter VII Palmer discusses what we know about alternatives in general and what remains to be considered. Emphasizing that alternatives may be complements as well as substitutes in a spectrum of care, he points out that the question of alternatives poses problems of cost comparisons.

Since their inception in 1966, Medicare and Medicaid have introduced such strong structural and incentive biases toward institutionalization and toward the medical model that there has been little experience with alternatives and even less information about them. Lack of experience hinders development of information which, in turn, further restricts the use of alternatives. Furthermore, insufficient insurance, limited incomes, and the regulations surrounding Supplemental Security Income (SSI), social security payments, and pensions also deter the use of alternatives. At an analytical and program level, lack of consistent criteria among patient assessors, lack of appropriate long-term care screening procedures for Professional Standards Review Organizations (PSROs), and lack of satisfactory process or outcome measures combine to hinder the planning, development, and evaluation of alternative long-term care systems. Theoretical knowledge of alternatives is limited, and more work on theories of comparative evaluation and on designing experiments to develop data for evaluations is needed.

Chapter VIII

In Chapter VIII, Sangl shows that the family continues to be the essential support system for the overwhelming majority of the elderly. She reports that families provide 80 percent of the personal and health-related care to the elderly who are chronically ill. There are two major indicators of the importance of the family: (1) the large percentage of bedfast and homebound elderly who still reside in the community, principally because of family support, and (2) the presence of family support for the elderly resident in the community, as opposed to the lack of family of those in institutions. While the caring burden on the family can be enormous, with the emotional strain generally greater than any financial strain, research has shown that families view institutionalization as a last resort. Presently, no incentives are offered to the family to retain the elderly in the community or to prevent unnecessary and premature institutionalization. In fact, certain programs, such as Supplemental Security Income (SSI) and food stamps, penalize the family support system.

The literature suggests several types of economic and service incentives to sustain family caregiving. With any incentive, cost is a major concern, and it is unclear whether such incentives may supplant rather than supplement family caregiving. Since the family is the major caregiver for the elderly, it is important that policy be formulated which views the elderly in the context of the family network, considering the caregivers' needs as well as those of the elderly. Public programs should be reviewed to determine any negative effect on the family support system. Moreover, policymakers must remain alert to changing demographics and family situations, especially the increased participation of women, who are the principal caregivers, in the labor force. Further research is needed on present family networks, emerging family forms (including family surrogates), and types of programs that would best support family caregiving.

Chapter IX

In Chapter IX, Palmer begins by distinguishing between two polar types of home care (HC). Home care is classified as "intensive" when it is aimed at reducing nursing home stays and features heavy medical/nursing involvement and high technology apparatus in the home. It is classified as "basic" (maintenance and/or personal) when it is designed to sustain dependents in the community and avoid custodial institutionalization. Currently, there are 2,900 Medicare/Medicaid-certified HC providers nationwide. In 1978, Medicare spent $427 million and Medicaid $211 million on home care; these expenditures are relatively low because under the Medicare/Medicaid regulations, only "medical" services prescribed by a physician (and usually services only to the home-bound) have qualified for reimbursement.

Home care research suffers from poor problem and outcome specification, lack of theoretical models linking inputs to outcomes, inability to ensure comparability of client groups, and the failure to identify secondary, tertiary, and family costs. Until now, comparisons of users and non-users of home care suggest few differences in physical functioning, institutionalization, or length of stay in institutions. Lastly, there seems to be a break-even point beyond which institutionalization is actually less costly than home care.

Chapter X

In Chapter X, Thomas examines housing and the dimensions of LTC dependency. He points out that the elderly are vulnerable to the environment in which they live and that "adequacy" (enough, but not too much, space) and "appropriateness" (usable space) must be the two major guideposts in housing for the elderly. Although income is the primary determinant of the living environment, there is currently no spectrum of housing for the elderly which accommodates a matching spectrum of their incomes or their needs. Moreover, present government policy subsidizes housing for the independent elderly rather than for the partially impaired elderly who do not need to be institutionalized. Thomas advocates eliminating the present institutional bias from income maintenance and health care financing programs. He concludes that the housing requirements of the elderly and chronically impaired must be studied further, especially to integrate various types of provision and support.

Chapter XI

Chapter XI considers adult day care (ADC) as part of a set of services provided to the dependent elderly to combine nursing, medical, and social services that may be difficult to administer at home and for which economies of scale may be realized in a central locale. Currently, there are about 600 ADC programs in 45 States, providing about 13,500 visits annually. Financial support for ADC is broadly based and fragmented. Medicare and Medicaid do not pay for ADC *per se,* but only for certain medical services in ADC programs, when prescribed by a physician.

As with other long-term care programs, ADC should be analyzed with respect to access, quality, and cost. Even though ADC programs in Massachusetts and California have been officially monitored at the State level, little is known about access, and even less is known about quality. Moreover, controversy still exists about the costs of ADC and their comparability to the costs of other forms of long-term care. More research is needed on the population that might benefit from ADC, on service packages offered in different day care programs, on labor force and space requirements for ADC, on appropriate safeguards or regulations, on useful costing methods, and on data systems.

Chapter XII

In Chapter XII, Palmer considers another alternative, domiciliary care. Domiciliary care facilities (DCFs) encompass a wide range of settings and services, including room, board, shelter, recreation, and sheltered work supervision. However, settings vary in number and amounts of services offered. Thus, the domiciliary care issue primarily relates to the provision of care for vulnerable, frail people needing only occasional medical assistance at about the same rate as the general population.

There are three factors responsible for the recent growth of DCFs: (1) a rapid increase in the number of persons 75 years and older; (2) the emergence of Federally financed income maintenance programs, especially Supplemental Security Income for the elderly, blind, and disabled; and (3) extensive deinstitutionalization from State mental hospitals. One of the key questions for the DCF revolves around the possibility of creating a humane and safe alternative to the mental hospital and intermediate care facility.

Little research has been done on DCFs, primarily because many are difficult to locate. As a potentially viable and less expensive alternative to the nursing home for the less severely disabled, there are many aspects about the DCF that we still need to study. Among these are (1) facts about possible candidates for deinstitutionalization who could be adequately served by DCFs, (2) the relative costs of DCFs and mental hospitals for comparable client groups, (3) the number of people who would never have been hospitalized had DCFs been available, and (4) the totality and types of dependence and their influence on the supply and demand for long-term care facilities, influences that include State Medicaid and social service policies.

Chapter XIII

Lack of transportation can create dependency, and, at the margin, push the elderly and impaired toward institutionalization. Chapter XIII shows how accessibility to transportation is difficult for the elderly and impaired both because of system and vehicular barriers.

Transportation problems also are intimately related to the housing problem and to the low income of the elderly. Given present living arrangements, transportation is simply not available for the majority of the elderly and disabled. For example, many of the elderly live in rural areas where no public transportation exists. Even where public transportation is available, it is often unreliable and poses problems for persons with physical handicaps. Perhaps the solution to LTC-related transport can only be achieved in conjunction with a solution to the housing and income problems of the elderly. Transportation difficulties emphasize the need for a total systems approach to enhance the well-being of the elderly and impaired and to address their LTC problems.

Chapter XIV

Another factor that enters into the demand for long-term care is the high incidence of mental illness in the elderly relative to the general population. In Chapter XIV, Hall reports that 15 percent to 20 percent of the elderly in the community have moderate to severe mental illness; she also finds that 50 percent to 65 percent of nursing home residents have serious mental problems. Despite their high vulnerability to mental health problems, the elderly are slower than other age groups to recognize mental problems. Even if they do define their symptoms in psychiatric terms, they encounter many barriers to treatment. Research has indicated that many mental illnesses of the elderly are treatable, but psychiatric treatment is expensive and is inadequately covered by Medicare and Medicaid. Changes in the financing of health care could encourage better mental health treatment for the elderly. Furthermore, early treatment could prevent deterioration which often results in institutionalization. One result of the incentives that Medicaid gives the States is that many of the elderly mentally ill have been transferred from State mental hospitals to nursing homes; however, mental health services do not follow the elderly into nursing homes. In light of these problems, both the Department of Health and Human Services and the Department of Housing and Urban Development are exploring alternative modes of treatment and living arrangements for the elderly who are mentally ill.

Part 3: The Nursing Home

Chapter XV

Chapter XV traces the evolution of the long-term care system through its legislative history. Although his focus is on nursing home care, Waldman shows how government support has both directly financed long-term care and provided income maintenance often used to purchase long-term care in various forms. Before the Depression, public support for the elderly and disabled was provided mainly at the local level in county poorhouses. The first significant piece of social legislation that helped to stimulate demand for nursing home care was Old Age Assistance, enacted in 1935. From that time until the enactment of Medicare and Medicaid in 1966, various benefits for the elderly, combined with subsidy programs for building nursing homes, nudged public provision toward institutional modes of care.

The Medicare and Medicaid programs further increased public demand for nursing home care. Public expenditures for this care rose dramatically to almost $18 billion in fiscal year 1979. Continued increases in social security benefits and the creation of the Supplemental Security Income (SSI) program in 1972 further enhanced the ability of the elderly to purchase nursing home care. Simultaneously, the structure of the Medicaid matching formula and its primarily medical orientation have provided incentives to the States to transfer patients from State mental institutions to nursing homes supported by Medicaid. We might also infer that the relatively high marginal "tax" rate placed upon the supplemental security income of those elderly living with their families has provided a further incentive to purchase nursing home services.

Waldman provides a descriptive analysis of the role of the voluntary nursing home sector in the Appendix to Chapter XV. These homes were primarily initiated by immigrant and religious groups and by voluntary hospitals and continue to be maintained by them, although much financial support now comes from patient-generated income as in nursing homes run for profit. As a result of the evolution of social programs supporting both types of homes, it appears that the modern-day voluntary home is not much different from the for-profit home in many respects. Differences in the behavior of non-profit homes are amenable to theoretical analysis, as Palmer and Vogel show in detail in Chapter XVI.

Chapter XVI

Palmer and Vogel analyze formal economic models of for-profit and non-profit nursing homes in Chapter XVI. One would expect pricing and output decisions in this industry to occur in the same fashion as they do in any monopolistically competitive industry. However, due to the Medicare and Medicaid programs, the provider faces peculiarly shaped demand functions. As a consequence, the provider becomes a price-setter for the private segment of the market and a price-taker from the public sector. Depending upon the level of costs and the level of demand curves that he/she faces, the provider may not wish to accept public-pay patients at all, or may not accept as many as might want entry at a given level of public payment and subsidized (to the users) prices. The authors analyze the question of subsidies between public and private patients and distinguish between internal and external subsidies. They then discuss "substandard care" and show that, theoretically, substandard care has both a quantitative and a qualitative dimension, although the data on this point are somewhat unclear. At bottom, substandard care for publicly supported patients may be all that taxpayers are willing to finance. The resolution of this policy dilemma may hinge on the discovery of alternative sources to public funding or more cost-effective means of providing care.

Chapter XVII

In Chapter XVII Vogel provides an industrial organization analysis of the nursing home industry, using the classical I–O paradigm. Such an analysis involves an investigation of the market structure, market conduct, and market performance of the industry. The market structure of the nursing home industry can be characterized as one having many sellers and many buyers, but buyers (or public-pay consumers) are both physically and mentally debilitated, and consequently lack information and mobility. Moreover, certificate-of-need regulations have created excess demand by public-pay patients. In light of demonstrated consumer behavior, the effects of certificate-of-need, the monopolistically competitive structure of the sellers' market, and the alleged abuses by nursing homes in the past, it would appear that nursing home operators have some measure of market power over consumers. Although government pays for 57 percent of all nursing home services, mainly through the Medicaid program, it cannot directly exercise monopsonistic countervailing power in the nursing home market because, legally, users have freedom of choice. It can, however, influence use and provision through regulation and eligibility determination. However, there has been considerable controversy about the effectiveness, usefulness, consistency and coordination of government regulation and enforcement in this market, which is composed of 54 Medicaid jurisdictions, each having different policies. Quality of the output of the industry, how to measure it (see Chapter IV) and what to do about it are also all matters of dispute.

Investment theory predicts certain outcomes in response to varying incentives provided by public policy. This chapter also outlines the relevant investment theory in some detail. Since the beginning of the Medicare and Medicaid programs, incentives have been weighted in favor of investments in nursing homes, to the virtual exclusion of investments in alternative modes of long-term care. Although the nursing home industry has grown rapidly, recent empirical evidence on the growth and profitability of the industry is equivocal. Growth has slowed, but this could result from lower profitability relative to other investments in the economy or from certificate-of-need regulations. The nursing home profitability question and the possibility of enhancing the profitability of alternatives to institutionalization need more careful research.

Chapter XVIII

Provider incentives under alternative nursing home reimbursement systems is the issue that Cotterill addresses in Chapter XVIII. In recent years, fiscal constraints have led individual States to strengthen the cost containment potential of their Medicaid reimbursement systems, typically by imposing various types of cost limits on cost-related systems. These changes might be expected to have worsened public patients' access to quality care. However, Cotterill shows that, even in the absence of cost containment pressures, the present cost-based reimbursement method provides weak access and quality incentives.

The disadvantages of cost-based reimbursement are particularly serious when the demand for nursing home care is so great that facilities can readily fill their beds with whatever severity of case-mix they choose. Under these circumstances, cost-based reimbursement subsidizes a more severe private case-mix and higher quality of care for private patients than does flat rate reimbursement. However, neither system gives providers any incentives to accept public patients who require more care or to provide more than minimal quality of care for public patients.

A possible solution to these problems is to modify flat rate systems to include quality and case-mix rate adjustments for public patients. However, systems of this type are complex and their effectiveness remains to be demonstrated. A critical issue is their ability to offset providers' preferences for patients requiring little care.

Chapter XIX

Chapter XIX provides a state-of-the-art analysis of the determinants of nursing home costs. Palmer surveys economic studies on the subject, in part using a framework developed by Christine Bishop. He finds that research results are equivocal as to scale effects arising from either size or occupancy rate. For-profit providers seem to have lower costs than non-profit providers; hospital-based homes have higher costs. Region of the country is also an important determinant of costs, with higher costs in the north and east. State regulatory activity also seems to increase costs, as does prospective reimbursement. Available services and patient condition appear to have a direct relation to level of costs, although research results are again equivocal. Public pay admissions have a strong positive effect on costs.

Structural analyses of nursing home costs have yielded some important results for public policy. Among these findings are that (1) cost control policies inhibit public-pay patient access, (2) lack of links between characteristics of patients and average operating costs may indicate that very debilitated patients are not receiving intense enough nursing and rehabilitative services, (3) certificate-of-need programs increase occupancy rates, (4) low occupancy penalties increase access for public patients, and (5) cost containment programs widen gaps between public and private-pay rates, implying either high private-pay profits or private internal subsidy of public patients (or both). Although all of the findings on nursing home costs have yet to be reconciled, and not as much sustained work has been done on these costs as has been done on hospital costs, the research community appears to be rapidly moving toward some general conclusions on the key elements of nursing home costs.

Chapter XX

In Chapter XX, Horen considers the labor supply question in long-term care, a major problem of current concern. Two-thirds of nursing home costs are labor costs. Labor costs account for an even larger proportion of the costs of alternative modes of long-term care provision. Unfortunately, labor-intensive industries share the common characteristic that productivity gains are difficult to achieve because capital is not easily substitutable for labor. Nurses' aides are the persons directly responsible for patient care, but they are difficult to find and to retain and cannot be replaced with capital goods. Labor market theory offers a certain amount of insight into these labor supply problems, since it argues that labor inputs will be hired to the point where their marginal revenue product equals their marginal cost. However, the minimum wage law makes it necessary to pay poorly trained and motivated aides more than their marginal revenue product. Thus, in effect, they do not "earn their keep." Moreover, public welfare programs or other low-skilled jobs offer financially attractive alternatives to the some-what unpleasant task of ministering to the basic needs of the elderly. As a consequence, labor turnover rates are high and job productivity low.

A similar circumstance arises in the market for nurses, although for different reasons. Apparently, nursing is a less attractive profession than it used to be, given the employment opportunities now available to women. Moreover, relatively large gains in hospital wage rates for nurses have helped siphon nursing labor power away from long-term care. This situation presents a pressing problem, and its resolution will not be easy. Capital substitutes are simply neither appropriate nor available. Thus, higher wages for long-term care workers seem to be the only way of attracting the needed skills into this industry and reducing labor turnover. This high-wage solution, however, implies higher long-term care costs, unless labor productivity grows and lower labor turnover costs are not offset by higher wages.

Planning shortages are not the same as economic shortages, but economic shortages may exist in the nursing home labor market due to dynamic lags in the wage adjustment process. Horen concludes with the observation that real labor shortages may not be as great as those that are alleged to exist, because the demand for nursing home care may be artificially inflated by various forms of subsidization. Elimination of some or all of these subsidies would, no doubt, lessen the pressure on labor demand.

Conclusion

One common theme running through all of these chapters is that long-term care is a unique and pervasive part of our society. However, fiscal and demographic realities have only recently forced us to try to articulate clear goals for it. The long-term care population is ill-defined on the spectrum of physical and mental debility and in terms of the supports it requires. Furthermore, we have barely captured the quality dimension of long-term care provision because of the chronic and regressive nature of the problems facing its clientele. We have not really stated what we wanted, nor have we had the means to know whether we have achieved it. Part of the need for LTC stems from processes inherent in the natural process of aging, so that long-term care implies meeting health care needs, as well as income, housing, and transportation needs, in a systemic framework. Until the last few years, little effort was spent on understanding provider responses to various incentive mechanisms. Major emphasis was placed upon a largely publicly-financed medical model that skewed incentives toward institutionalization; little thought was given to alternatives.

The popular press maintains that the United States idolizes youth and vigor, and thus prefers to hide its elderly and debilitated from sight. This may be true, but the inescapable fact is that we are an aging society and the problems of long-term care will loom ever larger if gains in economic productivity do not compensate for upward shifts in the dependency ratio. Such a potential outcome implies that we must learn to provide long-term care in an economically efficient manner, once we have specified societal goals for long-term care.

On one extreme, some would argue that more direct public financing is necessary because long-term care is basically a problem of social insurance and because the elderly cannot protect themselves adequately from providers. From a similar perspective, others would argue that long-term care is more an income problem than anything else and could be accommodated by an expanded social security system. At an opposite extreme, some would rely more on private financing for long-term care. These perspectives reveal basically normative issues about the proper role of the public versus the private sector. This book has not attempted to answer such questions. Rather, the authors of the individual chapters, while sensitive to parameters of policy, have addressed technical problems with respect to the state-of-the-art. They also hope to have pushed the state-of-the-art forward in a modest way in their respective areas of expertise. It is our hope that this research will add to the understanding of long-term care problems now facing the nation and contribute to their resolution. We also hope that our efforts will help to raise the quality of life for those who need long-term care.

Chapter I

The System of Provision

by Hans C. Palmer

This chapter will introduce the general problem of long-term care (LTC) and the analytical and research issues which must be addressed to understand it. We necessarily begin with definitions and proceed to questions of the role of time in LTC for the individual and for society. Since no evaluation of any service provision or system for making such provision can exist without some idea of desired outcomes, we also must raise questions about individual and social and public and private goals of LTC.

Similarly, we need to address questions about the influences of users, providers, and government on the demand for and supply of LTC services:

- To what extent are dependent individuals and their families truly responsible for the use of LTC services?
- Are health and social care professionals involved on both the demand and supply sides of the use and provision of LTC?
- What is the role of government support, public agencies, legislation, reimbursement provisions, and regulation in determining levels and configurations of LTC use?
- Do provider trade groups influence use of LTC?
- How do medical, nursing, social, and rehabilitative professionals, who manage the flow of dependent people, help determine patterns in use of LTC services?
- How are team approaches to LTC important?

We must also look at the system (or lack thereof) of LTC provision. What is a systems approach to LTC? Do we now have one? Why or why not? What would an ideal systems approach look like?

Before addressing these behavioral, organizational, and systemic issues, however, the following additional specific questions, posed by William Weissert (1979), should be considered:

- Which age groups are most likely to need LTC?
- Which medical conditions create the need for LTC?
- What are the near, medium, and longer-run projections about the requirement for LTC?

I wish to thank James Callahan for his useful suggestions for this chapter.

- What are the actual Federal objectives in LTC?
- What types of provision are appropriate to serve identifiable long-term care requirements, by type of requirement?
- What are the current shortfalls in the amount of provision, given the objectives of Federal policy?
- What are the determinants of provider behavior at both the micro and macro levels?
- How have private health insurance systems affected provider behavior, the types of care provided, and the amounts?
- How have Federal reimbursement programs affected provider behavior, the types of care provided, and the amounts?

Together, these sets of questions should guide the LTC analyst and the policymaker. Much of the analytical literature on LTC already addresses some of these issues, yet much of it never brings them together. Other parts of that literature, by contrast, frequently discuss the larger problems with no grounding in data or analytical specifics. Also, some analyses are rich in data, yet poor in analytical conclusions. Similar weaknesses exist in the formulation of policy.

What is Long-Term Care?

Millions of Americans suffer from physical and mental weaknesses which lead to impairment, handicap, and disability.[1] Their disabilities often necessitate a dependence on others, a need for care which often must be given for a long period of time. In our society, although many younger people require LTC, the aged, especially those 75 and older, constitute the great majority of people in such need.[2]

The incidence of chronic, degenerative, disabling conditions seems to increase with age. As a result, cancers, heart and vascular problems, and mental disturbances are the most common causes of death and disability among the elderly. Because of the time aspect of these conditions, more than one-half of all acute hospital bed days are devoted to these sources of morbidity, and it is not surprising that restricted activity days increase along with age. What is not necessarily to be expected is that the rate of bed confinement is also higher for older women than for older men and is also more common among members of lower socioeconomic groups. Overall, the cumulative effects of combined morbidities and the weaknesses

---

[1] For a discussion of the concepts of impairment, disability, and handicap, and of their interactions, see World Health Organization (1977).

[2] Recent medical developments ensuring the survival of birth-damaged children and severely injured younger adults have increased concern about these younger users of LTC services.

2

of age imply that perhaps 30 percent of the population 65 and older requires some assistance and that perhaps 5 percent is totally disabled and housebound. The magnitude of the LTC need may well be enormous, particularly since the number of people 65 and older, and especially those 85 and older, is growing so rapidly (Brody and Messinger, 1979).

Many of these disabled older people need support services rather than sophisticated medical technologies. Indeed, many dependent people need little other than routine types of help with the functions or activities of daily living (ADL) which they can no longer provide for themselves. Although such dependent people may not need highly technical support, the chances are that they will need many types of services, provided from different sources (Brody and Brody, 1980).

Requirements for LTC are thus seen to arise from disease, injury, and the inexorable processes of aging. Although aging is associated with the onset of certain diseases, many physical and mental weaknesses of older people emerge in the aging process itself. Additionally, disease and weaknesses often associated with aging can increase vulnerability to injury. Psychological and emotional weaknesses, as well as social and financial problems, also often contribute to the need for LTC. Moreover, proper care and support demand proper settings and appropriate transportation. Accordingly, the dependent person has to be adequately housed and, often, transported. Many types of support, ranging from high technology, acute medical interventions to the provision of personal services and household chores may thus be required in a given program of long-term care.[3]

The cited requirements reflect the need for a systematic program of support; they reinforce each other and usually appear together, although in different patterns and concentrations depending on individual and community circumstances. Thus, the supports to meet these requirements must be combined in systematically designed structures featuring differing resource mixes. For some dependent people, medical care or nursing is essential and sufficient, while for others "high tech" medicine must be systematically complemented with basic types of social and economic services. For still others, systems of economic or social and psychological support are all that is required.

Paul Grimaldi and Toni Sullivan (1981) have proposed a system for classifying potentially vulnerable people into four dependency

---

[3] An excellent summary of long-term care issues is contained in U.S. Department of Health, Education, and Welfare, Federal Council on Aging, "Key Issues in Long-Term Care—A Progress Report," Washington, D.C., December 1979.

categories. (These categories and their associated required services are shown in Appendix Figures I–A–1 and I–A–2.) Group I, the *Independent*, is essentially "young" old (people 65 to 74) or people who share attributes of that group, for example, having an advanced education, married, usually having a spouse and/or children present, and having infrequent contact with the health and/or social services helping systems. Group II, the *Independence Threatened*, requires high levels of self-care and care from providers. These people are vulnerable to declining health and may require episodes of intensive care.

Those in Group III, the *Independence Delegated*, depend on others for many of the activities of daily living (ADL) and, generally, have lower levels of health and other self-care ability than people in Groups I or II. Their health status is uncertain, possibly because of social situation, the processes of aging, or illness. They often require intensive services not available to them in their immediate environments.

Those in Group IV, the *Dependent*, are in poor health and have very limited self-care abilities. They are disproportionately very old (usually 85 and older), poor, and have little education. Their complex health problems are further compounded by a need for help with bathing, toileting, and walking. They constantly interact with, and require support from, medical, nursing, and other health professionals. Frequently, they are institutionalized (or should be) and/or require intensive home care. Financial and personal stresses accompanying their being at home can force their families to institutionalize them. Maintaining a dependent elder at home usually mandates temporary institutionalization (respite care) if families are to cope. Ideally, people in Group IV and their families should be assisted with adequate home care coupled with timely placements in nursing homes or other institutions.

As Grimaldi and Sullivan state, and as this chapter emphasizes, these varying dependency levels suggest differing types and systems of services. Appropriate linkages among formal health and social services, informally provided services, and capabilities for self-care are crucial to the success of these services. Unfortunately, the nature and functioning of these linkages is, as yet, unknown. All aspects require further theoretical and empirical work. Some linkages (perhaps 30 percent) are made by information and referral programs and transport. Peer groups, special interest groups, voluntary associations, and ombudsmen also match providers with dependent persons. Of course, no satisfactory meeting of requirements can occur unless there are sufficient and appropriate services available.

4

The Elements of Time

The very term "long-term care" suggests a time-related process, the outcomes of which emerge only with time's passage. Time, however, can be viewed in many senses which have implications for providers and users of LTC, the analysis of LTC, and for development of policy responses to the need for LTC.

Time and the Participants in LTC

At a personal level, time is an important dimension having various implications. For users (patients), time is implicated in the effects of long periods of dependency on their capacity to "get well" and on their sense of having to rely on others, often at the cost of their self-esteem. Paradoxically, LTC dependency may also feed on itself, in that the more time people spend in a heavy care environment, the less able they may be to care for themselves independently. Furthermore, the "time-centeredness" of LTC emphasizes the need for a continuity of care, which many caring situations do not provide.

For the caregiver, usually a family member, the time aspects of LTC imply a loss of control over the manner in which time is spent, a loss which increases with the passage of time. Also, this loss of control is matched by the increasing costs of care to the family with the passage of time. Earning opportunities which should expand with experience may be reduced or eliminated because the need to provide care prevents continuity of work. Alternatively, the cost of care provided at home or in a nursing home may rise over time because the patient's condition deteriorates.

Although some studies have shown that the average weekly allocation of time to the care of adults in the family can be measured in minutes, the impact of such time can be considerable. Much more research, however, is needed in this area (Szalai et al, 1972; Robinson, 1977).

To the health/social care professionals, the passage of time may imply different relationships with care receivers, as medical, mental or psycho-social conditions change.

Time as an Input and an Output

Time is additionally an element on both the input and output sides of the LTC process. Both of these aspects of time are important to analyze LTC and develop appropriate policy responses.

First, time serves as input to the caring process. Many of the diseases and conditions leading to the disabilities that create a need for LTC are chronic and/or degenerative. Even for those conditions amenable to "cure" (for example, cerebrovascular accidents, certain cancers, traumas), time is an input in the curing process. Necessary medical procedures may be time-consuming or demand lengthy recovery periods, as with strokes. Rehabilitation requires time, as in recovery from hip fractures. In those situations where a cure is not foreseen, maintaining a given functional level or slowing the rate of deterioration again usually occurs over long periods of time.

Time also figures as an output of LTC activities, since adequate support can lengthen life for the dependent person. Also, appropriate LTC may enhance the quality of life; thus time (added years to be productive or enjoy life) as an output is a key "product" of the caring process.

These roles for time in LTC contrast to the roles of time in acute medical processes. While additional (high quality) time usually is sought as an outcome of acute procedures, the ongoing nature of care, which is central to LTC, is lacking. This suggests that models of care appropriate to the acute and medical setting are not very suitable in LTC.

Time and Changes in Requirements

The requirement for long-term care is not static, either for a given individual or for the society. For some people, the need is clearly defined and emerges from a medical crisis such as a stroke, automobile accident, or nervous breakdown. In many instances, care is needed for a long time, yet there may be a predictable end point when individuals return to a normal level of functioning and ability to care for themselves. In other cases, the need for care ends when the person dies, also at some more or less predictable point. For others, the need for long-term support may continue for an indefinite time. For them, LTC need may reflect aging, possibly the onset of disabling disease, and increasing frailty as they become "frail elderly;" thus the passage of time brings the need for more care. In these last cases, the goal of a support system is to provide some form of maintenance, usually under the assumption that functional capacity will continue to deteriorate or cannot be significantly enhanced, either because of the severity of medical or psycho-social condition or because of aging processes.

It must be emphasized, however, that a gray area exists in which dependent individuals *may* be raised to higher levels of functional capability through service and rehabilitation programs which allow them a less restricted life situation and which may remove the need for many elements in a complex support system (heavy nursing care, for example). Conversely, many individuals given LTC continue to deteriorate over time in their ability to function, though more slowly than without care. Therefore, any consideration of the LTC problem has to recognize the potential of time-related rehabilitation for reducing the magnitude of needed LTC supports. Outcomes may be uncertain, however, and large expenditures for rehabilitation and care may yield few results. Further research is needed on the personal and technical links between outcomes and volumes and types of resources employed in LTC.

Society's overall need for long-term care also changes over time because of shifts in the age structure, disability incidence, and social needs of the population. Wars increase LTC needs because of major disabling injuries. The mean age of the population increases because of a falling birth rate. Changes in social mores and environmental conditions (for example, the increase in divorce, better diet, etc.) reduce or enhance vulnerability to certain medical and psychological difficulties. Obviously, we must consider the nature and effect on services of these potential changes in needs. We must also recognize that they will be affected by seemingly unrelated social policies. For example, more stringent environmental protection policies may reduce the incidence of many impairments, such as emphysema, while shifts in energy policy possibly increase the appearance of others, such as certain forms of cancer.

The Need for a Systemic View

Both the definition of LTC and the role of time in LTC indicate that a systemic view of long-term care is more appropriate than perspectives based on single outcomes or outputs. More importantly, LTC dependency requires a complex set of related services affecting users, families, and the community. Many types of professionals provide these services; many financial sources contribute to them, and many agencies administer them. In addition, current concerns with costs and alleged excessive institutionalization have prompted proposals for more comprehensive, often community-based, structures for care. These structures necessarily must function within a system of care if they are to be effective. Given these systemic imperatives, the following questions are appropriate:

- What are the ingredients of an LTC system?
- How much of an LTC system do we now have?
- What changes must be made to create a satisfactory LTC system?
- What policies are needed, especially at the Federal level, to help create the desired LTC system(s)?

LTC: Many Inputs, Many Outputs

It is a commonplace that the goals of LTC for an individual or a group are not simple nor, usually, readily identifiable. In the first place, those needing LTC are functionally limited because of chronic conditions, several of which occur simultaneously, frequently reinforcing one another. Because of the demographic and epidemiological dynamics discussed in subsequent chapters, major causes of death are no longer acute, infectious illnesses but rather chronic, disabling conditions, often degenerative in their effects. As Stanley Brody points out (1980), health planners, policymakers, and analysts must now be concerned with morbidity and disability rather than mortality. Unfortunately, our policy responses and private attitudes have not adjusted adequately to this reality.[4]

As shown by the list in Figure I–A–3 (taken from Brody, 1979), the range and number of needed supports can be formidable. Callahan (1980) also cites a long list, 70 items in all, which he breaks down into a) intramural, b) intermediate, and c) extramural. (See Figure I–A–4.) He boils the unwieldy plethora down to 15 essential categories: case management, meals on wheels, home health aide, homemaker assistance, physical therapy, physical protection, skilled nursing, telephone assurance, checking, transportation, living supervision, information and referral, emergency medical service, mental health services, and nursing home residential care.

As Brody and Messinger state (1979), the elderly user of these services can be a patient, client, resident, beneficiary, recipient, inmate, applicant, or consumer, depending on the type of service, the nature of the provider, the setting for delivery, or the source of payment. It is also clear from the structure of both of these lists that many dependent elderly need more than one service, orchestrated in a systematic manner, and provided in a true system of integrated provision. Only in a systemic framework, as both Brody and Callahan assert, can these LTC services be made available, adequate, and affordable in a comprehensive, continuous, and coordinated structure (Callahan, 1980).

Settings and Services

In considering the wide range of services and the many sites for provision of care, it is clear that service and setting must be jointly analyzed. Unfortunately, these aspects are too infrequently combined for analysis. For example, Brody and Woodfin (1979), in their analysis of 42 health systems agency plans (executed under the National Health Planning and Resources Development Act of 1974), found that few planners had considered services across a variety of settings. Rather, they had looked at each setting independently or they had considered a given service, nursing, for example, in a variety of settings without any distinctions as to the different roles of nursing in the different settings.

---

[4] As Brody observes, this perspective has been offered by a number of reports on aging and long-term care.

Figure I–1 illustrates one approach to the interaction of services and settings. From this matrix, it appears that certain services may be inherent in a setting, but that others may not naturally, or appropriately, be placed there (DiFederico, Scanlon, and Stassen, 1979). For example, totally independent housing is naturally a setting for shelter. Other services may be provided in the home, but these would usually result from an external contractual relationship or intervention by third parties, often family members living elsewhere. The Urban Institute's matrix also allows analysts and planners to identify those services which may have to be introduced into a setting to provide a given type, level, and quality of care. The matrix also facilitates distinguishing the type of service appropriate to a given setting, for example, the kinds of skilled nursing required as one moves from a hospital to a nursing home. (It should be noted that we have added the acute general hospital to the Urban Institute list of settings.)

The Urban Institute type of services/settings matrix can be usefully juxtaposed to a Veterans Administration matrix which relates disability level to placement alternatives.[5] (See Figure I–2.) Given the proper placement (setting), perhaps determined by the VA-type matrix, analysts and planners can then identify the types of services "naturally" occurring in the setting and move on to identify those services which may have to be added to support a given type of patient. It may be that multiple placements are appropriate or that a philosophy of care dictates a choice of a home setting when an institutional environment may be technically indicated. If so, the nature of the additional services required in the home to serve a given patient may be determined by comparing the naturally occurring services with those suggested by the placement matrix.

The next step would be to determine the amount of each type of service needed for each condition. Ideally, such calculations could be aggregated over categories of vulnerable individuals. Numbers of people in these categories could be determined by demographic and epidemiological techniques. This type of calculation might be effectively accomplished with operations research techniques.

Public Policy and the Lack of System

At present, it is arguable that there is no system of LTC provision in the United States. Although many LTC elements and structures exist, the various parts are not linked together in any systemic (or systematic) fashion, even at the State level. Most analysts of LTC in this country are alarmed at the rapidly rising costs of

---

[5] See Brody and Messinger (1979) for a discussion of the VA model.

FIGURE I-1
Array of Possible Housing Settings for the Elderly and Services Inherent in Each Setting

Housing Settings	Services										
	Shelter	Monitoring	Meal Preparation	Housekeeping and Chore Services	Shopping Errands	Personal Care Intermittent	Personal Care Continuous	Rehabilitation	Skilled Nursing	24-Hour Skilled Nursing	Technical Intervention
General Hospital	X	X	X	X	X	X	X	X	X	X	X
Nursing Homes											
• Skilled Nursing	X	X	X	X	X	X	X	X	X	X	
• Intermediate Care	X	X	X	X	X	X	X	X	X		
Personal Care and Other Homes											
• Personal Care	X	X	X	X	X	X					
• Domiciliary Care	X	X	X	X	X						
Caretaker Environment											
• Foster Home	X	X	X	X	X						
• With Relatives	X	X	X	X	X						
Congregate Housing	X	X	X								
Independent Housing											
• Self and Spouse	X										
• Self	X										

Note: The General Hospital setting has been inserted in the original matrix.

Key: X = Service inherent in a setting.
   Blank = Service not inherent but may be contracted.

Source: DiFederico, Elaine et al., Long-Term Care, Current Experience and a Framework for Analysis, Urban Institute, February 1979, p. 56.

FIGURE I-2
VA Placement Alternatives
by Level of Care Needed

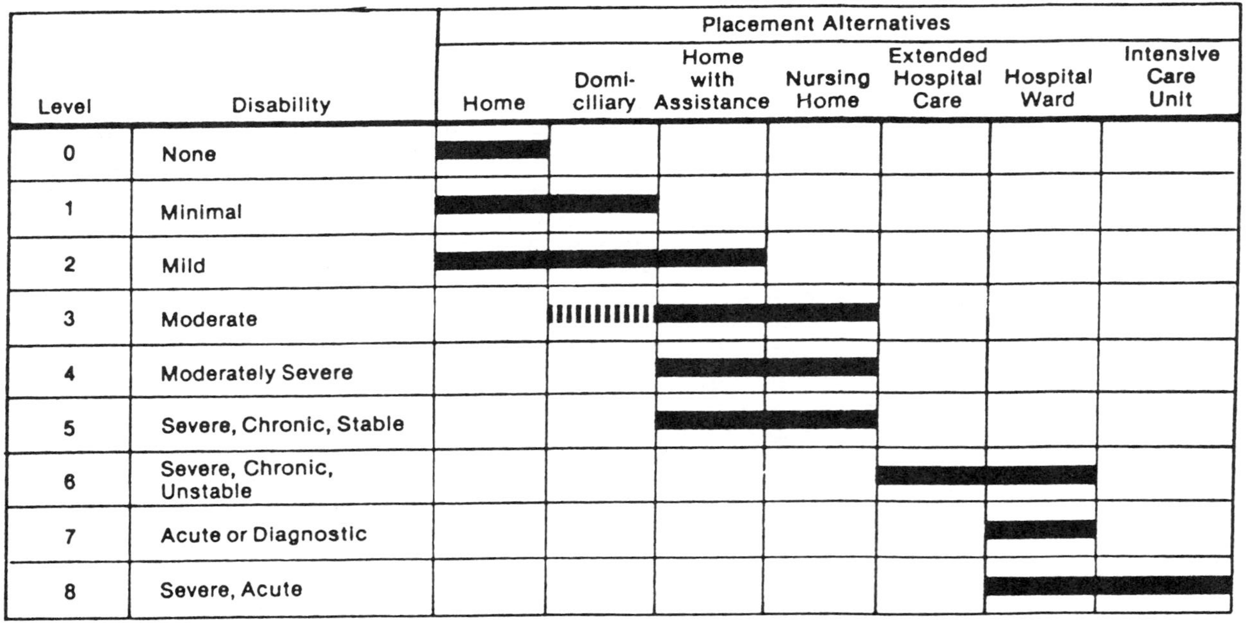

Level	Disability	Placement Alternatives						
		Home	Domiciliary	Home with Assistance	Nursing Home	Extended Hospital Care	Hospital Ward	Intensive Care Unit
0	None	▮						
1	Minimal	▮	▮					
2	Mild	▮	▮	▮				
3	Moderate		▮	▮	▮			
4	Moderately Severe			▮	▮			
5	Severe, Chronic, Stable			▮	▮			
6	Severe, Chronic, Unstable					▮	▮	
7	Acute or Diagnostic						▮	
8	Severe, Acute							▮

Source: Veterans Administration. *The Aging Veteran: Present and Future Medical Needs*, October 1977, Figure B-3, p. 12

nursing home and hospital provision; yet, although the common call is for community-based systems of care, they do not exist in a systemic sense.

These concerns about the lack of an LTC system reflect partial misconceptions about the various elements which could form such a system. Specifically, many observers believe that the relationship among modes of LTC is uniformly one of substitutability. Actually, it is better to think of the various types of care as forming a spectrum, in which services and settings may be complements as well as substitutes. One should consider nursing homes, for example, as sites of service in which skilled nursing care must be provided when the home environment can no longer stand the stress of such provision or when acute hospital interventions are not needed. In this large sense, it is necessary to conceive of modes of provision which together form a system of care. The appropriate sites for users would depend on personal, social, and health status circumstances. Obviously, the position of an individual and the associated appropriate service setting must change as the determinants of dependency change. These larger systemic aspects of LTC will be discussed further in Chapter VII on alternatives, but it is necessary to raise them here as well.

Unfortunately, current public policy seems to fragment, rather than build, an LTC system. To the extent that policy fosters systemic development, that development is highly biased toward institutions. Evidence for these assertions can be found in the very small expenditures of both Medicare and Medicaid on non-institutional medical and health care and social services. Indeed, as Stanley Brody emphasizes (1980), the pattern of Federal LTC programs (to the extent that they exist) suffers from an artificial dichotomy between health and social services, much to the disadvantage of the latter.

This split thinking hinders the development of a system of provision featuring the necessary combination of services. It also heavily influences thinking at the State level which necessarily follows the Federal lead because of the dominant Federal role in financing all programs (Brody and Woodfin, 1979). Furthermore, the heavy medical/institutional bias subverts the emergence of support structures which could help families maintain their dependent elders in the community. In fact, it may hasten institutionalization. Placing older relatives in nursing homes can be cheaper and easier than trying to maintain them at home, either because community-based services are unavailable or because the means tests determining eligibility for institutionalization are less stringent than those conferring a right to home, or other non-institutional, care. Frequently, both situations hold; nursing homes are used because they appear relatively cheap (to the user) and seem more readily available than non-institutional services.

The extent of Federal skewing of LTC provision is shown by the rules governing eligibility and sources of support under different Federal health and social services programs: Titles XVIII, XIX, and XX of the Social Security Act and Title III of the Older Americans Act. For example, homemaker services are most heavily financed under Title XX but in most cases only for those persons with incomes at or below 80 percent of the State median. Home health care is supported under Medicare (XVIII) and Medicaid (XIX) only if prescribed by a physician, and then often only to the homebound. Adult day care services can be provided as a set of individual, medically-related services under Medicaid and as a set of social services under Title XX. Again, as noted by Stanley Brody (1980), what results is a multi-tiered patchwork of programs, which appears even more motley when Title III, Community Mental Health Centers, and the Veterans Administration efforts are included. Ironically the approach to systemic care may lie in the programs of the VA, which may soon have to support a majority of elderly males, veterans of World War II, Korea, and Vietnam.

Many local and State initiatives are aggravating the lack of LTC systems. For example, under the 1974 act, as noted, most health systems agencies developed health services plans which are heavily institutional in nature, largely because incentives under the Act stress cost containment and institutional development (Brody and Woodfin, 1979). Although the Act emphasizes LTC, this mandate has been applied to the nursing home rather than the creation of a multi-faceted system of LTC. This focus reinforces the current assumption that LTC equals medical (institutional) care.

What Should the LTC System Be and Do?

Conceptualizing and then developing a systemic approach to LTC demands specification of system goals. Initially, this requires designation of the target population. The following groups appear to be the main candidates for LTC: the developmentally disabled (including the mentally retarded); those suffering from disabling physical, mental, or emotional trauma; and the frail elderly, mainly people 75 and older. For these people, the care should enhance their capacity to adapt to age and/or disease through prevention, modification, or maintenance of condition and ADL capabilities. Alternatively, it might ensure functional maintenance or enhancement in the least restrictive environment (Callahan, 1979). To produce these outcomes, a number of services and settings must be provided: adequate, supervised residential facilities; special services for the homebound (transportation, meals, personal care);

13

institutional skilled nursing and medical care; and compassionate terminal care.

Given the key role of the family in LTC, meeting these requirements can be linked to the need to help those families which seek to support their elders in a "normal" community setting and to provide high quality institutional and congregate care as needed when families cannot cope.

Goals and Objectives for Long-Term Care

To analyze provision of long-term care, one must relate the requirements for support of LTC to the goals and objectives of those needing care, to their families' goals, to policy goals, and to society's goals (which may not be the same as policy goals).

These goals and objectives of LTC should be clearly stated and understood. Otherwise, individuals, families, communities, and the overall society will not know what they wish to achieve, will have no way of knowing whether they have made any progress, and will have no way of comparing alternatives among care modes. Without explicitly stated goals, analysis of LTC is impossible.

Individual and Family Goals

Some dependent individuals seek full restoration of function, others, the reduction of dependency (however defined), and still others, the reduction of pain and the restoration of some human dignity. These goals, of course, are not mutually exclusive. Whatever the nature of individual objectives, they are obviously influenced by the sources of disability and associated physical and psychological outcomes and by the norms of their communities.

If adequate income were always available, if reliable information were present, and if competent sources of care were accessible, dependent individuals and their families could buy their care in the market. Without formal community or governmental support, however, dependents and their families, friends, and communities would have to rely on their own internal strengths and available income as they sought care and support. In that type of environment, the market can provide a set of outcomes for individuals and the community which will usually reflect the interaction of basic demand and supply conditions for long-term care services. Unless there are some externalities, or some continuing structural or economic reasons for the needed supply not to emerge in the marketplace, those with the information and money will be able to get the services they require at prices they are willing to pay. Of course, much the same can be said about any type of service.[6]

---

[6] In economic terms, an externality arises when one person's consumption or production of a given good affects another person's satisfaction or capacity to produce. Externalities may be positive or negative. Pollution

These ideal conditions do not always exist, however, and the community, the government, or some other collective agency may feel obliged to enter the LTC picture, either to provide the care itself or the financial support for its purchase and use. Society long ago decided that some market solutions, often involving much private agony, are uncivilized and, therefore, unacceptable.

Government Goals, Policy Goals, and Public Provisions

The perceived unacceptability of market solutions and the unwillingness of the community to allow certain needs to go unmet have led to the creation of formal systems of provision by the community and society. Some of these systems directly provide service, others finance it, and still others offer information and direction. Some handle more than one of these functions.

Individual need does not, by itself, justify a system of governmentally provided or financed long-term care. Making the provision of care a political matter and an object of public policy must rest on some assumptions about the prevalence of the need, the priority accorded to meeting LTC need, the political power of the needy and their relatives, humanitarian considerations, and the presumed incapacity of the needy to provide care for themselves, either because of their inadequate incomes or because of other constraints on access to care. (Such constraints may derive from conditions of market failure, but they may also reflect the public's preferences for other forms of consumption.[7] These preferences, of course, may underlie the reasons for inadequacy of income among the needy, that is, society has opted for a given type of income distribution.) We must also acknowledge that governmental provision of support may be considered a good thing in and of itself, a so-called merit good,

---

is a good example of a negative externality: my paper mill produces smells and pollutants which affect your nose and lungs even though you do not buy my paper or sell me any of the inputs I use in producing it. In LTC, a positive externality might arise when I build a ramp to allow my wheelchair to get over the curb and it permits other wheelchair users to get over the curb as well, at no cost to them.

[7] Market failures occur when private and social (marginal) valuations (benefits) and/or costs are not equal. In such cases, markets may fail to reflect all cost and benefit elements which should be part of the decision to produce or not produce. The failure of the market to lead to the production and sale of automobile exhaust devices because neither producers nor buyers want to pay for such devices might be a case of market failure, if exhaust devices are a good thing to have on other grounds (health reasons, for example). In LTC, market failure might occur if there is agreement that a system of home care might be desirable from a social standpoint, yet consumers will not (or cannot) pay for home care, while potential providers cannot (or will not) provide it either. In such situations, the government may step in to provide. These circumstances are discussed in the following sections on needs, wants, demands, and supplies.

like clean air or unpolluted water to the environmentalist. In general, political justifications for governmental support for long-term care usually rest on the inadequacy-of-income and merit-good arguments.

While being sensitive to the multiplicity of private choices, government goals in providing services necessarily have a more constricted range of objectives, if only for administrative simplicity. Often governmental objectives do not arise from the specifics of the problem area but from other considerations. They can be political, as in the desire to fulfill a given administrative objective or to make provision at the least cost to the public treasury. To the extent that governments pursue these other, often narrow objectives, governmental or policy goals may differ from societal goals which might emphasize quality of life.

If government is to exert significant policy influence as provider, financier, standard setter, and/or information disseminator, the purposes of intervention should be identified specifically for LTC.

Particular government objectives in long-term care might include the following:

- maintenance of life in a custodial environment
- restoration of maximum possible functional capacity
- restoration of functional ability in the least restrictive environment
- alleviation of acute medical distress followed by rapid return to the community when the individual is out of danger
- minimization of recurrence of the disabling condition
- reduction of dependency of the vulnerable population and subsequent reduction of costs
- minimization of administrative and legislative inconvenience and complexity
- creation of a system of provision where one does not now exist.

William Weissert (1979) has offered a policy statement about long-term care which succinctly combines many of these goals and also recognizes the multi-sided nature of the problem, while trying to stay within the realms of practicality. He says:

Ideally, a long-term care system would provide the most cost-effective care of the right level, at the right time, in the right setting, and at the maximum quality achievable within the state of the art (1979, p. 106).

His specification of the policy objective lets us develop a number of questions addressed to the existing policy framework, to the nature of the long-term care "system" (if one indeed exists), and to the body of analysis on long-term care.

16

Setting Standards Consistent With Goals

Having thus stated the goals and objectives of the long-term care system, we should establish criteria for the system that actually delivers the care. Brody and others argue that such a set of services should include all segments in the community as parts of an overall LTC system. The system should feature easy access for dependent people and their families, and it should leave individuals in their "natural" context as much and as long as possible, recognizing that families are the most common support institutions. Medical services, nursing care, health-related social services, residency programs, income maintenance programs, transportation, legal services, etc. should all be linked. Special programs for the specially disabled should also be provided. In all, the structure of the system should ensure continuity, accessibility, accountability, and affordability.

Such a system obviously must be managed to ensure provision of the right service, in the right place, at the right time, in an ongoing manner. Housing programs, the educational system, and vocational rehabilitation services must all cooperate with the health/social systems to ensure attainment of LTC system goals. This coordination, too, requires management. Just what the management structure should be is still a matter of debate. Some observers favor a single monitoring system to provide services on a catchment area basis. Other analysts favor a more centralized system for both provision and monitoring, while still others favor even more decentralization than Brody does. In short, this issue is still open for analysis and judgment. In any event, the functions of the managerial structure should permit the following administrative and organizational activities: reference and referral, assessment and reassessment, monitoring of use, client advocacy, maximization of available financial resources, coordination of timing of services, reporting of gaps in services, creation of cooperative agreements, purchasing of services, and case finding. How to ensure the appropriate combining of these services and their management in a system still remains an open question.

An LTC Systems Model

James Callahan (1979) has developed a model which addresses the nature of systems functions to be provided as well as the proper relation of those functions to each other. Although his analysis directly aims at the development of a community-based, non-institutional system for delivering LTC services to people with LTC needs, his concepts are applicable across a wide range of possible service and setting configurations.

Callahan bases his analysis on systems concepts developed by Churchman, Sayles and Chandler, and Parsons and Shils. His argu-

17

ment is essentially that LTC is characterized by two attributes noted by Sayles and Chandler in connection with the NASA space program: the collaboration of a large number of private and public institutions and an uncertain technology. Unlike the space program, however, LTC is not characterized by a single-valued outcome (for example, a moon landing) but rather has goals on at least two levels.

The Callahan model involves, first, a general model of inputs (the patients or clients), an LTC system, and a set of desired outcomes. Patients are described by variables in Figure I–3 (to which has been added income, evidently a significant determinant of institutionalization and other LTC circumstances). Outputs of the system are shown on the right-hand side of the diagram.

The functional aspects of the LTC system, which must be performed if the system is to attain its objectives, are divided into system management, operational management, and patient management, all shown in Figure I–A–5. Each of these functions is divided into the specific activities shown in Figures I–A–6 through I–A–8, which show the allocation of financial and organizational responsibilities (in the national context) to the Federal, State, and local levels of government. Most of the listed functions are self-evident and require little explanation of their nature or their appropriate levels of responsibility. Specific items, however, require amplification.

At the system management level, financial resources must be provided from various sources if the system is to exist, let alone serve. The planning function would include comprehensive (system-wide or nationwide) planning, identification of target population, and cataloguing of resources. System development involves ensuring an adequate supply of resources and their appropriate development. Included in system development might be capital equipment and structures, organization structures, labor force procurement, etc. Control implies management of activities which influence behavior among actors in the system, while evaluation relates to how the overall system functions. Evaluation might include analyses of the cost-effectiveness of alternative care modes, coordination of services, comprehensiveness of services, and efficient operation of programs. In one sense, these represent operational criteria for the system, as opposed to outputs which represent the outcomes criteria. Good evaluation considers both sets of criteria.

At the operational management level, the coordination function includes the integration of services, especially at the community, not the case, level. Quality control refers to such activities as performance monitoring, quality assurance, etc.

At the patient level, one of the most important functions is entry, that is, the mechanisms by which a patient enters the system. Ideally, entry points ease access to the system, most desirably at the community level. System entry can be "open" in the sense that no

18

FIGURE I-3

Long-Term Care System Input-Output Overview

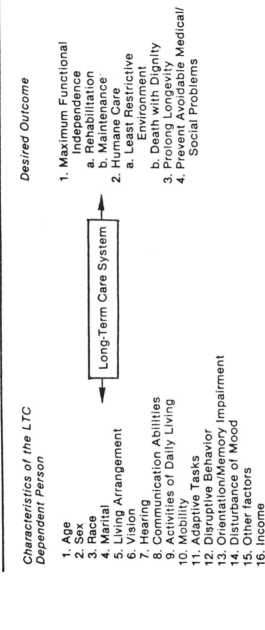

Characteristics of the LTC Dependent Person

1. Age
2. Sex
3. Race
4. Marital
5. Living Arrangement
6. Vision
7. Hearing
8. Communication Abilities
9. Activities of Daily Living
10. Mobility
11. Adaptive Tasks
12. Disruptive Behavior
13. Orientation/Memory Impairment
14. Disturbance of Mood
15. Other factors
16. Income

Long-Term Care System

Desired Outcome

1. Maximum Functional Independence
   a. Rehabilitation
   b. Maintenance
2. Humane Care
   a. Least Restrictive Environment
   b. Death with Dignity
3. Prolong Longevity
4. Prevent Avoidable Medical/Social Problems

Source: Callahan, James J. Jr., "The Organization of the Long Term Care System and the Potential for a Single Agency Option," Discussion Paper DP-16b, Brandeis University, University Health Policy Consortium, February 1979

formal requirements are posed; people may come through on their own, getting services directly from a provider if they wish. Users of closed entry systems would come through a designated gatekeeper, such as a physician. Entry points, open or closed, may be single or multiple, and could include institutions as well as official agencies. Among the most critical management functions at the patient level is needs assessment, which is a necessary basis for any plan of care. Some needs assessments are functional, while others are largely medical or, in a few instances, social.

When all of the other functions (including the provision of information) have been completed, the system can begin to provide service. Figure I–A–4 shows components of service provision (to which we add chiropody to ensure mobility).

Obviously, the Callahan framework is more of an analytical and structural construct than a dynamic, mathematical, analytical model; yet it illustrates how these key organizational elements fit together to provide LTC services to the target population.

A number of other observations about this Callahan formulation are in order. First, it is clear that the systems, as Callahan describes them, draw on many subsystems, both conceptually and organizationally. Second, although the personal services subsystem is postulated as the most important, it is unclear whether it really exists and/or can be brought into being. Third, if the LTC person is marginal to the concerns of health planners and analysts, to say nothing of those providers conventionally (or politically) judged to be most important in the system (physicians, nurses, home health providers), how can the various needed systems be brought into being? Fourth, if LTC systems must operate in the community, how can local parochialisms and territorial jealousies be overcome to permit the necessary coordination and integration of services?

To meet the last problem, Federal authorities might conceivably establish an alternative system, competitive with existing local structures and following the VA model, but this would be, in Callahan's view, hard to accomplish (Callahan, 1980). Modification of behavior, on the other hand, is very hard to attain at the local level because of Federal and State constraints and exogenous environmental factors. (See the list in Figure I–4.)

Although he provides no formulae for engineering changes at the local level, Callahan cites some potential sources of alteration which may shift the elements of provision in a desirable, systemic direction. (See Figure I–A–9.) Among them are increases in the numbers of the elderly and disabled, increases in the number of service professionals, emergence of a professional dynamic, which uses the energy of competing professional groups to generate changes, and the interactions of client groups and professionals which may raise client consciousness. Although these factors may produce change, there

20

is no assurance that the changes will be desirable. For example, the actions of professional groups may be self-serving and self-protective as well as ameliorative, while the actions of enlarged and politicized client groups may exclude the rights or entitlements of others.

Economic Theory and LTC: A Micro-Focus and a Macro-Focus

Economic theory conventionally analyzes the behavior of individual consuming units in terms of their want satisfaction and of the impact of scarcity and constraint on the ability to attain goals. The determinants of consumers' behavior are prices, consumer resources, and consumer preferences or tastes. The last reflect the objectives of consumers in defining their patterns of consumption and in choosing to consume (or not) given amounts of a particular good or service at differing prices and incomes.

Given the previously discussed goals for LTC, the sources of service provision could be the dependent individual, his/her immediate or extended family, neighbors, informal community supports, formal community non-profit supports, private providers operating on a profit-making basis, or some level of government. The behavior of proprietary providers can be analyzed conventionally by the same assumptions and techniques related to maximizing goals or outcomes, subject to constraints. Traditionally, a profit-maximizing assumption has applied: producers offer that amount of a given commodity at prices which will maximize profits subject to the constraints of costs of production. Prices are set by interaction of supply and users' demand, financed by themselves or someone else.

The analysis of consumers' and producers' behavior theoretically yields equilibrium outcomes of output and price reflecting the simultaneous effects of the desire for commodities with the producers' (and thus society's) capacities to produce those commodities.

Economists have for some time analyzed utilization of health and social services using the conventional models of supply and demand. For the most part, these analyses have produced no startling results (at least to economists), but they have not usually been applied to questions of LTC systems or of the interactions between the micro- and macro-levels of behavior. Analytical developments in health and welfare economics have thus increasingly shown the need for more sophisticated econometric and modeling techniques and for broader definitions of commodities, costs, and the utility functions of users, providers, and governments. The need to consider non-profit behaviors, on the one hand, and the need to assess the effects of government regulation and reimbursement, on the other, are examples of these new analytical imperatives.

21

FIGURE I-4

Factors Limiting Flexibility of Local Human Service Managers

1. The workings of the national economy as they affect the resources available to local policymakers
2. The deliverage results of national policy, such as strings and categorical grants or regulatory policies requiring environmental impact statements
3. The inadvertent effects of national policy such as a support for suburbanization in the tax structure which resulted from the Highway Act
4. The role of State government
5. The role of public opinion and constraining local actors
6. The views of outside political actors themselves, unions, interest groups and individual citizens
7. Geography of the city and region (for example, the degree to which the city's boundaries incorporate or are separate from the metropolitan economy, allowing linkage of local dollars outside the locality itself and in the region)
8. Demography since the make-up of the city's populations constrains its policy
9. The city's own resources in light of both actual fiscal strength and its taxpayers' perceptions of their tax burdens
10. Time as a constraint on short-range policymaking
11. Judicial decisions as they set the legal boundaries of local policy

Source: Taken by Callahan (1980) from Gardner, Sydney, "Poilcy Space. A Sharper Perspective on Local Decision Making," in *Human Services Management: Parameters for Research,* Michael J. Murphy and Thomas Glynn, editors, Washington, D.C.: International City Management Association, 1978, pp. 19-20.*

*Reprinted with permission.

Users and Providers

The LTC User As Demander and Provider

Users of LTC services most often are the dependent individuals themselves. In some instances, however, family caregivers may need LTC services to help with the caring function and to assist in coping with the stresses imposed by their obligations to the dependent person. For example, the family frequently requires help from social workers or needs to have homes modified to accommodate wheelchairs, hospital beds, etc. Services to the dependent person range from high-technology, acute hospital interventions to help with shopping or cooking. Furthermore, both goals and perceptions of service need may differ widely over time for the same individual and may diverge greatly between two individuals with the same disabilities and social circumstances. For each individual, the impact of the prices of services (including zero prices), their incomes, and their perceptions of their disabilities and the needs for services will be individually determined.

The essence of LTC vulnerability and dependency, of course, is that disabled individuals are not able to care for themselves at a level consistent with standards of decency and health. The core of the problem is that outside help is essential. The question then is who the provider should be and how the provision should be made.

As stated earlier, with adequate information and income vulnerable individuals could buy the services they needed. However, in many cases the vulnerables are psychologically, physically, or emotionally unable to gather necessary information about their own needs and about available services in the marketplace to make informed choices. Furthermore, commercial providers may not be available to them at affordable prices.

In large measure, the service/support requirements perceived by an individual will be powerfully conditioned by family situation (marital status, children, presence of relatives or friends) and by family income. Certainly, an individual's ability to cope with incapacities will depend on the availability of help from family, spouse, and/or children. In that context, family economic circumstances (income, assets) will influence purchase of health/social support services at different prices. Because an individual needing LTC will not always be able to decide on the nature of his/her own needs and on practicable means of satisfying them, families and friends must often make arrangements with providers or key interveners such as social workers, geriatric nurse practitioners, and physicians.

Families as Demanders of LTC

The role of the family members as providers and determiners of service needs, as finders of services, and as brokers for their elderly relatives in securing services has been analyzed in a number of research works and is examined in a succeeding chapter. Nonetheless, a few words on the family role in resource use are needed here.

Family goals in seeking LTC are frequently only speculative, but making their relatives get well, restoring their ADL capacity, and preventing further deterioration are all probable ingredients in family decisions. There must also be some family desire to reduce the burden on themselves, while still preserving the bonds of affection and devotion which are important in family life. Family burdens include not only direct institutional and/or home costs but also some very tangible dislocations produced by having a disabled elderly person in the home, requiring many services, often of a most personal nature. Economic burdens include not only the direct costs of buying services (medicine, nursing care, home modifications, etc.), but also the incomes foregone (time costs) by family members who may stay home from work to provide care and/or supervision.

From an economic, analytical standpoint, the behavior of families/friends in making resource decisions in LTC has yet to be examined. At this time, we can only surmise that the influences of prices, incomes, and preferences must all be involved in the analysis of family behavior. So also must family perceptions about the physical availability of services, as well as the financial and psychological supports evidenced by systems of third-party payers. Although these latter appear to reduce prices of services (often to zero) to users, their role may well be to provide an emotional cushion for the dependent individual and for families/friends who have to cope with the need for LTC.

The Family as Provider of LTC and as a System of Support

In light of family structure, tradition, etc., it has often been natural to assume that families would provide for their dependents. In some cases, provision can be made at home from internal resources, but in others, outside help is necessary. Sophisticated, acute-level, medical techniques may be essential, continuing nursing skills beyond family abilities may have to be mobilized, and professional rehabilitation therapists may be needed. For the vast majority of long-term care needs, however, the required level of sophistication is low; the essential need is for routine support with the functions of daily living: eating, dressing, bathing, and moving about. It would seem that these services are within the skills of the average healthy family member, provided that the individual has the physical, psychological, and emotional strength. More importantly, that individual must also be able to take time from income-producing work and other concerns. In many families, the needed strength and

24

time are not available, thus again creating the requirement for external intervention, either purchased in the market or conferred as a gift or transfer from outside the family.

One of the central conclusions derived from looking at dependent people and their need for services is that the family is a crucial subsystem in the total system of support. Elaine and Stanley Brody (1980) noted that families provide the majority of LTC health care services and homemaker services to their dependent elders. The GAO Cleveland study (1977) similarly found large proportions of family support under certain circumstances. Such levels of family support should not be surprising, since 80 percent of people 65 and older have children; 94 percent of those with children have grand-children, and 46 percent are great-grandparents. Viewed from the descendants' perspective, 25 percent of people 50 to 59 years of age have surviving parents, a proportion which will increase over the next 20 years.

These parent-child relationships obviously work two ways: the burden of dependency on those individual families which may be obligated to care for their elders will be very high, since so many families will have elders for at least the next 20 years. On the other hand, from a social perspective, it is possible that more caregivers may be available in those same years to minister to the needs of the dependent elderly. One crucial implication of these family developments is that the focus of public policy should shift increas-ingly to helping family systems support their elders through expanded home services and/or outpatient and outreach programs which facilitate home maintenance of dependent people (Brody and Brody, 1980).[8]

It is appropriate here to note key aspects of the question of family support. First, families do not appear to be "dumping" their elders into the institutional care structure. Elaine Brody's research (1979) shows that families at present will try to cope with highly dependent older relatives at home unless forced to shift them to institutions by medical stringency, unmanageable caring requirements (Stanley Brody suggests that continual fecal incontinence may be a crucial condition), and/or financial stringency, as Bruce Vladeck suggests.[9] Ironically, Federal and State policy and administrative decisions (embedded in Medicare/Medicaid regulations) may be instrumental in forcing a family to institutionalize a dependent elder for financial reasons.

---

[8] The implications of the different parent/child proportions for the period after the year 2000 are not clear, not just because of demographics but also because of rapidly changing family relationships and structures.

[9] See Vladeck (1980) on this point. Also, see Brody and Brody (1980) for comments to the same effect.

Within the family, it is often the presence of an adult daughter, married or unmarried, which is crucial. In some cases, a niece or granddaughter may substitute, but the attitudes of older parents, as well as strong filial bonds, may skew the choice in the daughter's direction, possibly at great career costs to her. (This finding is borne out in the British research of Peter Townsend and others.) Again, Elaine Brody, in her cross-generational studies of women's attitudes toward caring for elderly family members, has determined that many daughters and granddaughters believe that families should care for older, dependent family members and express their willingness to do so. Generational differences appear, however, in the greater demands by younger women for more male help in the caring process and in their greater willingness to accept formal public support in helping families to cope (Brody, 1979; Townsend, 1957; Isaacs, 1971).

A number of questions about crucial family support systems and use of resources remain. Overall, the American family is caught up in a series of massive social changes which may subvert its ability to cope. In the first place, many elders have no families or friends. For these unattached people, the alternatives may be neglect or high cost institutionalization, unless some sort of family surrogate can be found. In the Scandinavian countries, where a combination of massive internal migration and a housing policy favoring two-bedroom, nuclear family housing units left many elderly without close social support, the state has had to assume the role of substitute family. The question thus appears to be: Will public policy in the United States be willing or able to provide such substitutes?

Even when the family is intact, it may not be available. Recent research shows that most elderly with families see family members with regularity even if they live apart; yet the pressures affecting modern families may reduce even this type of support. Rising divorce rates, smaller family sizes associated with the Depression, increased numbers of single-parent families, and the increased frequency of non-marital and/or childless cohabitation may reduce the availability of supportive family members in the near future. Perhaps most important is the increased participation of women—particularly middle-aged women—in the labor force. The women's movement, expanding economic opportunity, and inflation-bred necessity have dramatically raised the proportion of married women, 45 to 64, now in the labor force to over 46 percent, high by historical standards (BLS, 1980). As a result, the "empty nests," which were being filled with older parents and grandparents after children left, are increasingly being abandoned by the middle-aged care givers. These dynamic changes pose some major questions for policy planners as they seek means to help families cope. Family surrogates and family reconstruction may be the big issues for family policy, especially in the context of expanded home care and related services. Such a prospect emphasizes the reality that family policy and elder policy must work together (Brody and Brody, 1980).

Much of the argument relevant to the family also applies to support from friends, the neighborhood, or the informal (as distinct from governmental or formally structured organizational) community. Again, assistance from the community is constrained by ability, capacity, and available time. If these are absent, there must be recourse to external sources of provision.

Gatekeeping and Access to the LTC System

Access to health and social services is not always direct, nor at the initiative of the user or the user's family. Frequently a professional intermediary must act as a "gatekeeper" or broker for the required services. Although patients (and their families) may often obtain LTC services on their own (for example, they may enter nursing homes or engage home services) more easily than they may enter an acute care hospital, gatekeeping is important for many parts of the LTC system.

Gatekeeping may include prescribing medications and services, certifying patients for entry to institutions, certifying eligibility for services (personal social services for example), and/or certifying delivery of services for reimbursement by third-party payers.

Gatekeeping has been studied by economists and sociologists (La Dou and Likens, 1977). It emerges from a combination of the nature of the goods and services provided, the professional qualifications of the providers (especially in the medical services), and the need for certification for payment by third-party payers.

Medical services and some social services, often of the type most common in LTC, fall in the category of "credence goods," that is, those goods about whose quality and proper use the consumer (demander) is not adequately knowledgeable. As a result, a professional (sometimes the supplier) must intervene to prescribe and/or certify their use to protect the health of the user.

Certification may also be necessary for LTC services if the product or service is scarce or must be rationed, especially if provision is public. In such cases, a representative of the government, usually a social worker, must prescribe or certify. Entry to public nursing homes, old age homes, or public day care centers may require certification or gatekeeping by both a social service worker and a physician.

Additionally, some form of gatekeeping is needed in third-party payment situations, to control utilization and level of expenditure by individual users and across all users. In such cases, the payer may require certification from a medical, health, and/or social services professional before services can be provided or reimbursed. Presumably, the certifying professional will know which services are reimbursable and at what level of payment. Of course, one gatekeeper's judgment about required type and intensity of service can conflict with that of another gatekeeper who is more attuned to the realities of regulation and reimbursement. Additionally, incentives for different gatekeepers may differ. In such cases, the users, their families and, often, providers have to choose which stipulations to follow.

Interventions by gatekeepers change the supply and demand characteristics in the markets for the goods and services provided. Since the gatekeeper's choices may be substituted for those of the users or their families, and since those choices reflect professional and regulatory influences, demand for LTC services is much more complicated than that for ordinary consumer goods. It is impossible to model this type of demand behavior without further theoretical and empirical analysis. One can only speculate on the possible offsetting effects of professional imperatives to prescribe much service in contrast with the service constraining influences of, say, reimbursement limits under third-party payment.

Supply and demand for certain LTC services can become intertwined (and hence difficult to analyze) because gatekeepers may also be providers. Because of this possibility, many proposals for LTC screening and case management emphasize the separation of gatekeeping, assessment, and case management from provision. Where gatekeeping and provision are combined in one agency, there may be a tendency for overutilization of services. The risk has been particularly noted in fee-for-service medical care, in which physicians earn fees from the services they prescribe. The problem is presumably aggravated when the physician knows that third-party payment is available. Coupled with these direct fee motives are technological imperatives to undertake sophisticated procedures and the doctors' desire to protect themselves from malpractice suits by using "best available" techniques (La Dou and Likens, 1977). These motivations may be reflected in excess institutionalization and lavish prescription of rehabilitative services.

These excess use imperatives may, however, be counteracted by a number of factors. First, most LTC requirement is for fairly routine personal service, not high technology medical care. The physician's involvement is not intense, although assignment to a nursing home for those services may mandate more frequent visits (and hence more fees) for the doctor. Second, much LTC service is provided by nurses not subject to the doctor's fee-for-service/ prescription imperatives. Third, some use of LTC service is determined by publicly paid professionals, who have no direct personal interest in providing service (although they may have a bureaucratic interest in enlarging their clientele). Fourth, reimbursement limits under public (Medicare/Medicaid) or private, third-party payment constrain the amount and type of services prescribed. In fact, these limits are often implicated in the alleged failure of the LTC system to provide home-based and other forms of non-institutional services.

The Physician as Gatekeeper

The role of the physician as an agent or broker permitting patients access to support systems has been considered in a number of studies of physician behavior (La Dou and Likens, 1977; Juba, 1979). For example, Mark Blumberg (1977) has attempted to isolate the proportionate influence of the physician in determining use of resources in treating medical problems. He concludes that, on average, about 70 percent of decisions about use of health care resources are dictated by the physician; in the care of geriatric patients, however, the proportion is much lower, perhaps 40 percent.[10] Studies such as Blumberg's highlight the fact that individuals and their families often must surrender their control over use of services to the doctor because of the latter's superior medical knowledge and/or because the doctor controls access to key elements of the support structure (for example, hospitals, prescription drugs, physical therapy, occupational therapy, speech therapy). Also, the physician must certify the necessity of certain services to establish eligibility for reimbursement from third-party payers— Medicare, Medicaid, private health insurance, etc. Unless the structure of the medical system is changed, the physician is an important gatekeeper for almost all who need LTC assistance. Physicians, therefore, can possibly exercise a degree of monopoly power in granting access to their own services and to the system.

These gatekeeping functions of the physician may produce conflict-of-interest situations. In some cases, as noted earlier, the physician prescribes a need for her/his own services, thus enhancing income. In other situations, the conflict of interest may be less obvious. For example, a physician can be woven into a net of referrals with fellow physicians so that they all keep making referrals to each other, often to their mutual benefit. In other cases, a physician may be indirectly benefited if on the staff of, or a proprietary partner in, an acute hospital or nursing home to which patients are referred.

A particularly vexing problem for government and other third-party payers or providers stems from possible conflicts of interest for MDs and other professionals certifying for service use or payment. The paying or providing agency cannot, *a priori,* be certain that the prescription of service is not designed to enrich the prescriber. To that end, elaborate control mechanisms (utilization review committees, Professional Standards Review Organizations, survey and

---

[10] Note that Blumberg's rough percentages cannot be extended to all LTC.

certification agencies) exist to guard against possible abuse. Similarly, the fiduciary agents who process claims for public authorities (often major insurance companies or health insurance providers) set up complicated review procedures.

Other Professionals as Managers

In LTC, more than in other types of medical provision, physicians share decisions about use of resources, as well as assessments of patients/clients, with other professionals. This situation exists partly because LTC need is not just a requirement for medical services but also a need for social and routine support services. In some instances, the only requirement is for supervision; in others, personal services, often of an intimate type, must be provided; in still others (probably a minority of cases) skilled nursing and medical interventions are required. Overall, it appears that the premium is on the systemic management of the patient and the patient's environment. As a result, the social worker and the nurse (or geriatric nurse practitioner) do, or should, have as much to say as the family or the physicians. In many instances, social service case workers are more attuned to individual patient and family circumstances and more aware of the realities of service provision and availability than are doctors. Additionally, a nursing professional can sometimes be more sensitive to the caring requirements, as distinct from the curing aspects, than can an MD. Of course, in many cases a physician may be as sensitive and aware as these other professionals, but demands on doctors' time may intervene in LTC provision. In any event, abundant folklore among LTC professionals indicates that the role of the MD for other than acute needs should be modest. Further research, however, is needed on this assertion.

The Interdisciplinary Team in LTC Management

Given the roles which other health/social professionals must play in LTC, and in light of the need for systemic patterns of provision, the appropriate caring and management agency may well be the interdisciplinary team rather than a single health care or social service entity. These teams may be found in many situations and be composed of differing mixes of professionals, perhaps including representatives of voluntary agencies. Overall, the general notion of an interdisciplinary team, operating as a cooperative unit, rather than as a hierarchical structure, appeals to many analysts. Some descriptions of these teams exist, but rigorous models and analytical studies of their behavior still await further investigation.

Professionals as Providers

In considering the uses and roles of differing types of health/social professionals, one should analyze their behavior not only as managers but also as individual providers and as members of teams. Again, the analytical issues of provider goals (or preference functions), alternate means of obtaining goals, and the constraints and obstacles of exploring alternatives and attaining goals are all relevant. Traditional economic theory has been applied to doctors who have been variously postulated as profit-maximizers or satisficers or as jointly maximizing members of physicians' cooperatives (La Dou and Likens, 1977). Although these models have provided us with key insights into physician behaviors, including choices of specialties, they have not yet provided us with close-ended solutions about physicians' actions and motives and the outcomes of their behavior for individual LTC patients. The current complex environment involving Medicare/Medicaid and private third-party payers, physicians' trade associations, and the relation between the physician and key institutions, especially the acute hospital and the nursing home, have not been adequately explored and offer numerous opportunities for productive research. Although extensive research is being done on physician behavior under Medicare/Medicaid, the *terra incognita* of physicians' actions and environments in LTC demands much more analytical attention. (Mitchell and Cromwell and Link *et al* are currently working on these issues.)

The complex situation of the physician is even more characteristic of social workers and the nursing professionals (who may have less formal power than the MD, however). Both of these groups may be private or public employees or work for voluntary agencies. Nurses (other than registry nurses) rarely are in business for themselves, often being in the employ of doctors, hospitals, nursing homes, visiting nurse associations (VNAs), or public or voluntary agencies. Although these professionals have their objectives, analytical models of their motivations and behaviors as LTC providers are, as yet, imperfect. We also have yet to develop good models and evidence for their actions as parts of LTC teams.

Institutions or Firms as LTC Providers

Thus far, we have focused on the actions of individuals as single or team member determiners of service supply and demand. Of equal importance is the set of behaviors of institutions or firms as LTC providers. Most prominent in the current setting are the acute hospitals and nursing homes, the most important institutional sources of LTC. Both have been extensively analyzed, though many questions remain.

Numerous other non-family sources of provision must also be considered in any comprehensive view of LTC. Adult day care (ADC) providers, home health agencies, providers of special therapies, domiciliary care facilities, and numerous others must all be analyzed to project a total picture of LTC and to develop models of an LTC

31

system. Objectives, alternatives, and constraints are all essential ingredients in any such analytical efforts. Unfortunately, the research has not gone far enough, and we are left with only qualitative and speculative analyses, coupled with much anecdotal evidence.

From the Individual Users/Providers to the Group and the System

Unfortunately, when analyzing the collective behavior of individual key decision units, the shortfalls are amplified. We are helped, however, by the econometric and sociological data concerning aggregate behavior and its outcomes. In the physician, nursing home, and hospital fields, research has now progressed to allow us to generalize about the effects of numbers of cases, reimbursement formulae, geographic aspects of input availability and input prices, etc. (Some of this research is discussed in following chapters.) Nonetheless, many gaps in the research and in our knowledge persist, hindering attempts to design and analyze any sort of system.

Just as we do not know enough about the behaviors of individual patients, families/friends, and other individuals as they influence both the demand and the supply of LTC services, we also lack an adequate picture of the interplay of disease, disability, social circumstance, and income across large segments of the population. We have studies of nursing home costs of physician reactions in certain situations, but we have not adequately considered time as a determining variable or the effects of changed circumstances. Nor have we made much headway with the equally ambitious task of analyzing behaviors at the subsystem level. For example, we have not tied the family response to LTC need to the actions of hospital discharge planners, nor have we linked the actions of both families and planners to the actions and availability of home care providers.

Analyses of associations of key interveners—social workers, consumer organizations, etc.—are crucial in understanding the provision and use of LTC. Despite many recent studies (for example, Vladeck, 1980), we need more institutional knowledge and analytical understanding about "industries," that is, all providers of a given service. Of equal importance are the actions of provider groups, such as medical associations at all levels, organizations of nursing homes, hospital associations, etc. These organizations help define standards and philosophies of care, mandating or enjoining certain actions, and they also interpret regulations. They act as advocates in determining reimbursement levels influencing official choices of reimbursement modes (prospective, retrospective, reasonable cost, flat rate, etc.), and shaping details of regulations promulgated by State and Federal authorities. Most visibly, trade organizations seek

32

to influence legislation at all levels. Again, we need models and analyses of this type of behavior as it helps define the need for LTC, the outcomes of various types of provision, and the nature of the LTC system.

Third-Party Payment and Access to LTC Provision

Many LTC users and their families do not pay directly for the services required. Rather, third-party agencies, the government, voluntary groups, or private insurance companies provide the financing and may thus act as interveners, a role parallel to gatekeepers. In some cases, as with private health insurance and some government programs, users and their families have paid insurance premiums, but actual payment is not perceived as out-of-pocket when services are used. In LTC, moreover, because of the large volume of social services required, the role of third-party payment or provision may be more important than in acute care. In 1979, approximately 68 percent of all health care services ($129 billion out of $189 billion) were paid for by third-party payers (Gibson, 1980). The percentage of all LTC services financed by third parties is not precisely known because of the large volume of social services involved; however, 57 percent of nursing home expenditures (the most rapidly growing category of health care expenditure) came from Federal and State (Medicare and Medicaid) sources.

At the Federal level, the major programs of acute and LTC support for elderly people are Medicare and Medicaid, although some services are provided under Title XX of the Social Security Act and Title III of the Older Americans Act. (Veterans Administration health care provides both acute and long-term care to former military personnel under certain circumstances.) The Medicare program, primarily an insurance system featuring individual and employer contributions to an insurance trust fund, as well as general fund allocations, provides benefits under two systems: Part A, Hospital Insurance, and Part B, Supplemental Medical Insurance (which pays for the services of physicians and other health professionals as prescribed by a physician). Some types of social services may be provided under home care provisions of both Parts A and B. (Details of eligibility, funding, costs, benefits, and utilization of various LTC services under different public programs are found in Chapter V.)

In 1979, Medicare did not support much LTC outside of acute hospitals. Although the skilled nursing facility (SNF) had originally been encouraged under Medicare as a cost-effective alternative to the acute hospital, the growth of Medicare SNF payments began to slow after 1969. Medicare nursing payments amounted to only $373 million in 1979. Other LTC-type Medicare expenditures for home care, etc. came to only $427 million in 1978 (*Health Care Financing Notes*, various issues).

Medicare contains copayment provisions so that users and families must provide part of the total costs. For example, Medicare will support 100 days maximum in an SNF after hospitalization for a Medicare-defined period of illness and if certified by local utilization review bodies. The first 20 days are wholly covered by Medicare, but days 21 through 100 require a copayment ($22.50 per day in 1980).

Medicaid, unlike Medicare, is not an insurance program. Instead, it is a means-tested form of support for persons defined as indigent, (that is, their incomes and/or asset levels fall below certain defined limits which vary by State). The program is financed by grants from the Federal government to the States, which then match on a formula-determined percentage basis reflecting State population and per capita income. The Federal contribution varies from 50 percent to 78 percent; the national average is 56 percent. The extent of public payment under Medicaid is determined by the willingness of individual States to pay. In short, the Federal authorities can only equal what the States are willing to pay. In 1981, there were 53 Medicaid jurisdictions (including the territories and the District of Columbia). Only Arizona did not have a Medicaid program.

In 1979, Medicaid expenditures for nursing homes came to $8.8 billion, about 41 percent of all of the program's costs for that year. The proportions varied widely across the States, however, as high as 68 percent in South Dakota and as low as 13 percent in the District of Columbia. In 1978, Medicaid also provided about 370,000 home health visits at a cost of $211 million, about 1.2 percent of all Medicaid expenditures in that year. It may well be that Medicaid provides more homemaker and personal care services than does Medicare under its home care programs.

Private health insurance payment for LTC is relatively modest, with only about $117 million going for nursing home care in 1979. Private plans vary from comprehensive coverage of all LTC services to supplemental add-ons to Medicare to cover extended nursing home stays.

Since Medicare and private coverage are both insurance programs, they share the characteristics of limiting amounts of service and the rates at which services will be paid. Medicare bills may be paid by users or families on a reimbursement basis or they may be paid directly to the provider if the providers accept "assignment" (agree to accept repayment at Medicare rates). Users or their families must absorb the difference between the official reimbursement rate and the full provider charges if assignment is not accepted. As noted earlier, Medicare also restricts the amount of coverage to 100 days of SNF service per defined benefit or illness period.

Medicaid, in contrast, does not limit the amount of service, but it does limit the rate for reimbursement of covered services. In some States, reimbursement is on a prospective basis; in others it is retro-

34

spective, while in still others, it is based on a flat rate. Some States have adopted Medicare reimbursement formulae, while others have developed separate Medicaid fee schedules.

Third-party payers constitute another set of interveners in the decision to seek and use LTC services. To the extent that they pay for services, they reduce the out-of-pocket expenditures of users and their families, thereby possibly increasing utilization. Of course, this expanded use may be offset by users' reluctance to pay the necessary insurance premiums to gain access to coverage. This reluctance may be important with respect to private health insurance but would be negligible in connection with Medicare, which is compulsory for most employed persons. On the other hand, to the extent that Medicare and Medicaid both limit amounts of service provided, the amounts of use may lie below those desired by users and/or health and social service professionals. If third-party payers limit reimbursement levels, they may also reduce the amount of service which providers may be willing to supply to the users. In the latter case, the amount of service utilization may lie below those levels desired by users and professionals.

In light of the key role of public and other third-party payment in all health care and in certain aspects of LTC, it is necessary to understand how the actions of government and the insurance industry affect use and provision of LTC. These agencies interact with individual users and providers, as noted earlier, and, in so doing, influence use and provision outcomes through legislation and regulation, including rate-setting. They also induce changes in user and provider actions in a feedback sense. Furthermore, governmental actions, in particular, may influence the well-being of entire industries and provider groups nationwide or in specific regions through reimbursement rate and/or eligibility decisions. Their effect on groups of patients is also critical. Many governmental actions have been extensively examined by political scientists employing models of bureaucratic politics and by health and public finance economists; yet our analytical understanding is spotty. Knowledge of the objectives of policymakers and regulators in LTC is also merely rudimentary, as is the impact of constraints on LTC policy decisions. We have not adequately calculated the impacts of LTC policy decisions on users, provider industries, or regional or national economic conditions, nor do we know enough of the actions and influences of private LTC insurers.

In the following chapters, both the micro and macro aspects of these questions will be analyzed to the extent made possible by the existing state of knowledge. Additionally, we will try to remain sensitive to the interactions between micro and macro conditions, while retaining an awareness of dynamics.

Need Versus Demand

Much of the discussion thus far has employed such terms as "needs", "requirements," and "wants." This is largely the language of health care professionals and their social service and analytical allies (social workers, sociologists, epidemiologists, demographers, political scientists, policymakers, etc.). Economists, however, prefer terms such as "demand," "supply," "utilization," and "price." Unfortunately, these differences are more than semantic; they emphasize differences in the analysis of LTC (and other social service provision) and in the approaches suitable for policy.

Needs and Wants

The concept of need reflects the opinions of professionals in the relevant fields—physicians, nurses, therapists, certain social science analysts, and, often, policymakers—as to the amount of LTC a given population "ought" to consume over a specified time span (Jeffers, Bognano, and Bartlett, 1971). Needs are usually defined in medical terms as the amount of service necessary to make or keep people as "healthy" as possible given the state of medical (and social service/ science) knowledge.[11] For LTC, need can be defined as "... a normative assessment of the long term care a person must receive in order to maintain or improve his/her health status, functional ability or postpone disability or death" (Grimaldi and Sullivan, 1981). As with other types of provision, defining needs in LTC demands information on existing health states, a clearly defined standard of "good" health and/or functioning, and perfect knowledge of what actions and services are necessary to achieve good health and functioning. These mandates are difficult enough to fulfill with respect to short-term interventions. In LTC they are even more problematical. As shown in following chapters, our knowledge of health and functional condition, mental status, social circumstances (presence or absence of family, spouse, etc.), economic situations, and availability of external supports for potentially vulnerable and dependent candidates for LTC is often scanty and imperfect; we do not measure what we think, nor do we measure what we should. Standards for good practice and good outcomes in LTC are even less well defined than for many medical procedures. The role of prevention is even less understood than for acute conditions. Lastly, we know very little about the effects of certain procedures, caring situations, diets, and drugs on LTC users; hence, we may not be able to produce desired outcomes even if we could define them.

---

[11] This definition of "need" applies to services other than LTC, that is, to the judgments of relevant professionals regarding the requirements of their specific client groups.

More important, however, LTC may be related to uncertain and delayed outcomes. As noted in the preceding section on the role of time, LTC outcomes may not be positive in the sense of removing a bad condition; rather they may be of a holding or deferring nature. They may also just be aimed at easing a painful transition, as with hospice care for the dying. They may be mundane as well as sophisticated.

Despite these informational and definitional difficulties, we do have some good ideas about what seems productive in certain situations. Particularly imaginative programs of LTC have yielded some positive results. The task now is to develop the information, often on an epidemiological basis, to analyze LTC and proposed procedures and policies. (These imperatives are discussed in Chapters III and VII.)

Wants derive from what the public would like to have rather than from the judgments of professionals. The public's wants for LTC may be as relevant to LTC problems as are needs defined by professionals. The relative merits of wants versus needs depends on whose judgments are more highly valued, the public's or the professionals'. Differences between needs and wants may derive from users' reluctance to receive certain types of service (for example, because of pejorative connotations). Ignorance is probably more important as a cause of this discrepancy. In LTC, this ignorance may afflict both the public and the professionals. In some cases, the public may want more LTC of a certain type, for example, that provided in nursing homes, because of perception about financial advantage and lack of service in the community. In other cases, the public may forego access to formal types of LTC provision because of misconceptions about the state of physical deterioration, etc., which might argue for institutionalization.

Wants may also be powerfully influenced by needs, in that the public comes to believe what it is told by the specialists in LTC. In such cases, wants and needs coincide more. Since wants, as we will see, compose a key element in defining tastes (preferences) and, thus, demand, this interaction may be very crucial in determining the amount of provision actually sought and, therefore, the amount and type of provision which policymakers seek to ensure.

The Economist's Concept of Demand

Demand, in contrast to need and want, is a behavioral concept expressing the linkages between what the public wants and what society can or desires to provide. As with other commodities, the demand for LTC is related to (is a function of) the price of LTC, the prices of alternatives to LTC, the financial abilities of the users of LTC, and the desire for all goods and services, not just LTC. Demands by all LTC consumers also are functions of the size of the population of potential users (in the case of LTC, especially the

37

numbers of people 85 and older) and of the collective consumer desires for all goods and services. (LTC users may include families, friends, or other agents for the client who may not be able to make self-interested "rational" choices.) The analysis of demand specifies the more important factors in the demand for a commodity and attempts to demonstrate that the quantity demanded of a service is affected by the listed factors individually. Conventionally, economists have started by considering the influence of price on quantity demanded, holding others things equal.

Symbolically, we may express the demand relationship as

$$Q_{LTC} = f(P_{LTC}, P_A, F, T, W)$$

where Q_{LTC} is the amount of LTC demanded by consumers,
       P_{LTC} is the price of LTC,
       P_A is the price of alternatives to LTC,
       F is financial resources,
       T is the population of potential users, and
       W is the collective desire of consumers for all types of goods and services.

As shown in Figure I-5, this specification can be expressed as a negatively sloped demand curve relating price and quantity. It also determines the position and slope (elasticity) of the curve. Changes in variables other than P_{LTC} would move the curve or change its slope (that is, shift the curve). Changes in P_{LTC} would, by themselves, cause a movement *along* the curve. The price-quantity relationship could be expressed as

$$Q_{LTC} = g(P_{LTC})$$

where P_A, F, T, and W are all held constant.

Grimaldi and Sullivan (1981) put LTC demand more explicitly in that they identify four major influences: physician-related, health-related, socio-demographic, and economic. Health-related factors appear quite straightforward. Physician influences reflect current medical practice, as well as doctors' understanding of alternative modes of care and willingness to use those alternatives. Socio-demographic factors include marital status, education, ethnicity, and users' preference for differing care modes. The economic element includes prices (of LTC, alternatives, etc.), income, and, particularly in LTC, the availability of third-party reimbursement, private and/or public.

Although one may discuss the concept of LTC demand in an abstract sense, it may be more appropriate to look at demands for various types of LTC. This is particularly true since different LTC services are often substitutes for each other as well for other types of medical/social services. They can also complement each other in

38

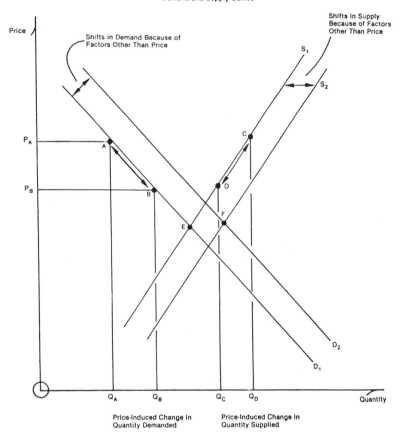

FIGURE I-5
Demand and Supply Curves

concert with other forms of service. For example, nursing home care may stand in for nursing care in a hospital, but it may also be added during periods of convalescence. Similarly, home care can substitute for either hospital or nursing home care and/or represent a less intensive stage of care as a patient progresses. (See Chapter VII.) For analytical and empirical purposes, it is imperative that these interactions be distinguished. Empirical work should be focused on the demand for one type of service but should simultaneously involve the substitutes and complements of the care or service under analysis. For example, analysis of the demand for nursing home service should include the availability of alternatives such as home care.

Paul Feldstein, in his 1979 analysis of the demand for medical care as the demand for treatments, asserts the importance of health status, cultural-demographic characteristics, and economic factors. He emphasizes that the relevant price is the net price to the user after payments for care from third-party payers. He also includes the cost of time as part of the price that users must pay. Those users with higher incomes will have higher opportunity costs of time lost to illness; hence they will seek care that saves them time. Their use of care at a given price may thus be higher than for lower paid potential users. Given that most individuals receiving LTC services are not in their most economically productive years, the time factor is not a very significant influence on LTC demand. Also, LTC provision may not, for most of them, represent an investment in enhancing or restoring productive powers (Grimaldi and Sullivan, 1981). On the other hand, while their time is not highly priced, that of their families may be quite valuable. For dependent elderly living at home and/or being cared for by members of their families, the amounts of family time necessary to provide services (even if only supervisory) can be considerable. That time cost, in addition to the personal stresses it implies, could be considerable. For LTC, therefore, the time factor in demand must explicitly reflect family time requirements.

Supply and Equilibrium in LTC

Supply must respond to demand if care is to be provided. As is clear from the earlier parts of this chapter, there are many types of LTC service and many types of providers. Some are commercial or proprietary; some are volunteers; some are family, and some are public. Each type of providers will have different motivations and be inspired by different incentives leading to the provision of varying amounts of service under widely divergent circumstances. To sharpen the focus on the demand-need interaction, it will be useful to focus on the supply emanating from proprietary providers. Their behavior can be presumed to reflect general assumptions about profit-maximizing behaviors among all commercial suppliers of any type of service. In addition, as stated earlier, the motives and

40

behaviors of volunteers, families, various types of health/social professionals, etc., are only imperfectly understood. Therefore, for abstract theoretical purposes, we can assume that a certain amount of supply will emanate from them anyway. The commercial provision will then be an additional source of supply.

If we assume profit maximization as a motive, then supply of a commodity is conventionally assumed to reflect the price of that commodity (P_{LTC}), the prices of inputs needed to produce the commodity (P_I), the market structure (M) within which the commodity is produced (purely competitive, monopolistic, oligopolistic, few sellers, etc.), and the technology available (R). These factors define the supply function which may be symbolically and graphically expressed in much the same manner as the demand function. (See Figure I–5.) Symbolically, we could write a supply function as

$$Q_{LTC} = \ominus (P_{LTC}, P_1, M, R)$$

We may also relate the quantity supplied to the price which is offered to the supplier(s), that is, $Q_{LTC} = \ominus (P_{LTC})$, where P_1, M, and R are all held constant. Again, note that one must distinguish between the supply and the quantity supplied. Normal supply curves slope upward, reflecting the law of diminishing returns in production. Obviously, changes in technology, input prices, and the other determinants of supply will affect the position of the curve, just as prices will affect the quantity supplied.

As with the demand for LTC, it is probably the case that the analyst should focus on one element in the pattern of provision, for example, the supply of nursing home services or of home care, rather than on the whole of LTC.

Equilibrium in prices and quantities in most markets is defined as occurring at the intersection of the demand and supply curves or at a position reflecting consistency between the behavior of demanders and suppliers. At equilibrium, the quantity the demanders wish to purchase at a given price equals the quantity of the commodity the suppliers wish to provide at that price. Other price-quantity combinations cannot be sustained without some external influences (governmental price fixing, for example), since they will generate excess demands or supplies which will bring the market back into equilibrium. For example, if demanders want more at a given price than suppliers wish to provide, prices will be bid up until consumers wish to buy less and sellers wish to provide more. The converse is also true.

The equilibrium attained may not be satisfactory in the opinions of some observers. For example, the equilibrium price, which may reflect society's capacity to produce LTC, may also be so high that it precludes most people from buying in the open market.

41

Under normal circumstances, an excess demand for a commodity will be corrected by appropriate price and quantity adjustments in the short run (that is, both will increase). In the long run, if the equilibrium price leads to profits or losses, suppliers will expand their production (profits) or reduce it (losses). Also, new suppliers may enter the industry, or existing suppliers may leave it. Economists refer to these adjustments in supplies in terms of the elasticities of supply. If suppliers increase or decrease quantity supplied by proportionally more than price changes, then supply is said to be elastic, that is, it has a value greater than 1.0. In such a case, the market may respond very rapidly to changes in demand which alter prices. If the response is slower, then the short-run elasticity is "low," and the industry may not so rapidly adjust to changed demand conditions. It may be elastically higher in the long run, however. In the case of LTC, there has been much speculation about the private market's short-run and long-run elasticities of supply, especially since Medicaid provisions contributed so signally to the expansion of demand by reducing net costs to consumers and increasing the public's want for LTC.

Market Equilibrium and Need

Obviously, there is no necessary relationship between the amount of LTC provided at equilibrium in the market and the amount which experts say is needed. The latter reflects best judgments, the former, behavior of consumers and suppliers as influenced by market forces and the determinants of demand and supply. If, for example, the amount of LTC provided and used at equilibrium in the market falls short of what experts say is needed, then the latter will say that there is a shortage or that there is "unmet need." Take the case of provision for nursing care for LTC-dependent people. Relatives, volunteers, and others may provide a fixed amount of care, determined by their presumably non-market motivations.[12] This amount of supply can be shown by the vertical line, V, in Figure I–6. Similarly, the amount of need as determined by expert opinion can be shown by the vertical line, N, on the same figure. Now assume the demand for LTC nursing is shown by the line DD, and the supply of such care by the line SS. SS and DD intersect at point E, with equilibrium price P_e and quantity Q_e. Medical experts might argue that this results in unmet need, since provision is not equal to Q_n, that level set by their need determination. Were a price P_1, lower than P_e, to appear in the market, there would be excess market demand, a market "shortage" equal to the gap between Q_d (the amount demanded at P_1) and Q_s (the amount supplied at P_1). Presumably market forces would correct

---

[12] Actually, both market forces and government policies may affect the supply behavior of non-market, non-proprietary suppliers. We do not deal with this factor here, however.

this shortage by adjusting both price and quantity. According to the experts, however, a "normative shortage" comprised of (Q_dQ_s) plus (Q_dQ_n) would also exist. Even if the market shortage were eliminated by increasing supply, some normative shortage (Q_dQ_n) would remain by expert reckoning.

The existence of this normative shortage has evoked public policy responses affecting both the demand and supply of LTC and other types of social services provision. In part, these policy responses reflect the belief that the public "should" want and have more LTC and "should" be able to afford it. This set of beliefs has led to educational campaigns about nursing home care, etc., but, more importantly, it has led to Federal programs to reduce to near zero the prices which LTC consumers must pay. Not only have these programs increased the quantity demanded by lowering price, they have also expanded demand (moved the demand curve outward). Additionally, they have skewed the demand away from and toward various types of care, depending on the nature of the financial incentive involved. Current Federal LTC financing policy and reimbursements stimulate the use of nursing home care but tend to discourage (move the demand curve to the left for) home care and/or adult day care.

On the supply side, Federal policy in the health care field has increased the supply of doctors, nurses, and other health care professionals. The nation's hospital beds have been augmented under the Hill-Burton Act, while nursing homes have been built under both Federal agricultural and housing programs. In some instances, Federal reimbursement of LTC costs has indirectly led to the expansion of the supply of LTC facilities, at least to the extent that reimbursement systems have provided a profit incentive for such expansion.

In many cases, the combination of Federal enhancement of demand and reimbursement policy has only added to the shortage problem. Refer again to Figure I–6. Assume that Federal policies have had two effects on the demand for LTC: they have lowered net price to users and families through third-party payments, and they have expanded demand, as has the increasing size of the older population. Even without increased demand, the reduction in prices would expand the quantity demanded. If Federal reimbursement policy compensated for this expanded amount of provision by allowing higher Federal repayments as costs rose (as shown by the positively sloped supply curve) with expanding output, then lowering net prices to users would not, by itself, aggravate the shortage problem. Suppliers would get what they would need to cover costs to offer the desired amount of provision, and the public would move nearer to receiving the amounts of LTC which experts believe that they should have. On the other hand, if there is, or can be, no supply side response, then the shortage problem may well be aggravated. If Fed-

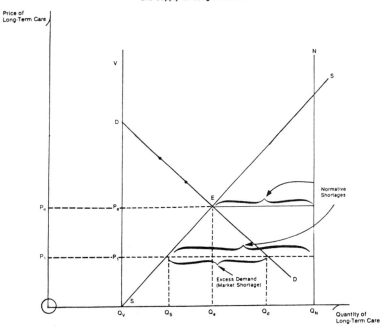

FIGURE I-6
Needs, Wants, Demand,
and Supply for Long-Term Care

Source: Adapted from Jeffers, James R., Mario Bognanno, and John Bartlett, "On the Demand Versus Need for Medical Services and the Concept of 'Shortage'," *American Journal of Public Health*, January 1971, pp. 46-63.*

*Reprinted with permission.

eral reimbursement levels are set too low to allow for cost recovery and/or inducements to private providers to expand the availability of services, it is possible that Federal programs may actually exacerbate the normative shortage problems.

Does Supply Create Its Own Demand for LTC?

Many analysts have asserted that, in the health field in particular, suppliers have been seeking to augment the demand for their services. As noted in the section on gatekeeping, it can be argued that physicians, faced with competition or other forces, may prescribe more treatment and tests than are medically necessary to augment their own incomes. This behavior, it is often claimed, is more prevalent when third-party payers pick up most of the cost, since users presumably will not be so price sensitive as when they must pay out of their own pockets. Similar arguments have surfaced in connection with LTC provision, especially that offered by nursing homes. In the case of doctors, however, Paul Feldstein (1979) has noted that the expansion of demand may have arisen as much from the intervention of other factors (increased public awareness of medical problems and therapies, changes in age structure increasing health vulnerability, etc.) as from the zeal of doctors in prescribing excessive amounts of treatment, especially surgery. He does note, however, that an unresolved problem is found in the steady expansion of demand for medical services somewhat after, rather than before, there has been an expansion in the supply of professionals and available services. Citing extensive evidence, La Dou and Likens (1977) also argue that supply may indeed create its own demand because of competition, the technological imperative, and third-party payment. In the LTC situation, however, it is difficult to imagine that suppliers could exercise much direct influence on the decision to use LTC services, particularly since most nursing homes and other LTC providers control neither the prescription of services nor, directly, the level of reimbursement. On the other hand, the existence of a large supply of nursing homes, for example, may skew policy in the direction of favoring the use of those facilities to the exclusion of other types of service. (These issues will be discussed in Chapter VII.) Again, more research is needed in these areas.

The Economic Approach Applied to Home Care

To illustrate the application of the economic model just set forth, let us examine a hypothetical case of home care (HC) provision. HC is an amalgam of home chore and home health services.

Assume that a given jurisdiction has an elderly (65+) population of one million. Expert judgment about that population suggests that perhaps 6 percent of the elderly "should have" or "could use" HC. This implies a "need" for 60,000 units of HC per day if provided

45

daily. The assessment of need is a normative conclusion which would serve as a reference point for estimating unmet need and would be reflected in the position of line N in Figure I–6. Assume also that all segments of the public agree with this estimate of "need."

Assume now that family and friends of the dependent elderly would provide 10,000 units of HC per day under all circumstances. This baseline provision would be reflected in line V in Figure I–6. There would now remain an unmet need of 50,000 units of HC per day. How would that be provided?

If users and their families could buy HC, they might react to a set of prices in the manner shown in the following table.

P_{HC}	Amount (Q_D) of HC they would purchase
$50 per unit	0 units
40 per unit	10,000 units
30 per unit	20,000 units
20 per unit	30,000 units
10 per unit	40,000 units

It is clear that in this example the buyers of HC behave in an expected fashion. As the price drops, other things (income, tastes, etc.) remaining constant, they will purchase more. Even at a low price of $10 per unit, there would still be an unmet need of 10,000 units. In other words, the purchase of 40,000 units added to the baseline 10,000 units does not add up to the estimated need for 60,000 units.

Thus far, we have not determined whether users and their families could get the amount of HC they would buy at the various prices. We also need to know how much HC will be provided at various prices in the market by suppliers. To know this, we have to look at suppliers' behaviors at various prices as follows.

P_{HC}	Amount (Q_s) suppliers would provide	Difference between Q_S and Q_D ($Q_S - Q_D$)
$50 per unit	40,000	+40,000
40 per unit	30,000	+20,000
30 per unit	20,000	0
20 per unit	10,000	−20,000
10 per unit	0	−40,000

From bringing the demanders' and suppliers' schedules together, it is clear that the market equilibrium price is $30 per HC unit, because at that price, the quantity demanders want equals the amount suppliers will provide. At any price higher than $30, there will be an excess supply. That is, suppliers will try to produce more than consumers want at that price, and the price will tend to fall back to the equilibrium because of competition among sellers. The reverse is also true: at prices below $30 there will be excess demand; consumers will want more than is available at those prices, and prices will be bid up by competition among consumers.

Even though an equilibrium may be established in the market, thus eliminating any market shortage or oversupply, there may still be "unmet need" because at equilibrium the purchased HC plus the contributed baseline HC only add up to 30,000 units (30,000 shy of the 60,000 estimated to be necessary). If the expert judgments are accepted by the public and the policymakers, various options may be adopted to fill the unmet need.

The authorities may choose to provide the HC required, thus increasing supply (moving the supply curve to the right). In the United States and many European countries, however, direct provision by public authorities has been limited. The preferred mode has been to finance the purchase of care by consumers in the marketplace, either on a reimbursable basis (the consumer pays and then collects from the government) or through direct government payment to the providers. Whether the government is a provider of care or of finance, the effect is to reduce the price to the consumer, often to zero, and thus to increase the quantity demanded (utilization or utilization rate).

Not only may the quantity demanded increase, but also users and their families above the projected 6 percent may come to believe that they also need HC. Additionally, present users may think that they need more HC. These changes in tastes may be translated into shifts in demand and a movement outward of the demand curve. In our example, consumers may be induced to increase their utilization if their net price is dropped to $10 per unit because the government finances all or part of the care. Existing users or new users may also increase their desire for HC so that even at the old equilibrium price of $30 they will want to buy more than the 20,000 HC units originally demanded.

Government attempts to expand HC use may not succeed unless the price to the supplier is raised, especially if the supply curve is positively sloped as in our example. In that instance, the production of more HC means higher costs to suppliers and subsequent increases in prices that they must charge. If the government pays the higher prices, there may be no problem, but if cost-containment or other political/economic pressures make the government unwilling

47

to pay higher prices, expanded financial support may just induce a market shortage which will augment the unmet need. Consumers, in that case, will desire more cheap (to them) care, but if the government does not raise the HC price it pays, suppliers may provide only the amount of care they made available at the old price, $30. Excess demand conditions may develop, waiting lists for HC may appear, and a black market may develop. Users may make under-the-table payments to HC providers or find other ways to jump their place in line. This situation is aggravated if the elasticity of HC supply is low. Suppose that consumers now want 40,000 HC units because the price to them is only $10. If an expansion of supply to 40,000 units runs into rapidly increasing costs and requires a corresponding increase in price to $60 (rather than $50), the government may have to pay a great deal more for HC than may be politically possible. If, at the same time, the consumers' responsiveness (the price elasticity of demand) is very high, the government may face a huge increase in quantity demanded which can only be met with a huge increase in outlays to induce the needed expansion of supply.

Of course, the government may also be fortunate in encountering a very high elasticity of supply (the supply curve may be almost flat), so that more HC does not cost a great deal more per unit of care. Nevertheless, at subsidized prices, the total number of HC units demanded may still increase significantly, thus greatly increasing the size of the government's bill. In the example, if the government reduces the users' price of care to $20, the public will want to buy 30,000 units of care. Even if the unit cost or price of HC does not go up, the cost to the government will be 30,000 units times $30 per unit ($900,000), minus the amount the public pays ($20 per HC unit or $600,000), equalling $300,000. If the price to the public is reduced further, to $10 per HC unit, quantity demanded will go to 40,000 units, the net government cost of which will be $800,000 (40,000 times $30 per unit minus 40,000 times $10 per unit).

The government may attempt to develop sources of HC supply to curtail rises in costs. In effect, it may seek to increase the elasticity of supply by financing or underwriting the training of HC operatives or the establishment of HC agencies. It may also encourage or coerce local governments to establish or subsidize HC agencies and providers. If these efforts are successful, they may yield more HC at little or no increase in unit price to the government, particularly if enough time has elapsed to allow supply to increase (that is, to shift the supply curve to the right). Nonetheless, the government still encounters increased costs from these efforts, costs which may preclude offering other types of services and/or which may require higher taxes. At the same time, other health and social care costs may increase because of the competition for inputs by an expanding

HC sector. This externality of HC may cause additional costs to the government. The problem gets even worse if families and friends reduce their baseline HC provision (below 10,000 units) because of government provision. Of course, if families can therefore earn more, they may be able to pay more of HC costs themselves, thus reducing government outlays somewhat. Politically, choices may be difficult to make.

In any event, even after stimulating increased use of HC and increasing its supply, the government may find that there is still unmet need in the eyes of the experts and, possibly, the public. Whether that need can ever be met or whether it just expands as provision expands is uncertain. Even if the need can be met, however, the government still has to decide whether it wants to do so and at what cost.

The Issues and the Research Agenda

Long-term care presents both the analyst and the policymaker with a complex of causes, requirements, and policy responses. LTC needs arise from a multiplicity of causes, call forth a variety of services, and depend on a wide spectrum of private and public supports.

The problem of LTC in American society has increased because of a changing age structure, changing family situations, and increased costs of health and social services, themselves a result of demographics, inflation, and higher expectations. These complexities confront the student of LTC with extremely difficult analytical and policy problems which provide abundant opportunities for analytical development and creative policy responses.

Analyzing the problems of LTC requires a systemic and systematic approach to the analysis, the manner of making provision, and the pattern of financial support. At present, this systemic approach is lacking. A systems approach requires a statement of goals for outcomes of LTC provision, a set of standards by which to monitor the performance of the system, and a system design. Goals appear on the individual, family, and system levels and largely relate to the maintenance or enhancement of functional performance with as much independence as possible. Standards for the system imply understanding the links between system components and system outcomes as linked to goals of the system. As Brody (1980) and Callahan (1980) emphasize, the system must provide care that is adequate, available, and affordable in a comprehensive, continuous, and coordinated structure.

Unfortunately, at present there is no system of LTC in the United States. Furthermore, public policy appears to hinder rather than enhance a systems approach. As Stanley Brody and others have emphasized, Federal Medicare and Medicaid programs favor insti-

49

tutions, while overall Federal LTC approaches aggravate the split between health and social care, a split which subverts the concept of an LTC system.

Evaluation of present LTC provision, as well as the design of an LTC system, requires the specification of goals. At the individual and family level many goals may appear: full functional restoration, death with dignity, maintenance of function in the most independent environment possible. Pursuit of LTC goals may not be feasible in the market because of economic and organizational difficulties. Consequently, the government may feel obliged to intervene in support of LTC. Again, the government's goals are manifold: administrative simplicity, creation of an LTC system or sources of provision, cost-effectiveness, satisfying a vocal constituency, etc. Unfortunately, government goals in LTC rarely are explicated at any level.

Obviously LTC is a complicated subject demanding much theorizing and research. Among the more significant definitional, organizational, and systemic topics for an LTC research agenda would be the following:

- What are the important linkages among identification of disability, information and referral, service use, and the management of individuals with specific dependency problems?
- How do families influence the use and pattern of LTC services?
- When does an investment in rehabilitation pay off?
- Do LTC providers create demand for their own or related services?
- Which disabled people need to be managed by some outside agency in their access to and use of LTC services and who can handle their needs through the market?
- What are the time-related changes in the need for LTC services for dependent individuals and across groups of such individuals?
- What is the role of the physician as a gatekeeper to LTC? What are the roles of other professionals as gatekeepers?
- How do interdisciplinary teams affect the form, use, and success of LTC provision?
- What are the most important hindrances to the development of LTC systems?
- How might public policy be changed to facilitate the development of more systemic approaches to LTC provision?
- What is the impact of proprietary provider behavior on the effectiveness of LTC provision and on the development of a systemic approach to LTC? What is the impact of other provider behavior?
- How do trade associations and professional associations

influence the use, effectiveness, and systemic characteristics of LTC provision?

- How do families behave as public LTC provision expands?

This list is not exhaustive, even for the topics considered in this chapter, and it must be considered complementary to the issues and questions set forth at various points in the preceding pages. Nevertheless, we argue that it offers a useful beginning in considering crucial questions of definition, organization, systemic development, and the applicability of economic analysis to the problems of long-term care.

FIGURE I A-1
Continuum of Long-Term Care Services, by Level of Independence

Patient Characteristic	Level of Independence	Potentially Needed Services
Wide range of options Most are married Kin and peers available Activities and social involvement readily available Mobile as desired Socioeconomic resources adequate Environment unaltered	I Independent	Health assessment/maintenance/promotion services Health education programs/education for self-care Physical fitness programs Information and referral Multipurpose senior centers Nursing services
Less wide range of options Most are married but widowed are increasing Kin and peers beginning to be unavailable Activities and social involvement less available Mobile with supports Socioeconomic resources less adequate Physical environment altered, such as senior citizen housing	II Independence Threatened	All of the above selectively plus: Health restoration services Nutrition center (congregate meals) Occasional requirement for community health nurse, home help such as chore services Community mental health center
Limited range of options Widowed increasing Kin and peers are increasingly unavailable Activities and social involvement increasingly unavailable Less mobile, even with supports Socioeconomic resources are increasingly depleted Physical environment altered more than above (such as congregate housing)	III Independence Delegated	All of the above selectively plus: Rehabilitation services Day care/day hospital In-home services--community health nurse, home health aide, homemaker chore services Escort and transportation services Friendly visiting/telephone reassurance Meals on wheels Sitting services
Severely curtailed range of options Most widowed Kin and peers largely unavailable Activities and social involvement unavailable Largely immobile Socioeconomic resources depleted Physical environment transformed, such as nursing home	IV Dependent	All of the above selectively plus: Life maintenance services Institutional care, such as nursing home or acute hospital Hospice care

Source: Grimaldi, Paul and Toni Sullivan, *Broadening Federal Coverage of Noninstitutional Long-Term Care* (Washington D.C., American Health Care Association, 1981).*

*Reprinted with permission.

FIGURE I A-2
Possible Health and Social Services Interventions,
by Level of Independence

Level I: Independent
1. Use of time in meaningful, health-promoting, self-care activities; work, volunteerism, education, self-advocacy, consumerism, political action, recreation, social involvement, hobbies, and community revitalization
2. Attitude development: consciousness raising and peer counseling, assertiveness training
3. Assistance to cope with turning points, anticipatory guidance—coping with life review
4. Physical fitness: nutrition and weight control, exercise and sexual functioning
5. Use of health care system: health maintenance/promotion checkups, health education
6. Referral assistance
7. Support clients' decisions and the right to make them
8. Education for self-care

Level II: Independence Threatened
All of the above selectively plus:
1. Health and social services, program for managing activities of daily living, periodic guidance and validation of self-care behavior
2. Living with diminished capacity and impairments, teaching self-management of necessary regimens, maintaining self-esteem, coping with losses
3. Supporting family and peers as they assist client

Level III: Independence Delegated
All of the above selectively plus:
1. Frequent monitoring of self-care activities in home or health care facilities
2. Direct illness care: therapeutic and rehabilitation services
3. Living with diminished capacity and chronicity; promoting self-esteem, assisting with planning for use of time and energy, remotivation
4. Assistance with performing activities of daily living
5. Advocacy by providers, social workers, and family
6. Assistance with environment modifications

Level IV: Dependent
All of the above selectively plus:
1. Continuous direct care
2. Continuous assistance with and monitoring of activities of daily living
3. Acceptance and coping with dying and death/terminal illness
4. Continuous, direct management of necessary regimens
5. Provide a therapeutic milieu
6. Sensory stimulation and reality orientation

Source: Grimaldi, Paul and Toni Sullivan, *Broadening Federal Coverage of Noninstitutional Long-Term Care* (Washington, D.C., American Health Care Association, 1981).*

*Reprinted with permission.

53

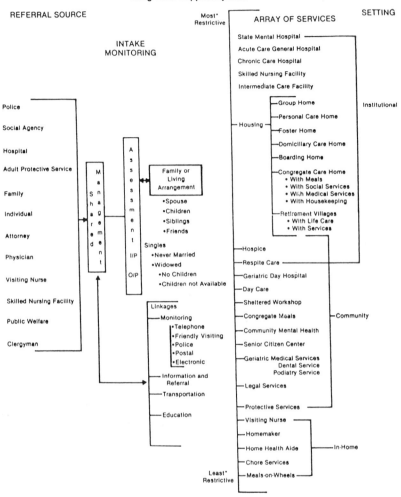

FIGURE I A-3
Long-Term Support System

REFERRAL SOURCE

INTAKE
MONITORING

Most* Restrictive

ARRAY OF SERVICES

SETTING

Police

Social Agency

Hospital

Adult Protective Service

Family

Individual

Attorney

Physician

Visiting Nurse

Skilled Nursing Facility

Public Welfare

Clergyman

Management
I/P
O/P

Assessment

Family or Living Arrangement
• Spouse
• Children
• Siblings
• Friends

Singles
• Never Married
• Widowed
• No Children
• Children not Available

Linkages
— Monitoring
  • Telephone
  • Friendly Visiting
  • Police
  • Postal
  • Electronic
— Information and Referral
— Transportation
— Education

State Mental Hospital
Acute Care General Hospital
Chronic Care Hospital
Skilled Nursing Facility
Intermediate Care Facility

— Housing
  — Group Home
  — Personal Care Home
  — Foster Home
  — Domiciliary Care Home
  — Boarding Home
  — Congregate Care Home
    • With Meals
    • With Social Services
    • With Medical Services
    • With Housekeeping
  — Retirement Villages
    • With Life Care
    • With Services

— Hospice
— Respite Care
— Geriatric Day Hospital
— Day Care
— Sheltered Workshop
— Congregate Meals
— Community Mental Health
— Senior Citizen Center
— Geriatric Medical Services
    Dental Service
    Podiatry Service
— Legal Services
— Protective Services
— Visiting Nurse
— Homemaker
— Home Health Aide
— Chore Services
— Meals-on-Wheels

Institutional

Community

In-Home

Least* Restrictive

---

* The classification of from most to least restrictive is a general view of services and may vary within each service.

Source: Brody, Stanley *et al,* "Planning for the Long-Term Support/Care System: The Array of Services To Be Considered." Prepared for Region III Center for Health Planning, Philadelphia, June 1979

FIGURE I A-4
Long-Term Care Services and Provider Agencies

Long-Term Care Services	*Providers of Services*
Homemaker/Chore	General Hospital
Home Health	Specialty Hospital
Transportation	Nursing Home
	Residential Facility
Social Services	Hospice
Personal Care (ADL)	Mental Health Center
Nursing	Home Health Agency
Legal Assistance	Homemaker Agency
Nutritionist/Dietician	Day Hospital
Telephone Reassurance	Day Care Center
	Sheltered Workshop
MD-DO Services	Hospital Emergency Room
Other Medical (Dentists,	
Optometrists)	Neighborhood Health Center
Counseling	Multipurpose Senior Center
Information and Referral	HMO
	Public Social Service Agency
Physical Therapy	Public Health Agency
Occupational Therapy	Individual Practitioners
Chiropody	Voluntary Social Service Agency
Nursing Home	Vocational Rehabilitation
	Agency
Residential Care	Employment Agency
	Adult Activity Center for
	Handicapped
Day Care	Library
Friendly Visiting	Recreation Agency
Recreation	Public Housing Authority
Protective Service	Public/Private Transportation
	Company
Speech and Hearing	Halfway House
Assessment Service	Foster Home
Foster Care	Church/Synogogue
Meals on Wheels	Community Long-Term Care
	Center
Congregate Meals	Outreach
Case Management	Sitting Service
Mental Health	Escort Service
Job Assistance	Laundry Service
Housing Assistance	Placement Service
Sheltered Employment	Special Support Group
Emergency Care	Hospice Care
Pre-retirement Counseling	Night/Day Partial Hospital or
Equipment Loan	Residential Care
Shopping Assistance	Family Member
Congregate Housing	
Day Health Care	

Source: Callahan, James Jr., "The Organization of the Long Term Care System and the Potential for a Single Agency Option," Discussion Paper DP-16b, Brandeis University, University Health Policy Consortium, February 1979

55

FIGURE I A-5
Long-Term Care System Array of Functions

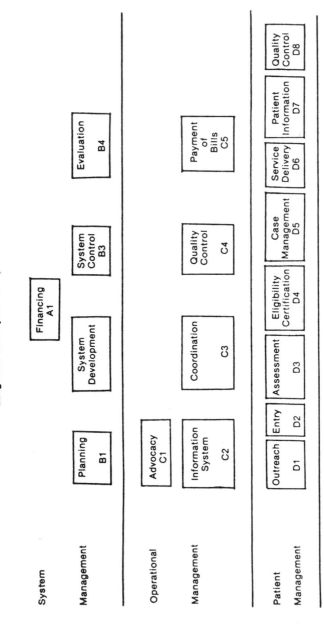

'Capital letters refer to management levels

Source: Callahan, James J., Jr., "The Organization of the Long Term Care System and the Potential for a Single Agency Option," Discussion Paper DP–16b, Brandeis University, University Health Policy Consortium February, 1979

FIGURE I A-6
Long-Term Care System Agencies Providing System Management Components

Financing
HCFA OHDS
AoA HUD VA
State Medicaid and
Title XX Agencies
State Mental Health
County Institutions
Local Matching

A1

Planning
HCFA OHDS AoA
State HSA
State DoN
State A95
State TXX
Regional HSA
Local Councils

B1

System Development
HCFA OHDS
State Health Department

B2

System Control
HCFA OHOS
AoA
State TXX
State Rate Setting
State Health

B3

Evaluation
HCFA
OHDS
NIA

B4

Source: Callahan, James J., Jr., "The Organization of the Long Term Care System and the Potential for a Single Agency Option," Discussion Paper DP-16b, Brandeis University Health Policy Consortium, February 1979

FIGURE I A-7
Long-Term Care System Agencies Providing Operational Management Components

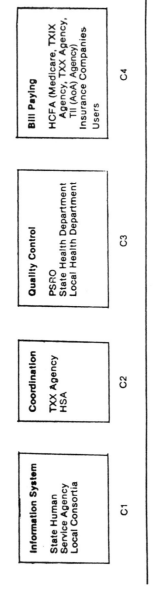

Information System	Coordination	Quality Control	Bill Paying
State Human Service Agency Local Consortia	TXX Agency HSA	PSRO State Health Department Local Health Department	HCFA (Medicare, TXIX Agency, TXX Agency, TII (AoA) Agency) Insurance Companies Users
C1	C2	C3	C4

Source: Callahan, James J. Jr., "The Organization of the Long Term Care System and the Potential for a Single Agency Option," Discussion Paper DP-16b, Brandeis University, University Health Policy Consortium, February 1979

FIGURE I A-8

Long-Term Care System Agencies Providing Patient Management Components

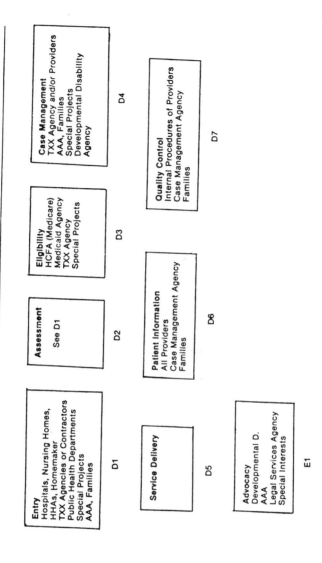

Entry
Hospitals, Nursing Homes,
HHAs, Homemaker
TXX Agencies or Contractors
Public Health Departments
Special Projects
AAA, Families

D1

Assessment
See D1

D2

Eligibility
HCFA (Medicare)
Medicaid Agency
TXX Agency
Special Projects

D3

Case Management
TXX Agency and/or Providers
AAA, Families
Special Projects
Developmental Disability
Agency

D4

Service Delivery

D5

Patient Information
All Providers
Case Management Agency
Families

D6

Quality Control
Internal Procedures of Providers
Case Management Agency
Families

D7

Advocacy
Developmental D.
AAA
Legal Services Agency
Special Interests

E1

Source: Callahan, James J. Jr., "The Organization of the Long Term Care System and the Potential for a Single Agency Option," Discussion Paper DP-16b, Brandeis University, University Health Policy Consortium, February 1979

FIGURE I A-9
Sources of Change and Sectors of Service in Long-Term Care

Sector	Demography	Manpower Growth	Professional Dynamics	Client Consciousness
		Source of Change		
Child	Large population growing both absolutely and proportionally	Apparently still growing; huge education sector in existence	Special education rising within the profession	Parent groups; strong Education of the Handicapped Act
Handicapped Young Adult	Small population not growing fast	Growing; expansion area for universities	Work with handicapped becoming more	Very high; new Rehabilitation Amendment
Disabled Adult	Moderately large, moderate increase	Unknown; may not be large	Unknown; apparently not important	Not very visible
Elderly	Moderate population growing absolutely and proportionately	Expanding substantially	Many professional sub-groups moving into this area	Very high

Source: Callahan, James J., "Delivery of Services to Persons with Long-Term Care Needs," AoA Symposium, Williamsburg, Virginia, June 12, 1980

References

Blumberg, Mark, "Control of Health Care Utilization and Costs," Kaiser Foundation, Oakland, California, March 9, 1977, mimeo.

Brody, Elaine M., "Woman's Changing Roles: The Aged Family and Long Term Care of Older People," *National Journal*, October 27, 1979, pp. 1828–1833.

Brody, Elaine M. and Stanley J. Brody, "New Directions in Health and Social Supports for the Aging," paper delivered to the Anglo-American Conference on New Patterns of Medical and Social Supports for the Aging, Fordham University, New York, May 12–13, 1980.

Brody, Stanley J., "The Formal Long-Term Support System for the Dependent Elderly," paper presented to the American College of Physicians, Washington, D.C., June 12, 1980.

Brody, Stanley J., with the assistance of Karlyn Messinger, "Planning for the Long-Term Support/Care System: The Array of Services to be Considered," prepared for Region III Center for Health Planning, Philadelphia, Pennsylvania, June 1979, mimeo.

Brody, Stanley J. and Anna Bell Woodfin, *Long-Term Support Systems: An Analysis of Health Systems Agency Plans*, Issue Paper No. 5, University of Pennsylvania, National Health Care Management Center, November 1979.

Callahan, James J. Jr., "Delivery of Services to Persons with Long-Term Care Needs," paper delivered at Administration on Aging Symposium on Long Term Care, Williamsburg, Virginia, June 12, 1980 (paper dated October 5, 1979).

Callahan, James J. Jr., "The Organization of the Long Term Care System and the Potential for a Single Agency Option," Discussion Paper DP–16b, Brandeis University, University Health Policy Consortium, February 1979.

Chapin, F. Stuart, *Human Activity Patterns in the City: Things People Do In Time and In Space*, (New York: John Wiley and Sons, 1974).

DiFederico, Elaine, William Scanlon, and Margaret Stassen, *Long-Term Care, Current Experience and a Framework for Analysis*, Working Paper 1215-10, Washington, D.C., The Urban Institute, February 1979.

Feldstein, Paul J., *Health Care Economics* (New York: John Wiley and Sons, 1979).

Gibson, Robert M., "National Health Expenditures, 1979," *Health Care Financing Review,* Summer 1980.

Grimaldi, Paul L. and Toni Sullivan, *Broadening Federal Coverage of Non-Institutional Long Term Care* (Washington, D.C., American Health Care Association and National Foundation for Long Term Health Care, 1981).

Isaacs, Bernard, "Geriatric Patients: Do Their Families Care?" *British Medical Journal*, 30, October 1971, pp. 282–286.

Jeffers, James R., Mario F. Bognanno, and John Barlett, "On the Demand Versus Need for Medical Services and the Concept of 'Shortage'," *American Journal of Public Health*, January 1971, pp. 46–63.

Juba, David A., *Price Setting in the Market for Physicians' Services, A Review of the Literature*, Research Report 79–1 (Camp Hill, Pa.: Pennsylvania Blue Shield, January 1979).

61

La Dou, Joseph and James Likens, *Medicine and Money: Physicians as Businessmen* (Cambridge, Mass.: Ballinger Publishing Co., 1977).

Robinson, John P., *How Americans Use Time, A Social-Psychological Analysis of Everyday Behavior* (New York and London: Praeger Publishers, 1977).

Sherwood, Sylvia, ed., *Long-Term Care: A Handbook for Researchers, Planners and Providers*, (New York: Spectrum Publications, 1975).

Szalai, Alexander, in collaboration with Philip E. Converse, Pierre Feldheim, Erwin K. Scheuch, and Philip J. Stone, *The Use of Time, Daily Activities of Urban and Suburban Populations in Twelve Countries* (The Hague and Paris: Mouton, 1972).

Townsend, Peter, *The Family Life of Older People* (London: Routledge and Kegan Paul, 1957).

United States Comptroller General, General Accounting Office, *The Well-Being of Older People in Cleveland, Ohio* (Washington, D.C., April 19, 1977).

United States Department of Health, Education and Welfare, Federal Council On Aging, "Key Issues in Long-Term Care—A Progress Report," Washington, D.C., December 1979.

United States Department of Health and Human Services, Health Care Financing Administration, *Health Care Financing Notes*, various issues covering financing of health care services.

United States Department of Labor, Bureau of Labor Statistics, Bulletin 2070, Washington, D.C., December 1980.

Vladeck, Bruce C., *Unloving Care: The Nursing Home Tragedy* (New York: Basic Books, 1980).

Weissert, William G., "Long-Term Care: An Overview," in U.S. Public Health Service, *Health United States 1978* (Washington: U.S. Government Printing Office, 1979).

World Health Organization, *Manual of the International Statistical Classification of Disease, Injury and the Causes of Death* (Geneva: WHO, 1977).

Chapter II

Operations Research

by Jeffrey H. Horen

Introduction

Thus far we have discussed problems in long-term care from the perspective of the public policymaker. In this chapter, we shall discuss operations research, a methodology designed to analyze decision problems, and its uses in long-term care.

Why should we be interested in operations research? The previous chapter asserts the need for a systemic view of long-term care. As in other fields, the formulation of a system can yield decision problems that were previously obscured within other issues.

For example, a public policymaker may already be aware of the decision of whether to place a patient in a nursing home or a private home. Suppose, however, that under a systemic view the policymaker envisions nursing homes and private homes as two components of a system of long-term care. In addition to the question of where to place a certain patient, there arise questions of resource allocation among the components. For example, the government could provide subsides to families to expand home care. The policymaker may not have considered this alternative unless the systemic view enabled him or her to view home care not as a fixed entity, but as one component of a system that could be altered and controlled.

Thus a systemic view can show us new decision problems, problems that can be analyzed with operations research. As we shall see, the modeling approach can enhance the creative scope of the public policymaker.

The following section defines operations research and provides a brief background on the subject. The next two sections discuss its applications to long-term care at the macro and institutional levels, respectively. The final section assesses the likelihood and direction of future applications.

What is Operations Research?

A succinct definition of operations research is offered by Harvey M. Wagner (1976) as a "scientific approach of problem solving for executive management." Application of operations research, also termed *management sciene,* involves: (1) constructing mathematical and statistical models of decision problems to treat complex and uncertain situations and (2) analyzing the relationships that determine the probable future consequences and devising appropriate

63

measures of effectiveness to evaluate the relative merit of alternative actions.

Although its scientific origins and mathematical development of some areas started in the late 1800s, operations research (OR) was first named and considered as a separate field in World War II. (The term originated with the development of radar in the Battle of Britain; a team of scientists conducted *research* to make radar *operational*.) After World War II, mathematical models for decision making spread from defense to other sectors of government and to business. This spread was accelerated by theoretical advances and by the rapid development of high-speed digital computers.

The environment most conducive to the application of OR is one that is complex in nature, producing interesting problems, but centrally controlled, allowing effective implementation of solutions. As we shall see, this description applies to some, but not all, health care systems.

In the development of OR, certain typical decision problems have been identified and linked with appropriate models. These "classical" models often serve as starting points for analyzing new situations. Some common types of models include:

(1) simulation—representing the behavior of a system over time by experimenting with a numerical model,

(2) linear programing—calculating the mix of activities which best contributes to a quantifiable objective while satisfying certain constraints,

(3) combinatorial models—dealing with situations where there are many combinations of decisions from which to choose,

(4) stochastic models—dealing with probabilities, and

(5) decision analysis—statistically analyzing decisions in uncertain environments.

In the Appendix to this chapter, we very briefly describe the general linear programing model that is applied in some examples below. However, complete description of any of the types of models just cited is beyond the scope of this chapter. We refer the interested reader to any standard OR textbook.[1]

Operations Research in Long-Term Care

Operations research was first applied to the health care field in the late 1950s. Models were developed for such diverse areas as blood banks, hospital staffs and ambulance deployment. Since 1970, OR in health care has grown rapidly for several reasons. (More than 75 percent of the published OR studies in health care have been done since 1970, according to Marshall and Richards, 1978.)

---

[1] See, for example, Budnick, Mojena, and Vollmann (1978), Hillier and Lieberman (1967), or Wagner (1976).

First, the health care field has greatly increased in complexity and size and is currently the second largest industry in the U.S. Second, there has been a trend toward greater organization. The shift has been away from the concept of a single physician operating his or her practice to a broader view of a system of aggregated and interacting health facilities.

Third, the predominance of payment for health services by third parties has changed the dealing from between a provider and single consumers to a provider and large government or large health insurance companies. These purchasing organizations, reacting to growing costs, are using their bargaining power to require new levels of efficiency by the providers. Furthermore, the organizations have also collected data that can form the basis for new management science techniques. Thus we see a trend toward large systems that are more centrally controlled and thereby more conducive to OR.

All of these reasons for the growth of OR in health care are particularly valid for long-term care. As outlined in Chapter XVII, long-term care facilities have grown rapidly in number since 1960 and are operated on a larger scale than ever before. Third-party payments, notably under Medicaid, have consolidated the concern for cutting costs, and the power to do so, to single groups—State and Federal governments. (One may, of course, note that the last reason, the growth of payments by third parties, is a major cause of the other phenomena—larger scale operations and increasing concern for cutting costs.)

In the following sections we shall consider OR models at both the macro level and the micro, or institutional, level. For each level we shall look at OR studies that have been done and then suggest other OR applications. Finally, we shall discuss the necessary prerequisites for more applications of OR in long-term care.

Macro Models

Models in long-term care at the macro level focus on the system of long-term care as a whole—its inputs and outputs and its relation to the overall system of health care. Most OR studies at the macro level consider long-term care as part of an overall system of health care for the community. Generally, these models analyze allocation of resources among competing types of care and groups of patients.

Linear Programing—Balance of Care

One advantage of a systemic approach to a problem is that decision-makers become aware not only of the effects of their decisions on their own areas but also on related components of the system. For example, one may consider different types of long-term care to best meet the needs of a group of elderly patients. Obviously, de-

65

TABLE II-1
Alternative Care Options and Resource Requirements
for One Category[1] of Elderly Patients

	Alternative Care Options (j)					
Location	1	2	3	4	5	6
Special Housing Place	X	X	X			
Own Home				X	X	X
Resource (k)						
1. Nurse (visits per week)	4	4	5	4	4	5
2. Part-Time Domestic Help (hours per week)	3	3	4	4	4	5
3. Meals Delivered to Patient's Home (per week)	1	1	4	1	1	4
4. Attendance at Psychiatric Day Hospital (times per week)	3			3		
5. Attendance at Geriatric Day Hospital (times per week)			3			3

[1] The category contains those who live with others and have poor housing, physical handicaps, and moderate to severe dementia.

Source: McDonald, Cuddeford, and Beale (1974).*

*Reprinted with permission.

voting more resources to one type of care draws resources from other types. But in a systemic view, one realizes also that devoting more resources to one or all types of long-term care can also take resources from, and therefore detract from, other areas of health care. For example, more nurses in nursing homes may mean fewer nurses in hospitals to tend younger patients.

One example of a systems model that includes long-term care as a component is a linear programing model by McDonald, Cuddeford, and Beale (1974), used in a project for the Department of Health and Social Security in Great Britain. This model is a typical resource-allocation model, in that alternative options of care are envisioned as competing for a fixed set of resources. The model measures the costs of alternative patterns of care and finds a minimum-cost combination.

In reality, each patient in a health care system may require individually specified quantities of resources for a given option of care at a given time. Furthermore, the set of options of care may depend on the individual. To simplify this setting, McDonald's model categorizes health care users into 150 groups. Each group represents a set of related patient types and has certain alternative options of care. Each option of care requires certain quantities of any of 38 specified resources. Thus, McDonald's model reduces the set of patients into a manageable number of groups and reduces a continuum of treatments into a specified set of options of care.

Thirty-four of McDonald's 150 categories are for elderly patients. Table II–1 shows six options of care for one category of elderly patients that requires five of the resources. In this example, three options involve a nursing home, and three options involve the patient's own home. The numbers in Table II–1 are the units of each relevant resource that a week of care requires under each care option. For example, Table II–1 shows that the weekly needs of a patient using Option 2 are four nurse visits, three hours of part-time domestic help, one meal delivered, and three visits to a geriatric day hospital. The model assumes that the consumption of resources in each category is linear with respect to the number of patients in the category. For example, five patients using Option 3 will require 5×4 nurse visits, 5×3 hours of part-time domestic help, 5×1 meals delivered, and 5×3 visits to a geriatric day hospital.

Below is McDonald's formulation of the decision problem of finding a least-cost allocation of patients to types of care.

$$\text{minimize } z = \sum_k C_k \sum_i \sum_j U_{ijk} \, x_{ij} \tag{1}$$

$$\text{subject to} \quad \sum_j x_{ij} \geqq D_i \text{ for all } i,$$

$$\sum_i \sum_j U_{ijk} \, x_{ij} \leqq B_k \text{ for all } k, \text{ and}$$

$$x_{ij} \geqq 0 \text{ for all } i, j,$$

where $i = 1, 2, \ldots, 150$ is a category of patient,
j is an alternative option for care,
$k = 1, 2, \ldots, 38$ is a resource,
x_{ij} is the number of patients from category i to be treated with alternative j,
C_k is the unit cost of resource k,
U_{ijk} is the usage of resource k per patient from category i under alternative j,
D_i is the number of patients in category i, and
B_k is the amount of resource k available.

The decision variable is x_{ij}. The unit costs per resource C_k were taken from previous studies or estimates by regression analysis. The U_{ijk}s are the unit resource requirements for the options of care; Table II–1 lists some of these values. For example, suppose that we index the patient category in Table II–1 as $i = 1$, the care options as $j = 1, 2, \ldots, 6$, and the resources as $k = 1, 2, \ldots, 5$. Then according to Table II–1, $U_{123} = 1$.

The first constraint in (1) ensures that all patients in all categories receive care. The second constraint limits any possible decision not to exceed the supply of available resources.

The solution to the linear program (1) gives values of x_{ij} that specify the appropriate patterns of care. McDonald *et al* (1974) found that their data did not yield a feasible solution to (1); that is, available resources *cannot* satisfy the "potential" demand for health care. Accordingly, McDonald *et al* subsequently modified the problem by reducing the resource usage factors to smaller but still "acceptable" levels of care and also reducing the demand levels by uniform percentages until a feasible solution was reached. The resulting solutions showed that, for example, 100 percent of the original level of care could be provided for 40 percent of the patients; alternatively, 50 percent of the original level of care could be provided for 50 percent of the patients. OR models frequently produce such information as by-products of their main objectives.

Expanding on this concept of flexible patient requirements, McDonald *et al* (1974) propose (but do not solve) an expansion of model (1) by replacing the fixed parameters D_i representing patient demand with decision variables d_i. They introduce an inferred-worth function $g_i(d_i)$, defined as the value of meeting demand of d_i patients in category i. The resulting non-linear program[2] is

$$\text{maximize } V = \sum_i g_i(d_i) - \sum_k C_k \sum_i \sum_j U_{ijk} \, x_{ij} \qquad (2)$$

$$\text{subject to } \sum_j x_{ij} = d_i \text{ for all } i,$$

$$\sum_i \sum_j U_{ijk} \, x_{ij} \leqq B_k \text{ for all } k, \text{ and}$$

$$x_{ij} \geqq 0, \, d_i \leqq 0 \text{ for } i, j.$$

The objective V represents the net inferred worth—value minus cost—of a given allocation of patients. Unlike D_i in (1), d_i is now a decision variable. This approach is interesting because it regards the demand for health care (including long-term care) not as an absolute "need" but as a goal that can be met in varying degrees, depending on the costs and benefits.

As one might suppose, the functions $g_i(d_i)$ would be difficult to estimate. McDonald *et al* propose to fit each g_i to the data by (a) assuming that g_i has constant elasticity with respect to satisfied demand and therefore is of the form:

$$g_i(d_i) = \alpha_i \, d_i^\beta, \text{ where } \alpha_i \text{ and } \beta \text{ are constants} \qquad (3)$$

---

[2] A *non-linear program* is a generalization of a linear program. It is formulated as the maximization or minimization of an arbitrary function of many variables subject to any number of arbitrary equality or inequality constraints involving these variables. Problem (1) is not a linear program unless the functions $g_i(d_i)$ are linear.

and (b) fixing a value $g_i(D_i) = \pi_i$, where π_i is the value of the LaGrange multiplier in the ith equation of (1).[3]

Assumption (a) is rather restrictive. The authors specify the functional form of g_i and also must state a numerical value of elasticity [given by the parameters α_i and β in (3)] to solve (2). However, the model is of interest because one can use it to infer the "ideal" levels d_i of health care demand to be met from the decisions of patterns of care made for the current levels D_i of demand.

The linear programing approach in problems involving allocation of resources is a powerful tool. Without it, problems such as (1) with an infinite number of possible decisions (patterns of care) would not be solvable. A decision-maker may be able to choose the "best" option of care for one class of patients, such as that shown in Table II–1, given a fixed set of resources. But only through linear programing can he or she model and solve a problem where the same resources cover many groups of patients. Because it accounts for this interaction of patient groups, the LP method is particularly well suited to modeling a systems approach.

Institutional Models

Institutional, or micro, models of long-term care focus on the operations of an economic unit such as a nursing home or a part-time domestic help program in a community. In this section, we suggest two OR models that can be adapted to describe institutions in long-term care. The first concerns allocation of nursing staffs in hospitals and can also apply to nursing staffs in nursing homes. The second model, used to compare efficiency of educational units, can also be used to compare the efficacy of long-term care institutions.

Referring to the systemic point of view, a micro model does not explicitly cover the interdependence of the relevant economic unit with other units in the system. However, this interdependence must be considered and, as we will show, it can be implicitly incorporated into a micro model.

Integer Programing—Personnel Staffing

An *integer program* is a linear program with the additional restriction that some or all of the decision variables be integer values. The following example is an integer programing model of a personnel staffing decision problem.

---

[3] The LaGrange multiplier or "shadow price" π_i is the marginal change in the minimum cost linear programing (LP) solution resulting from a change in the value of the right-hand side of the ith constraint. The values of the LaGrange multipliers can be obtained as a by-product of the LP solution. For more information on LaGrange multipliers, we refer the reader to any standard OR or LP textbook.

TABLE II-2
Classification of Nursing Tasks

Task Type	Description
1	Highly technical tasks for high care patients
2	Highly technical tasks for intermediate care patients
3	Highly technical tasks for self care patients
4	Less highly technical tasks for high care patients
5	Less highly technical tasks for intermediate care patients
6	Less highly technical tasks for self care patients
7	Evaluation of patient need and assignment
8	Supervising and teaching
9	Tasks preparatory to highly technical tasks
10	Tasks preparatory to less highly technical tasks
11	Clerical tasks directly related to patient care
12	Clerical tasks less directly related to patient care
13	Medical record notation
14	Housekeeping
15	Escorting and emergency checks
16	Maintenance, checking, ordering

Source: Wolfe and Young (1965).[*]

[*]Reprinted with permission from *Nursing Research*.

The staffing of nursing personnel is important to hospital administrators because their salary cost is approximately one-third of the total hospital budget. The following model was used by Wolfe and Young (1965) for hospitals and can also be applied to nursing homes, where salary costs are even larger.[4]

The work of different skill levels of nurses overlaps in some areas. For example, both a registered nurse (RN) and a licensed practical nurse (LPN) may be able to keep medical records for a patient, although the RN may do it more efficiently. With this in mind, the hospital (or nursing home) administrator may want to change his/her staffing to reduce staffing costs while adequately meeting the patients' needs.

To model this problem, we assume that there are three skill levels: registered nurse (RN), licensed practical nurse (LPN), and nurse's aide (AIDE) that can be scheduled in an eight hour shift. To represent the fact that different skill levels can do different sets of tasks, Wolfe and Young classify the patient care tasks into 16 categories, as shown in Table II-2.

We shall formulate constraints that represent the requirement that all tasks be covered. Let i denote the skill class with values

$$i = \begin{cases} 1 & \text{if RN} \\ 2 & \text{if LPN} \\ 3 & \text{if AIDE} \end{cases}$$

---

[4] According to the 1977 National Nursing Home Survey (National Center for Health Statistics, 1979), salary costs constituted 60 percent of all nursing home costs.

and let $j = 1, 2, \ldots, 16$ denote the categories of tasks listed in Table II–2. The decision variable given by X_{ij} represents the number of nurse shifts (a nurse shift is eight nurse-hours) of skill class i performing task j. The X_{ij}s can be fractions. Let B_j be the total number of nurse shifts needed for task j over an eight-hour period. (B_j is not a decision variable.) Then the coverage requirement is represented by

$$\sum_{i=1}^{3} X_{ij} \geq B_j, \text{ for } j = 1, 2, \ldots, 16 \qquad (4)$$

Since nurses can only be hired in whole numbers, we also require that

$$\sum_{j=1}^{16} X_{ij} = 0, 1, 2, \ldots, \text{ for } i = 1, 2, 3 \qquad (5)$$

Because some skill classes may perform certain tasks better than other classes, Wolfe and Young assign a "cost" c_{ij} representing the dollar value in the loss of quality of a nurse of skill class i performing task j over one shift. For example, if RNs can perform task 1 statisfactorily, $C_{11} = 0$. If LPNs can perform the task with some difficulty and AIDEs cannot do it at all, C_{21} may be positive and C_{31} may be very high.

As with McDonald's model, this model has some simplifying assumptions. For example, the tasks for a nurse are numerous and varied; the model puts them in 16 groups. The capability of doing any task almost certainly varies with the individual; the model assumes that all personnel in a given skill level perform the same task equally. As with any other OR model, such assumptions make it possible to formulate the staffing problem. The researcher and administrator must judge the plausibility of these assumptions.

Let S_i be the salary cost of a skill i nurse for one shift. The formulation is then:

$$\text{minimize} \sum_{i=1}^{3} \sum_{j=1}^{16} (S_i + C_{ij}) X_{ij} \qquad (6)$$

subject to (4), (5), and

$$X_{ij} \geq 0 \qquad (7)$$

The problem is an integer programing problem because of (5). The resulting solution will give values of X_{ij} that describe the amounts of each skill level to assign to each task.

Of course, the costs C_{ij} must be estimated by staff and administrators. As Wolfe and Young suggest, we can solve the problem for

71

"cautious" C_{ij} (where, for example, only RNs can do all tasks) and then more "liberal" C_{ij}, and then observe the change in the resulting schedules.

As stated before, the institutional model cannot fully represent the interdependence between the institution and other units. For example, the administrator of a nursing home has some control over the patient load. From a systemic view, any change in the patient load of the nursing home affects the other components of the long-term care system. The micro model does not account for the other components. Instead, we assume that the patient load is fixed and therefore the requirements B_j are also fixed.

If the model is solved for a given set of requirements B_j, and the health care planner considers a different patient load, he or she can make an alternative set of requirements B_j and solve the altered problem. By comparing solutions, he/she can measure the effect of the change in the patient load. Thus the micro model can be used in analyzing the system.

Mathematical Programing—Measuring Efficiency of Institutions

Various studies in health care focus on the "efficiency" or "productivity" of individuals, programs, or institutions. These analyses relate quantities of "outputs" (for example, patient days, caseloads, trained nurses) to inputs (such as man hours, operations, meals). Two major problems often arise in such studies. First, some desired outputs such as "quality of care" may be difficult to measure. Second, it is necessary to compare different kinds of outputs. For example, for the same quantities of inputs, is it better to have one nursing home with 100 happy patients or 200 unhappy patients?

Most analyses treat the latter problem either by narrowing the scope to one output or objective or by aggregating the outputs into one objective. Reducing the analysis to one output may facilitate comparison, but such a restriction can be misleading. Alternatively, aggregating the outputs requires that the outputs be numerically weighted. Usually such weights are arbitrary. Charnes, Cooper, and Rhodes (1978) developed a model for measuring efficiency of decision-making units that avoids both problems. The model evaluates activities of non-profit entities participating in public programs. Charnes and Cooper (1979) applied the model to public school systems. We can also apply it to long-term care facilities (and other health care decision-making units). Below we outline the general model.

Suppose that there are n long-term care facilities that we wish to evaluate, each with s different inputs and m different outputs. Charnes et al define and justify the following measures of efficiency. Let Y_{rj} denote the quantity of the rth output and X_{ij} the quantity of the ith input for facility j. If 0 is the index of the unit to evaluate, then the value h_o of 0's efficiency is the solution to the mathematical program.[5]

$$\text{Maximize } h_o = \sum_{r=1}^{s} U_r Y_{ro} \Bigg/ \sum_{i=1}^{m} V_i X_{io}$$

$$\text{subject to } \sum_{r=1}^{s} U_r Y_{rj} - \sum_{i=1}^{m} V_i X_{ij} \leq 0, \text{ for } j = 1, 2, \ldots, n, \qquad (8)$$

$$\text{and } U_r \geq 0, V_i \geq 0 \qquad \text{for all } r \text{ and } i$$

This definition of efficiency, which Charnes *et al* discuss in detail, yields values of h_o between 0 and 1. Essentially, (8) shows the ratio of outputs to inputs for unit 0 relative to the best linear combination of the other units.

To illustrate the meaning of (8), we use a simple example with two inputs and one output. Consider a set of community programs of non-institutional care with inputs X_1, part-time domestic help (in man hours per week), and X_2, meals delivered to the patient's own home (per week), and one output, Y, home care (in "units"). Figure II–1 shows inputs for five programs of care. Each vector P_j represents the quantity of each input required to produce *one* unit of care. For example, $P_5 = \binom{2}{8}$ means that one unit of output for program 5 requires two hours per week of domestic help and eight meals delivered.

The heavy broken line in Figure II–1 is the "lower envelope" of points.[6] This line relates to formulation (8) as follows. One can show that the points on this curve P_1, P_3, and P_5 have values of efficiency $h_1 = h_3 = h_5 = 1$. That is, they are the most efficient. The values of h_2 and h_4 are less than 1. In particular, one can show from (8) that P_2 has efficiency

$$h_2 = \frac{\text{distance from } A \text{ to } P_2'}{\text{distance from } A \text{ to } P_2}$$

We can also show that $h_2 = 14/15$ either by the geometry in Figure II–1 or by solving (8) and interpret this value as follows: One unit of care from program 2 currently requires three hours of domestic help and one meal per week. By taking a certain linear combination of units of care from programs 1 and 3 in a manner that gives the input vector P_2' in Figure II–1 (on the straight line connecting P_1 and P_3), we can produce one unit of care with only 14/15 of the resources

---

[5] Formulation (8) is not a linear program because the objective function h_o is a quotient. However, Charnes *et al* show how to transform (8) into an equivalent problem that is an LP. Thus we can find h_o by using the methodology for solving linear programs.

[6] We can envision the *lower envelope* as the shape that a flexible string would take if it were pulled tightly under the points in Figure II–1 without crossing any point.

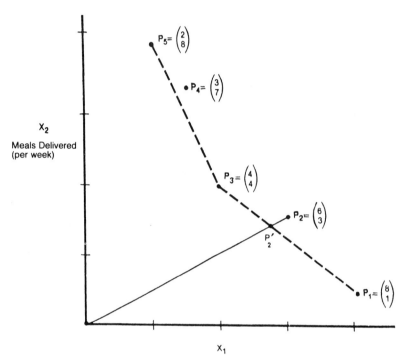

FIGURE II-1
Efficiency Points

$P_5 = \begin{pmatrix} 2 \\ 8 \end{pmatrix}$

$P_4 = \begin{pmatrix} 3 \\ 7 \end{pmatrix}$

X_2

Meals Delivered
(per week)

$P_3 = \begin{pmatrix} 4 \\ 4 \end{pmatrix}$

$P_2 = \begin{pmatrix} 6 \\ 3 \end{pmatrix}$

P_2'

$P_1 = \begin{pmatrix} 8 \\ 1 \end{pmatrix}$

X_1

Part Time Domestic Help
(hours per week)

74

needed by program 2, that is, 5.6 hours of domestic help and 2.8 meals. Therefore, we can send all of the patients in program 2 to programs 1 and 3 and require fewer resources. In this manner we can consider program 2 as being less than maximally efficient.

Thus far, we have avoided a major question in our formulation of efficiency: How are "units" of long-term care defined? Finding a quantifiable measure of outcome is a major bottleneck for applying OR to long-term care and more generally in applying quantitative analysis to health care. For this model, we suggest a change in health status of the nursing home patients over a specified period of time, say a year, where the health status is measured by an index. For example, Mitchell (1978) uses a change in a behavioral index of health status to compare the outcomes of three alternative long-term care settings in the Veterans Administration. This approach is comparable to Charnes *et al* using changes in test scores as a measure of outcome for educational institutions. Developing an adequate index of health status, however, is still a topic of considerable discussion among health planners.[7]

Other Studies

The studies discussed earlier are examples of complete OR analyses. For each problem, we formulate the model, specify the set of alternative decisions, quantify the consequences of the decisions, and obtain a solution.

There are many studies which go through some, but not all, of these steps. These are grouped under the more general term "quantitative analysis." For example, Mitchell (1978) assesses the change in health status for Veterans Administration patients who are transferred to three alternative long-term care settings. This comparison would be useful in a decision model of assigning patients to settings in which costs were incorporated. Kane *et al* (1981) model the level-of-care decisions of physicians and nurses who place patients in nursing homes. The two descriptive models are an algorithm and a linear regression. Either model could be used to develop a more complete normative model to optimize or improve the placement of long-term care patients.

Operations Research and Long-Term Care— Summary and Outlook

In view of the growing importance of long-term care within the field of health care, and the many successful applications of OR in

---

[7] For example, the Winter 1976 issue of *Health Services Research* is devoted to studies of such indexes.

other areas of health care, we may ask why there are not more OR studies in long-term care. We attribute this relative paucity to the nature of long-term care.

On the the macro level, long-term care should be viewed as one component of an overall system of health care. As stated before, then, any macro level study involving long-term care would not be restricted to this field. Alternatively, on the institutional, or micro, level, a nursing home is similar in structure to a ward in a hospital. Therefore, we can model many features in the operation of a nursing home, such as staffing and inventory of supplies, by directly applying OR models for hospitals. No conceptual change is needed. Also, a nursing home is simpler than a hospital and is easier to run, so it is less likely to require analysis of systems.

We interject that, although we may not need *new* methodology on the institutional level, nursing homes may yet benefit from more widespread application of the standard OR models for hospitals. At present, there are no published studies measuring the extent of OR practice in nursing homes. However, analysts in nursing homes are reported to be using OR techniques to solve problems such as scheduling of nurses.

A second reason for the lack of OR studies is that systems of long-term care are in general not centrally controlled. As was previously mentioned, central control is more conducive to application of OR. Therefore, decision models of systems are not as relevant in long-term care as in other fields.

A final and major reason is that the outcome of long-term care is difficult to evaluate, as we mentioned in the previous section. As useful indexes of health status are developed, we can expect more OR studies.

We have offered justifications for not having more OR research in long-term care. However, the benefits of an OR approach often extend beyond the intended benefits of solving the stated problem. The modeling process can often illuminate aspects of the problem that were previously overlooked.

For example, the OR approach forces a formal setting of goals. An agent of a State granting the certificate of need to a nursing home may apply a queuing model with the intended goals of high occupancy and low costs from service and empty beds. But the model may also suggest that reducing time on a waiting list is a desirable goal.

As another example, the modeling process forces the planner to enumerate resources. In home health care, part-time domestic help and meals delivered to the home are obvious resources. But one must also allow for services of administrators. The planner of a

76

community program may overlook this resource, but an OR model would draw attention to it.

In addition, the OR approach may enhance the creative scope of the planner of long-term care, as it often does for managers in other areas. For example, as we discussed for macro models, McDonald *et al* (1974) first conceived of the balance of care problem as a decision of allocating scarce resources to fixed demands. But the formulation led them to change the demands from fixed parameters to decision variables and also to alter the previously fixed quantities of resources. Therefore, the modeling process of OR may yield useful insights into problems in long-term care.

Reiterating our assessment of future studies, the development of good health status indexes, combined with the growing interest in long-term care, should produce a greater number of successful applications of operations research in long-term care.

Appendix
Linear Programing

This Appendix gives a very brief description of linear programing (LP) and defines the common terms. For a more complete description we refer the reader to any standard operations research text.

Linear programing is an operations research technique that models problems involving allocation of resources or activities as the mathematical problem of maximizing or minimizing a linear function, called the objective function, of a set of variables.

The variables can have integer or non-integer values and are usually restricted to being non-negative. In addition, the variables must satisfy a set of linear equalities and/or inequalities, called constraints. Below is an example of an LP problem with three variables x_1, x_2, and x_3 and two constraints.

$$\text{Minimize} \quad z = 4x_1 + 2x_2 + x_3 \quad (9)$$
$$\text{subject to} \quad x_1 + x_2 + x_3 \leq 10$$
$$2x_1 + x_2 + 0.5x_3 \geq 10$$
$$x_1, x_2, x_3 \geq 0$$

The function z to be minimized is the objective function. A set of values of the variables that satisfy the constraints of an LP problem is called a *feasible solution.* In the example given here, the values $x_1 = 4$, $x_2 = 3$, $x_3 = 0$ make a feasible solution because they satisfy both inequality constraints. The value of the objective z for this feasible solution is $z = 4x_1 + 2x_2 + x_3 = 4 \times 4 + 2 \times 3 + 0 = 22$.

To solve an LP, we must find the feasible solution with the lowest value of z of all feasible solutions. This solution is called the *optimal solution*. The optimal solution of (9) is $x_1 = 5$, $x_2 = 0$, $x_3 = 0$. For this solution, $z = 20$, which is the lowest z of any feasible solution. In practice, most LP problems have many more variables and constraints than shown here. The optimal solution is usually not easy to see at first. However, there is a well-developed methodology for solving LP problems, called the *simplex method*. Variations of the simplex method can be programed on a computer and handle LP problems with hundreds of constraints and thousands of variables.

References

Berg, Robert L., Francis E. Browing, John G. Hill, and Walter Wenkert, "Assessing the Health Care Needs of the Aged," *Health Services Research*, Spring 1970, pp. 36–59.

Bishop, C.E., A.L. Plough, and Thomas W. Willemain, "Nursing Home Levels of Care: Problems and Alternatives," *Health Care Financing Review*, Vol. 2, 1980, pp. 33–46.

Bithell, J.F., "A Class of Discrete Time Models for the Study of Hospital Admission Systems," *Operations Research*, Vol. 17, 1969, pp. 48–69.

Budnick, Frank S., R. Mojena, and T.E. Vollmann, *Principles of Operations Research for Management* (Homewood, IL: Richard D. Irwin, Inc., 1978).

Charnes, A. and W.W. Cooper, "Management Science Relations for Evaluation and Management Accountability," Plenary address for The Institute of Management Sciences XXIV International Meeting, June 1979.

Charnes, A., W.W. Cooper, and E. Rhodes, "Measuring the Efficiency of Decision Making Units," *European Journal of Operational Research*, Vol. 2, 1978, pp. 429–444.

Flagle, Charles D., "Operations Research in the Health Services," *Operations Research*, Vol. 10, 1962, pp. 591–603.

Fries, Brant E., "Bibliography of Operations Research in Health Care Systems," *Operations Research*, Vol. 24, 1976, pp. 801–814.

Hillier, F.S. and G.J. Lieberman, *Introduction to Operations Research* (San Francisco: Holden-Day Inc., 1967).

Kahn, Alfred E., *The Economics of Regulation: Principles and Institutions*, Vol. 1 (New York: Wiley, 1970).

Kane, R.L., L.Z. Rubenstein, R.H. Brook, J. Van Ryzin, P. Masthay, E. Schoenrich, and B. Harrell, "Utilization Review in Nursing Homes: Making Implicit Level-of-Care Judgments Explicit," *Medical Care*, Vol. XIX, 1981, pp. 3–13.

Luckman, J. and J. Stringer, "The Operational Research Approach to Problem Solving," *British Medical Bulletin*, Vol. 30, September 1974, pp. 257–261.

McDonald, A.G., G.C. Cuddeford, and E.M.L. Beale, "Balance of Care: Some Mathematical Models of the National Health Service," *British Medical Bulletin*, Vol. 30, September 1974, pp. 262–271.

Marshall, Kneale T. and F.R. Richards, *The OR/MS Index 1952–1976* (Providence: The Institute of Management Sciences, 1978).

Mitchell, J.B., "Patient Outcomes in Alternative Long-Term Care Settings," *Medical Care*, Vol. XVI, 1978; pp. 439–452.

Wagner, Harvey M., *Principles of Operations Research*, 2nd Ed. (Englewood Cliffs, NJ: Prentice-Hall, Inc., 1976).

Warner, D.M. and D.C. Holloway, *Decision Making and Control for Health Administration—The Management of Quantitative Analysis*, Health Administration Press, 1978.

Willemain, T.R. and R.B. Mark, "The Distribution of Intervals Between Visits as a Basis for Assessing and Regulating Physician Services in Nursing Homes," *Medical Care,* Vol. XVIII, 1980, pp. 427–441.

Willemain, T.R., "Nursing Home Levels of Care: Reimbursement of Resident-Specific Costs," *Health Care Financing Review,* Vol. 2, 1980, pp. 47–52.

Wolfe, H. and J.P. Young, "Staffing the Nursing Unit: Part I," *Nursing Research,* Vol. 14, 1965, pp. 236–243.

Wolfe, H. and J.P. Young, "Staffing the Nursing Unit: Part II," *Nursing Research,* Vol. 14, 1965, pp. 299–303.

Chapter III

Demographic and Epidemiologic Determinants of Expenditures

by Korbin Liu, Kenneth Manton, and Wiley Alliston

Introduction

Increases in expenditures for long-term care in the United States can be anticipated as a result of the rapid growth of the elderly population. Accurate projections of the magnitude of these increases, however, are not available to either policymakers or the general public. This problem was recognized by a recent Congressional Budget Office (CBO) report on long-term care for the elderly and disabled:

If one conclusion may be drawn from this paper, it is that much further research should be undertaken to assemble the data base necessary to prepare more precise estimates. The estimates contained here should be viewed as gross orders of magnitude rather than precise levels of expenditures (CBO, 1977).

There are many factors which ultimately affect long-term care expenditures. These include the characteristics of potential users of long-term care (for example, age composition, socioeconomic status, health status), the types and levels of services available (such as numbers and geographic distribution of nursing homes and home health providers), and governmental policies and programs (expanding or contracting entitlements, reimbursement policies, etc.).

Studies to forecast long-term care expenditures have produced an overly broad range of estimates due to limitations of available data and the lack of adequate projection strategies. As implied by the CBO, there is no ideal data base with which to make these important projections. In addition, the roles and interrelationships of essential determinants of long-term care expenditures have not been adequately conceptualized, in part because of the complexity of the problem and in part because of the urgency of reaching conclusions.

To obtain improved estimates of future long-term care expenditures, it will be necessary to carefully examine the extensive number and variety of determinants of such expenditures. Careful study will also minimize oversight of important interactions which can result in gross or erroneous conclusions. In this vein, this chapter addresses one set of factors important in determining long-term care expenditures—the demographic and epidemiologic characteristics of the elderly population. Specifically, we review the fertility and mortality processes which have determined the size and composition

81

of the U.S. elderly population and explore prospects for change in the future. In light of the relatively straightforward information available on this aspect of the problem, our intent was to describe the role of demographic processes in determining potential long-term care requirements. In contrast, information on the epidemiologic characteristics of the elderly population—morbidity and disability—is much more elusive. Morbidity can be defined as both the underlying degenerative processes (which may be clinically latent) and more critical acute manifestations of such processes. Disability, on the other hand, is the functional impairment that generally results from morbid processes. Since appropriate data are less readily available on these dimensions of the elderly population, our discussion of them is directed toward the various sources and potential utility of representative data for use in forecasting long-term care expenditures. In bringing together the demographic and epidemiologic characteristics of the elderly, in the final section, we describe how conventional projection strategies employ data on these factors and address the shortcomings of such approaches. As we will show, both the available data and the projection strategies have led to the overly broad range of currently available estimates of expenditures for long-term care. In recommending new approaches to obtain improved estimates, we delineate a set of criteria for employing demographic and epidemiologic variables in long-term care forecasting models.

Requirements for Long-Term Care
Resulting from Demographic Processes

Long-term care requirements are determined, in large part, by the size and composition of the elderly population (65+). As a result of prior fertility and mortality trends, we have witnessed a rapid growth in recent decades of the number of older Americans. The elderly population has doubled in the 30 years since 1950 and is presently estimated to be 25 million (Table III–1). In addition to growth in absolute numbers, this group has increased at a faster rate than the U.S. population in general. While those age 65 and over composed 8.1 percent of the total population in 1950, they now constitute 11.2 percent. Finally, the divergence in age-specific death rates by sex since 1900 has increased the proportion of females to males in the elderly population. Among those 85 and older, for example, there are approximately two females for every male.

The recent rapid growth of the elderly population is primarily a function of the historical rise in the numbers of births up to the early 1920s. Changes in mortality, however, have also contributed significantly to the survival of these cohorts to old age. Table III–2 indicates that life expectancy has been increasing steadily since the

82

TABLE III-1
U.S. Population from 65 Years of Age and Older:
Number and Percent of Total U.S. Population for Selected Years

Year	Number (in thousands)	Percent of U.S. Population[1]
1950	12,397	8.1
1960	16,675	9.3
1970	20,087	9.9
1976	22,934	10.7
1980	24,927	11.2 (11.1 − 11.3)
1990	29,824	12.2 (11.7 − 12.6)
2000	31,822	12.2 (11.3 − 12.9)
2010	34,837	12.7 (11.1 − 13.9)
2020	45,102	15.5 (12.7 − 17.8)
2030	55,024	18.3 (14.0 − 22.1)
2040	54,925	17.8 (12.5 − 22.8)

[1] Estimates for 1980 and later employ the Census Bureau's fertility assumption series II; numbers in parentheses are based on fertility assumption series I and III, respectively.

Source: Bureau of the Census, Series P–23, No. 78.

beginning of the 20th century. Most of the increase in the first half of this century is attributable to the reduction of the mortality risk of infectious diseases and to reductions in infant and maternal mortality. Recent increases in life expectancy, on the other hand, stem from reductions in mortality associated with chronic diseases. The age-specific implications of these trends may be illustrated by observing that life expectancy at birth for the total population increased 48.8 percent (24 years) during the period 1900 to 1977, while life expectancy at age 65 increased only 38.9 percent (4.4 years) over the same period. However, in recent years there appears to have been a greater proportional increase in life expectancy at advanced ages. Since 1965, life expectancy at birth has increased only 4.3 percent (3 years), while life expectancy at age 65 has increased 11.6 percent (1.1 years). In assessing mortality trends by cause of death, researchers have observed that substantial reductions in age-adjusted mortality rates are due to declines in heart and cerebrovascular diseases, both of which are particularly prevalent among the elderly.

The recent positive growth of the elderly population is expected to continue. However, the rate of increase will probably not be as rapid as before. On the basis of Census Bureau estimates (Siegel, 1979), for example, the next doubling of the population in that age group will require approximately 45 years. Once again, prior fertility patterns will be a major determinant of future changes in the proportion

Years	Total Population	White Males	White Females	Non-White Males	Non-White Females
At Birth:					
1900–02	49.2	48.2	51.1	32.5	35.0
1929–31	59.3	59.1	62.7	47.6	49.5
1939–41	63.6	62.8	67.3	52.3	55.6
1949–51	68.1	66.3	72.0	58.9	62.7
1955	69.5	67.3	73.6	61.2	65.9
1959–61	69.9	67.6	74.2	61.5	66.5
1965	70.2	67.6	74.7	61.1	67.4
1969–71	70.8	68.0	75.4	61.0	69.0
1974	71.9	68.9	76.6	62.9	71.2
1977[1]	73.2	70.0	77.7	64.6	73.1
At Age 65:					
1900–02	11.9	11.5	12.2	10.4	11.4
1929–31	12.3	11.8	12.8	10.9	12.2
1939–41	12.8	12.1	13.6	12.2	13.9
1949–51	13.8	12.8	15.0	12.8	14.5
1955	14.2	12.9	15.5	13.2	15.5
1959–61	14.4	13.0	15.9	12.8	15.1
1965	14.6	12.9	16.3	12.6	15.5
1969–71	15.0	13.1	16.9	12.9	16.1
1974	15.6	13.4	17.6	13.4	16.7
1977[1]	16.3	13.9	18.4	14.0	17.8

[1] U.S. Public Health Service, *Health, 1979.*

Source: Bureau of the Census, Current Population Reports, Series P–23, No. 59.

of the elderly relative to the total U.S. population. These changes will be characterized by two phases. In the next three decades, the proportion age 65 and over will grow slowly as a result of the depressed fertility rates of the 1920s and 1930s; about 2015, however, the proportion of the elderly will increase dramatically as a function of the entry of the post-World War II "baby boom" cohorts into the 65 and over age group. By 2030, the elderly will compose more than 18 percent of the total U.S. population, given the current fertility rate schedule. Moreover, we can expect significant changes in the mean age of the individuals who compose the 65+ population in the coming decades. Table III–3 shows, for example, that while the 65 to 74 "young-olds" will increase at about the same rate

TABLE III-3
Decennial Percent Increase of Population
by Selected Age Groups: 1950–2010

Year	All Ages	65–74	75–84	85+
1950–1960	18.7	30.1	41.2	59.3
1960–1970	13.4	13.0	31.7	52.3
1970–1980[1]	8.7	23.4	14.2	44.6
1980–1990[1]	10.0	13.8	26.6	20.1
1990–2000[1]	7.1	−2.6	15.6	29.4
2000–2010[1]	6.2	13.3	−2.4	19.4

[1] Estimates for these years employ the Census Bureau's fertility assumption Series II.

Source: Bureau of the Census, Series P–23, No. 59.

as the general population in the 1980s, the 75 to 84 and 85+ "old-olds" will increase at twice the rate of the general population.

Although both fertility and mortality will determine the proportion of elderly in the general population in the future, the actual number of people to reach old age in the next 65 years will be a function solely of mortality, since these individuals have already been born. Since 1968, mortality has been declining steadily, and recent data from the National Center for Health Statistics (NCHS) suggest that this trend will continue. While the rates of change and limits for mortality reduction in the future cannot be determined, any further declines in mortality will probably add to the number of elderly requiring long-term care.

An idea of the potential decline in U.S. mortality can be derived by comparing the life expectancy in the U.S. with that of other countries (Siegel, 1978). Table III–4 presents comparisons for 1973 in which life expectancies at birth and at age 65 are compared for the U.S. and Sweden, the country with the longest life expectancy, and between the U.S. and a best country composite, derived from combining the lowest age-specific mortality rates of all countries. Table III–4 suggests that if changes in mortality patterns are to be governed by the experience of other national populations, the greater potential gain among the elderly (65+) will be made for males (2.1 years), and a smaller increase in life expectancy (0.8) can be expected for elderly females.

Moreover, recent empirical evidence (for example, provisional mortality statistics for 1979), raises questions about whether intrinsic mortality limits, as embodied in comparisons between U.S. mortality and the best country composite, have been reached. There have been, for example, continuing major reductions in mortality at extreme ages in the U.S. (85+) which may shortly exceed expectations

TABLE III-4
Comparison of Life Expectancies for the U.S., Sweden, and
Best-Country Composite: 1973

Area	Males		Females		Excess of Females Over Males	
	e_0	$e65$	e_0	$e65$	e_0	$e65$
U.S., 1973	67.6	13.1	75.3	17.2	7.7	4.1
Sweden, 1973	72.1	14.0	77.7	17.1	5.6	3.1
Best Country Composite	73.5	15.2	78.7	18.0	5.2	2.8
Difference, U.S. and Best Country Composite	5.9	2.1	3.4	0.8	−2.5	−1.3

Source: Bureau of the Census, Current Population Reports, Series P–23, No. 59.

based on age-specific mortality rates in other countries. It is apparent that the present state of the art in predicting mortality has not developed enough to accurately predict future mortality trends. One reason for this deficiency may be the failure to adequately represent underlying health states of the population. The problem is further compounded by the potential impact of more effective medical management of chronic diseases than is anticipated in the future, as well as continuing changes in life styles, both of which can prolong life.

In light of the demographic patterns discussed above, general changes in the size and composition of the elderly population can be confidently predicted for the future. However, the accuracy of estimates of the magnitude of these changes will reflect the quality of population and mortality data—each of which has particular measurement characteristics that can affect results in important ways. Population counts, for example, are subject to differential under- and over-enumeration by race and sex. Partial adjustments can be made to these data across race, age, and sex—adjustments largely derivative of the demographic analyses of Coale and Zelnick (1973) and Coale and Rives (1973). Adjustments have not been derived, however, for other variables likely to be associated with enumeration errors (for example, urban versus rural residence). To obtain short-range population projections of the elderly, the adjusted or unadjusted population counts are decremented by projected mortality trends. The mortality trends are based on present cause specific mortality data which have been subject to concerns about failure to completely match census records (Kitagawa and Hauser, 1973). Perhaps more important, however, are the effects on mortality estimates of the unreliability of death certificate diagnosis of specific conditions and the questionable validity of the underlying cause of death concept on which the death certificate and the national mortality statistics are based. The reliability issue can be addressed in part by a review of the limited literature on the differentials in reliability of death certificate diagnoses. The validity of the underlying cause of death is probably the more critical issue since there is a high prevalence of chronic conditions at the older ages. Resolution of the validity question is problematic, but its effects can be reduced by using multiple cause mortality data, (that is, mortality data where all causes listed on the death certificate are reported). Naturally, such multiple cause data will require specialized analytic procedures. Because of the multiplicity of data quality issues, in addition to conceptual difficulties in the models used to project mortality trends, projections of elderly populations have not been totally successful.

In the next two sections, we address chronic disease and disability, the health status determinants of long-term care expenditures. Distributions of these characteristics among the elderly determine the probable need for long-term care within the broad boundaries established by the demographic effects just discussed. While future mortality trends are difficult to predict, the distributions of morbidity and disability are even more elusive.

The Distribution of Chronic Disease in the U.S. Elderly Population

Numerous data sources and an extensive literature (Singer and Levinson, 1976) exist on chronic disease morbidity in the U.S. population. National estimates of the magnitude of these problems, however, are not normally available from these sources. One reason for this gap is that many of the data sources and epidemiological studies are very restricted in their coverage of the population; they are often limited to populations of convenience or those for which a "natural experiment" affecting health state has occurred. A more basic reason for the limited information is the nature of chronic diseases themselves. Unlike acute illness, chronic disease frequently entails pre-clinical stages which may be long-lasting. Detection of the disease in these stages is difficult and estimates of the prevalence of the disease in national level distributions tend to be biased downward.

In this section, we review some of the major data sources on chronic disease, and discuss weaknesses in their ability to obtain accurate distributions of chronic illness in the population. Rather than presenting findings from the multiplicity of data sources, we focus on their basic characteristics and potential application in strategies that can yield more accurate estimations of chronic disease in the U.S. Five general categories of information sources on chronic diseases are: (1) nationally representative health surveys, (2) enumeration systems, (3) statistical systems on insured populations, (4) epidemiological studies, and (5) clinical studies.

Perhaps the best known of the nationally representative health surveys is the Health Interiew Survey (HIS), which collects self-reported data on acute and chronic diseases, health care utilization, and disability for the non-institutionalized population. The HIS is conducted annually by the NCHS, and public use tapes of HIS data are available for a reasonably lengthy time series. Despite these advantages, studies of the completeness and reliability of the self-reporting of chronic disease in the HIS indicate that it may be hazardous to use this survey to generate disease prevalence and incidence rates (NCHS, 1965, 1973). The HIS seems to perform better in assessing health care utilization and providing measures of disability than in measuring the prevalence and incidence of specific diseases.

In addition to the HIS, NCHS has conducted several health examination surveys (HES, HANES I and II). These surveys differ in methodology from the HIS in that information on the health states of individuals is derived from physical examinations rather than solely from self-reports. As a consequence, these surveys contain some information on the distribution of certain basic pathophysiologic parameters in the population (hypertension, for example). Although physical examinations increase the reliability of the medical data, these surveys have several difficulties: (1) they have a smaller sample size than HIS, (2) they are not conducted annually, and most important, (3) the very old population is not examined. (In HANES I, for example, no persons over age 75 were examined.)

To complement the surveys of the health status of the non-institutionalized population, NCHS has periodically conducted surveys of the institutionalized population. The most recent of these were the National Nursing Home Surveys in 1974 and 1977, which collected data on the health status of nursing home residents—in particular the prevalence of chronic conditions and primary diagnoses. In addition to the various general purpose health surveys sponsored by NCHS, there have been periodic disease-specific surveys. For example, the National Cancer Institute has periodically sponsored national surveys of cancer incidence and prevalence. The latest of these surveys, the Third National Cancer Survey of 1969–71, has been used as a baseline to determine if there have been recent increases in cancer incidence. However, the representativeness of this survey, which is conducted primarily in major metropolitan areas, has been questioned (Smith, 1980).

Data collected through surveys of individuals, such as the HIS, are subject to methodological difficulties, beyond the understatement of pre-clinical stages of chronic diseases. For example, it is difficult to elicit accurate and complete responses to questions about major chronic illnesses (for example, Chambers *et al*, 1976). As a result, estimates of the prevalence and incidence of chronic illness from such surveys tend to be lower than prevalence and incidence estimates derived from medical records (NCHS, 1965, 1973). Moreover, disability among elderly respondents (especially the very old who are at highest risk of chronic illness) may increase response errors in surveys of health status.

Apart from the problem of obtaining accurate and complete responses, most sample surveys on chronic illness are quite limited in their coverage over time (for example, to control for seasonal effects of influenza on morbidity and mortality) and space (for example, to control for important regional differences). In addition, sample surveys cannot provide a cohort time series that is long enough to reflect the progression of individuals through the chronic disease processes. It is this type of data base (one that represents at least overlapping partial experiences of cohorts) that is needed to estimate the prevalence of chronic disease in the population, stratified by stages of severity.

Enumeration systems constitute a second major source of data on the population distribution of chronic conditions. Probably the most frequently employed data sources of this type are the national cause-specific mortality data produced by NCHS. For example, recent declines in the risk of developing circulatory diseases have been inferred from recent declines in their mortality rates. Cause-specific data have also shown consistent geographic differentials in cerebrovascular mortality rates, revealing the existence of a mortality stroke "belt" in southeastern States—a finding confirmed by specially designed epidemiological studies (Kuller *et al*, 1969, a,b,c,d). A third type of morbidity differential inferred from cause-specific mortality data is the increase of cancer mortality among U.S. non-white males. These examples suggest that the primary advantage of the data from the mortality registration system is their scope—temporally, geographically and medically—which makes them particularly useful for monitoring the health of the national population. The present cause-specific mortality data produced for public release by NCHS, however, have the limitation of reporting only one medical condition, (that is, the "underlying cause of death") for each death, even though the physician usually reports additional medical conditions.

While the "underlying cause" may be the most significant medical condition causing death, it is clear that, especially for elderly persons, the health state at death often cannot be represented by a single medical condition. The utility of the mortality data system will be enhanced in the near future because NCHS is implementing release of a multiple cause of death tape (Rosenberg, 1978). In multiple cause data all medical conditions listed on the death certificate are reported. In 1969 for example, 5.2 million medical conditions were reported in connection with the 1.9 million deaths; hence, underlying causes of death data for that year were supplemented by information on 3.3 million contributing causes of death.

This additional information is particularly important for monitoring the health state of the elderly, in that many of the non-underlying causes of medical conditions were chronic diseases such as diabetes mellitus and generalized atherosclerosis—conditions whose onset occurs relatively late in life. Although mortality data have important properties for estimating long-term care requirements, it is clear that they are not sufficient in themselves, since they (a) do not directly represent the health effects of non-lethal diseases; (b) do not contain direct information on the temporal aspects of the morbid process leading to death; and (c) do not contain information on a variety of relevant health covariates.

Two other types of enumeration systems are surveillance programs for specific diseases and population based registries for specific diseases. An example of the former is the Center for Disease Control's (CDC) system for collecting information on a variety of "reportable" infectious diseases and on mortality from selected U.S. cities. The mortality data are used by CDC to construct its pneumonia and influenza index. Analyses of this index show that the elderly compose one of the population subgroups most susceptible to elevated death rates from a variety of chronic illnesses during influenza epidemics. The CDC system also demonstrates that mortality data can be used as an *index* of underlying health changes in the population.

Illustrative of population based registries are the tumor registries which are operated as part of the Surveillance, Epidemiology, and End Results (SEER) program of the National Cancer Institute. While SEER data have been used to generate incidence rates of clinically diagnosed cancer, the representativeness of the registry areas has been questioned, as has the adequacy of the time series to make reliable estimates of incidence changes (Smith, 1980).

The third major data source that is frequently employed to assess the health of the population comprises the statistical systems of privately and publicly insured populations. In interpreting the results from studies of such populations, it is necessary to be aware of the effects of selection factors (for example, criteria for participation under the various programs). The nature of selection is likely to be different for public versus private insurance programs. For example, private insurance programs may require a screen for pre-existing medical conditions. Also, entitlement for private insurance will be based on ability to pay premiums. Consequently, populations which are privately insured are likely to be higher in socioeconomic status and thus are likely to use medical care both more intensively and

90

earlier in the disease process. Entitlement to public insurance programs is not contingent upon screening or pre-existing medical conditions and requires less payment.

A data base derived from a public program, and one that is nearly as comprehensive as the mortality registration system, is the 20 percent sample of acute care hospitalizations (MEDPAR) administered under the Medicare program. This file represents elderly people who used hospitalization services, and it has sufficient cases (1.5 million per year) to investigate detailed diagnostic categories. The fact that the file is generally restricted to persons over age 65 is not a critical problem since this is the population of greatest interest in identifying the requirements for long-term care. The file is available for each year since 1971, so it represents a significant amount of temporal variation of population health characteristics. Also, the information in this file is different from the NCHS mortality files in many respects. For example, hospitalization for an individual over time can be linked, allowing development of longitudinal information on an individual's morbidity. In addition, the file contains information on non-lethal conditions, such as fractures, arthritis, and joint conditions, which are seldom reported in the mortality files.

As with MEDPAR, hospital utilization data containing disease-specific information are available at other geographic levels. For example, recent state-wide studies have been conducted, using diagnostic related groups (DRGs) to measure hospital costs. Regardless of the geographic level of analysis, the critical feature of these statistical systems is the availability of data to trace segments of chronic disease histories in individuals.

The fourth important source of information on the health status of the U.S. population comprises the special purpose "epidemiological studies." These studies, which as a group have used a variety of study designs and methodologies, deal with populations of convenience or for which a natural "health" experiment has occurred. The primary purpose of such studies is not to produce national estimates of prevalence or incidence rates but to determine the association of suspected risk factors with disease and the behavior of the disease within individuals. For example, the Framingham longitudinal study of coronary heart disease followed intensively, over a 20 year period, a large proportion of the adults in the community of Framingham, Massachusetts. Not only was Framingham not representative of large segments of the national population (for example, there were no blacks in Framingham), but a number of selection factors operated to determine who participated in the study (Kessler and Levin, 1970). This selection did not detract, however, from the value of the Framingham data in identifying possible risk factors or in characterizing disease etiology.

The last major source of information on chronic illness in the U.S. are "clinical" studies. There are many different types of clinical studies, such as the human experimental data gathered on physiological responses to various types of pollutants. The course of chronic disease is followed in clinical populations. For example, there are many studies (Steel and Lamerton, 1966; Archambeau, 1970) on the rate of tumor growth and metastasis which used sequential X-ray evaluations of tumor size and distribution. Other studies, such as those from the SEER program (Axtell et al, 1976), evaluated the effects of different clinical interventions on survival of patients with varying characteristics. The clinical characteristics of "aging" and disease are determined in intensive longitudinal studies of selected aging populations. The distinctive feature of such studies is that they collectively examine clinical aspects of the "natural history" of chronic disease processes in individuals. They may also provide a scientific basis on which to theoretically extrapolate the behavior of the disease in its pre-clinical stage. They do not provide a basis for estimating population incidence and prevalence rates and thus are most valuable if they can be linked to other data sources on the population distribution of disease.

With national surveys, enumeration systems, and health insurance statistical systems, chronic diseases are generally reported in terms of incidence or prevalence rates. Other dimensions of chronic diseases, such as duration, progression, or severity, are determined less often. To derive data that are useful in determining long-term care requirements, concepts appropriate to the "natural history" of a chronic disease—the identification, ordering, and rate of progression of the stages of a chronic illness—must be developed and then implemented in appropriately designed studies and projection strategies.

Examination of the various types of data sources on morbidity suggests that no single source of data is adequate to simultaneously determine, for a broad range of chronic diseases, (a) the distribution of morbidity in the national population, (b) the natural history of the chronic disease process, and (c) the change in the health state of individuals in various cohort groups as those individuals progress through the natural history of the chronic disease. Clearly it will be necessary to use data of several different types to fulfill these three criteria. One strategy is to augment epidemiological data with biological theory and clinical data in a structure that can relate this information to the health effects of the population. For example, mortality data can be augmented by information from epidemiological and clinical sources in a model which reflects population dynamics to project long-term care requirements. We explore these alternate strategies later in the chapter.

92

The Distribution of Disability in the U.S.

The second component of health status among the elderly which will determine expenditures for long-term care comprises specific types and levels of functional disability. Disability is naturally associated with morbidity, since it is generally a product of one or more chronic diseases. While there is usually a clear link between morbidity and disability, there is also a clear distinction between the types of services required by disease and disability. This requires that they be analyzed separately. For example, morbidity may be treated in acute care hospitals or at home, for conditions such as hypertension, diabetes, or leukemia. Disability, on the other hand, requires expenditures for services necessary to cope with functional impairments from morbid processes. Examples of services required to deal with disability are those which overcome sensory deficiency (for example, hearing aids or glasses) or restrictions on mobility (such as wheelchairs). Although generally a result of morbidity (for example, restrictions on mobility due to degenerative bone and joint disease), disability may continue in the absence of the morbid condition.

The studies of disability in the population that are used to assess the magnitude of long-term care problems in the U.S. have usually employed surrogate measures of disability, such as limitations in activities of daily living. Considerable effort has been invested in producing such measures, since they provide a more practical and parsimonious means of estimating general long-term care requirements than coping with the complex of morbid conditions and disabilities that actually characterize an individual's health state. We examined several health assessment studies which yielded estimates of population disability. They seem to constitute a representative sample of the survey techniques that have been used to derive general estimates of the disability of the elderly in the United States. Specifically, we examined findings from five of the most frequently cited surveys:

(1) 1975 Survey of Well Being of Older People in Cleveland, Ohio (GAO, 1977)
(2) 1976 Health Interview Survey (Butler and Newacheck, 1980)
(3) 1976 Survey of Income and Education (Okada *et al*, 1979)
(4) 1972 Survey of Disability Among Adults (Saad Z. Nagi, 1976)
(5) 1964 Survey of the Health Needs of the Aged in Monroe County (Berg *et al*, 1970).

With the exception of the Berg study, data were derived from interviews with elderly respondents. In the Berg study, distributions of need for long-term care were determined on the basis of professional assessments. Table III–5 summarizes selected findings from

93

TABLE III-5
Distribution of Functional Limitations in the U.S. Elderly Population: Findings from Five Major Surveys

Survey of Well Being of Older People in Cleveland, Ohio (GAO)[1] 1975	Health Interview Survey (NCHS) 1976	Survey of Income and Education (Census Bureau) 1976	Survey of Disability Among Adults (Nagi) 1972	Survey of the Health Needs of the Aged in Monroe Co. (Berg et al) 1964
Excellent/good — 41%	No limitations — 57%	No problems working around house — 62%	No limitations — 71.8%	Need neither physical care nor supervision because of impaired mental status — 75.5%
Mildly or moderately impaired — 53%	Limited, but not in major activity — 5.7%	Having problems working around house — 38%	Limited but independent — 12%	Need physical care only — 8.6%
Severely or completely impaired — 5%	Limited in kind or amount of major activity — 20.1%	—	Mobility assistance required — 9.0%	Need supervision due to mental impairment — 8.8%
—	Unable to conduct major activity — 17.2%	—	Personal care assistance required — 6.9%	Both physical and mental care needs — 7.4%

[1] Response to items on physical health only.

the five studies. Although the criteria used to classify functional status vary from study to study, there are a few similarities which permit limited interstudy comparisons. It is apparent from Table III–5, for example, that estimates of the proportion of elderly people with minimal to no need for assistance range from 41 to 76 percent across the five studies. Additional comparisons can be made about other segments of the distributions, but the obvious variations in definitions in response categories make such comparisons tenuous. The studies of activity limitations of the elderly population, such as those noted above, provide important information for estimating the general magnitude of need for long-term care services. These data are typically used to forecast long-term care expenditures for the elderly and disabled. To derive a more precise estimate of the magnitude of long-term care expenditures, or to estimate the costs for specific health services, the summary indexes of activity limitations are not adequate. The derivation of population distributions through surveys employing these measures relies heavily on respondents' subjective evaluations of their own limitations. Hence, they are asked to develop reasonably objective scales to determine degrees of their disability. In addition, with the exception of the HIS, most health assessment surveys are limited in time and scope, calling into question their general applicability. Most important perhaps, changes in the health status of the national population cannot be monitored over time with spot surveys.

The limitations of disability assessment surveys in providing input for forecasting long-term care expenditures reflect the expense involved in their implementation and general survey research problems. Consequently, alternative strategies for estimating the types and levels of disability in the population are required. For example, given our previous discussion that disability is generally the result of chronic disease, one alternative approach is to implement a two-stage estimation process: (1) determine the relation of specific types of disability to chronic disease processes (through sample surveys), and (2) estimate the distribution of disability by using the relationships determined in (1) with estimates of the population distribution of chronic diseases.

Strategies for Estimating the Effect of Population and Morbidity on Long-Term Care Expenditures

The assessment of our knowledge about the demographic and epidemiologic determinants of long-term care expenditures suggests that new approaches for using data are required to enhance formulation of long-term care policy. The organization of such data in a "full information" model, for example, has not been attempted. In this section, we review the basic strategies that have produced current estimates of the population at risk for long-term care and discuss major conceptual and data deficiencies of these models.

The conventional approach for projecting demographic and epidemiologic determinants of long-term care expenditures is characterized by static component models. Basically, estimates of disease or disability rates for different demographic groups are applied to population projections for some future time. A usual refinement is the addition of stratifications for socioeconomic subgroups when data are available. The population projection involves data on census counts and mortality—each of which has particular measurement characteristics that can affect results in important ways. For example, population count data are subject to differential under- and over-enumeration by a number of variables of interest. In addition, projections of the elderly population are based on census counts decreased by extrapolated mortality trends. As noted earlier, the extrapolations of mortality trends have underestimated the survival rates of this population.

The second component of the basic model is "morbidity." Considering this component involves estimating morbidity or disability rates from survey data as discussed earlier. In light of the definitional and response problems in health surveys that are based on self reports, their results must be interpreted cautiously. Health surveys involving medical examinations or medical record reviews are not as subject to concerns about diagnostic reliability but are subject to the effects of selection (for example, of individuals or conditions that have already been diagnosed).

Some of the deficiencies of these models have been noted in preceding discussions about the types and quality of data that are available as inputs. Of equal importance are conceptual issues which are generally not addressed satisfactorily. First, the models actually describe only population changes because period morbidity or disability rates for specific demographic groups are fixed over the course of the projection interval. This procedure ignores the presence of potentially important simultaneities between population change and the health of the population. Specifically, the primary force of decrement—cause-specific mortality—will be correlated with the underlying morbidity patterns. Furthermore, it is reasonable to expect that long-term care expenditures and other forces (lifestyle change, for example) will affect morbidity and disability and therefore population mortality risks. Finally, changes in patterns of morbidity and mortality affect the size and composition of the elderly population. Thus, there are interactions which cannot be represented in the model structure if morbidity and disability rates are static model components.

Second, the conceptual and operational point not addressed by the basic model is that, because of the mixture of acute and chronic morbid conditions and the cross-temporal relation of disability to morbidity, the modeling of demographic and epidemiologic determinants is necessarily longitudinal in nature. Chronic diseases cannot be effectively modeled as events, since their effects unfold over time. The fact that chronic diseases progress (and with that progression the likelihood of severe disability increases) also implies that we need to examine the health characteristics of identifiable cohorts. A simple period assessment of the instantaneous health state of an array of cohorts, because it does not provide information on the prior health characteristics of individuals, will not be adequate to determine the future distributions of chronic disease by stage or the associated disabilities. Dealing appropriately with the time dimension will require much conceptual clarification and technical innovation in existing models for projecting long-term care expenditures.

Third, the search for disease risk factors in individuals and the fact that considerable variation in risk for many diseases remains unexplained suggest that, at birth, human populations are quite heterogeneous with respect to factors affecting health and survival. Most forecasting models (with the exception of stratification) do not represent the potentially dramatic effects of differential rates of mortality and morbidity selection on a heterogeneous population (Vaupel *et al*, 1979).

Fourth, at advanced ages the individual is at high risk for many different diseases, so that alteration of the mortality or morbidity risk of one disease may greatly affect the risk of another disease. For example, reductions in the mortality risk of cardiovascular disease and stroke imply a compensating increase in cancer mortality at greater ages (Manton *et al*, 1980). Implicit in this phenomenon of "competing risk" are two additional conceptual complications. First, though standard competing risk theory assumes that diseases operate independently (Manton and Poss, 1979), they in fact interact in a variety of ways. Second, because of the increasing likelihood of accumulating one or more chronic conditions at advanced ages (Manton *et al,* 1980), and because the onset of one chronic disease will frequently increase the risk of onset of a second, the prevalence of individuals with multiple chronic diseases will increase as the population ages. For example, diabetes mellitus is a chronic, degenerative diseases which increases the age-specific risk of cerebrovascular disease. Therefore diabetes, as a long-term health problem, can affect health and disability not only directly, but also indirectly, through the increased risk of more lethal and disabling conditions such as stroke. Since persons with multiple chronic diseases may represent very different health needs than persons with only one condition, it will be important to develop concepts and data forms appropriate to identify the coexistent occurrences of chronic diseases in individuals.

Fifth, physiological changes and risk of disease increase rapidly at advanced ages. This makes study of the critical advanced ages difficult because, while more age detail is required to accurately document the rapid changes, the surviving population is small and rapidly decreasing.

Finally, statistical issues arise when information from different data sources are mixed. For example, systematic sample designs can make it difficult to mix results from different surveys. In addition, it appears that standard statistical procedures tend to underestimate the variance of survey results due to systematic and possibly unmeasured heterogeneity of the populations from which the samples are drawn.

In light of the technical difficulties in developing forecasting models for long-term care, it is not surprising that the estimates of future expenditures vary so broadly. From our review of data sources and projection strategies for the demographic and epidemiologic determinants, it is apparent that more accurate projections are feasible if additional research is directed toward applying the multiplicity of available information to more sophisticated models. Moreover, it will be important to estimate the level of expenditures for specific health services, in addition to the general levels of expenditures. Since such models are extremely complex and currently not available, we have focused our discussion only on the population and health status components. On the basis of our review, we determined the probable requirements for improved projection models which are particularly suited for the demographic and epidemiologic determinants of long-term care. The following is a list of criteria which constitute, we believe, a starting point for future research in this area:

- The model should be biologically realistic. That is, it should be representative of a population aging through time, heterogeneous in risk, and undergoing systematic mortality selection. The conceptual and mathematical structure of this model should reflect available theoretical knowledge from various relevant disciplines (for example, medical science and epidemiology), as well as being consistent with an underlying stochastic process.
- The model should reflect aspects of disease dynamics that are important to policy concerns. Thus, it should identify clinically latent periods, the rate of disease progression, and the distribution of differential risks in the population. This, too, requires care to ensure that the representation of the natural history of a chronic disease is biologically realistic.

98

- The model should permit the introduction of etiologically relevant covariates as drivers of morbidity and mortality. The inclusion of variables affecting morbidity and mortality risks, when available, would enhance the success of the model. For example, changes in the amount and type of smoking could affect both population structure, by altering the force of decrement, and the physiological health state of the surviving population, by affecting the amount of chronic obstructive lung disease.
- The model should use longitudinal information. It is difficult to see how successful predictions can be made from cross-sectional data alone. This suggests that the model should be based on data with reasonable time series information.
- The model should integrate multiple data sources so that their joint information can be used to investigate and resolve some of the data reliability and validity issues raised earlier.
- The model should provide a reasonable estimate of uncertainty. With such estimates, the costs of different policy actions can be more precisely assessed. This is an area in which available models are inadequate since they do not identify the non-sampling error variance in the data from which parameters are estimated (for example, model specification error, variance due to population heterogeneity, and mortality selection).
- The model must be able to determine the simultaneous interaction of population change, morbidity, disability, and the effects of health care expenditures.
- Each of the model components must be readily reviewable by experts in each of the relevant fields. Since many different data sources may be employed, each with its attendant level of uncertainty, it seems appropriate that the model produce quantitative results that can be reviewed for consistency and reasonableness. Thus, in addition to overall reasonableness and consistency, each model component should be developed to reflect the current state of knowledge.

Summary and Conclusion

We have discussed demographic and epidemiologic determinants of the magnitude of long-term care expenditures. Our concern has been on the inadequacy of currently available forecasts which is due to deficiencies in avaliable data and weaknesses in standard projection strategies. It is apparent that the roles and interactions of essential components of forecasting models have not been adequately conceptualized, in large part because of time constraints on the researchers and policy analysts who generate estimates.

To supplement the traditional, rapid turnaround projections normally demanded from policy analysts, we believe that considerably more research should be directed toward crystallizing the individual roles and interrelationships of the determinants of long-term care expenditures. In this regard, we have focused on only one component, the demographic and epidemiologic characteristics of the elderly population. In addition, we feel that new strategies should be contemplated to optimize the use of current knowledge and available data sources. Pursuing a more scientific approach to this problem will yield a better understanding of long-term care requirements, as well as more accurate estimates of the magnitude of future long-term care expenditures.

References

Archambeau, J.O., M.B. Heller, A. Akanuma, and D. Lubell, "Biologic and Clinical Implications Obtained from the Analysis of Cancer Growth Curves," *Clinical Obstetrics and Gynecology* 13: 831–856, 1970.

Axtell, L., A. Asire, and M. Myers, *Cancer Patient Survival, Report No. Five,* DHEW Pub. No. (NIH) 77-992, PHS, NIH, NCI, Bethesda, MD, 1976.

Berg, Robert L., Francis E. Browing, John G. Hill, and Walter Wenkert, "Assessing the Health Care Needs of the Aged," *Health Services Research* Spring, 1970, pp. 36–59.

Butler, Lewis H. and Paul W. Newacheck, "Health and Social Factors Relevant to Long-Term Care Policy," Presented at the Symposium on Long-Term Care Policy, Williamsburg, Virginia, June 11–15, 1980.

Chambers, Larry W., Walter O. Spitzer, Gerry B. Hill, and Barbara E. Helliwell, "Underreporting of Cancer in Medical Surveys: A Source of Systematic Error in Cancer Research," *American Journal of Epidemiology* 104, 1976, pp. 141–145.

Coale, Ansley J. and Melvin Zelnick, *New Estimates of Fertility and Population in the United States.* Princeton, N.J.: Princeton University Press, 1963.

Coale, Ansley J. and Norfleet W. Rives, "A Statistical Reconstruction of the Black Population of the United States: 1880–1970," *Population Index* 39, 1973, pp. 3–36.

Congressional Budget Office, *Long-Term Care For the Elderly and Disabled,* Washington, D.C.: U.S. Government Printing Office, 1977.

Kessler, Irving I. and Morton L. Levin, "The Community As an Epidemiologic Laboratory," in *The Community As An Epidemiologic Laboratory: A Casebook of Community Studies* (Kessler and Levin, eds.). Baltimore: Johns Hopkins University Press, 1970.

Kitagawa, Evelyn M. and Philip M. Hauser, *Differential Mortality in the United States: A Study in Socioeconomic Epidemiology,* Cambridge: Harvard University Press, 1973.

Kuller, Lewis H., Abraham Bolker, Milton S. Saslaw, Bertha L. Paegel, Charles Sisk, Nemat Borhani, JoAnn Wray, Herbert Anderson, Donald Peterson, Warren Winkelstein, John Cassel, Philip Spiers, Allen G. Robinson, Hiram Curry, Abraham M. Lilienfeld, and Raymond Seltser, "Nationwide Cerebrovascular Disease Mortality Study: I. Methods and Analysis of Death Certificates," *American Journal of Epidemiology* 90, 1969a, pp. 536–544.

Kuller, Lewis H., Abraham Bolker, Milton S. Saslaw, Bertha L. Paegel, Charles Sisk, Nemat Borhani, JoAnn Wray, Herbert Anderson, Donald Peterson, Warren Winkelstein, John Cassel, Philip Spiers, Allen G. Robinson, Hiram

Curry, Abraham M. Lilienfeld, and Raymond Seltser, "Nationwide Cerebrovascular Disease Mortality Study: II. Comparison of Clinical Records and Death Certificates," *American Journal of Epidemiology* 90, 1969b, pp. 545–555.

Kuller, Lewis H., Abraham Bolker, Milton S. Saslaw, Bertha L. Paegel, Charles Sisk, Nemat Borhani, JoAnn Wray, Herbert Anderson, Donald Peterson, Warren Winkelstein, John Cassel, Philip Spiers, Allen G. Robinson, Hiram Curry, Abraham M. Lilienfeld, and Raymond Seltser, "Nationwide Cerebrovascular Disease Mortality Study: III. Accuracy of the Clinical Diagnosis of Cerebrovascular Disease," *American Journal of Epidemiol* 90, 1969c, pp. 556–566.

Kuller, Lewis H., Abraham Bolker, Milton S. Saslaw, Bertha L. Paegel, Charles Sisk, Nemat Borhani, JoAnn Wray, Herbert Anderson, Donald Peterson, Warren Winkelstein, John Cassel, Philip Spiers, Allen G. Robinson, Hiram Curry, Abraham M. Lilienfeld, and Raymond Seltser, "Nationwide Cerebrovascular Disease Mortality Study: IV. Comparison of Different Clinical Types of Cerebrovascular Disease," *American Journal of Epidemiol* 90, 1969d, pp. 567–578.

Manton, Kenneth G. and Sharon S. Poss, "Effects of Dependency Among Causes of Death for Cause Elimination Life Table Strategies," *Demography* 16, 1979, pp. 313–327.

Manton, Kenneth G., Eric Stallard, and Sharon S. Poss, "Estimates of U.S. Multiple Cause Life Tables," *Demography*, 1980, pp. 85–102.

Nagi, Saad Z., "An Epidemiology of Disability Among Adults in the United States," *Milbank Memorial Fund Quarterly*, Fall, 1976, pp. 439–466.

National Center for Health Statistics, "Health Interview Responses Compared with Medical Records," *Vital and Health Statistics: Data Evaluation and Methods of Research*, Series 2, No. 7, Washington, D.C. 1965.

National Center for Health Statistics, *Net Differences in Interview Data on Chronic Conditions and Information Derived from Medical Records*, HSMHA Publication No. (HSM) 73-1331, Rockville, MD., 1973.

Okada, Louise M., William F. Stewart, and Mary E. Lafferty, "An Index of Need: Functional Disability, Living Arrangement and Poverty Among the Elderly," Presented at the Annual Meeting of the American Public Health Association, November 7, 1979, New York City.

Rosenberg, Harry M., "National Multiple Cause of Death Statistics," Presented at the 17th Biennial Meeting of the Public Health Conference on Records and Statistics, Washington, D.C., June 5–7, 1978.

Siegel, Jacob S., "Demographic Aspects of Aging and the Older Population in the United States," *Current Population Reports*, Series P-23, No. 59, January 1978.

Siegel, Jacob S., "Prospective Trends in the Size and Structure of the Elderly Population, Impact of Mortality Trends, and Some Implications," *Current Population Reports*, Series P-23, No. 78, January 1979.

Singer, Richard B. and Louis L. Levinson, *Medical Risks: Patterns of Mortality and Survival,* Lexington, Massachusetts: Lexington Books and DC Heath, 1976.

Smith, R. Jeffrey, "Government Says Cancer Rate is Increasing," *Science* 209, 1980, pp. 998–1002.

Steel, G. and L. Lamerton, "The Growth Rate of Human Tumors," *British Journal of Cancer*, Vol. 20, 1966.

101

United States General Accounting Office, *The Well-Being of Older People in Cleveland, Ohio,* Washington, D.C.: U.S. Government Printing Office, 1977.

United States Public Health Service, *Health United States: 1979.* Washington, D.C.: U.S. Government Printing Office, 1980.

Vaupel, James W., Kenneth G. Manton, and Eric Stallard, "The Impact of Heterogeneity in Individual Frailty on the Dynamics of Mortality," *Demography* 16, 1979, pp. 439–454.

Chapter IV

The Measurement and Assurance of Quality

by Bettina D. Kurowski and Peter W. Shaughnessy

Introduction

When faced with the problem of expanding the availability of long-term care services to meet the needs of a growing elderly and disabled population and simultaneously containing costs, one predictable area of conflict is the quality of care. Although cost overruns can be explained away, there is no acceptable rationale that justifies residents dying in nursing home fires or home health workers abusing their clients. The quality of care is a visible, undeniable reflection of the resources we are willing to invest in long-term care services, one that warrants more attention than it has heretofore received.

The many definitions (and resulting measures) of the quality of long-term care demonstrate its complexity and multidimensionality. It has been viewed both normatively and comparatively, from the patient's, provider's, or system's viewpoint. It can include such components as the provision of preventive services, coordination of care, privacy, safety, outcomes of care, satisfaction, and medical and nursing services that meet recognized standards of care.

Because the quality of long-term care can be defined and measured in so many ways, the diversity of current efforts to assure that care meets accepted standards is not surprising. Quality assurance is not identical to the measurement of quality. This distinction is important, because quality assurance generally includes both the measurement of the quality of care provided and efforts to improve it. Operationally, quality assurance entails an ongoing system which yields reliable information about the delivery of health services and is also designed to induce beneficial change in those practices, maintaining and/or increasing conformance with established standards.

The most popular approach to quality assurance in the last 10 years has been through direct regulatory mechanisms, including facility (and personnel) licensure and certification, legal remedies, and mandatory peer review. Recent reports have questioned the effectiveness of these programs in long-term care. Department of Health and Human Services (DHHS) audits indicate widespread failures of the utilization review standards to ensure that patients receive the appropriate level of care. Congressional reports indicate that many Medicaid patients do not receive the required periodic medical review to ensure adequacy of care. Other reports have noted non-compliance with conditions of participation dealing with required

103

services, life safety code requirements, and patients' rights (U.S. Congress, House, 1978; U.S. Congress, Senate, 1976; U.S. Congress, Senate, 1975; U.S. General Accounting Office, 1979).

There are several explanations for the limited success of Federal, State, and peer review efforts to improve the quality of long-term care. Basically, these explanations all stem from an inadequate knowledge of the measurement and assurance of the quality of long-term care. This chapter reviews the state of the art in measuring and assuring the quality of long-term care to identify major knowledge gaps which might benefit from further research. In so doing, the following sections (1) describe many of the significant research contributions to the field, (2) summarize the overall conclusions of the research evidence, and (3) identify major information gaps which obstruct refinement of policies to ensure the quality of long-term care.

Although there may be relevant lessons to be learned from the literature on acute care and chronic disease, this chapter is limited in its scope to a review of research (both applied and basic) which focuses on the long-term care delivery system. To place relevant research in perspective, the chapter will briefly describe a wide array of research rather than discussing a few efforts in detail. In-depth discussions of many of the studies mentioned hereafter can be found in other chapters of this volume. It is our intention to place these studies and others within a framework to assist the reader in evaluating future work in the field.

Measuring the Quality of Long-Term Care

To develop measures which adequately assess the quality of long-term care, it is necessary to begin with a common understanding of the concept. Quality of care includes a wide range of concepts associated with professionally recognized standards of care.

To ascertain the level of compliance with recognized standards of care, standards must first be developed and then the care provided measured in relationship to those standards. In the case of long-term care patients, who often suffer from multiple chronic diseases, standards of care are often intended to maintain or slow deterioration of patients and reduce exacerbations and acute episodes. For these patients more than others, the relationship between the improvement of health status and the receipt of care is very difficult to establish. Thus, it becomes especially important to measure the quality of care not only in terms of its effect on patient status, but also with respect to the provision of services which meet professionally recognized standards for the appropriateness of provider responses to patient need.

Professionally recognized standards of care may be measured by the capacity of the provider to respond to patient needs (structure), by activities with respect to that need (process), or by the observed consequences of the activities (outcomes). These three kinds of measures correspond to the classification scheme proposed by Donabedian (1966, 1980), which groups the objectives associated with the quality of care into three categories: structure, process, and outcome. Human, organizational, and material resources are the basis for structural components of care. Availability of an adequately trained administrator, buildings which meet life safety codes, and minimal levels of nursing staff are all examples of structural aspects of care. Procedures, activities, or services (and the resources they use) are process components of care (such as diagnostic testing, physical examinations, and therapeutic interventions). Changes in the physical, functional, and psychosocial status of the patient (which were the intended result of care) are outcome components of quality. Death, disability, disease, discomfort, and dissatisfaction of the patient are often suggested as appropriate for the development of outcome measures.

Because they are more objective, reliable, and easily measurable than other criteria, structural measures of quality have been the most commonly used. Process measures of quality have been studied less often, in part because they are more difficult to agree upon and validate than structural measures. Outcome measures are the most elusive and have only recently been used in long-term care. The development of appropriate outcome measures which consider the combinations of diseases and disabilities of long-term care patients is extremely difficult. Different from process measures, outcome measures require that standards be derived from a knowledge of potential outcomes under optimal conditions (although outcome measures themselves need not be expressed relative to ideal outcomes). Such knowledge is not currently available for most long-term care patients.

Institutional capacity (structure), activities (process), and consequences (outcome) are attributes of care which may or may not be associated. Although capacity may exist, it may not be used or may be used inappropriately. Even if used appropriately, it may be applied in insufficient quantities or with less skill than is needed to produce a positive effect. In fact, the relatively undeveloped state of the art of long-term patient care may result in inherently ineffectual standards of care. Thus, it is important to this review to include studies which have dealt with measures of each kind. The following section describes key studies using a structural measures of quality. Thereafter, we summarize studies using process and outcome measures. Finally, we discuss special problems in specifying outcome measures.

Studies Using Structure and Process Measures of Quality

Early approaches to measuring the quality of care usually focused on structural measures. On the assumption that these criteria represent necessary, albeit minimal, conditions for the delivery of adequate care, they have formed the basis for much of the research and program emphasis in assuring the quality of long-term care. In general, few significant associations have been consistently found across studies between structural measures of the quality of care and the process or outcome of nursing home care. There is little or no empirical evidence with respect to these issues for non-institutional long-term care services (that is, home health or adult day care).

The early evidence on structural characteristics of nursing homes was mixed. For example, Gottesman and Bourestom (1974) studied 1,144 residents of 40 Detroit nursing homes, focusing largely on hours of (various types of) service per patient day as their primary measure of quality. They found that more care was associated with facilities that (1) required aides to be experienced in patient care and (2) permitted patients to keep personal possessions in their rooms.

Later studies which investigated the relationship of general structural measures of quality to the process of care have not found many strong links between them. An evaluation of skilled nursing facilities in Massachusetts by Connelly et al (1977) used a qualitative estimate of the adequacy of three components of nursing home services (medical care, nursing care, and social services) for review teams to assign a score of excellent through poor to each patient. When these estimates (of process measures) of the quality of care were aggregated to the facility level, none of the structural measures used in the study exhibited a significant relationship to the quality of care.

Most recently, these results were supported by preliminary findings of a three-year study of 74 Colorado nursing homes (Shaughnessy, Schlenker, et al, 1980), where facility size and overall level of certification were not related to the process measures of quality used in the study. Greenberg (1980) completed a companion study of Minnesota nursing homes and found no significant difference in the quality of care, measured by numbers of administrative (process) certification violations in a facility on the basis of any of the structural characteristics measured.

Another study by Linn et al (1977) compared similar structural measures of quality to the outcome of care for a sample of 1,000 male nursing home patients. Using multivariate analyses to control for differences in their initial characteristics and prognoses, they found that only a few of their structural measures of quality were consistently related to the outcome of care (measured by mortality

106

and change in functional status). Of the structural variables, staff size and staff-to-patient ratios, only the number of registered nursing hours per patient day (a measure which is sometimes classified as a general process measure) was consistently and positively related to good outcome.

In spite of the mixed evidence with respect to structural measures of quality, they warrant further study for two reasons. First, they are relatively easy to measure. Second, there is limited evidence to suggest that in particular circumstances, structural criteria directly affect the process of care. For example, Ray et al (1980) reported one study of 6,000 Medicaid intermediate care facility (ICF) patients in Tennessee where they investigated the relationship between the use of antipsychotic drugs (a process measure of care) and various characteristics of physicians and nursing homes (structural measures of quality). Their findings indicated that a strong correlate of drug usage was direct care staff-to-patient ratios (that is, patients treated by facilities with less direct care received more drugs than patients in other facilities). These findings suggest that nursing homes which are understaffed may overutilize antipsychotic drugs as a substitute for adequate nursing staff.

The University of Colorado (Shaughnessy, Tynan, et al, 1980) studied the quality of care using patient level, problem-oriented, process quality scores in its evaluation of the swing-bed experiments in Texas, Iowa, and South Dakota. In that study, several structural measures of quality were found to be significantly related to the process of care. For example, the availability of social services was a consistent positive indicator of process quality at the facility level, while availability of dental services and physical therapy were positive determinants of process quality at the patient and problem levels.

One example of an effort to further refine structural measures of quality is a study recently begun by Abt Associates, Inc. (1980) entitled "Study of Appropriate Staffing Ratios of Daily Nursing Hours for the Purpose of Establishing Federal Requirements in Nursing Homes." Using a sample of 20 facilities in 10 different States, the study will measure the effects of alternative staffing arrangements on the process and outcome of long-term care. Based on study findings, Abt will recommend Federal requirements regarding appropriate nurse staffing ratios in nursing homes.

In spite of a few examples to the contrary, most structural, facility-based measures of the quality of care have not been shown to be directly related to overall quality (measured by the process and outcome of care). This is because they are intended to measure the capacity for the provision of quality of care but do not necessarily measure whether the capacity is actually used. It may also be due to the fact that wide variations in structural measures have not, and perhaps cannot, be studied. For example, violations of certification standards are likely to be strongly related to quality if they fall well below certain limits, but regulations (and even common sense) prevent this. In the areas of life safety codes and the physical characteristics of the facility, structural measures of quality are useful because capacity is virtually identical with performance. On the other hand, structural criteria are least likely to measure the quality of care in the areas of patient activities, social services, and rehabilitative services, since they merely measure whether providers demonstrate the capacity to give services should a patient need them, not that they actually provide such services. For this reason, recent efforts to assess the quality of long-term care have focused more intensely on process and outcome measures of quality. These efforts are summarized in the next section.

Studies Using Process and Outcome Measures of Quality

Process measures of quality assess quality in terms of the resources actually consumed and procedures (services) performed during the provision of care. Both collecting data and defining criteria are more difficult in process measurement than in structural analysis of the quality of care. However, process measures generally have greater validity, since they are more directly related to patient health status. Yet problems with the reliability and general applicability of process measures persist. When process analyses use medical records as their primary source of data, it is difficult to differentiate between procedures that were performed but not recorded and procedures that were never performed; when verbal reports are used, faulty memories can cause similar problems. Thus it becomes important to use several sources to collect data on process measures of quality—an expensive and time-consuming effort.

In all areas of health care, the most prevalent technique for evaluating the process quality of care is comparing process data to explicit criteria (or service standards) which have been generated by panels of experts. Inclusion of "exception" categories for each service permits the criteria to be applied individually to each long-term care patient.

Like structural criteria, process criteria represent a useful tool for evaluating the quality of care. However, the use of either structural or process measures is based upon the assumption that there is a positive causal relationship between them and the outcome of care, as expressed in the final condition of the patient. As indicated, this relationship has not yet been empirically demonstrated with much consistency.

Studies which have found the weakest relationships between the process and outcome of the quality of care have been those using relatively insensitive measures of the process and outcome of care, for example, use of services (a process or outcome measure, depending on the acuity level of the services) and mortality (outcome). An implicit assumption within the framework of such studies is that the care is provided (measured by number of services of different types) in a way which meets accepted standards with respect to the needs of each patient. Because these measures of process quality (utilization) are so loosely linked to the actual process of care, it is not surprising that most such studies find weak relationships between process and outcome measures of quality.

One study which tested the relationship between the use of homemaker and adult day care services (process) and the use of nursing home or acute care services (outcome) was reported by Weissert et al (1980). It analyzed two groups of adult day care patients and concluded that only the adult day care experimental group had significantly lower utilization of nursing home care than the control group (which received the usual array of services). Neither experimental group had lower hospital utilization. Although the study showed that both homemaker and day care programs helped to improve the functioning and lower the mortality rates of the patients participating in the study, the significance of the differences over time was uncertain due to reported methodological weaknesses in the study.

Another study that is testing the impact of community-based services for the elderly appears to substantiate the findings of lower mortality in the group receiving services. Skellie and Coan (1980) report that, under a Medicaid waiver, the State of Georgia is offering three types of community-based services (day care, home health care, and alternative living services) to all Medicaid clients over the age of 50 who would otherwise be eligible for nursing home placement. One-quarter of all clients judged eligible for community-based services are randomly assigned to a control group (which receives traditional Medicaid/Medicare services). Reports of the effect of the project on 267 clients indicate that, although the experimental and control groups are not significantly different on key baseline measures, use of project services appears to have decreased mortality rates by two-thirds in the first six months of the project. Differences in mortality rates in the second six-month period were not significantly different between the groups. Overall, during the program's first year, 15 percent of the experimental group died compared to 29 percent of the control group. These findings suggest there may be a stronger positive influence on mortality rates in the early period of a community-based service program, tapering off as length of participation in the program increases. Whether the impact on mortality (and life expectancy) will remain significant over time remains to be seen. In addition, whether the experimental services will affect more sensitive outcome measures (functional status) is unknown.

Another group of studies comprises those which use components of services as process measures and change in functional status or the use of more intensive levels of care as outcome measures. These studies generally find few significant relationships between process and outcome measures. They also conclude that initial patient characteristics are a much stronger determinant of outcome of care than is the process of care. Mitchell (1978) conducted one such study of 318 patients in three different Veterans Administration long-term care programs (home health care, community-based nursing home care, and hospital-based nursing home care). Although criticized by some for her approach, her finding that almost 60 percent of the variation in patient outcomes (measured by functional status at discharge and mortality) was accounted for by the initial disability level of the patients (rather than the process of care) seems well-founded. The relationships found between process and outcome were not strong.

Similar findings resulted from a study of home health care patients by Kurowski et al (1979). The authors evaluated the outcomes of care (measured by change in functional status) in over 2,000 episodes of illness. They found that the functional status of the patients at admission was the primary determinant of outcome of care (not the process of care, measured by utilization of services).

Another example of such a study is one of 101 elderly patients in a Canadian, hospital-based nursing home by Chekryn and Roos (1979). The purpose of their evaluation was to determine the relationship between process and outcome measures of care for a wide array of patient diagnoses. Process measures were: a multidisciplinary patient assessment, specified diagnostic procedures as part of the initial workup, problem-oriented care plans, and contact with the patient's family. Outcome measures included changes in functional and mental status from admission to discharge, changes in life satisfaction, and length of stay. The major finding of their study was that only weak or insignificant relationships existed between individual outcome measures and the process measures of care. The only significant correlations with outcomes were with functional and mental status and life satisfaction at admission. These findings are not surprising, since the researchers evaluated the care provided to patients with diverse needs with a generic set of process measures, using outcome measures that were no more specific to the problems of the patients.

It is certain that many factors, in addition to specific treatment and services, affect health status in long-term care. Major influences can include the interaction of multiple diagnoses, emotional status, environmental adequacy, intervening life events, and attitude toward, knowledge about, and willingness to comply with the prescribed plan of care. Thus, although the measurement of outcome appears valid as a measure of effectiveness, the degree to which the outcome in any particular case is actually attributable to the treatment is questionable. Indeed, McAuliffe (1979) argues that the myriad of factors which intervene between the process and outcome of care make the relationship(s) almost impossible to demonstrate empirically.

Studies that use highly specific process measures linked directly (and based on solid conceptual grounds) to specific outcomes of care intuitively seem to offer the greatest potential for uncovering the actual relationships between the process and outcome of care. Although few long-term studies have thus far demonstrated strong relationships between the two, there is reason to believe that current research efforts will be able to determine the true nature of these relationships. This expectation is based, in part, on the findings of several small experiments intended to assess the effects of a particular treatment(s) on the outcome of patient care.

One such study was conducted by Langer and Rodin (1976) in a nursing home in Connecticut, where the impact on psychosocial functioning over time was tested by giving patients greater choice and control over their own environment. The findings of this study indicate that there is a stronger relationship between the process and outcome of care than detected previously, and they highlight the importance of process and outcome measures which are specific to the problem under study.

Another in-progress research effort cited earlier is using highly specific measures to evaluate the quality of care in Colorado nursing homes (Shaughnessy, Schlenker et al, 1980; Harley et al, 1981). This investigates the relationship between problem-specific process criteria (forced fluids, for example) and changes in patient status over time, measured by outcomes which are conceptually linked to a particular problem and the process of care appropriate to that problem (for example, improvement in the problem of dehydration). Changes in selected problems expected to exhibit varying degrees of association between process and outcome quality measures will be evaluated over a three-month period. Findings of this study should provide some information on discernible relationships between the process and outcome of care controlling for certain intervening events.

A second study (Shaughnessy and Kurowski, 1980a) will expand this methodology to assess the quality, including the process and outcome, of care provided to patients of four different long-term care modalities: hospital-based nursing homes, free-standing nursing homes, hospital-based home health agencies, and free-standing home health agencies. This study is intended to provide policy recommendations with respect to appropriate placement and quality assurance activities in home health and nursing home care.

Another study was recently developed by the intramural research staff of the National Center for Health Services Research (Weissert and Wan, 1980), to provide incentive payments to nursing homes in two cities in order to encourage more appropriate care on the basis of process measures of quality and better outcomes. The experiment is intended to determine whether nursing homes can be encouraged to admit severely dependent patients and provide them with quality care. This study should also provide information with respect to potential relationships between care provided on the basis of highly specific patient care plans (process criteria) and positive outcomes in health status.

Refining Outcome Measures

Outcome evaluation in patient care has received a great deal of attention recently as the most appropriate way to approach the concept of quality. Conceptually, attaining appropriate outcome represents the ultimate validation of the effectiveness of the care process. However, it is extremely difficult to specify appropriate outcomes of care and to empirically demonstrate their relationship to the process of care.

Specifying appropriate outcomes of long-term care requires prior knowledge in two related aspects of health: the general course of health status expected of individuals at a given level of physical and mental status or age and the expected response of particular problems (or disease states) to treatment. Because of the wide variation in patient problems, outcome criteria (if they are to be sensitive) must be specified in relationship to the particular problem which produces dysfunction, not only in terms of final outcomes, but more importantly, in terms of intermediate outcomes. For example, degenerative joint disease may cause mobility restrictions which will never show improvement on an activities of daily living (ADL) scale. Nonetheless, appropriate treatment may produce measurable results in relief of pain, ability to engage in more social activities, and increased well-being. Such expected outcomes have been determined for only a limited number of conditions. Stroke and hip fracture are two such conditions that have been studied in detail (Granger *et al*, 1977; Lehman *et al*, 1975; Miglietta *et al*, 1976).

Establishing outcomes from a purely empirical base is both difficult and expensive. It requires that large quantities of data be collected and analyzed and that the variation in the quality of care be controlled. One recent study by Wan *et al* (1979) highlights this difficulty. Based on a comparison of expected changes in functional status compared to actual changes over three months, they found that prognostic judgments were accurate only 50 percent of the time. One important drawback of the study methodology was its inability to control for variations in the quality and appropriateness of services provided. In other words, implicit in the judgment about expected outcomes is an estimate of the expected quality of services provided (process quality). If these implicit expectations are unmet, then conceptually expected outcomes will also be unmet. Since the nature of the relationship between the outcome and process of care is unclear, how it affects prognosis is also unclear. This is why, as stated earlier, it is often best to base outcome standards on the assumption that optimal or totally appropriate care is provided. Outcome measures can then be expressed relative to such standards.

An example of current efforts to address the issue of prognosis is being conducted by the Rand Corporation in Los Angeles (Kane, 1980). In that study, actual changes in the outcomes of 500 patients will be compared to multidisciplinary, prognostic judgments. Quality of services provided will, in theory, be held relatively constant by using data collected only in high quality nursing homes. The study by Weissert and Wan (1980), described earlier, will pay nursing homes for achieving optimal outcomes. Findings of such studies should permit a comparison of actual outcomes to those possible under optimal circumstances, thereby advancing our capacity to interpret the meaning of quality of care measured in patient outcomes.

Due partly to greater difficulties in controlling for intervening factors which confound the process-outcome relationship, appropriate outcomes for home health care are less well-specified than those for nursing home care. In fact, only within the past few years have home health care providers begun to develop outcome criteria at all for evaluating the quality of home health care. One recent example is a system (Daubert, 1977) developed entirely on the basis of professional opinions. It provides an example of an attempt at patient classification by prognosis and translation of patient assessment into a tool for care planning and analysis of outcomes. Another example, reported by Decker et al (1979), is a voluntary, statewide program in Minnesota to improve patient assessment, the process of care, and the outcome of care. That system was developed on the basis of expert opinion and focuses solely on outcome criteria because, as the authors report, auditing patient records to develop process criteria was extremely time consuming and costly. One hundred twenty sets of outcome criteria covering 33 different conditions were eventually developed. The vast majority of the 510 patients reviewed during pilot testing of the criteria did not meet their outcomes, primarily due to the presence of unavoidable and unexpected complications. In spite of this, the authors anticipate

113

that by focusing the nurses' attention on the desired outcomes, patient care processes will improve.

One group that has specified exceptions to outcome criteria is the Pennsylvania Assembly of Home Agencies, which began a state-wide quality assurance project in 1974 (Berkoben, 1977). Using expert opinion, the group developed outcome criteria sets for 12 problems (including arthritis, cardiovascular disease, hip fracture, and mental illness). Up to 13 outcomes for each problem were specified. The criteria were used to compare outcome quality scores across providers for 2,500 patients treated in two years. Thus far, the criteria sets have not been actually used to evaluate the outcomes of care as they relate to process or structural measures of quality.

To tailor outcome measures to the prognosis of the patient, the Visiting Nurse Association of New Haven also developed a set of outcome criteria for patients grouped according to their rehabilitative potential (Daubert, 1979). For example, one group includes patients with acute diseases who are expected to recover fully; their outcome objective is complete elimination of existing health problems.

One project which uses an empirical approach (rather than one based solely on expert opinion) is being conducted by the Visiting Nurse Association of Omaha (Martin *et al,* 1979). By analyzing problem and outcome data for patients in four agencies in Nebraska, Iowa, Delaware, and Texas, the Association developed specific outcome criteria for each of the most common home health problems. Outcomes were then clustered by problem group to identify those which were met in the majority of cases. At this writing, these outcome criteria are still being field-tested.

None of the outcome measures developed specifically for home care have been well tested. Thus, it is difficult to say which, if any, will be valid and reliable for assessing the relationship of process or structural measures of quality to the outcome of care.

In summary, these concerns have led to the continuing debate over the relative advantage of using process measures, as opposed to outcome measures, to assess the quality of care (or as a basis for corrective actions and policy decisions). What is becoming clear is the presence of a "threshold" level of process or structural quality below which a poor outcome is much more likely and above which the relationship between process (or structure) and outcome is less predictable. Furthermore, the studies cited make a strong argument that attempts to compare the outcome of long-term care should take into account the initial characteristics and overall individual potential (that is, initial health status) of the patient. In other words, each patient possesses a unique combination of disabilities, accompanying complications, subjective expectations, beliefs, and specific

114

demographic characteristics. The subsequent use of services is partly determined by this and by the decisions and practices of providers. Measures used to categorize patients with respect to the process or outcome of treatment must incorporate this uniqueness, or they run the risk of being invalid.

Summary of the Evidence

Results of long-term care research generally support the conclusion that the relationship between structural measures of quality and the process of care, and between the process of care and its outcome, is not well established. In spite of this, we know a reasonable amount about certain aspects of such relationships and therefore about specific issues related to the measurement of the quality of long-term care. First, structural criteria are least likely to measure process and outcome quality in the areas such as patient activities, social services, and rehabilitative services because they merely measure whether a provider demonstrates the capacity to provide services should a patient need them. They do not indicate whether the organization actually has a functioning program, and least of all, if it actually provides services to patients who need them.

Second, process criteria generally constitute a useful tool for evaluating the quality of care. The use of either structural or process measures is usually based upon the assumption that there is a causal relationship between them and the outcome of care as expressed in the patient's final condition. However, this relationship has not yet been consistently demonstrated. Third, although conceptually the attainment of outcome represents the ultimate validation of the effectiveness of the care process, it is difficult to specify appropriate outcomes of care and to empirically relate individual outcomes to the process of care. Thus, expert opinion (not outcomes) may be the best way to validate process measures of care.

Fourth, those assessing the outcome of long-term care must consider the initial characteristics and overall potential of the individual patients. Fifth, in addition to validated measures and accurate data, other necessary conditions for the determination of the true relationships between the three types of measures of the quality of care are adequate sample sizes, financial resources, and time. In part because of the effect of intervening events on the health status of long-term care patients, thorough and practical studies require substantial resources. This situation suggests the necessity of committing further resources to the effort, rather than abandoning it.

Assuring the Quality of Long-Term Care

Although there are various approaches to quality assurance, they generally may be classified as market and non-market mechanisms.

The obvious market mechanism for ensuring quality is the exercise of freedom of choice (most often on the part of private patients) to purchase services in the marketplace. The indirect effects of reimbursement (a second market mechanism) on the quality of long-term care and the incorporation of quality assurance incentives into reimbursement schemes have only begun to be studied (Shaughnessy and Kurowski, 1980b).

Non-market methods include both direct and indirect efforts to ensure quality. Indirect efforts include approaches such as certificate-of-need requirements that services be of demonstrated quality and appropriateness. Another indirect quality-enhancing effort is the imposition of educational requirements on long-term care personnel. Yet the most common approach to ensuring the quality of long-term care, and the one to which most research evidence pertains, has been the use of direct non-market (regulatory) efforts. Thus, direct non-market or regulatory approaches serve as the focus of this section.

Licensure

Formal programs intended to directly ensure the quality of long-term care were instituted in the early 1930s, when States developed the licensure survey process which all nursing homes must undergo before providing services. The licensure of health professionals and the organizations in which they provide care is a basic quality assurance mechanism found in most health care settings. Licensure occurs primarily at the State level and is intended to ensure a minimal level of organizational capacity (or professional competence). It is the process by which a governmental agency grants permission to individuals or organizations meeting predetermined qualifications to provide given services or engage in a given occupation.

Facility licensure standards are generally based on structural measures of quality, although some States have recently expanded patient care/service requirements. Nursing homes in all States must be licensed (for a specific number of beds at a particular level of care) in order to treat patients (regardless of their desire to receive Medicare or Medicaid funding); 22 States currently have licensure laws for home health agencies; three States license adult day care programs. Personnel licensure standards are also typically based on structural requirements, for example, minimal levels of education, internships, and examinations. All clinical personnel (for example, physicians, nurses, therapists) working in long-term care programs are required by their State practice laws to be licensed. Furthermore, the nursing home administrator is the only type of health care administrator required by all States to be licensed.

116

Certification

With the passage of the Social Security Act Amendments of 1965, which established the Medicare and Medicaid programs, providers were required to undergo a certification survey before being reimbursed by either program. To be certified eligible to receive reimbursement for care rendered to Medicare and Medicaid beneficiaries, nursing homes (providing skilled and/or intermediate levels of care), home health agencies, and adult day care programs must meet certain "conditions of participation." These conditions are generally based on "structural" requirements intended to ensure the capacity to provide adequate care. They focus on the availability of certain services, educational requirements of the staff, minimal staffing patterns, fire and safety codes, etc. The conditions for home health agencies are similar, but fewer in number, to those currently in effect for nursing homes. They emphasize management structure rather than actual patient care. Certification requirements for adult day care exist in only two of the eight States which currently reimburse for the services under the Medicaid program. It is important to keep in mind that certification requirements pertain only to providers reimbursed by Medicare or Medicaid.

Mandatory Medical Care Review

One part of the certification requirements calls for Medicaid and Medicare programs to provide yearly medical care reviews of all publicly funded nursing home patients to ensure a minimum-level quality of care. This review is conducted by the departments of health or social services in each State for Medicaid patients and by the Federal regional agencies for Medicare patients (although often contracted to the States thereafter).

Medicare requires that the appropriateness of services and the quality of care be reviewed by a utilization review committee (within a skilled nursing home). Similar, but broader, requirements imposed upon facilities by Medicaid are called Utilization Control and Inspection of Care (IoC). The Medicaid requirements applicable to intermediate care are limited to IoCs. Both types of reviews (previously called Periodic Medical Review and Independent Professional Review) assess the adequacy of services provided (generally using process criteria and, sometimes, outcome criteria) and the necessity of continued placement.

Voluntary Peer Review

In the mid-1940s, the nursing home industry itself began an informal system to review the types of care provided and the outcome of that care. Such voluntary peer review began at about the same time for home health providers. Peer review is performed by practicing health professionals (nursing home or home health agency administrators) to assess the adequacy of services provided by other members of the same profession. In long-term care, peer review usually takes the form of accreditation. Requirements focus on structural criteria, such as the education or experience of the administrator, and the quality of the recordkeeping, rather than on the actual provision of services.

A recent report on long-term care quality assurance programs to the Undersecretary of DHHS (1980) summarizes the general goals of such programs:

(1) Providers must meet minimum structural standards (for example, certification, licensure, voluntary peer review).
(2) Client placement is appropriate, with respect to the level and site of care (for example, mandatory medical review/PSRO).
(3) Care meets professional standards of quality (for example, mandatory medical review/PSRO, voluntary peer review).
(4) Care reflects changes in the quality and need for care (for example, mandatory medical review/PSRO).

The extent to which these goals are met is related to the state of the art of quality measurement (discussed earlier) and to the effectiveness of the quality assurance programs (as discussed in the following four sections).

Certification and Licensure Programs

Because there are so many components of long-term care quality, it has been impossible to emphasize all components and programs equally. Partly because of early scandals involving fatal nursing home fires, licensure and certification standards have emphasized physical plant and equipment requirements (which are often costly to the facility owner), possibly diverting funds which might have been invested in other aspects of the quality of care. This emphasis was not surprising given that much was known about building construction, educational requirements, etc., while there was little agreement about the specific components, programs, and measures appropriate for nursing and medical care, social services, etc. Now that the possibility of major disasters due to structural deficiencies has been reduced dramatically, it is easy for critics to focus on other deficiencies in long-term care, pointing to the failure of structural standards to improve the care in these other areas.

The foundation for structural standards was described previously. In essence, structural measures of quality concentrate on evaluating the physical plant, the written procedures, and the internal documents which detail procedures for complying with standards, among other things. They focus on the capacity to provide care,

118

rather than on the actual provision of care itself. Very little attention is given to the quality of care or life. Thus far, researchers have not succeeded in empirically validating many specific facts about which of the structural measures of quality are most important. Thus, those involved in implementing these programs have been forced to refine the process of certification and licensure largely on the basis of conceptually appealing arguments.

In recent years, several States have attempted to refine the certification process to concentrate their resources on nursing homes with histories of poor quality of care. In theory, this restructuring of the review process is intended to obtain the greatest improvement in patient care for a fixed sum of money. Examples of States trying to streamline the certification process include Wisconsin (Wisconsin Department of Health and Social Services, 1979), Colorado (Colorado Department of Health, 1980), New York (Schneider and O'Sullivan, 1980), Ohio (Ohio Nursing Home Commission, 1979), and Illinois (Medicus System Corp., 1976). Generally, their approach has been to focus on the key certification standards which appear to be most directly related to patient care and to review facilities with a history of violations in greater depth than those without such histories.

Two examples are illustrative of these efforts. Wisconsin has published an evaluation of its experience with a focused review process. The 1978–79 annual report of the Nursing Home Quality Assurance Project (Wisconsin Department of Health and Social Services, 1979) reports that in the first year of operation, about the same number of deficiencies which directly threaten the health, safety, or welfare of residents were detected in those homes assigned to the new review process as in the facilities reviewed with the full process. Further, they detected fewer deficiencies which were not directly threatening to the health, safety, or welfare of residents. The conclusion of the Department of Health and Social Services after one year of operation was that the focused survey detects serious deficiencies in the quality of nursing home care as well as the full survey process. An independent evaluation of the program began in July of 1980.

Using certification non-compliance data, the Colorado Department of Health has taken a similar approach to evaluate nursing homes (Colorado Department of Health, 1980). Thirty-six out of 541 Federal survey elements were selected on the basis of their (a) importance to some aspect of patient care, (b) potential impact on the safety of patients, (c) compliance not affected by "intervening issues" such as area-wide manpower or reimbursement shortages, or (d) pertinence to patient rights. An overall score for each nursing home was computed, based on the number of deficiencies in the prior year. This measure was found to be highest for State-run facilities and lowest for county-based nursing homes. (Statistical tests of significance were not reported.) Colorado has not yet had the opportunity to review nursing homes for certification using this approach, although State regulators are hopeful that their experiences will be similar to those of Wisconsin. Such similarity would suggest that the certification process could be streamlined without sacrificing its ability to detect the more important (patient care related) violations of quality of care standards.

New York is developing an innovative approach to long-term care quality assurance and has received Federal waivers to begin implementing the program throughout the State. New York will use a screening mechanism based on patient conditions or outcomes to identify facilities which require further review. This allows the reviewers to assess process quality only in selected facilities. The system is currently being field-tested. Early findings suggest that the system is workable, using regular field surveyors (Schneider and O'Sullivan, 1980).

To the best of our knowledge, no such revision of the licensure and/or certification processes for home health agencies has taken place at the State level. Even though 22 States currently license such agencies, no studies have compared the quality of care offered by licensed providers to that offered by unlicensed providers. Since there is no reason to expect licensure to be any more effective for home health than nursing home care, such studies might shed some light on reviews for both programs. Revised conditions of participation were published for comment at the Federal level, but their scope or purpose was not appreciably altered from existing standards. Although some providers argue on the basis of anecdotal evidence, no studies thus far have directly investigated the effectiveness of certification standards in ensuring the quality of home health care.

Regulations in the area of adult day care are in the developmental stage and vary considerably by State. An internal study currently being conducted by the Health Care Financing Administration, DHHS, indicates that, of the eight States which reimburse for adult day care services under Medicaid (California, Georgia, Kansas, Maryland, Massachusetts, New Jersey, New York, and Washington), only four have either licensure or certification programs. Of these, Massachusetts and California review individual patient care procedures in addition to evaluating structural measures of care. The other States use a variety of less structured mechanisms for monitoring adult day care programs. As indicated previously, there is no evidence yet on the effectiveness of these programs.

Another component of the certification/licensure review process which strongly influences the success of the programs is enforcement. A review by the Ohio Nursing Home Commission (1979) found a wide disparity among the various professionals involved in the survey process (for example, nurses, sanitarians, and life safety code inspectors) with respect to sanctions recommended and violations judged important. The Commission concluded that their "consultative" model of enforcement (with education and consultation as the primary method of response to violations) promotes too close a relationship between inspectors and nursing homes, which results in unreported violations year after year. Therefore the Commission recommended the adoption of interim sanctions (receivership, fines, etc.) recently made possible at the State level through Federal regulations.

Until recently, the only generally available option to a State when it found violations of certification requirements was the termination of certification. States viewed this as a severe punishment, a difficult and time-consuming process, and one that was potentially damaging to residents' health. As a result, facilities continued to provide care until violations become so pervasive that decertification was the only appropriate sanction. But Federal regulations provided no allowance for the due process requirements of the States, so the State Medicaid agency was at risk to assume the total cost of services for patients in facilities which were no longer certified. If the facility's certification revocation was upheld on appeal, the Federal share of Medicaid nursing home costs incurred during the litigation process was not paid to the State. The result was that nursing homes were often allowed to continue treating patients for years while violations went uncorrected.

Following in the footsteps of Ohio, six States have adopted systems which allow for the licensing agency to issue fines for violations of nursing home standards. Upon determining a deficiency, an inspector issues a citation which gives the facility a certain period of time (often one month) to correct it. If the deficiency has not been corrected within the appropriate time, a fine is levied, from $250 to $1,000 per day, until the violation is corrected. Unfortunately, any fine has the potential of reducing funds available for patient care, thus possibly promoting additional violations.

Another possible sanction is civil receivership which legally transfers control of the management of the facility to another individual or organization. Six States now currently grant their licensing authority this option. Receivership has several advantages in that it does not move residents, it is easier to impose than removal of a license, and the receiver has freedom of action to correct deficiencies. Receivership is not without its problems, however. Some States have had difficulty in finding individuals or organizations willing to be receivers. Other enforcement tools which have been discussed include malpractice suits and requirements in professional licensure that observed violations be reported to authorities (Butler, 1979).

Clearly, there is no easy solution to the question of enforcement. It will be especially important to evaluate the impact of the procedural and enforcement changes in the licensure-certification process, at the same time improving our understanding of the important structural measures of quality which serve as their bases.

Mandatory Medical Care Review Programs

As discussed earlier, mandatory medical care (sometimes called quality of care) reviews are studies to evaluate and improve the quality of long-term care. Although there are several types, they generally are performed by multidisciplinary teams using specific criteria. Generally based on process criteria of quality, these reviews are required by Federal law for all publicly-financed nursing home patients (and for a sample of home health patients) and are the responsibility of the Medicaid (and Medicare) agency.

Medical care should be reviewed for all Medicare/Medicaid admissions to nursing homes prior to the expiration of the length of stay which is assigned at the time of pre-admission certification. This is concurrent assessment of the necessity for placement, the appropriateness of the care provided, and the quality of that care. The actual quality of care portion of the review process is intended to evaluate the appropriateness and quality of several aspects of care provided to Medicare/Medicaid patients. It is often composed of two types of review: a broad screen and the in-depth (focused) review. (These same types of reviews are typically completed internally by home health agency utilization review or audit committees.)

Medical care evaluation studies are usually intended to be educational mechanisms to ensure the quality of care, frequently by studying the process and outcome of care retrospectively. Such studies may include (1) administrative audits which concentrate on the adequacy of structural measures of quality (for example, hospital transfer agreements, nursing care records, frequency of physician visits); (2) medical audits which can entail focused diagnostic studies to evaluate the process of care for particular medical conditions (such as diabetes or skin ulcers) based upon explicit professional criteria; and (3) outcome indicator studies which evaluate problem-specific outcomes of care for various patient groups. Like certification and licensure efforts to improve the quality of care, medical care evaluation studies are only as good as the measures and the enforcement process they use.

Whether concurrent quality assurance reviews or retrospective medical care evaluations (performed externally by PSROs or State agencies and internally by utilization review committees) actually improve the process or outcome of care is uncertain. Several studies

122

have contended that their impact is substantial (Allison-Cooke and Ellis, 1979; Bronx PSRO, 1979; Kahn *et al,* 1975; Kahn *et al,* 1977), while a major evaluation effort funded by DHHS concluded that there was much more to be done (Kane *et al,* 1979a and b).

A study completed by Allison-Cooke and Ellis (1979) examined the San Joacquin Valley PSRO (SJPSRO) using measures of nursing home quality that were developed using a checklist of 43 non-specific process quality measures (such as admission/transfer information, nursing care plans, availability of special services, etc.). Each facility was assigned a final score based upon the weighted average of non-compliance with the items on the checklist. The control group of nursing homes was not subject to the PSRO review; a second group was subject to major PSRO interventions (including frequent continued stay reviews and follow-up audits), while a third study group was reviewed in the SJPSRO's traditional manner. Comparison of pre- and post-test measures at six-month intervals revealed that, on the basis of changes in the process measures of quality, the control group quality of care significantly deteriorated, while the study group subject to traditional PSRO review exhibited the greatest improvement. The authors concluded that concurrent review procedures using medical care evaluations significantly improved the process quality of care in nursing homes.

The study of PSRO quality assurance programs which found them insufficient was reported by Kane *et al* (1979a and b). In that study, researchers retrospectively assessed the operation of 10 PSRO demonstration sites during 1976–1978, using a case study approach. With respect to the general quality assurance components of the PSRO review programs studied, the authors recommended several areas for improvement, including (1) the addition of bedside patient assessment to the review process, (2) increased attention to criteria development, especially for drug use, (3) the addition of more outcome criteria, (4) increased participation of non-physicians in the review process, and (5) improvement in the capacity for feedback to and from nursing homes to determine which recommendations were accepted.

Their findings concerning concurrent PSRO quality review suggest that the process was able to identify deficiencies, although evidence of effectiveness was primarily anecdotal. Furthermore, at least six of the PSROs took an active role in promoting quality, by educating and consulting with nursing home personnel. The study concluded that, in general, the PSROs lacked effective follow-up systems.

With respect to in-depth medical care evaluation studies, the authors suggested that these studies be used only to supplement overall concurrent quality assurance programs for several reasons:

(1) There was great difficulty in developing appropriate process and outcome criteria.
(2) There was disagreement about the scope and content of the studies.
(3) Delegation of studies to nursing homes was not effective.

To improve the effectiveness of medical reviews, several new projects have just begun. The Health Care Financing Administration recently awarded a contract to develop a nursing home PSRO evaluation protocol which will provide design specifications for the conduct of PSRO quality assurance programs. The final product of the contract will permit analyses of the impact of PSROs on the quality, utilization, and cost of long-term care review. The same agency recently distributed a request for proposals to research organizations to develop quality assurance guidelines for PSRO review of home health care. The contract was awarded to the Orkand Corporation in 1981 and should provide valuable information about appropriate procedures and measures to ensure the quality of home care. Regardless of which agency eventually performs the reviews, the contracts should provide valuable information.

Voluntary Peer Review

Both the American Health Care Association and the American Association of Homes for the Aged (national organizations representing the nursing home industry) and the Joint Commission on Accreditation of Hospitals (JCAH; largely representing hospital-based facilities) have established guidelines for peer review. Some State affiliates of the first two groups link peer review to continued membership in the association; the same is true of JCAH accreditation at the national level. Sanctions can be severe; in Louisiana and California, peer review committees have recommended the revocation of nursing home licenses. It is important to note that vigorous, voluntary, peer review efforts in the nursing home industry are not common, however. Although there are some States with effective programs, they are the exception and not the rule.

For example, a few State nursing home associations, such as those in Minnesota and Maryland, have sponsored active peer review programs for several years. These programs generally have site visit teams composed of administrators and other health care professionals who review dietary, nursing, and social services, in addition to general administration and building maintenance. Such efforts are intended to incorporate continuing education as well as quality assurance activities into one process. In Maryland, if a facility does not meet the standards of the association, it is given time to correct deficiencies but denied continued membership if corrections are not made in a specified time period. If violations affect the safety of patients, the association reports its findings directly to the health department for remedial action.

Several voluntary peer review programs exist for home health agencies. These include those of JCAH (which applies to hospital-based programs), the National League for Nursing, and the National Council for Homemaker-Home Health Aid Services (CHHHAS). CHHHAS has developed a list of structurally-oriented, quality of care measures by which a home health agency can measure its compliance with accepted standards of care. Another national agency representing member home health agencies, the National League for Nursing, established a voluntary accreditation program in 1977. Thus far, few home health programs (106 to date) have taken advantage of this accreditation program, and no studies are known which compare the quality of care provided by accredited and unaccredited providers.

In general, in spite of isolated instances, peer review programs in nursing homes and home health agencies have received little attention from the industries. Thus, their impact has been essentially untested.

Summary of the Evidence

Results of the evaluation of long-term care quality assurance programs generally support the conclusion that prior efforts have not been effective in maintaining or improving the quality of care provided. However, recent attempts to improve such programs indicate that modifications to the programs may be having a positive impact on their effectiveness.

Specifically, the evaluation of current quality assurance efforts supports the following findings. First, current licensure and certification standards for home health and nursing home care are not sufficient to ensure high quality care. Second, preliminary conclusions from the several States that are experimenting with "streamlined" certification and licensure surveys suggest that serious deficiencies can be as well detected using such surveys as with the full survey process. Third, additional interim enforcement options in the licensure and certification areas improve the probability that standards will be enforced. To the extent that lack of enforcement has negatively affected the quality of care, these new options should improve the care of patients. Fourth, evidence on the effectiveness of quality of care and medical care evaluation studies is mixed. Evidence of positive effects is largely anecdotal. Finally, there are no available empirical studies on the effectiveness of voluntary peer review as an approach to long-term care quality assurance.

Summary

Measuring and ensuring the quality of long-term care are not simple tasks. The field is characterized by features which make these tasks especially difficult, including the presence of (1) a large number of different types of programs and settings (that is, nursing homes, home health agencies, adult day care programs), (2) multi-disciplinary teams of providers representing diverse and sometimes conflicting points of view, and (3) patients who are often not expected to improve. Thus, existing analytic approaches and methods must be refined to specifically address the idiosyncratic nature of long-term care.

It is clear that although there is much to be learned from existing research, there is much more to be learned from future efforts to develop the state of the art of measurement and assurance of the quality of long-term care. These efforts should be guided by two principles. First, the temptation to *summarily discard efforts* to measure or ensure the quality of care because of their imperfections *should be resisted.* As described earlier in this chapter, several approaches to evaluating and ensuring the quality of long-term care have been attempted during the past decade. Depending on how the effectiveness of such efforts are judged, it is safe to say that all have been imperfect, and several have been relatively unsuccessful. The tendency to argue that these efforts have been tried and judged lacking and should not be further investigated could be termed "research annihilism." In fact, many have strengths, and additional study of these efforts could reveal features on which we should build as well as those approaches which should be discarded. This might be termed "research incrementalism" and warrants strong consideration if we expect to provide practical results upon which to base long-term care quality assurance policies.

Second, because of cost limitations, as well as the breadth of potential approaches to quality measurement and assurance, it is essential to develop priorities indicating the areas of patient care in strongest need of attention. This would involve developing expert opinion-based lists of patient care services or patient typologies where quality problems are most serious and frequent, as well as developing priorities about which settings or provider types have the most serious quality problems. Research resources are limited, and efforts cannot be uniformly distributed across all potential areas. The above two principles may serve as guidelines in developing specific research projects to measure and ensure the quality of long-term care.

Several specific areas requiring research are listed below.

• Refined Measures of the Quality of Care: The refinement of the specificity, sensitivity, reliability, and relevance of process and outcome (and even structural) measures of the quality of care is a continuing need. This need is particularly acute with respect to home health care. If these types of measures are to be incorporated into quality assurance systems, the data upon which they are based should not be extremely difficult to collect. Yet the measures must be refined enough to adequately capture the patient status, process, and outcome relationships within the care process.

- Relationship of Process and Outcome Measures of Quality: Further research is essential to determine the nature of the process-outcome relationships in health care to validate acceptable process measures. Evaluation of these relationships must be undertaken in various care settings, for different problems, diagnoses, and procedures, and under varying provider types and durations of care. It is imperative to recognize and determine, if possible, the point at which increases in the numbers of types of services provided produce diminishing marginal utility with respect to improvements in patient status (outcomes).

- Optimal Outcomes/Effectiveness: Conceptual and empirical research is needed to further determine the optimal outcomes possible for patients with various health impairments. Quality standards can be defined in terms of maximum rather than optimal outcomes, but it is difficult to evaluate the level of outcome attained unless knowledge exists about the possible levels of outcome under the best of circumstances (controlling for differences in initial patient status).

- Case-Mix Measures: At a theoretical level, quality cannot be separated from case-mix since patient outcomes are dependent on, and defined in, terms of patient conditions or health problems. To define quality using changes in patient status or outcomes, it is necessary to initially specify the patient condition or patient status. Empirical refinement of case-mix measures and classification schemes which lend themselves to quality measurement is needed. Since descriptors of patient status are used both as measures of patient needs and measures of patient outcomes over time, such descriptors form a key component of any long-term care placement, utilization review, and quality assurance system.

- Incentives to Change Provider Behavior: A fundamental purpose associated with quality assurance is to provide a remedial mechanism to increase the quality of care in those areas where it is wanting. This emphasizes the need for continued research into ways of changing provider behavior through increased

awareness, incentives, and, where appropriate, disincentives.
- Relationship(s) Between Quality and Cost: A major gap in our knowledge is the relationship between measures of case-mix, quality of care, and cost of care. Since quality incentives can be incorporated into reimbursement only if the relationships between (various types of) quality measures and (various types of) costs are known or accurately estimated, such relationships should form the focus of empirical studies. Furthermore, additional conceptual refinement is needed on whether (and how) definitions of quality should include cost, or at least implicitly refer to cost.
- Quality Assurance and Reimbursement: The issue of where lines should be drawn in attempting to link quality assurance and reimbursement needs considerable study. It is doubtful that a complete unification of the two objectives can be attained by a single program. Further, the possibility of subjecting only portions of institutions (cost centers, specific patient categories, etc.) to a unified quality assurance/reimbursement approach needs to be researched.

In conclusion, the refinement of approaches to quality measurement and assurance is, without doubt, an essential goal from the perspective of an efficient and effective long-term care delivery system. However, in view of the apparent methodological and operational impediments, it is necessary to recognize that the attainment of such a goal will require a substantial investment of resources and take place in a gradual and evolutionary manner.

The authors wish to acknowledge the invaluable assistance of their associate, Linda Breed, who obtained much of the background material for this paper. Alan Rosenfeld and Christine Bishop of Brandeis University and Mark Meiners of the National Center for Health Services Research, DHHS, provided valuable comments and suggestions on earlier drafts of this manuscript.

References

Abt Associates, Inc., *Study of Appropriate Staffing Ratios of Daily Nursing Hours for the Purpose of Establishing Federal Requirements in Nursing Homes,* Cambridge, MA: Abt Associates, Inc., 1980.

Allison-Cooke, Sherry and Susan E. Ellis, *An Assessment of the Impact of SJPSRO Concurrent Quality Assurance Review on Quality of Care in LTC Facilities, Part I: A Final Report,* report submitted to DHEW under Contract Nos. 240-76-0075 and 104-74-179, Providence, RI: Rhode Island Health Services Research, Inc., 1979.

Berkoben, Rita, "Home Health Care and Quality Assurance: The Experience of the Pennsylvania Assembly Project," *Quality Review Bulletin* (October 1977): 25–28.

Bronx PSRO, *The Bronx PSRO Long-Term Care Demonstration Project: Final Report,* report submitted to HCFA, DHEW under Contract No. HSA-105-74-165, Bronx, NY: May 1979.

128

Butler, Patricia A., "Nursing Home Quality of Care Enforcement, Part II—State Agency Enforcement Remedies," Research Institute, Legal Services Corporation, 1979 (mimeograph).

Chekryn, Joanne and Leslie L. Roos, "Auditing the Process of Care in a New Geriatric Unit," *Journal of the American Geriatrics Society* 27 (1979): 107–11.

Colorado Department of Health, Medical Care Licensing and Certification Division, *"QC" Factors, A Relationship Between Computerization, Patient Care and the Regulatory Process*, Denver, CO: Colorado Department of Health, 1980.

Connelly, Kathleen, Philip K. Cohen, and Diana Chapman Walsh, "Periodic Medical Review: Assessing the Quality and Appropriateness of Care in Skilled Nursing Facilities," *The New England Journal of Medicine* (April 1977): 878–80.

Daubert, Elizabeth A., "A System to Evaluate Home Health Care Services," *Nursing Outlook* 25 (March 1977): 168–71.

Daubert, Elizabeth A., "Patient Classification System and Outcome Criteria," *Nursing Outlook* (July 1979): 450–54.

Decker, Frances, Linda Stevens, Margaret Vancini, and Lorene Wedeking, "Using Patient Outcomes to Evaluate Community Health Nursing," *Nursing Outlook* (April 1979): 278–82.

Donabedian, Avedis, "Evaluating the Quality of Medical Care," *Milbank Memorial Fund Quarterly* 44 (1966): 166–206.

Donabedian, Avedis, *Explorations in Quality Assessment and Monitoring, Volume I: The Definition of Quality and Approaches to its Assessment*, Ann Arbor, MI: Health Administration Press, 1980.

Gottesman, Leonard E., "Nursing Home Performance as Related to Resident Traits, Ownership, Size and Source of Payment," *American Journal of Public Health* 64 (March 1974): 269–76.

Gottesman, Leonard E. and Norman C. Bourestom, "Why Nursing Homes Do What They Do," *The Gerontologist* (December 1974): 501–06.

Granger, Carl V., Clarence Sherwood, and David Greer, "Functional Status Measures in a Comprehensive Stroke Care Program," *Archives of Physical Medicine and Rehabilitation* 58 (1977): 555–61.

Greenberg, Jay, *Cost, Case Mix, Quality, and Facility Characteristics in Minnesota's Nursing Homes: An Exploratory Analysis,* First Year Progress Report, Minneapolis, MN: Center for Health Services Research, University of Minnesota, 1980.

Harley, Barbara, David Landes, and Bettina D. Kurowski, Working Paper 10: *Case Mix and Quality: Design and Development of a Methodology for Data Collection*, Denver, CO: Center for Health Services Research, University of Colorado Health Sciences Center, 1981.

Holmberg, Hopkins R. and Nancy N. Anderson, "Implications of Ownership for Nursing Care," *Medical Care* 6 (July-August 1968): 300–07.

Kahn, Kenneth A., William Hines, Arlene S. Woodson, and Gabrielle Burkham-Armstrong, "A Multidisciplinary Approach to Assessing the Quality of Care in Long-Term Care Facilities," *The Gerontologist* 17 (1977): 1–65.

Kahn, Kenneth A., William Hines, Arlene S. Woodson, Gabrielle Burkham-Armstrong, and Charles Holtz, *A Multi-Disciplinary Approach to Assessing the Quality of Life and Services in Long Term Care Facilities, Research Report*, report submitted to EMCRO, DHEW under Contract

No. 5-R18-HS-01243-02, Denver, CO: Colorado Foundation for Medical Care, November 1975.

Kane, Robert L., "Progress on Prognosis: Report on Prognosing the Course of Nursing Home Patients Project," Santa Monica, CA: Rand Corporation, 1980 (mimeograph).

Kane, Rosalie A., Robert L. Kane, Dorothy Kleffel, Robert H. Brook, Charles Eby, George A. Goldberg, Laurence Z. Rubenstein, and John Van Ryzin, *The PSRO and the Nursing Home, Vol. I, An Assessment of PSRO Long-Term Care Review*, report submitted to HCFA, DHEW under Contract No. 500-78-0040, Santa Monica, CA: Rand, 1979a.

Kane, Rosalie, Robert L. Kane, Dorothy Kleffel, Robert H. Brook, Charles Eby, and George A. Goldberg, *The PSRO and the Nursing Home, Vol. II, Ten Demonstration Projects in PSRO Long-Term Care Review*, report submitted to HCFA, DHEW under Contract No. 500-78-0040, Santa Monica, CA: Rand, 1979b.

Kurowski, Bettina, Working Paper 3: *Programs to Assure Quality of Care in Colorado Nursing Homes*, Denver, CO: Center for Health Services Research, University of Colorado Health Sciences Center, 1979.

Kurowski, Bettina *et al*, *Applied Research in Home Health Services, Volume II: Cost Per Episode*, Denver, CO: Center for Health Services Research, University of Colorado Health Sciences Center, 1979.

Langer, Ellen J. and Judith Rodin, "The Effects of Choice and Enhanced Personal Responsibility for the Aged: A Field Experiment in an Institutional Setting," *Journal of Personality and Social Psychology* 34 (1976): 191–98.

Lehman, J.F. *et al*, "Stroke: Does Rehabilitation Affect Outcome?" *Archives of Physical Medicine and Rehabilitation* 56 (1975): 375–82.

Linn, Margaret W., Lee Gurel, and Bernard S. Linn, "Patient Outcome as a Measure of Quality of Nursing Home Care," *American Journal of Public Health* 67 (April 1977): 337–44.

Martin, Karen *et al*, "Field Testing of a Problem Classification Scheme and Development of an Expected Outcome Scheme with a Methodology for Use," Draft Executive Summary, Omaha: Visiting Nurse Association of Omaha, September 1979 (mimeograph).

McAuliffe, William E., "Measuring the Quality of Medical Care: Process Versus Outcome," *Milbank Memorial Fund Quarterly* 57 (No. 1, 1979): 118–52.

Medicus System Corporation, *Regulatory Use of a Quality Evaluation System for Long-Term Care, Part 3, Analyses: Design and Results, Final Report*, report submitted to NCHSR, DHEW under Contract No. HSM 110-73-499, Springfield, IL: Illinois Department of Public Health, November 1976.

Miglietta, Osvaldo, Tae-Soo Chung, and Vemireddi Rajeswaramma, "Fate of Stroke Patients Transferred to a Long-Term Rehabilitation Hospital," *Stroke* 7 (1976): 76–77.

Mitchell, Janet B. "Patient Outcomes in Alternative Long-Term Care Settings," *Medical Care* 16 (June 1978): 439–52.

Ohio Nursing Home Commission, *A Program in Crisis: Blueprint for Action, Final Report of the Ohio Nursing Home Commission*, Columbus, OH: October 1979.

Ray, Wayne A., Charles F. Federspiel, and William Schaffner, "A Study of Antipsychotic Drug Use in Nursing Homes: Epidemiological Evidence

130

Suggesting Misuse," *American Journal of Public Health* 70 (May 1980): 485–91.

Schneider, Don and Anne O'Sullivan, "Quality Assurance for Long-Term Care: Revising the Periodic Review," Troy, NY: Schneider and Associates, 1980 (mimeograph).

Shaughnessy, Peter W. and Bettina D. Kurowski, "A Comparison of the Cost and Quality of Home Health and Nursing Home Care Provided by Free-Standing and Hospital-Based Organizations, Project Narrative," a proposal submitted to HCFA, DHEW, Denver, CO: Center for Health Services Research, April 1980a.

Shaughnessy, Peter W. and Bettina D. Kurowski, Working Paper 8: *Quality Assurance Through Reimbursement*, Denver, CO: Center for Health Services Research, University of Colorado Health Sciences Center, 1980b.

Shaughnessy, Peter W., Robert Schlenker, Barbara Harley, Nancy Shanks, Gerri Tricarico, Vann Perry, Bettina D. Kurowski, and Arlene Woodson, *Long-Term Care Reimbursement and Regulation: A Study of Cost, Case Mix, and Quality: Working Paper 4, First Year Analysis Report*, Denver, CO: Center for Health Services Research, University of Colorado Health Sciences Center, 1980.

Shaughnessy, Peter W., Eileen Tynan, David Landes, Charles Huggs, Daniel Holub, and Linda Breed, *An Evaluation of Swing-Bed Experiments to Provide Long-Term Care in Rural Hospitals, Vol. II: Final Technical Report*, Denver, CO: Center for Health Services Research, University of Colorado Health Sciences Center, 1980.

Skellie, F. Albert and Ruth E. Coan, "Community-Based Long-Term Care and Mortality: Preliminary Findings of Georgia's Alternative Health Services Project," *The Gerontologist* 20 (1980): 372–79.

U.S. Comptroller General, General Accounting Office, *Report to the Congress of the United States: Entering a Nursing Home—Costly Implications for Medicaid and the Elderly*, Washington, D.C.: November 1979.

U.S. Congress, House, Select Committee on Aging, *New York Home Care Abuse* (Publication No. 95-145), Washington, D.C.: Government Printing Office, 1978.

U.S. Congress, Senate, Committee on Government Operations, Subcommittee on Federal Spending Practices, Efficiency and Open Government, *Problems Associated with Home Health Agencies and the Medicare Program in the State of Florida*, Washington, D.C.: Government Printing Office, August 1976.

U.S. Congress, Senate, Special Committee on Aging, *Nursing Home Care in the United States: Failure in Public Policy* (No. 1-4, 94th Congress, 1st Session), Washington, D.C.: Government Printing Office, April 1975.

Wan, Thomas T.H., William G. Weissert, and Barbara B. Livieratos, "The Accuracy of Prognostic Judgments of Elderly Long-Term Care Patients," paper presented at the American Public Health Association Meeting in New York, November 1979.

Weissert, William G. and Thomas T.H. Wan, "Encouraging Appropriate Care for the Chronically Ill: Design of the NCHSR Experiment in Nursing Home Incentive Payments," paper presented at the APHA annual meeting in Detroit, MI, October 1980.

Weissert, William G., Thomas T.H. Wan, and Barbara B. Livieratos, *Effects and Costs of Day Care and Homemaker Services for the Chronically Ill:*

131

A Randomized Experiment, NCHSR Research Report Series, Hyattsville, MD: NCHSR, February 1980.

Willemain, Thomas R. and Roger G. Mark, "The Distribution of Intervals Between Visits as a Basis for Assessing and Regulating Physician Services in Nursing Homes," *Medical Care* 18 (April 1980): 427–41.

Winn, Sharon, "Analysis of Selected Characteristics of a Matched Sample of Nonprofit and Proprietary Nursing Homes in the State of Washington," *Medical Care* 12 (1974): 221–28.

Wisconsin Department of Health and Social Services, Division of Health, *Annual Report: Nursing Home Quality Assurance Project, FY 1978–79,* Madison, WI: 1979.

Chapter V

Nursing Homes, Home Health Services, and Adult Day Care

by Susan Lloyd and Nancy T. Greenspan

Introduction

This chapter discusses the levels of supply, utilization, and expenditures for the delivery of three modes of long-term care services: nursing homes, home health-homemaker services, and adult day care. Because of the lack of unity in the collection of long-term care data, truly comparable data are not available. The data presented here represent our best efforts to obtain the most recent figures.

This chapter will address, in three parts, the available data on nursing homes, home health services, and adult day care. Part I, which concerns nursing homes, presents data on the entire nursing home industry (gleaned mainly from the 1977 National Nursing Home Survey) and describes the conditions for and the scope of government subsidization of nursing home care under the Medicare and Medicaid programs. Because there are no data with which to draw a picture of the *total* home health service industry, Part II will examine only the home health services that are publicly funded (through Medicare, Medicaid, Title XX, and Title III–B–OAA). Part III uses the limited 1980 data to describe adult day care nationally, with ensuing sections on the adult day care services funded by Medicaid, SSA Title XX, and Title III–B–OAA.

Part I—Nursing Home Sector

Total Nursing Home Sector (SNF, ICF, Non-Certified)

Supply

In the 1977 National Nursing Home Survey (NNHS), the National Center for Health Statistics defines a nursing home as a facility offering living accommodations, personal care, and, in most instances, some degree of health care to the elderly and disabled. The NNHS then subcategorizes nursing homes into four groups: nursing care homes (nurses are employed and at least 50 percent of the residents receive nursing care), personal care homes with nursing (nurses may or may not be employed, but there is some nursing care and health supervision), personal care homes (there is no nursing care of residents although there is some health care supervision), and domiciliary homes (only personal care is provided).

TABLE V-1

Ratio of Nursing Home Beds to Elderly, 1977

Age	1977 U.S. Population	Number of Nursing Home Beds per 1,000 Elderly	Ratio Beds: Elderly
65 Years or Older	23,494,000	60 Beds per 1,000 Elderly	1:17
75 Years or Older	8,910,000	157 Beds per 1,000 Elderly	1:6
85 Years or Older	2,079,000	673 Beds per 1,000 Elderly	2:3

Source: National Center for Health Statistics, *The National Nursing Home Survey: Summary for the United States 1977* (Washington: U.S. Government Printing Office, 1979). adapted from Tables 1 and 18.

According to the 1977 NNHS, there were 18,900 nursing homes in the country, with 1,402,400 beds and 1,303,100 residents. During this same time, the population of elderly Americans (defined as 65 years or older) was 23,494,000; therefore, there were approximately 60 nursing home beds for every 1,000 elderly, with the ratios for older age cohorts, 75 to 84 and 85+ years, far higher, as shown in Table V–1. An important consideration when analyzing nursing home bed supply is the wide variation among and within States.

TABLE V-2
Number and Distribution of Nursing Homes, Beds, and Residents by Type of Facility, 1977

Nursing Home Characteristics	Nursing Homes		Beds		Residents	
	Number	Percent	Number	Percent	Number	Percent
All Nursing Homes	18,900	100%	1,402,400	100%	1,303,100	100%
Nursing Care Homes	12,300	65%	1,105,100	79%	1,113,300	85%
Personal Care and Domiciliary Homes	6,600	35%	297,300	21%	189,800	15%

Source: National Center for Health Statistics, *The National Nursing Home Survey: Summary for the United States 1977*, (Washington: U.S. Government Printing Office, 1979) Table 1.

134

Data collected for 1978 show that, although the average national bed supply was approximately 56 beds per 1,000 elderly, the range in bed supply extended from a high of approximately 97 beds per 1,000 elderly in South Dakota to a low of 23 beds per 1,000 elderly in Florida (Strahan, 1979). Seventy-nine percent of beds and 85 percent of residents were in nursing care homes; 65 percent of institutions were classified as nursing care homes. (See Table V-2.)

The 1977 NNHS shows that the predominant ownership pattern for nursing homes is proprietary (77 percent). This contrasts sharply to the ownership pattern of acute care hospitals, where 85 percent are primarily non-profit. (See Table V-3.) According to Burton Dunlop (1979), proprietary ownership of the majority of nursing home beds has been characteristic of the industry at least since the 1940s. On the average, proprietary nursing homes are somewhat smaller than non-profit homes.

The 1977 NNHS also indicates that three out of four nursing homes in the country were Federally certified to accept Medicare and/or Medicaid patients at the skilled and/or intermediate level. Although 4,700 nursing homes (25 percent of all nursing homes nationally) did not participate in Federal certification programs, they possessed only 12 percent of the beds. (See Table V-4.)

All nursing homes, regardless of ownership or certification status, had a uniformly high occupancy rate of 89 percent. (See Tables V-5 and V-6.) One consequence of high occupancy rates is that they can inhibit effective regulation. Authorities vacillate in the enforce-

TABLE V-3
Number and Distribution of Nursing Homes,
Beds, and Residents by Ownership, 1977

Nursing Home Characteristics	Nursing Homes		Beds		Residents	
	Number	Percent[1]	Number	Percent	Number	Percent
All Nursing Homes	18,900	100%	1,402,400	100%	1,303,100	100%
Proprietary	14,500	77%	971,200	69%	888,800	68%
Non-Profit	4,400	23%	431,300	31%	414,300	32%
Voluntary	3,400	18%	295,600	21%	281,800	22%
Government	1,000	6%	135,700	10%	132,500	10%

[1] Figures do not add to total due to rounding.

Source: National Center for Health Statistics, *The National Nursing Home Survey: Summary for the United States 1977* (Washington: U.S. Government Printing Office, 1979), adapted from Table 1.

TABLE V-4

**Number and Distribution of Nursing Homes,
Beds, and Residents by Certification Status, 1977**

Nursing Home Characteristics	Nursing Homes		Beds		Residents	
	Number	Percent	Number	Percent	Number	Percent[1]
All Nursing Homes	18,900	100%	1,402,400	100%	1,303,100	100%
Certified Nursing Homes	14,200	75%	1,235,000	88%	1,165,600	90%
SNF only	3,600	19%	294,000	21%	269,600	21%
SNF and ICF	4,600	24%	549,400	39%	527,800	41%
ICF only	6,000	32%	391,600	28%	368,200	28%
Non-Certified Nursing Homes	4,700	25%	167,400	12%	137,500	11%

[1] Figures do not add to total due to rounding.
Source: National Center for Health Statistics, *The National Nursing Home Survey: Summary for the United States 1977* (Washington: U.S. Government Printing Office, 1979), adapted from Table 1.

ment of licensure or certification standards for substandard institutions if there is no better place to transfer the residents.

The 1977 NNHS shows the mode for nursing home size to be small facilities of fewer than 50 beds. However, the majority (87 percent) of nursing home beds were located in larger nursing homes of more than 50 beds (Table V–7). In 1977, the average size of nursing

TABLE V-5

**Number and Distribution of Residents by Ownership of
Nursing Home and Occupancy Rate, 1977**

Ownership	Number of Residents	Percent of Distribution	Occupancy Rate
All Nursing Homes	1,303,100	100%	89%
Proprietary	889,000	68%	90%
Non-Profit	415,000	32%	87%
Voluntary	282,000	22%	87%
Government	133,000	10%	87%

Source: National Center for Health Statistics, *The National Nursing Home Survey: Summary for the United States 1977* (Washington: U.S. Government Printing Office, 1979), adapted from Tables 1 and 2.

TABLE V-6

Number and Distribution of Residents by Certification Status of Nursing Homes and Occupancy Rate, 1977

Certification Status[1]	Number of Residents	Percent of Distribution[2]	Occupancy Rate
All Nursing Homes	1,303,100	100%	89%
SNF Only	270,000	21%	92%
SNF + ICF	528,000	41%	89%
ICF Only	368,000	28%	87%
Non-Certified	137,000	11%	89%

[1] This does not indicate that all patients were at the level of care for which the institution is certified. Private pay patients are not officially classified by level of care.

[2] Figures do not add to total due to rounding.

Source: National Center for Health Statistics, *The National Nursing Home Survey: Summary for the United States 1977* (Washington: U.S. Government Printing Office, 1979), adapted from Tables 1 and 2.

homes, according to ownership, was 67 beds for proprietary institutions, 87 beds for voluntary institutions, and 136 beds for government institutions (derived from Table V–3).

Utilization

The typical nursing home resident is described in the 1977 National Nursing Home Survey as an 80 year-old, widowed, white

TABLE V-7

Number and Distribution of Nursing Homes According to Bed Size, 1977

Size	Nursing Homes		Beds	
	Number	Percent	Number	Percent
All Nursing Homes	18,900	100%	1,402,400	100%
Less than 50 Beds	8,000	42%	182,900	13%
50–99 Beds	5,800	31%	417,800	30%
100–199 Beds	4,200	22%	546,400	39%
200 Beds or More	900	5%	255,300	18%

Source: National Center for Health Statistics, *The National Nursing Home Survey: Summary for the United States 1977* (Washington: U.S. Government Printing Office, 1979), adapted from Table 1.

137

woman, suffering from approximately three chronic health problems. She had been in the nursing home 1.6 years at the point of the survey. General characteristics by demographic variable from the NNHS 1977 indicate the following:

- Approximately 86 percent of the residents of nursing homes are 65 years of age or older, with 35 percent of the total 75 years and over.
- Seventy-one percent of nursing home residents are female.[1] When age is held constant, it would be expected that there would be approximately the same rate of institutionalization for both sexes. However, this is not the case; women still have a higher rate of institutionalization than do men.
- Twelve percent of nursing home residents were married. In the elderly, non-institutionalized population age 65 to 74 years, 81 percent of the men and 48 percent of the women were married. In the elderly population age 75 years and older, 70 percent of the men and 23 percent of the women were married (Bureau of Census, 1980). It therefore appears that a major variance between the elderly in nursing homes and the non-institutionalized elderly is marital status, with a higher percentage of the unmarried residing in nursing homes.

Interestingly, when age *and* marital status are both standardized, the rate of institutionalization for unmarried women is consistently lower than the rate of institutionalization for unmarried men, except in the 85 years and older category. However, married women in all age brackets have a higher rate of institutionalization than do married men. This may be partially explained by the cultural convention that there is an age differential between spouses, with the husband likely to have a somewhat younger spouse to care for him should he fall ill.

- Ninety-two percent of the residents of nursing homes were white Americans; another 6 percent were black, and 1 percent were Hispanic. Blacks were under-represented in nursing homes, since they compose 8.3 percent of the nation's elderly population (Administration on Aging, 1980). However, when nursing home utilization is disaggregated by primary source of payment, blacks are only under-represented in the category of nursing home residents primarily supported by private funds.

---

[1] Figures from a personal communication with the State and National Estimate Branch, Population Division, Bureau of the Census, show that in 1977, of the U.S. population age 65 years and older, 59 percent were female. Of the population age 75 years and older, 64 percent were female. Of the population 85 years and older, 69 percent were female.

- Nursing home residents had an average of 3.5 burdensome chronic ailments. The most prevalent illnesses and disabilities among nursing home residents were arteriosclerosis (49 percent), heart trouble (34 percent), and senility (32 percent).
- The NNHS showed that in 1977, 37 percent of nursing home residents had lengths of stay less than one year; another 33 percent had stays between one and three years, and 31 percent were there three or more years at the point of the survey. The median number of days of nursing home residence was 597, or approximately 1⅔ years.

The majority of admissions to nursing homes (54 percent) were patients transferred from another health facility primarily general or short-stay hospitals (32 percent). However, a sizable proportion of the nursing home admissions (40 percent) came directly from a private residence, mostly from homes that they shared with others (24 percent). (See Table V–8.)

As shown in Table V–9, 56 percent of nursing home residents listed a government program as their *primary* source of support. This does not necessarily mean that 100 percent of these residents' nursing home charges were paid by a government program. The Medicaid program requires a copayment from the nursing home recipient whenever the recipient has resources (pensions, insurance benefits, private income sources) to contribute, and the Medicare program requires a copayment of $22.50 from its beneficiaries for day 21 to day 100 of nursing home care.

Thirty-eight percent of the residents of nursing homes listed private funds as their primary source of support. Note that this category of nursing home residents does not necessarily exclude Medicaid-supported residents because a Medicaid recipient in a nursing home could personally contribute 51 percent or more to the cost of his/her care (say through a pension), with Medicaid picking up the remaining 49 percent or less.

Expenditures

In 1979, the U.S. population spent an estimated $17.8 billion on nursing home care (Gibson, 1980).[2] This represents 9.4 percent of the estimated $118.6 billion spent on personal health care in 1979 and is only surpassed by expenditures on hospital care ($85.3 billion) and physicians' services ($40.6 billion). The 1979 figures for nursing home care represent a 15 percent increase in expenditures over 1978 and almost a 470 percent increase for the decade 1969–

---

[2] The Division of National Cost Estimates defines nursing home care more restrictively than the NNHS and only includes in its cost estimate figures for "nursing care home."

TABLE V-8
Living Arrangements Prior to Nursing Home Admission,
by Primary Source of Payment, 1977

Living Arrangements	All Residents of All Nursing Homes (1,303,300)	All Privately Supported Residents in All Nursing Homes (500,900)	Medicaid SNF Residents (260,700)	Medicaid ICF Residents (362,600)
All Living Arrangements	100% [1]	100%	100%	100%
Another Health Facility	54% [1]	49%	66% [1]	52% [1]
General or Short- Stay Hospital	32%	31%	44%	24%
Another Nursing Home	13%	12%	14%	13%
Mental Hospital	6%	3%	3%	10%
Other Health Facility or Unknown	4%	2%	4%	4%
Private Residence	40% [1]	46%	30%	42% [1]
Alone	14%	18%	8%	12%
With Others	24% [1]	25% [1]	19% [1]	26% [1]
Children	10%	10%	10%	13%
Spouse	6%	9%	3%	4%
Other Relative	6%	5%	5%	8%
Unrelated Persons	3%	3%	3%	2%
Unknown if With Others	3%	3%	3%	3%
Unknown or Other Arrangement	5%	5%	4%	6%

[1] Figures do not add to total due to rounding.

Source: National Center for Health Statistics, *The National Nursing Home Survey: Summary for the United States 1977* (Washington: U.S. Government Printing Office, 1979), adapted from Table 40.

1979. As Gibson reported, nursing home input price increases alone rose 8 percent per year in the period 1970–1978, which can be partially attributed to increases in food and fuel prices and to increases in the national minimum wage. Other factors advanced to explain the overall increase in expenditures for nursing home care include the changing demography of the U.S. population (both the sizable growth in the number of elderly and their advancing aging) and also the increased costs associated with more stringent licensure standards on the State and Federal levels.

140

TABLE V-9
Utilization of Nursing Homes by Primary Source of Payment, 1977

Primary Source of Payment	Number of Nursing Home Residents	Percent[1]
All Sources	1,303,100	100%
Public Support	732,900	56%
Medicare	26,200	2%
Medicaid SNF and ICF	623,300	48%
Other Government Assistance or Welfare	83,400	6%
Private Support—Own Income or Family Support	500,900	38%
All Other Sources	69,200	5%

[1] Figures do not add to total due to rounding.
Source: National Center for Health Statistics, *The National Nursing Home Survey: Summary for the United States 1977* (Washington: U.S. Government Printing Office, 1979), adapted from Tables 19 and 40.

TABLE V-10
Public/Private Financing of Nursing Home Care, Calendar Year 1979

Total Nursing Home Care	$17.8 billion	100%
Private Payments	$ 7.7 billion	43.3%
Consumer Payments	$ 7.6 billion	42.7%
Direct Payments	$ 7.5 billion	42.1%
Insurance Benefits	$ .1 billion	.6%
Other Private Funds	$ .1 billion	.6%
Business/In-Plant Philanthropy	$ .1 billion	.6%
Public Programs	$10.1 billion	56.7%
Federal Programs	$ 5.5 billion	30.9%
Medicare	$ .4 billion	2.1%
Public Assistance	$ 4.8 billion	27.0%
Medicaid	$ 4.8 billion	27.0%
Non-XIX Assistance	–0–	
Veterans' Administration	$ .3 billion	1.7%
State and Local Programs	$ 4.6 billion	25.8%
Public Assistance	$ 4.6 billion	25.8%
Medicaid	$ 4.0 billion	22.5%
Non-XIX Assistance	$ .6 billion	3.4%

Source: Gibson, Robert M., "National Health Expenditures, 1979," *Health Care Financing Review*, Summer 1980, adapted from Tables 6 and 7.

As seen in Table V–10, of the estimated $17.8 billion spent on nursing home care in 1979, $7.7 billion (43.3 percent) was paid privately (almost entirely "out-of-pocket"), and $10.1 billion (56.7 percent) was paid through public programs (primarily Medicaid). The private insurance industry has little involvement in its financing. Public funds accounted for only 25 percent of the financing of nursing homes six years before the enactment of Medicare and Medicaid. Now the nursing home sector is the health component most heavily supported by public funds, with more than 25 percent of all nursing home expenditures paid by the States and localities, primarily through the States' contributions to the Medicaid program. (See Table V–11.)

As indicated in Table V–12, nursing homes certified as skilled nursing facilities (SNFs), intermediate care facilities (ICFs), or both received 92 percent of the revenue. Proprietary nursing homes, which housed 68 percent of the residents, received 66 percent of the revenues, showing that nursing home care in the United States is, in the main, a for-profit enterprise. (See Table V–13.)

TABLE V-11
Percentages of Federal and State/Local Spending
by Health Sector, Calendar Year 1979

Major Health Sectors	$ Amount	Public Percent of Amount[1]	
All Health Sectors	$188.6 billion	40.2%	
		28.3%	Federal
		12.0%	State/Local
Nursing Homes	$ 17.8 billion	56.7%	
		30.7%	Federal
		26.1%	State/Local
Hospital Care	$ 85.3 billion	55.9%	
		40.9%	Federal
		15.0%	State/Local
Physicians' Services	$ 40.6 billion	26.2%	
		19.7%	Federal
		6.5%	State/Local
Dentists' Services	$ 13.6 billion	4.0%	
		2.2%	Federal
		1.8%	State/Local

[1] Figures do not add to total due to rounding.
Source: Gibson, Robert M., "National Health Expenditures, 1979," *Health Care Financing Review,* Summer 1980, Table 2A.

TABLE V-12
Amount and Distribution of Nursing Home Revenue
by Federal Certification, 1976

	Nursing Home Revenues, 1976	Percent Distribution of Revenues, 1976	Percent Distribution of Nursing Home Residents, 1977
All Nursing Homes	$10.8 billion	100%	100% [1]
Certified			
(SNF and/or ICF) [2]	$ 9.9 billion	92%	90%
SNF Only	$ 3.0 billion	28%	21%
SNF and ICF	$ 4.6 billion	43%	41%
ICF Only	$ 2.3 billion	21%	28%
Non-Certified			
Nursing Homes	$ 0.9 billion	8%	11%

[1] Figures do not add to total due to rounding.

[2] This does not indicate that all patients were at the level of care for which the institution is certified. Private pay patients are not officially classified by level of care.

Source: National Center for Health Statistics, *The National Nursing Home Survey: Summary for the United States 1977* (Washington: U.S. Government Printing Office, 1979), adapted from Tables 1 and 17.

TABLE V-13
Amount and Distribution of Nursing Home Revenue
by Ownership Status, 1976

	Nursing Home Revenues, 1976	Percent Distribution of Revenues, 1976	Percent Distribution of Nursing Home Residents, 1977
All Nursing Homes	$10.82 billion	100%	100%
Proprietary Nursing Homes	$ 7.16 billion	66%	68%
Non-Profit Nursing Homes	$ 3.65 billion	34%	32%
Government Nursing Homes	$ 1.14 billion	11%	10%
Voluntary Nursing Homes	$ 2.51 billion	23%	22%

Source: National Center for Health Statistics, *The National Nursing Home Survey: Summary for the United States 1977* (Washington: U.S. Government Printing Office, 1979), adapted from Tables 1 and 17.

TABLE V-14

Average *per Diem* Charges and Average Amount Paid by Primary Source for Residents of Nursing Homes in 1977, and Estimates for 1979

(Figures rounded to the Nearest Dollar)

Source of Support	1977[1]		1979 (Estimate)[2]	
	Per Diem Charge	Paid by Primary Source	*Per Diem* Charge	Paid by Primary Source
All Sources	$23	$20	$28	$24
Own Income or Family Support	$23	$22	$28	$25
Medicare	$38	$33	$45	$39
Medicaid (SNF)	$29	$24	$35	$29
Medicaid (ICF)	$20	$16	$24	$19

[1] National Center for Health Statistics, *The National Nursing Home Survey: Summary for the United States 1977* (Washington: U.S. Government Printing Office, 1979), adapted from Table 36.

[2] Calculations were made from the National Nursing Home Input Price Index. See *Health Care Financing Trends,* Winter 1981, Table C–1.

The 1977 National Nursing Home Survey presents average charges for nursing home care, disaggregated by primary source of payment. For Medicaid, there is a further breakdown by level of care. In Table V–14, the least discrepancy between the *per diem* charge and the proportion of that charge paid by the primary source is for those nursing home residents who list their own or their families' incomes as the primary source of financial support. The *per diem* charges not covered by the Medicare program can be attributed to be the copayment required of Medicare beneficiaries after the 20th day of nursing home institutionalization and the 20 percent copayment required for items furnished under Part B of Medicare. Nursing home charges not paid by the Medicaid program are generally paid by the Medicaid recipient's pension, insurance, or other personal income that he/she is required to contribute toward nursing home support. By 1979, average charges had risen approximately 21.7 percent over 1977 levels, while the amount paid by the primary source had risen 20 percent.

Medicare: Skilled Nursing Facilities

Skilled nursing facility benefits are established for all Medicare beneficiaries under SSA-Title XVIII. A beneficiary is defined as a

[3] The program descriptions include changes due to the 1980 Omnibus Reconciliation Act but not the 1981 Omnibus Reconciliation Act.

person who is eligible through Social Security/Railroad Retirement benefits (over 64 or disabled), through the end-stage renal disease program, or through special circumstances (birth year and/or work record). Under Title XVIII, a physician must certify the need for skilled nursing or rehabilitation services on a daily basis for a condition for which the beneficiary was hospitalized for a minimum of three days, or for a condition which developed while in an SNF, subsequent to the initial condition for which the beneficiary was hospitalized. Placement within an SNF generally must occur within 30 days of discharge from the hospital, although this requirement can be waived in particular circumstances. (Prior to 1980, placement must have occurred within 14 days of discharge.) Medicare, which specifically does not pay for any sort of custodial care within any nursing facility, will support 100 days maximum of skilled nursing and/or rehabilitation in an SNF, as long as the local PSRO (or sometimes the Medicare intermediary) certifies the patient's need for such service. However, the average length of stay of Medicare beneficiaries was only 27 days in 1977. The first 20 days are financed fully by the Medicare program, but days 21 to 100 demand a copayment of $22.50 per day from the beneficiary.

SNFs are Federally administered either through private insurers acting as fiscal agents of the Health Care Financing Administration (HCFA) and Social Security Administration or directly through HCFA's Office of Direct Reimbursement. Nursing homes wishing to contract with HCFA to provide such services must satisfy a number of Federal standards known as "conditions of participation."

Supply

As of December 1979, there were 5,399 SNFs participating in the Medicare program, with approximately 460,715 certified beds.[4] However, of the total of 5,399 SNFs, there are only 373 SNFs that were exclusively certified for Medicare patients, with the remainder Federally certified to also care for Medicaid patients. Furthermore, the 373 Medicare-only SNFs have only a potential bed supply of 27,000, whereas the 5,026 Medicare-Medicaid certified SNFs have 433,715 beds. HCFA's Health Standards and Quality Bureau states that there is a decreasing number of nursing homes seeking Medicare-only SNF certification and an increasing number of nursing homes with the combined certification status. For 1977, approximately 67 percent of the Medicare-certified SNF beds were located in proprietary nursing homes, which closely parallels the fact that 69 percent of *all* nursing home beds are located there (NCHS, 1979; Table V–3).

---

[4] Figures are from the Division of Long Term Care, Health Standards and Quality Bureau, Health Care Financing Administration.

TABLE V-15
Medicare Expenditures for Nursing Home (SNF) Care as a Percent of Total Medicare Payments, Selected Years

	Medicare $ for Nursing Home Care (Column 1)	Total Medicare Expenditures (Column 2)	Column 1 Divided by Column 2
1967[1]	$282 million	$ 4.6 billion	6.0%
1970[1]	$246 million	$ 7.1 billion	3.6%
1975[1]	$278 million	$15.6 billion	1.9%
1979[2]	$373 million	$30.3 billion	1.2%

[1] Figures are from the Division of Information Services, Office of Statistics and Data Management, Office of Research, Demonstrations, and Statistics, HCFA.

[2] Gibson, Robert M., "National Health Expenditures, 1979," *Health Care Financing Review,* Summer 1980, adapted from Tables 6 and 7.

Utilization

In 1977, Medicare paid SNF charges for close to 300,000 beneficiaries (282,540 aged and 9,520 disabled) and approved claims for 9.6 million days of SNF care.[5]

Expenditures

Medicare is estimated to have financed $373 million in SNF care in 1979, which accounts for a mere 2 percent of the $17.8 billion spent on nursing home care and 12 percent of the $30.3 billion in Medicare expenditures. Expenditures for nursing home care have not been a large portion of the total Medicare budget, since the Medicare program was basically set up to alleviate the financial burden on the elderly of acute (not chronic) medical care. As illustrated in Table V–15, expenditures for nursing home care through the years have become an increasingly smaller proportion of total Medicare expenditures.

Medicaid: Skilled Nursing Facilities (SNF) and Intermediate Care Facilities

Under Title XIX, Medicaid funds two types of long-term care facilities with monies contributed both by the Federal government and the States. They are SNFs, which compose one of nine basic services

[5] Figures are from the Division of Information Services, Office of Statistics and Data Management, Office of Research, Demonstrations, and Statistics, HCFA.

mandated for all State Medicaid programs, and ICFs, which constitute an optional service in State Medicaid programs. States must include all persons over 21 years of age receiving AFDC cash benefits from the Federal government and either all persons receiving SSI cash benefits or those persons meeting additional, more restrictive, State-defined standards of Medicaid eligibility. Furthermore, States may include additional groups (with higher incomes than AFDC and SSI maximums) as Medicaid-eligible. For patients to qualify for SNF benefits, a physician must certify their need for intermittent health-related services that are more than custodial care but less than the intensity of services offered in a general hospital or an SNF.

Medicaid will support an eligible individual in an SNF or ICF indefinitely as long as the local PSRO certifies the patient's need for such service. The Medicaid recipient must contribute any personal income over $25 per month as a copayment.

Supply

Data for 1980 show that Medicaid has certified 7,685 nursing homes as SNFs. Of these, 2,659 were exclusively certified for Medicaid, and 5,026 were certified for both Medicaid and Medicare patients with approximately 140,000 and 431,000 beds, respectively.[6]

The same data show that Medicaid has ICF provider agreements with 11,837 nursing homes. (SNF and ICF figures are *not* mutually exclusive.) Of these ICFs, 954 were designated exclusively for the mentally retarded (ICF-MR). Excluding this number, ICFs had about 905,000 certified beds. The scant information on the bed supply of the ICFs-MR shows that the vast majority are small facilities of between 15 and 20 beds. For 1977, the latest year for which data are available, 69 percent of the SNF beds and 71 percent of the ICF beds were located in proprietary nursing homes, with the remainder located in voluntary non-profit or government facilities. The modal size for both Medicaid-certified SNFs and ICFs was 100 to 199 beds (NCHS, 1979; Table V–3).

Utilization

In 1977, there were close to 1.5 million Medicaid *admissions* to nursing homes, with 57 percent of these into ICFs and the remainder into SNFs. Many of these were multiple admissions of the same individuals, because about 14 percent of Medicaid nursing home admissions came from other nursing homes (see Table V–8), and an indeterminate number of admissions are the result of transfers

---

[6] All figures on bed supply and utilization are from the Medicaid Program Data Branch, Division of Beneficiaries Studies, Office of Research, Demonstrations, and Statistics, HCFA.

back and forth between general hospitals and nursing homes. No figures were available on the individuals who received nursing home care, but 1977 figures do show that there were 296.3 million days of nursing home care (excluding ICF-MR care) provided to Medicaid recipients.

In 1976, Medicaid recipients were estimated to be using at least 44 percent of all nursing home beds in every State with a Medicaid program. In six States, Medicaid recipients used as much as 75 percent of the total nursing home beds.[7]

Two out of three Medicaid SNF residents were admitted from another health facility, generally a short-stay hospital (NCHS, 1979). Only about 30 percent of Medicaid SNF residents had been admitted into the nursing home directly from a private residence; those that were had usually been living with others prior to the nursing home admission. For Medicaid ICF residents, slightly over half (52 percent) were admitted to a nursing home from another health facility, generally from a short-stay hospital. Ten percent of Medicaid residents were admitted to the nursing home directly from a mental hospital. Of those individuals admitted to a nursing home from a private residence (42 percent), most came from homes they shared with others.

About a third of Medicaid SNF residents had been institutionalized in a nursing home for less than one year, another third for one to three years, and a final third for more than three years. Approximately the same length of stay since admission was noted for Medicaid ICF residents as for Medicaid SNF residents, with a somewhat higher proportion of the Medicaid ICF residents in nursing homes for over three years. In comparison to privately supported residents, both SNFs and ICFs recorded longer lengths of stay (NCHS, 1979).

A 1977 Congressional Budget Office report stated that almost half of the patients who were at least partially supported by Medicaid in nursing homes were not initially poor enough for Medicaid eligibility as defined by the States. Once they depleted their savings and assets for privately financed nursing home care, they then qualified as "medically needy" under Medicaid (CBO, 1977a).

Expenditures

Medicaid is estimated to have financed $8.8 billion in SNF and ICF (including ICF-MR) care in 1979, which accounts for 49 percent of the $17.8 billion spent on nursing home care in that year (Gibson,

---

[7] This information is from the Division of Long-Term Care Experimentation, Office of Research, Demonstrations, and Statistics, Health Care Financing Administration.

TABLE V-16
Amount and Distribution of Medicaid Nursing Home Expenditures as a Percent of Total ($15.1 Billion) Nursing Home Expenditures, 1978

Level of Care	1978 Medicaid Expenditures	Percent of Total Nursing Home Expenditures
SNF + ICF	$7.6 billion	50%
SNF	$3.2 billion	21%
ICF	$4.4 billion	29%
ICF (Excluding ICF-MR)	$3.0 billion	20%
ICF-MR	$1.3 billion	9%

Source: *Preliminary National Medicaid Estimates, Fiscal Year 1978*, Table E, Health Care Financing Administration.

1980). In 1978, Medicaid financed $7.6 billion of nursing home care for Medicaid beneficiaries, representing approximately 42 percent of total Medicaid expenditures for that year, with SNFs and ICFs accounting for $3.2 billion and $4.4 billion, respectively. (See Table V–16.) Expenditures for nursing home care have always been a large component of Medicaid payments; since 1972, nursing home care has accounted for increasing amounts, rising from 28 percent to 49 percent of total expenditures (HCFA, 1978). If one looks only at the cohort 65 years and older, however, the proportion of Medicaid funds spent for nursing home care is even higher. In 1976 for example, 72 percent of the Medicaid money spent to provide health care services for the elderly went to pay for nursing home care (Medicaid-Medicare Management Institute, 1979).

The range of Medicaid expenditures for nursing home care within individual States went from a high of 68 percent to a low of 23 percent (Table V–17). Of equal interest is that although some States balanced Medicaid nursing home expenditures evenly between SNF and ICF institutions, most appeared to favor the financing of one or the other. (Definitions of ICFs and SNFs vary across States.)

Part II—Home Health Services Sector

Medicare: Home Health Services

Home health is generally defined as health care services (such as nursing care and physical, speech, and occupational therapy) provided to individuals in their homes. A physician is responsible for establishing and periodically reviewing the patient's plan of care but would rarely be directly involved in providing services.

TABLE V-17

State Variation in the Distribution of Amounts of Medicaid Payments for Nursing Home Care as Percent of Total State Expenditures for the Medicaid Program, Fiscal Year 1978

State	SNF + ICF	SNF	ICF (Total)	ICF-MR (Only)
Total: U.S. $	$7.6 billion	$3.2 billion	$4.3 billion	$1.3 billion
Percent	41.9%	17.7%	24.3%	7.4%
South Dakota	68 %	8 %	60 %	20 %
Minnesota	64 %	26 %	38 %	19 %
Alaska	63 %	13 %	50 %	21 %
New Hampshire	62 %	2 %	60 %	5 %
Wyoming	61 %	19 %	42 %	—
Colorado	61 %	15 %	46 %	24 %
Texas	58 %	5 %	54 %	10 %
Iowa	58 %	1 %	58 %	16 %
Nebraska	58 %	9 %	49 %	12 %
Idaho	57 %	16 %	41 %	16 %
Wisconsin	57 %	41 %	16 %	—
Arkansas	56 %	8 %	48 %	16 %
Montana	54 %	6 %	48 %	6 %
North Dakota	54 %	35 %	19 %	—
Connecticut	53 %	44 %	9 %	4 %
Indiana	53 %	12 %	41 %	3 %
Oklahoma	53 %	—	53 %	12 %
Utah	53 %	15 %	38 %	16 %
Nevada	51 %	22 %	29 %	5 %
Oregon	49 %	3 %	46 %	19 %
Maine	48 %	2 %	46 %	—
Pennsylvania	48 %	26 %	22 %	15 %
Louisiana	47 %	1 %	46 %	13 %
Virginia	46 %	3 %	44 %	13 %
Tennessee	46 %	1 %	45 %	11 %
Alabama	46 %	24 %	22 %	—
Vermont	45 %	2 %	43 %	12 %
South Carolina	45 %	25 %	19 %	8 %
Georgia	45 %	14 %	30 %	8 %
New York	44 %	26 %	18 %	6 %
Kansas	44 %	1 %	43 %	13 %
Hawaii	44 %	24 %	20 %	—
Rhode Island	43 %	7 %	37 %	14 %
Kentucky	42 %	12 %	29 %	7 %
Mississippi	41 %	30 %	11 %	4 %

150

TABLE V-17

State Variation in the Distribution of Amounts of Medicaid Payments for Nursing Home Care as Percent of Total State Expenditures for the Medicaid Program, Fiscal Year 1978

State	SNF + ICF	SNF	ICF (Total)	ICF-MR (Only)
Florida	40 %	18 %	22 %	2 %
Ohio	40 %	21 %	19 %	7 %
North Carolina	40 %	15 %	25 %	9 %
Delaware	40 %	1 %	39 %	15 %
Michigan	39 %	17 %	22 %	10 %
Massachusetts	39 %	13 %	26 %	10 %
Missouri	39 %	1 %	38 %	9 %
Washington	38 %	28 %	10 %	2 %
New Jersey	36 %	2 %	35 %	6 %
Maryland	34 %	13 %	21 %	—
New Mexico	31 %	1 %	30 %	7 %
Illinois	30 %	7 %	23 %	6 %
California	24 %	23 %	1 %	—
West Virginia	22.5%	.1%	22.4%	—
Washington, D.C.	13 %	1 %	12 %	—

Source: *Preliminary National Medicaid Estimates, Fiscal Year 1978*, Table F, Health Care Financing Administration.

To qualify for home health benefits under either Part A or Part B of the program, a beneficiary must be eligible for Social Security/ Railroad Retirement benefits (over 64 or disabled), an end-stage renal disease enrollee, or in special circumstances (birth year and/or work record) entitling him or her to be deemed Medicare eligible. A beneficiary must be homebound and certified by a physician as needing skilled nursing, physical, or speech therapy. Prior to July 1, 1981, there was the additional stipulation for Part A that the beneficiary must have been hospitalized three days for the condition for which the home health service was ordered. Once a beneficiary qualifies, he/she may also receive the other home health services specified in the law. These services include medical and social services, the use of medical supplies and medical appliances, and the part-time or intermittent services of home health aides. After July 1, 1981, a beneficiary may also qualify for home health services based on the need for occupational therapy.

HCFA directly administers the Federally funded, open-ended program through private insurers acting as fiscal agents.[8] The Federal

---

[8] Part B of Medicare is partially financed through monthly premiums paid by the beneficiary.

government sets "conditions of participation" for certifying home health agencies (HHAs) to care for Medicare (and Medicaid) beneficiaries. Primary among these is the requirement that HHAs offer at least skilled nursing and one other therapeutic home health service (such as physical, speech, or occupational therapy, medical social work, or home health aide care). Medicare (unlike Medicaid) contracts only with agencies, not individual providers, to render home health services.

Supply

As of January 1981, 3,014 HHAs were Medicare-certified.[9] Several types of HHAs provide services to Medicare (and Medicaid) beneficiaries. The most prevalent of these are official agencies (most often city and county public health departments; 44 percent), visiting nurse associations (18 percent), private non-profit agencies (16 percent), hospital-based programs (12 percent), proprietary agencies (6 percent), SNF-based programs (.3 percent), rehabilitation programs (.2 percent), and other (2 percent). In addition to this known supply, there is an uncertain number of home health agencies which are not Medicare-Medicaid certified and so do not participate in the programs unless they are subcontractors to certified agencies.

An HHA's lack of certification can emerge from a variety of factors; for example, a home health agency may be a small operation and not offer both skilled nursing and other approved home health services necessary for certification. Furthermore, prior to May 1981, Federal statutes prohibited Medicare-Medicaid certification for proprietary HHAs unless they were State-licensed. It was a State prerogative as to whether to license HHAs.[10]

Individual providers also furnish some services, although enumeration of the providers and the scope of their work is, thus far, unexplored.

Whereas the private non-profit agencies received only 19 percent of total Medicare payments for home health services in 1975, by 1977 their share had risen to 31 percent of the market. This increase is not only attributable to actual multiplication of the numbers of private, non-profit HHAs, but also to particularly rapidly increasing costs of visits provided by private non-profit HHAs.

---

[9] Office of Standards and Certification, Health Standards and Quality Bureau, Health Care Financing Administration

[10] Proprietaries had been excluded by law in States that do not have licensure laws. With the Omnibus Reconciliation Act of 1980, all HHAs are eligible for Medicare-Medicaid certification, regardless of whether the States in which they operate have licensure laws.

152

Utilization

About 700,000 Medicare beneficiaries received a total of 15.5 million home health services through the Medicare program in 1977.[11] These recipients accounted for approximately 2½ percent of the total Medicare population. In 1976, the five most common diagnoses of Medicare beneficiaries receiving home health visits were (in order) stroke, malignant neoplasms, diabetes, arteriosclerotic heart disease, and fractured hips.

Figures for 1977 show nursing visits as the major type of home health visit financed by the Medicare program (57 percent of total Medicare home health visits), followed by home health aide visits (29 percent of total) and physical therapy visits (10 percent of total). The average number of visits per beneficiary was 22.5. (See Table V–18.)

Medicare bills indicate that nursing visits as a proportion of total Medicare home health visits have decreased from 71 percent in 1971 to 56 percent in 1978. Associated with this change, home health aide visits increased, at least during a portion of this period, going from 26 percent of the total in 1974 to 30 percent of the total in 1977 (HCFA, 1977). It has been suggested that, although official HHAs and visiting nurse associations have themselves somewhat increased the proportion of home health aide visits made, it is principally the proliferation of proprietary and private non-profit HHAs, and their apparent partiality for the high volume-low cost home health aide visit, that has caused the overall increase in home health aide visits and the decrease in nursing visits.

Expenditures

Total Medicare reimbursement for home health services in 1978 is estimated at $427 million. This is 1.8 percent of total Medicare reimbursement for all health services for that year, a slightly higher proportion than in prior years. Whereas Medicare reimbursement for all health services increased 13.8 percent between 1977 and 1978, Medicare reimbursement for home health services increased more rapidly at 16.5 percent. In 1978, expenditures for home health care under Part A/Medicare ($312 million) were more than 2½ times the expenditures for home health care under Part B/Medicare ($116 million; HCFA, 1978a).

Average charge per Medicare-covered home health visit in 1978 was $27, ranging from a low of $14 in South Dakota and Iowa to a

---

[11] The number of visits in 1977 increased 85 percent from the 8.5 million visits in 1969. During the same period, the number of Medicare enrollees rose 35 percent.

153

Type of Service	Total Number of Clients[1]	Total Number of Visits	Distri- bution of Visits	Average Number of Visits per Beneficiary
Total	689,700	15.5 million	100%	22.5
Nursing Care	660,500	8.9 million	57%	12.9
Home Health Aide	224,400	4.6 million	29%	20.5
Physical Therapy	155,000	1.5 million	10%	9.9
Other (including speech and occupational therapy; medical social work; other health disciplines like inhalation therapist)	90,500	.5 million	3%	5.8

[1] Detail does not add to total since persons may receive more than one type of service.

Source: *Health Care Financing Program Statistics: Medicare: Use of Home Health Services, 1977,* Table 9, Health Care Financing Administration.

high of $35 in Alaska and Illinois (HCFA, 1978a). Medicare billing data show a 124 percent increase in average charge per Medicare-covered home health visit in the seven year period 1971–1978 (Table V–19). Data for 1977 reveal that an average of $559 was spent per Medicare beneficiary receiving home health care in that year (HCFA, 1977).

Medicaid Home Health and Personal Care Services

Home health services have been a mandated Medicaid benefit since 1970 (SSA-Title XIX). States must minimally offer nursing, home health aide services, and medical equipment, supplies, and appliances to Medicaid recipients. States *may* include physical, occupational, and speech pathology therapies if they wish to expand the variety of home services available. In addition, a separate option exists under Medicaid that allows for personal care in the home. Personal care services consist of assistance to disabled individuals in activities of daily living. Since the total number of units of home health services are not restricted by Federal law, the number of units per Medicaid recipient is entirely dependent upon the State, which usually limits the number of services by funding only the mandated

TABLE V-19
Average Charge per Home Health Visit and Average Interim Reimbursement per Home Health Visit, 1971–1978

Year Ending June	Charge per Visit		Interim Reimbursement per Visit	
	Amount	Percent Change	Amount	Percent Change
1971	$12.10	—	$10.90	—
1972	$13.36	10.4%	$12.19	11.8%
1973	$13.97	4.5%	$12.76	4.7%
1974	$15.93	14.0%	$15.31	20.0%
1975	$19.14	20.2%	$18.29	19.5%
1976	$21.76	13.7%	$20.49	12.0%
1977	$24.24	11.4%	$22.23	8.5%
1978	$27.09	11.8%	$23.93	7.7%

Source: Personal communication from Charles Fisher, Division of National Cost Estimates, Office of Research, Demonstrations and Statistics, Health Care Financing Administration.

home health services (nursing, home health aide, and medical equipment) and/or restricting the number of units of home health services per Medicaid recipient.

Any adult over 21 years of age who is categorically eligible (for cash payments) and who meets his/her State's income/assets criteria can receive home care under Medicaid. In States where SNF care is offered to youths under 21, the State plan must include youths as eligible for home health services. The same is true for those States which opt to provide personal care. For home health services and personal care, the Medicaid recipient needs authorization from both a caseworker and a physician. In 23 States, there is a prior authorization stipulation. A different cross section of 23 States has added a homebound requirement (which differs from Medicare, where the recipient must be homebound to receive benefits.)

The Federal government's share of funding for this program ranges from 50 percent to 83 percent, depending on the State. The State contributes the remainder. HCFA supervises various State administrations (Departments of Welfare or Health), which in turn may administer directly or delegate to counties the provision or the purchase of health services for Medicaid recipients.

Supply

All 3,014 HHAs certified by Medicare are automatically eligible for Medicaid certification. However, not all Medicare-certified HHAs seek Medicaid certification or Medicaid clients. At least 104 HHAs refused Medicaid certification, according to a 1978 HCFA survey.[12] Presumably, this occurs because of the low, fixed reimbursement rates which are set independently in each State. The number of HHAs which accept Medicaid certification status but severely limit the amount of Medicaid home service provided (or number of clients accepted) is unknown.

As with Medicare, prior to the 1980 Omnibus Reconciliation Act proprietary HHAs could only be Medicaid-certified in the 25 States that licensed them. Unlike Medicare, which only recognizes agencies as providers of home health services, Medicaid may contract with registered nurses to provide nursing services in areas where there are no certified HHAs.

Utilization

Approximately 370,000 persons (5 percent of the estimated 24 million Medicaid recipients) received home health services under the Medicaid program in 1977.[13] Of the total, 300,000 aged accounted for the bulk of service recipients (81 percent). Since Medicare is the health program first called upon to finance health services for the aged who are eligible under both programs, the high proportion of aged Medicaid home service recipients probably indicates that the Medicaid program is providing services either not covered under Medicare or only covered in conjunction with a need for skilled nursing or therapy services.

The inclusions of Medicaid home health benefits are Federally-mandated service inclusions for all categorically needy adults in all State Medicaid programs. However, in 1977 the majority (54 percent) of actual home health service recipients were residents of one State, New York, which has 12 percent of the national Medicaid population.[14] These figures indicate that most States must have restrictive (if unwritten) policies concerning the provision of home health services to the Medicaid population, and that the home health benefit is not equally accessible to Medicaid recipients in every locale.

One way for the States to curb utilization of home health services is to set the reimbursement rates below market levels. Hence, home health service providers find it economically unattractive to accept Medicaid clients and frequently refuse to accept more than a certain

---

[12] Bureau of Program Policy, HCFA, *Home Health Care Services: State Descriptions, 1978*

[13] Figures are from the Medicaid Program Data Branch, Division of Beneficiary Studies, Office of Research, Demonstrations, and Statistics, Health Care Financing Administration.

[14] Figures are from the Medicaid Program Data Branch, Division of Beneficiary Studies, Office of Research, Demonstrations, and Statistics, Health Care Financing Administration.

number of them, accept none at all, or set a limit on the total number of services rendered to Medicaid recipients.

Medicaid data are not available to describe proportionately the types of home services and personal care rendered, the total number of visits made, or the health conditions of the Medicaid recipients.

Expenditures

Preliminary 1978 figures on Medicaid financing of home health services estimate that $211 million was spent. This figure represents 1.2 percent of total 1978 Medicaid expenditures of $18.1 billion. In 33 States, expenditures for home health services are actually less than .5 percent of State Medicaid expenditures (HCFA, 1980).

As noted, the Medicaid home health program is not inappropriately described as a predominantly New York State program. In 1978, $164 million went to finance home health services in New York, representing 78 percent of the total $211 million spent on Medicaid home health services in that year. Likewise, of the $247 million spent on personal care in the 14 States with established programs, $220 milliion was spent in New York in 1979.

Title XX Home-Based Services

Title XX is a Federal-State program that, since its inception in 1974, has funded social services throughout the country. The program was designed to permit the individual States wide latitude in determining the social service needs of their specific populations. Consequently, limits on the number of units of service an individual receives are entirely based upon what the State and the caseworker deem appropriate. Federal law demands that Title XX social service recipients with incomes between 80 percent and 115 percent of the State median contribute to the cost of the service. Additionally, 40 States choose to demand fees (for all or for particular services) from recipients with incomes less than 80 percent of the State median. In most cases, fees asked of social service recipients are calculated on an income-related, sliding scale basis and by type of service.

Home-based services are included in every State program to some degree. By far the most generously funded home-based services nationally are "homemaker" (general household tasks) and "chore" (general home maintenance) services. Other services described as home-based are "home health aide," "personal care attendent," "home management," "consumer education," and "financial counseling." All home-based services support Title XX goals of increased self-sufficiency, decreased institutionalization, and provision of protective services for those unable to care for themselves. Health care is clearly limited in Title XX funding to only those health services intrinsically tied, but subordinate, to a social service.

157

Individuals of any age (children as well as adults) who meet their States' income/assets criterion for social services and whose caseworkers authorize their need for services are eligible. Federal law sets an upper limit of 115 percent of the State median income as qualifying for most social services (including home-based services), but a State may choose to restrict eligibility below the 115 percent income maximum for all or for particular services. Income eligibility levels are *not* at the maximum level of 115 percent of the State median income in most States for most services.

Public funding is 75 percent Federal, matched by 25 percent State/local monies. A Federal ceiling is imposed by statute ($2.9 billion in 1979), and money is apportioned to the States based on their populations. There is Federal oversight (Administration for Public Services/DHHS) of various State administrations, which in turn authorize counties to provide or purchase services. Each State must prepare an annual plan, subject to Federal approval, delineating how its Title XX allotment will be spent and to whom the services will be targeted.

Supply

Home-based services under Title XX are either provided directly by county welfare or human services departments or are purchased by these departments from other public agencies, private non-profit agencies/organizations, proprietary agencies, or individuals. Information available only on the two major, home-based services, homemaker and chore, indicates that homemaker services are most frequently provided directly by welfare or human resources departments, but chore services are generally purchased from private agencies and/or individuals (Table V–20).

Utilization

Title XX utilization data are collected on a quarterly basis by service type and by category of income eligibility, but not by age. Therefore, the most that can be ascertained about use of Title XX home-based services is the number of individuals (by category of income eligibility) who received a particular service in a particular quarter. (One cannot aggregate the quarterly reports for a yearly total, because service recipients may need and receive a home-based service for a longer time period than three months.) For the two major home-based services, homemaker and chore, the average numbers of primary service recipients per quarter in fiscal year 1978 were 224,100 and 158,400, respectively (Administration for Public Services, 1978). These are not separate cohorts of individuals, since a disabled person may certainly require more than one home-based service. Title XX data list homemaker and chore services as eighth

158

TABLE V-20
Source of Provision of Title XX Home-Based Services

Source of Service Provisions	Percent of Home-Based Service Provided Under Title XX	
	Homemaker	Chore
Direct Provision by Welfare/ Human Resource Department	53%	36%
Purchased from Public Agencies	10%	4%
Purchased from Private Organizations, Agencies, or Individuals	37%	60%

Source: Office of the Secretary/DHEW (1980).

and tenth in terms of number of primary recipients served by a particular Title XX service in 1978.

Expenditures

The most recent data on planned expenditures for home-based services in 1979 cover only the two most funded services, homemaker and chore. In 1979, planned Federal expenditures for these two services were $568.5 million, up 19 percent from $479 million in 1978. This amount represents almost 20 percent of the total Federal contribution into the Title XX program of $2.9 billion.[15] Of the expenditure of $479 million on homemaker and chore services in 1978, 68 percent ($323.4 million) went to provide homemaker services, and 32 percent ($115.6 million) went to provide chore services (Administration for Public Services, 1978).

Expenditures for home-based services take approximately 18 percent of all Federal, State, local, and private funds used to finance Title XX services. Because data are not collected by age cohort, we do not know what proportion of the home-based services go to the aged or to younger adults and children.

Title III-B and C Older Americans Act:
In-Home Services and Home-Delivered Meals

In-home services and home-delivered meals are funded through the Older Americans Act (OAA) of 1965. Federal funds are available to States to develop, support, and administer social services (Title III–B, OAA), which include such in-home services as "homemaker," "home health aide," "chore or maintenance," and "visiting and telephone reassurance." The Federal government also appropriates funds annually for a nutrition program (Title III–C, OAA),

---

[15] Office of the Secretary, Department of Health, Education, and Welfare

which includes "home-delivered meals." Federal allotment of funds to the States is based upon the percentage of the population over age 60.

Prior to fiscal year 1981, the Federal government paid up to 90 per-- cent of the cost of social service and nutrition programs, with the States and localities contributing the remainder. As of fiscal year 1981, the Federal share changed to 85 percent. There are two separate, close-ended, Federal allotments. Under Title III–B, $196.3 million was allotted in 1979 for the States to provide social services, operate multipurpose senior centers, and administer costs of area agencies on aging. Under Title III–C, $262.8 million in Federal support was designated in 1979 to support nutrition programs for the elderly and administer costs of area agencies on aging.

The State Administrations on Aging (AoA) and the area agencies on aging decide the number of units of in-home service they will fund. As for "home-delivered meals," the duration is dependent upon the scope of the area agency on aging's nutrition program and upon the home-bound status of the recipient.

Although in principle all social services under OAA are provided without charge, area agencies on aging frequently solicit contribu- tions from the elderly in accordance with their means. Voluntary contributions from the elderly toward meal costs of nutrition pro- grams are also encouraged (with contributions made in various forms, such as food stamps).

Recipients of social services, including in-home services, must be at least 60 years old and have a need for service certified by the local area agency on aging. Technically, by statute, there is no means test for the provision of social services to the elderly. How- ever, following a 1978 amendment to the OAA, States must give preference in social service provision to those elderly in the greatest economic and/or social need. Additionally, 1978 amendments ordered that States spend additional sums above the amount re- quired prior to 1978 to provide services to the rural elderly.

Eligibility for the nutrition program is simply based upon age (60 years or older) or kinship (a spouse of an individual 60 years of age or older is eligible regardless of his/her age). For "home- delivered meals," the area agency on aging certifies that the recip- ient is homebound and in need of meals.

The Administration on Aging/DHHS supervises individual State administrations (Department of Human Services, Aging, or Welfare) which, in turn, authorize area agencies on aging to purchase services for the local elderly. Each State is required to submit a three-year plan to the Administration on Aging at the Federal level, outlining the State's intended use of its share of formula grant OAA funds. Approval of the State plan is necessary before the State's AoA funds are released.

160

Supply

Area agencies on aging purchase services from other public agencies, visiting nurse associations, private non-profit agencies, proprietary agencies or individual providers. No data are available as to the proportion of services provided by provider type. Area agencies on aging are prohibited from providing services directly unless there are no qualified service providers in the area.

In 1979, there were 11,771 OAA nutrition programs. However, there are no data describing the number of nutrition sites providing "home-delivered meals" as well as congregate meals (AoA, 1979b).

Utilization

Federal law stipulates that the area agencies on aging must ensure that a minimum of 50 percent of Title III–B funds (social service provision, senior centers, and area agencies on aging administrative costs) are used to provide in-home, access, and legal services for the local elderly.

Data collected by the Administration on Aging (AoA, 1979c) indicate that, in 1979, 106,300 elderly persons received home health services, 153,287 received homemaker services, and 291,360 received other services (such as chore or maintenance). Since an individual may receive more than one type of in-home service, the numbers cannot be aggregated. AoA estimates that, altogether, 9.7 million elderly received some form of social service funded through the OAA Title III–B in 1979. We do not know the total number of units of in-home services provided under Title III–B OAA, nor is there information on the average number of units of in-home service received per elderly recipient.

Although 1979 AoA data show 2.9 million aged participating in the Title III–C OAA nutrition program, we do not know how many of these participants are receiving meals in the home (AoA, 1979c). AoA estimates that, in 1979, 20 percent of meals prepared went to shut-in elderly (30.6 million meals out of a total figure of 155.1 million; AoA, 1979c). However, since the shut-in person would probably receive meals more regularly than the ambulatory elderly who might go out only occasionally to the congregate meal site, there would seem to be less than 20 percent of the 2.9 million nutrition program participants receiving home-delivered meals. No data are available on the average number of meals served per week per elderly person, either at the congregate meal site or in the home.

Expenditures

Total Federal funds allocated under Title III–B for social service provision, senior centers, and administrative costs of area agencies on aging were $196 million in 1979. This amount represents 35 percent of all Federal OAA allotments of $543 million for 1979.[16] The individual States' annual financial status reports submitted to the Administration on Aging for fiscal year 1979 show approximately $19 million in Federal and non-Federal funds used specifically to provide in-home services to the elderly. Of this amount, approximately one-quarter was contributed by non-Federal sources (State/local and private funds), well above the 10 percent match required by Federal statute (AoA, 1979a).[17]

Financial data are not disaggregated for specific types of in-home services and, therefore, it is unknown which services are most prevalent under OAA funding and/or for which services there were the greatest expenditures. There is no information available regarding total charges per recipient of in-home services, nor is there information concerning the average charge per type of in-home service.

Total Federal funds allocated under Title III–C for the nutrition program were $262.8 million in 1979, representing 48 percent of all OAA Federal funding ($543 million) that year.[18] No data are collected concerning the proportion of the nutrition program funds used for home-delivered meals. However, because 20 percent of the meals in 1979 are estimated to have gone to homebound elderly, in light of transportation costs, one may gauge that at least 20 percent of the expenditures were connected with meal preparation and delivery to shut-in elderly (AoA, 1979c). No data are available presenting charges per participant in the nutrition program.

There are only dated estimates of costs per meal in the AoA nutrition program. Estimates from an AoA survey in the fall of 1976 set the price of meal preparation alone at an average of $1.80 per meal (ranging from $.59 to $2.73). Other estimates from the survey gave total expenditures for meal preparation *and* delivery (including those meals delivered to shut-ins) at an average of $2.82 per meal (ranging from $1.07 to $6.03). The survey indicated that that there were economies of scale, with medium and large nutrition projects furnishing meals less expensively than small projects.[19]

Part III—Adult Day Care Sector

Adult day care (ADC) is a broad term that describes a variety of programs to prevent, delay, or reduce institutionalization. Restora-

---

[16] Figures are from the Administration on Aging, Department of Health and Human Services.

[17] Two States, Hawaii and Arizona, had not reported financial data for fiscal year 1979 by June 1980. Thus the $19 million excludes the expenditures of these two States for in-home services.

[18] Figures are from the Administration on Aging, Department of Health and Human Services.

[19] The survey was conducted by the Administration on Aging, 1976.

162

tive programs, maintenance programs, and social programs are all designated as adult day care. All of these programs offer disabled individuals varying degrees of health and social services, assistance with activities of daily living (ADL), opportunity for social interaction, at least one congregate meal per session, and transportation to and from the adult day care site.

Of the total 617 adult day care programs, there are approximately 467 adult day care programs in 46 States (1980) funded by Title XIX and Title XX of the Social Security Act and Title III of the Older Americans Act. Other forms of financing, such as revenue sharing, United Way, mental health departments, philanthropic funds, and private financing, support clients in the 150 adult day care programs which receive no funds from Medicaid, Title XX–SSA, or Title III–OAA. Medicare, as a general rule, does not fund ADC.

The only utilization figures available for adult day care are from the 1980 average *daily* census count for the 617 ADC programs. This shows 13,426, or an average of 22 persons per program per day.[20] The figure, however, gives no idea of the total number of individuals enrolled in adult day care, since enrollees frequently come to ADC sessions a few times per week. No figures are available from the three Federal programs (Medicaid, Title XX–SSA, Title III–OAA) on the total number of persons enrolled in ADC, nor on the average number of sessions per enrollee per month or per year. There are no national utilization data describing personal or disability characteristics of ADC enrollees, although some States (for example, California and Massachusetts) have begun to collect this information.

There are no national expenditure data for ADC, although some States (California, New York, and New Jersey) do collect such figures. The three Federal programs presently supporting ADC do not sort expenditure information on adult day care use of specific services.

Medicaid: Adult Day Care

Adult day care, an option under Medicaid, is reimbursed under SSA-Title XIX as an "adult day health care service," for services such as an outpatient hospital service (the provider is licensed and certified as a hospital), a clinic service (the provider is any licensed and certified health facility), or a rehabilitation service. The District of Columbia and Pennsylvania reimburse for ADC under the Medicaid provision for mental health. The medical focus is frequently rehabilitation therapy, often coupled with a social service scope.

Although Medicaid is an open-ended, Federal-State program

---

[20] Division of Long-Term Care, Health Standards and Quality Bureau, Health Care Financing Administration (1980).

(with Federal funding of 50–83 percent, matched by 50–17 percent State monies), the decision of how many units of service will be funded for all, or for categories of, Medicaid recipients characteristically rests with the State. For those States with programs, any individual who meets the income/assets test for Medicaid eligibility in his/her particular State and has the need for ADC authorized by a caseworker and a physician is eligible, regardless of age.

Federal authorities supervise individual State administrations, which in turn delegate the authority to counties to provide or purchase service.

Supply

Presently, 10 States cover ADC as a Medicaid service, supporting recipients in 118 ADC programs. Of these, 95 are funded by Title XIX only, and 23 have joint funding with either Title XX or OAA–Title III.[21]

Title XX—Social Services: Adult Day Care

Adult day care is financed under Title XX as a social service which provides a protective setting to promote self-sufficiency and to decrease institutionalization. The benefits and eligibility are identical to those previously described under Title XX—Home-Based Services.

Supply

Presently, 38 States include ADC in the State Title XX annual plan, supporting social service recipients in some 291 programs. Title XX alone funds 225 of these programs, and the remainder are funded jointly by Title XIX and OAA–Title III.[22]

Utilization

The only ADC utilization data available from the Administration for Public Services estimated that approximately 12,000 persons *per month* were receiving services in 1978, that 45 percent of the recipients were SSI beneficiaries, and that 36 percent were classified as "income eligibles" (DHEW, 1980).

Expenditures

The Administration for Public Services estimated the Federal Title XX program costs for ADC to be $42.6 million in 1979. This sum was 1.5 percent of total Federal Title XX expenditures of $2.9 billion in 1979 (DHEW, 1980).

---

[21] Division of Long-Term Care, Health Standards and Quality Bureau, Health Care Financing Administration (1980).

[22] Division of Long-Term Care, Health Standards and Quality Bureau, Health Care Financing Administration.

164

Older Americans Act, Title III: Adult Day Care

Title III-B of the Older Americans Act funds the development, administration, and support of ADC in States which include this service in the State Administration on Aging social service plans. Adult day care funded under the OAA can be either medically or socially oriented. Title III-C of the Older Americans Act can fund the nutrition component (congregate meals and nutrition education) of ADC. The benefits and other eligibility requirments are similar to those described under Title III B and C, Older Americans Act: In-Home Services and Home Delivered Meals.

Supply

Nineteen States that include ADC programs in their annual plans support elderly people in 136 programs. Title III funds 72 of these alone, and Titles XIX and XX fund the remainder jointly.[23]

References

American Health Care Association, *Long Term Care Facts, 1975* (Washington: A.H.C.A., 1976).

Congressional Budget Office, *Long Term Care: Actuarial Cost Estimates,* (Washington: U.S. Government Printing Office, August 1977a).

Congressional Budget Office, *Long Term Care for the Elderly and Disabled* (Washington: U.S. Government Printing Office, February 1977b).

Dunlop, Burton, *The Growth of the Nursing Home Industry* (Lexington: D.C. Heath and Company, 1979).

Fisher, Charles R., "Differences by Age Groups in Health Care Spending," *Health Care Financing Review,* Spring 1980.

Gibson, Robert M., "National Health Expenditures, 1979," *Health Care Financing Review,* Summer 1980.

National Center for Health Statistics, *The National Nursing Home Survey: Summary for the United States, 1977* (Washington: U.S. Government Printing Office, 1979).

National Center for Health Statistics, *The National Nursing Home Survey: Summary for the United States, 1974* (Washington: U.S. Government Printing Office, 1976).

Pollak, William, "Utilization of Alternative Care Settings by the Elderly," in M. Powell Lawton *et al,* eds., *Community Planning for An Aging Society* (Strousburg, PA: Dowden, Hutchington & Rose, Inc., 1976).

Strahan, Genevieve, "Inpatient Health Facility Statistics: United States, 1978," *Vital Health Statistics,* Series 14, No. 24 (Washington: U.S. Government Printing Office, 1980).

U.S. Department of Commerce, Bureau of the Census, *Estimates of the Population of States, by Age: July 1, 1971 to 1979,* Current Population Reports, Series P-25, No. 825 (Washington: U.S. Government Printing Office, 1980).

---

[23] Division of Long-Term Care, Health Standards and Quality Bureau, Health Care Financing Administration.

U.S. Department of Commerce, Bureau of the Census, *1976 Survey of Institutionalized Persons*, Current Population Reports, Special Studies Series, P-23, No. 69 (Washington: U.S. Government Printing Office, 1978).

U.S. Department of Health, Education, and Welfare, Administration on Aging, *Financial Status Reports, Part B: Social Services for Individual States*, 1979a.

U.S. Department of Health, Education, and Welfare, Administration on Aging, *Nutritional Services: Projects and Sites*, 1979b.

U.S. Department of Health, Education, and Welfare, Administration on Aging, *Title III Social Services Under Area Plans*, 1979c.

U.S. Department of Health, Education, and Welfare, Administration for Public Services, *Quarterly and Annual Costs of Social Services Under Title XX, October 1977-September 1978*.

U.S. Department of Health, Education, and Welfare, Health Care Financing Administration, Bureau of Program Policy, *Home Health Care Services: State Descriptions*, 1978.

U.S. Department of Health, Education, and Welfare, Health Care Financing Administration, Medicaid-Medicare Management Institute, *Data on the Medicaid Program: Eligibility, Services and Expenditures*, 1979 Edition.

U.S. Department of Health, Education, and Welfare, Health Care Financing Administration, Office of Research, Demonstrations, and Statistics, *Health Care Financing Program Statistics: Preliminary National Medicaid Statistics, Fiscal Year 1978*, April 1980.

U.S. Department of Health, Education, and Welfare, Health Care Financing Administration, Office of Research, Demonstrations, and Statistics, *Medicare: Use of Home Health Services, 1978a*.

U.S. Department of Health, Education, and Welfare, Health Care Financing Administration, Office of Research, Demonstrations, and Statistics, *Medicare: Use of Home Health Services, 1977*.

U.S. Department of Health, Education, and Welfare, Office of the Secretary, *Annual Report to the Congress on Title XX of the Social Security Act, Fiscal Year 1979*, February 1980.

U.S. Department of Health, Education, and Welfare, Public Health Service, *Vital Statistics of the United States, 1977*, Life Tables, Volume II (Washington: U.S. Government Printing Office, 1979).

U.S. Department of Health and Human Services, Administration on Aging, *Characteristics of the Black Elderly*, Statistical Reports on Older Americans (Washington: U.S. Government Printing Office, 1980).

U.S. Department of Health and Human Services, Administration on Aging, Quarterly Program Performance Report, current data.

U.S. Department of Health and Human Services, Administration on Aging, Quarterly Financial Status Report, current data.

U.S. Department of Health and Human Services, Health Care Financing Administration, Office of Research, Demonstrations, and Statistics, *Health Care Financing Trends, Winter 1981*.

Chapter VI

Research, Demonstrations, and Evaluations

by Linda V. Hamm, Thomas M. Kickham, and Dolores A. Cutler

Introduction

Because the Health Care Financing Administration (HCFA) is the primary source of funding for long-term care services in the United States, it has an inherent interest in seeking alternative approaches to the delivery and financing of this care. The Medicaid program is the principal payer of long-term care services, with Federal and State payments in fiscal year 1979 of approximately $7.1 billion for skilled nursing and intermediate care facility (ICF) services and an estimated $263.5 million for home health services. That same year, the Medicare program spent approximately $358 million for skilled nursing facility (SNF) services and $624 million for home health services (National Annual State Medicaid Statistical Report, 1981; Budget of the United States Government, Fiscal Year 1981: Appendix, 1980).

The purpose of this chapter is two-fold: to briefly outline the major policy and analytical issues in long-term care faced by HCFA and to discuss the demonstrations which HCFA has implemented to investigate how these issues have affected the Medicare and Medicaid programs.

Background

The population at risk of long-term care services is small but growing. In 1980, about one out of nine persons was 65 and over. However, in the next 50 years, nearly one in five persons will be elderly. Expressed in absolute terms, the 25.5 million elderly in 1980 will become 55 million in 2030 (U.S. Bureau of the Census, 1977 and 1981). Data also indicate that currently three-fourths of all nursing home residents are 75 and over, and more than one-third are 85 years and older (Statistical Reports on Older Americans, 1978). However, the aged are only one segment of the long-term care population.

The adult disabled constitute a substantial element of the population with long-term care needs. Approximately 23 percent of the population over the age of 18 has at least some limitation in physical functioning (Center for the Study of Welfare Policy, 1980). Data also indicate that the number of adult disabled under age 65 who have severe impairments is equal to the number of impaired persons over 65 (Congressional Budget Office, 1977).

The mentally retarded and developmentally disabled compose still another segment of the long-term care population. Developmental disabilities are those conditions attributable to mental retardation, cerebral palsy, epilepsy, or other related conditions. Mental retardation is defined on the basis of IQ as well as adaptive behavior. Recent estimates set the number of mentally retarded persons of all ages in the United States at six million, of whom 670,000 are diagnosed as severely handicapped. Of the remaining developmentally disabled population, 580,000 have cerebral palsy, 206,000 are epileptics, and 600,000 have other neurological disorders, including muscular dystrophy and speech and hearing disorders (LaVor, 1979). Within this segment of the long-term care population alone, there are several levels of impairment, from the profoundly retarded who require total and constant care, to the moderately retarded who might be able to manage some personal tasks with supervision, to the mildly retarded, who are often able to care for themselves and hold jobs. This latter subgroup is often able to live in a sheltered environment or alone (LaPorte and Rubin, 1979).

The adult chronically mentally ill make up another growing portion of the long-term care population. Mental disorders affect up to 15 percent of the population in the United States during any given year (Archives of General Psychiatry, 1978). The President's Commission on Mental Health reports that the direct cost of mental health services in the mid-1970s exceeded $17 billion per year, representing 12 percent of total national health care expenditures. In addition, the mentally ill have higher than average rates of physical illness, using medical services at almost twice the rate of the non-mentally ill population (National Institutes of Mental Health, 1974). Primary diagnosis data from 1976 and 1977 reveal that 800,000 mentally ill people were residents in nursing homes during that time. This accounts for over two-thirds of the total nursing home population (Wallack, 1979).

The terminally ill who require care for an extended period of time, such as persons suffering from certain terminal forms of cancer, also fall within the long-term care population.

It is generally agreed that there is some overlap between these groups in their long term care needs, but we know little about their characteristics and how their needs intersect or how they might be unique. This raises the issue that is at the core of the policymaking dilemma in long-term care: the lack of a precise definition of long-term care in terms of what constitutes such care and who should receive it.

The distinguishing feature of the long-term care population has been its inability to carry out certain routine daily tasks. Under the current service delivery system, the severity of the condition, combined with personal characteristics such as age, income, living

168

arrangements, and availability of an informal support system, are the factors which often arbitrarily determine the type of care received and who should receive it. However, it has become increasingly evident that these factors are interrelated. No single aspect— diagnoses, age, income, etc.—can easily determine the need for one type of care or treatment over another.

A good deal of interest has recently been directed at the financial and human implications of an inadequate service delivery system and the resulting placement of patients in inappropriate levels of care, especially those who have been inappropriately institutionalized. Various studies have indicated that anywhere from 15 to 50 percent of institutional residents could be better served at a lower level of care. (For a discussion of these studies, see General Accounting Office: Report to the Congress, 1979.) However, because of the multifaceted nature of the long-term care populations, levels of care cannot be easily quantified or determined, regardless of whether the care is provided in an institutional setting or in the patient's home. The challenge has been to develop a delivery system that can strike a balance between meeting dependency needs of the long-term care patient and maintaining opportunities for rehabilitation and independent living (Center for the Study of Welfare Policy, 1980).

During the past several years, public opinion and professional concern have focused on the availability and appropriateness of community-based, long-term care. Specific efforts have been directed at the organization and delivery of community-based, long-term care services, their financing and reimbursement, control of quality, the definition of eligibility, and coordination of services.

A major motive behind this increased governmental interest is the desire to control escalating long-term care costs. Community-based care has been advanced as an economy measure; however, the cost-effectiveness of community alternatives to institutionalization has not yet been proven in the aggregate. True costs of delivering long term care in the community have been difficult to measure or predict (Center for the Study of Welfare Policy, 1980). The costs per unit of service are only now becoming available, but from a public policy perspective, it may be equally important to learn the total (system) cost of caring for a given individual with certain characteristics over a period of time.

In determining the appropriate type and level of care for an individual, various value considerations come into play, not all of which are mutually compatible. For example, independence, self-determination, individualization and normalization may clash with the goals of equity, economy, right to treatment, protection from harm, and the protection of society (Center for the Study of Welfare Policy, 1980). None of these factors is easily measured, but from the consumer's and the general public's perception, they are the

169

key determinants of whether long-term care is effective or responsive to needs. In the final analysis, these factors may be as important as cost in developing a comprehensive long-term care strategy.

Policy and Analytical Issues

The major debates in the field of long-term care revolve around the following three policy and analytical issues: (1) the long-term care population, especially the group at risk of institutionalization, will continue to grow, (2) publicly-supported costs of long-term care are growing rapidly and currently represent a response only to institutional long-term care needs, and (3) the current mix of long-term care services and financing is neither the most efficient nor the most responsive to the needs of the groups that compose the long-term care population.

Many groups both in the private and public sector are investigating the implications of these issues for society and the health care system. HCFA's research and demonstration activities in long-term care examine several aspects of these issues as they relate to the Medicare and Medicaid programs.

Research

Research activities within HCFA have focused on describing and explaining the demand for long-term care and the basic economic underpinnings of the long term care industry. In addition, considerable effort has been devoted to developing a methodology to measure the quality of long-term care provided in different settings.

The purpose of these activities is to construct a model (understanding) of the long-term health care delivery, reimbursement, and financing systems to provide some direction for private and public policymaking and to identify promising areas for demonstration activities. In large part, the other chapters in this book draw upon the knowledge gained through research either directly supported or undertaken by the Federal and State governments.

Demonstrations

From the Federal perspective, HCFA's demonstration and experimental projects generally have the following two roles: feasibility testing and formal experimentation.

In many instances, State Medicaid agencies wish to implement a change in their operating systems (coverage, procedures, reimbursement) for a limited time and geographic region to see if the changes will achieve certain objectives. For the most part, HCFA has encouraged States to experiment with their present Medicaid programs when changes appear to improve the program in some way and when the results might benefit other State programs. Through waivers of Title XIX and the granting of special Federal funds, HCFA encourages States to explore, on their own initiatives, interesting and innovative concepts in health care delivery and financing.

On the other hand, HCFA engages in formal experimentation, in part based on the results of its own research activities and on special initiatives generated by Congress or the Secretary. Under this type of demonstration program, HCFA tests a certain number of hypotheses by introducing an intervention into an ongoing system and observing the result(s). The Agency establishes experimental and control (or comparison) groups and collects sufficient data on characteristics of both groups to control for external events.

The purpose of this type of demonstration is to answer specific questions about present and future policy for the Medicare and Medicaid programs specifically and for the health care system (providers, consumers, and insurers) generally. These activities take place in one or more States, and, to the extent possible, national inferences are made from the demonstration data.

HCFA is supporting demonstrations that focus on (1) alternatives to institutional long-term care, the population which is best served by these alternatives, and the costs of providing them and (2) alternative reimbursement strategies which offer incentives for long-term care providers to be efficient in delivering services and responsive to the needs of long-term care patients.

In general, the demonstrations emphasize the following areas:

- the coordination and management of an appropriate mix of health and social services directed at individual client needs with the goal of reducing institutionalization and costs without sacrificing quality of care
- Medicare and Medicaid coverage of long-term care services in which payment for certain quasi-medical services, or changes in the location of services, may reduce the overall costs of long-term care
- innovative reimbursement methods which test whether costs are reduced without adversely affecting patient outcomes
- the impact of changes in the current survey and certification methods for determining quality of care in long-term care institutional settings.

The following discussion provides an overview of HCFA's demonstration activities. For readers who wish a more complete description of the demonstrations, project summaries and current findings can be found in the appendix of this chapter. The demonstration summaries are organized in the Appendix to correspond to the four areas of emphasis mentioned earlier.

Coordination and Management

A major part of HCFA's demonstration efforts has been directed toward developing the concept of organized community care. The following describes the history of this concept and HCFA's current demonstration involvement.

The community-long term care concept can be traced to the middle 1950s, when the National Commission on Chronic Illness pointed out the importance of coordination and integration of services for the long-term patient with interrelated needs. The study advanced the notion of a single, community-based agency concerned with the complex needs of long term patients, noting that "without some central organization concerned with (long-term care) needs, gaps and overlap in long term care are almost inevitable" (Commission on Chronic Illness, 1956).

In the 1960s, long-term care again became the focus of interest with the "deinstitutionalization" movement in the mental health field. At that time, many mental health professionals believed that the large mental hospital was not the most appropriate setting for a good percentage of these, primarily elderly, long-stay patients. (One deinstitutionalization study found that, of the patients recommended for transfer from Texas State mental hospitals, more than half were over 60 years of age, and 24 percent were between ages 50 and 60; Sheehan and Craft, 1974). The enactment of Medicaid during this period made large amounts of matching funds available to States that provided certain services. While coverage for patients in State mental hospitals was limited to persons under 21 and over 65 needing medical care for a physical ailment, nursing home requirements under Medicaid were more flexible. The growing nursing home industry could absorb many of the "deinstitutionalized" patients, be reimbursed by Medicaid, and the States could receive matching funds.

Thus the resident population in State mental hospitals dropped by half (from 490,000 in 1964 to 249,000 in 1973) in just under a decade. The population of nursing homes grew by 53 percent from 1963 to 1973, reaching one million (LaPorte and Rubin, 1979). Although not all of the increase in nursing home admissions was due to transfer from State mental hospitals, the interrelationship of the data illustrates the trend. In many cases, elderly, long-stay patients were shifted from one institutional setting to another because they were unable to cope in the community and there were few available, community-based care or treatment alternatives—and none that were organized to meet all of the long-term care needs of this population.

The focus of deinstitutionalization changed in the early 1970s to reflect concerns about the fragmented and duplicative nature of the social service delivery system and the growing awareness of the rising costs of nursing home care under Medicaid and Medicare.

172

Government policymakers began to explore the possibilities of services integration to rationalize service delivery and avoid inappropriate placement of patients in nursing homes. Services integration is defined as the building of service systems in the community, either through voluntary interagency/provider cooperation or the use of specific authority which promotes the coordination of a range of community services. Contracting authority, case management, and pooled funding were some of the integrative mechanisms that were attempted in over 30 services integration research and demonstration projects funded by the Department of Health, Education, and Welfare in the early 1970s. These projects raised interesting possibilities but were never thoroughly evaluated. Much of the literature dealing with the services integration efforts focuses on social services delivery.

In 1971, the single community agency concept referred to earlier was revived with the personal care organization (PCO) concept developed by Robert Morris of Brandeis University. The PCO was seen as an organization which would fill the gap between available home-delivered medical services (home health agency) and the combination of medical, room and board, and social services of an institution. It was based on the assumption that a significant number of older people were institutionalized because they required nonmedical services which were unavailable in the community on an organized basis. The services that were considered necessary included homemaker, chore, home repair, meals, laundry, legal advice, etc. (Callahan, 1979). The Home Care Program for the elderly in Massachusetts is a state-wide system based primarily on the PCO model. A demonstration of the concept, called a community care organization (CCO), began to be tested in Wisconsin in 1974 under a Section 1115 grant from the former Social Rehabilitation Service (The grant was transferred to HCFA and expanded to include health services in 1977.) The Wisconsin CCO published its final report in 1980.

Several other variations on the CCO theme are being tested by HCFA in current demonstrations. Each of the demonstrations provides similar case management functions, including centralized intake/screening, client assessment and reassessment, care planning, and follow up. The manner in which these tasks are carried out reflects the differing organizational structures of the various projects and the adjustments that each one makes to its own State or local socio-political environment. The projects also share similar research goals and objectives which reflect the basic concerns of Federal, State, and local administrators and policymakers about:

- the medical and personal characteristics of the long-term care population being served and how the services provided affect the client's functioning, health, and quality of life

173

- the costs of providing community-based, long-term care versus the costs of care provided in institutional settings
- the most efficient and effective organization of community-based services to meet the needs of the long-term care client.

Some examples of the different Medicaid and Medicare demonstration projects and the extent of State or local involvement and support are illustrative:

- The Wisconsin CCO project was a State-supported, Medicaid waiver project, operated through three county sites. Each site was relatively autonomous, using separate and distinct assessment instruments and organizational structures. Although the State did not implement the program when the demonstration period ended, each of the local communities in which the sites were located retained components of the respective site's organizational and program structure. Only one site, Milwaukee, retained and continued all elements of the demonstration.
- The Georgia Alternative Health Services Medicaid waiver project operated in 17 counties of the State with uniform case management functions carried out by State employees. Georgia is currently phasing the program in on a state-wide basis, under the State Medicaid agency.
- After two years of operation of the Oregon Flexible Intergovernmental Grant (FIG) project, the State is implementing portions of the project state-wide. The demonstration involved five counties. One county provided case management which emphasized community-based alternatives to coordinate the provision of services from existing county resources. A second county combined the same case management with an expanded set of services made possible by waivers. Two counties provided only expanded services with traditional case-management, and the fifth county operated within the traditional service structure. The State has created a new division to implement the portions of the project which emphasized community-based alternatives and case management throughout the State. It will be administered by local governments through area agencies on aging.

Further examples of these and other CCO-type demonstrations are summarized in the appendix.

In addition to the HCFA supported projects, in 1980 Congress appropriated $20.5 million to further test community-based, long-term care on a research-oriented basis. The effort is known as the National Long-Term Care Channeling Demonstration Program.

The goal of channeling is to efficiently use the entire spectrum of community services that a client needing long-term care may require. Channeling is intended to coordinate and manage the use

174

of such services so that they fit each client's needs. It includes formally organized medical, mental health, social, and personal care services, as well as a wide array of informal services.

The program is an intradepartmental effort which includes the close cooperation of HCFA, the Administration on Aging (AoA), and the Office of the Assistant Secretary for Planning and Evaluation (ASPE), which was designated the lead agency in the effort.

On September 30, 1980, the Department announced implementation of the program, which includes the following four components:

Channeling Demonstrations

The 12 States that were awarded contracts to conduct channeling demonstrations are Maryland, Maine, Pennsylvania, Kentucky, Texas, Hawaii, Florida, Massachusetts, Missouri, New York, New Jersey, and Ohio.

The term channeling refers to the organizational structures and operating systems required in a community to make sure that a client receives needed long-term care services. The primary elements of this concept are outreach/case finding, screening, comprehensive client assessment, and case management.

As part of the demonstration program, each State is required to establish an inter-agency long-term care planning group to prepare a State long-term care plan. Members of the planning group are designated by the governor of each State.

Evaluation Contract

A contract was awarded to Mathematica Policy Research, Inc., to evaluate the 12 demonstrations.

Technical Assistance Contract

The Department of Health and Human Services (DHHS) awarded a technical assistance contract to the Temple University Institute of Gerontology to provide support to the 12 demonstrations in developing uniform assessment and data collection procedures.

State System Development Grants

Fifteen States received 1-year system development grants. These grants will help States build their capacity to plan, coordinate, and manage the allocation of long term-care resources.

AoA is monitoring the system development grants. Teams of representatives from ASPE, HCFA, and AoA are monitoring the evaluation and technical assistance contracts.

Of the 12 channeling demonstrations, HCFA is monitoring six (Maryland, Maine, Pennsylvania, Kentucky, Texas and Hawaii), and the Administration on Aging is monitoring the remaining six (Florida, Massachusetts, Missouri, New Jersey, New York, and Ohio).

175

All of these community-based, long-term care efforts have generated increasing Congressional interest. One result of this interest has been the inclusion of Section 2176 in the Omnibus Reconciliation Act of 1981. This provision allows the Secretary to approve State plans that include home and community-based services (other than room and board) as medical assistance by waiver. Such services must be provided under a written plan of care to individuals who would otherwise require the level of care which is covered by the State when provided in an SNF or ICF. These services may include case management, homemaker/home health aide services, personal care services, adult day health, rehabilitative services, respite care, and other services, as approved by the Secretary. To be granted a waiver, the State must provide assurances to the Secretary that, among other things, the average *per capita* expenditure it estimates for Medicaid individuals who are provided services under the waiver will not exceed the average *per capita* expenditures for such individuals if no waiver was granted. The waivers will be for a three-year period and may be renewed.

Medicare and Medicaid Coverage

HCFA implemented two major initiatives in 1980 to test whether the coverage of additional services not strictly medical in nature would reduce the cost of long-term care.

The national hospice demonstration permits the waiver of certain statutory and regulatory requirements to allow coverage of hospice services to terminally ill Medicare beneficiaries and Medicaid recipients. Participating hospices may be reimbursed under the demonstration for a number of items and services not currently covered by Medicare and Medicaid. Examples include outpatient prescription drugs, institutional respite and home respite services (primary care giver relief), visits by dieticians and homemakers, supportive and counseling visits to hospice patients during occasional hospital stays, continuous care (by nurses, home health aides, or homemakers) on a shift basis in the home, certain self-help devices, inpatient hospice care, and bereavement services to family members. The evaluation of demonstration data will focus on the cost and use of hospice care and will attempt to determine the difference (if any) between the quality of care provided by hospices and the quality of life experienced by patients receiving hospice care and the quality of care and life for patients who receive services from conventional health providers.

The other initiative, funded by the Departments of Housing and Urban Development and Health and Human Services, is a demonstration to test whether the chronically mentally ill can be deinstitutionalized and integrated into the community if provided with housing

176

support and Medicaid coverage of services such as life skills, transportation, and supervision.

The Department of Housing and Urban Development (HUD) is providing direct Federal loans to assist private, non-profit corporations in the development of new or substantially rehabilitated housing. Over a three-year period, HUD has set aside loan reservations for 229 sites in 39 States, including the District of Columbia and Puerto Rico. These sites will house from 3,500 to 4,000 residents. In addition, HUD will provide Section 8 rental assistance for all of the units.

The Department of Health and Human Services is waiving specific sections of Title XIX to authorize Federal matching funds for presently non-covered services such as case management, supervision, training in life skills, and transportation. Four States (Minnesota, Georgia, Tennessee, and Vermont) have received Title XIX waivers, and another 22 are expected to request Federal matching funds.

Innovative Reimbursement Methods

HCFA is engaged in several activities that test alternative reimbursement systems. For the past five years, selected hospitals in four predominantly rural States (Texas, Iowa, Utah, and South Dakota) have been permitted to provide long-term care using the "swing-bed" concept of care. Under this concept, a designated number of hospital beds can be "swung" from acute care to extended care use and back again as the needs of patients change. Reimbursement for swing-bed care differed from Medicare's traditional methodology. Hospitals were reimbursed for providing long-term care on the basis of the State Medicaid rate per day paid to SNFs or ICFs. Reimbursement for acute care was based on the hospital's total allowable costs minus its long-term care revenues.

Evaluation (Shaughnessy, 1981) indicated that the swing-bed approach appears to be the most cost-effective means to provide long-term care. The approach also represented a method of rural hospital diversification. Hospitals in rural areas are highly regarded by the residents in their communities not only in terms of the hospitals' ability to take care of the residents' acute health care needs but also in their importance to the economic health of the community. Because many small rural hospitals are financially threatened due to low occupancy rates, the ability to provide additional needed services under the swing-bed approach strengthened these institutions.

In the social/HMO project, Brandeis University is testing the concept of providing a continuum of medical and health services to an elderly population within an HMO. This three-year project will develop a demonstration and evaluation protocol for the social/HMO

177

concept, select and developmentally assist three sites, and implement the demonstration.

Together with the West Virginia Department of Welfare, HCFA is testing an alternative method of reimbursing nursing home capital costs (interest on debt, depreciation, and a return on equity capital). Currently, the West Virginia Medicaid program reimburses nursing homes for their *routine* costs on the basis of a prospective rate setting methodology. Under waivers from HCFA, West Virginia will reimburse nursing home *capital* costs using a standard appraisal value approach. Each year, the physical structure of the nursing home is appraised to determine its current replacement value. The State reduces this amount by the home's estimated physical and functional depreciation. A rate established by West Virginia is applied to the difference and serves as the reimbursement for the reasonable costs of investment in long term care facilities. The reimbursement for capital costs is independent of the owner's book value of the home and thereby attempts to prevent the frequent sale and resale of nursing homes.

In southern California, the National Center for Health Services Research and HCFA are jointly testing the effects of an incentive payment to nursing homes on the appropriateness of care and the efficient use of resources. Approximately 20 proprietary nursing homes in the San Diego area will receive payments to encourage them to (1) admit "heavy care" patients who might otherwise remain inappropriately hospitalized, (2) improve resident outcomes by using resident-specific goal setting and care planning, and (3) discharge patients who might be better served in a home setting. The experimental phase is expected to last two years.

Survey and Certification

Projects which streamline the nursing home survey and certification process are currently underway in Wisconsin, Massachusetts, and New York.

In Wisconsin and New York, the goal is to move from a single "paper review" of patient care and a facility's ability to meet Federal/State standards to a screening approach which focuses surveyor time on the actual care provided to patients and the facility's ability to provide that care.

While the Massachusetts project does not change the current medical review (MR)/independent professional review (IPR) requirements, it does concentrate surveyor time on identifying nursing homes which have had difficulty in complying with Federal/State conditions of participation.

It is anticipated that findings from these three projects will be instrumental in developing more effective nursing home survey and certification methods in which surveyor time is better used.

178

Appendix

All project information contained in this appendix is current as of July, 1981.

Table of Contents

179

Innovative Reimbursement Methods

Survey and Certification

Triage: Comprehensive, Coordinated Care of the Elderly

The Triage model is based upon a single entry access point to the health delivery system for elderly persons. The project tests the feasibility and effectiveness of service coordination for elderly and disabled individuals living in a seven town area in central Connecticut. The project establishes a liaison between clients and multiple service agencies so that care is organized around the client and the available resources.

Connecticut initiated Triage in 1974, with State funding and a grant from the Administration on Aging. In 1975, the State received Section 222 Medicare waivers together with funding from the National Center for Health Services Research, Public Health Service, for the research component of the project. These initial years of the project are referred to as Triage I.

On April 1, 1979, HCFA approved a two year project using the same demonstration and research design to obtain needed longitudinal data on the utilization and cost of services provided to this group of patients from the inception of the project. This project is known as Triage II.

The project is targeted at an eligible population of 19,526 people, 65 years and over, who are entitled to Medicare parts A and B. The service delivery system has been developed around individual needs rather than tailored to fit existing reimbursable sources. The delivery model includes the following features: patient assessment and individual plans of care; coordination of all available health-related services; creation of new services in the demonstration area; monitoring of the plans of care; and evaluation of pertinent data in accordance with a research design so that patient outcomes and costs of services can be studied.

The project serves 1,500 participants.

The objectives of the project are:

- to increase the effectiveness of health services,
- to develop necessary preventive and support services and demonstrate their value to the target population,
- to provide a single entry, assessment mechanism to coordinate delivery of institutional, ambulatory, and in-home services which will result in cost containment,
- to demonstrate the effectiveness of coordinated care, including a) care to prevent illness, compensate for disability, and support independent living at home, b) care prescribed to answer need rather than to accomodate third-party payer service restrictions, and c) use of professional nurse-clinician/social service coordinator teams to assess needs of individuals, arrange for appropriate services, and provide case management, and

181

- to reduce expenditures for health care delivered to the target population.

The Triage model operates through a clinical process of care developed and monitored by interdisciplinary teams, each of which consists of a nurse-clinician and a social service coordinator (social worker). The clinical process of care includes the following four stages:

Referral—Most frequent sources of referral have been self-referral, family, friends, visiting nurses, hospital discharge planners, physicians, and social workers.

Assessment—The team visits the client's home to fully assess client needs, using a comprehensive assessment form. This form was developed and refined by project clinical staff, the project research team, and a geriatric physician consultant. The assessment consists of a modified physical examination and an extensive interview eliciting a complete health history and information on client functional status, nutrition, physical environment, and an informal support system. Functional status is assessed by the use of three standardized instruments—the Activities of Daily Living (Katz *et al*), the Instrumental Activities of Daily Living (Lawton and Brody), and the Mental Status Questionnaire (Goldfarb, Kahn, *et al*). This process provides the data base upon which the plan of care is developed for each client.

Coordinating the Care Plan—Based on the assessment data, the team develops a plan of care. The Triage team works with the client and his or her family to select services appropriate to the client's needs and the providers that will be asked to deliver the authorized services.

Monitoring—After service delivery commences, the Triage team maintains ongoing contact with the client to ensure that services continue to be consistent with the care plan in quality and quantity. In addition, the team consults frequently with providers, meets on a monthly basis with home health agencies in the region, and consults with other providers as needed. A medical-dental advisory committee is available to Triage staff for consultation and review of client status. The committee consists of five physicians (with different specialities), two dentists, a podiatrist, and a pharmacist.

The Section 222 Medicare waivers have made it possible for Triage to authorize payment for many ancillary and support services not traditionally covered by Medicare and to waive specific Medicare requirements such as coinsurance, deductibles, and restrictions on home health care.

182

The following table identifies the services available to Triage clients, including waived services and traditional Medicare services.

Service Category	Traditional Medicare Services	Waived Services
Institutional	Hospital Skilled Nursing Facility	Intermediate Care Facility Home for the Aged Day Care
Home Care	Visiting Nurse Home Health Aide	Homemaker Chore Companion Meals and Meal Delivery
Ambulatory	Physician Outpatient Service Diagnostic Services (X-ray and laboratory) Therapies (Speech Physical, Occupational) Dentist (selected medical conditions) Podiatrist (selected medical conditions)	Optometrist Dentist (routine and preventive) Podiatrist (routine and preventive) Mental Health Counseling
Products	Medical Equipment Supplies	Pharmaceuticals Hearing Aids Glasses
Transportation	Ambulance	Chair Car Taxi

Traditional Medicare services are reimbursed according to the procedures and rates of that program. For other services not normally included under Medicare, the method of reimbursement varies according to service type. Homemaker and ICFs, for example, are reimbursed on a cost reporting basis; pharmaceuticals and optical care are reimbursed using Medicaid rates established by the State Department of Social Services. For other services, Triage obtained schedules from government and industry sources (for example, Connecticut Public Utilities Commission rates used for transportation). Rates were negotiated with each provider for services such as meals and meal delivery, companions, and chore service.

Triage has provided training opportunities for providers and students in health professions programs throughout the life of the project.

Preliminary data from Triage I indicate that 72 percent of participants improved or maintained their ability to conduct activities of daily living and their mental status scores. However, the overall performance of the participant group on assessment scores decreased with advancing age. The total cost per participant for 1978 was $3,620, or an average *per diem* cost of $12.63 per day. Data from Triage II are not yet available.

Alternative Health Services

In July 1976, under the authority of Section 1115 of the Social Security Act, the Georgia Department of Medical Assistance embarked on a demonstration project in two of the State's human resources districts (covering 17 counties). The project offers alternatives to nursing home care for persons who would otherwise be placed in institutions. The model is built on a centralized single point of entry into all service systems. In addition to regular Medicaid-financed health services, the demonstration offers three alternative services; adult day rehabilitation, home delivered services, and alternative living services (for example, personal care, adult foster care, boarding services, and congregate living arrangements). The program serves 1,385 clients; approximately 1,040 have been referred to the experimental group and 345 to the control group for research purposes.

All potential Alternative Health Services (AHS) clients receive a health and social needs assessment prior to enrollment. Along with self-referrals, the project receives referrals from hospitals, the county Department of Family and Children's Services, and the Georgia Medical Care Foundation, the project's independent utilization review contractor. Clients who appear to be eligible for services are interviewed by county caseworkers who collect health and social information. Following the interview, the caseworker obtains the relevant medical data from the client's physicians and additional information on family and support systems.

The information gathered by the caseworker is reviewed by a team consisting of an AHS nurse, social worker, and the caseworker. The team uses the State maximum units of service guidelines to identify patients who require more intensive care than the project can provide. After the conference, the caseworker notifies the client of service recommendation or control assignments. (Three out of every four clients determined appropriate for the project are randomly assigned to AHS service groups, with the fourth assigned to a control group. Clients in both groups are tracked for the duration of the project.)

Once a patient is accepted, he or she is referred to appropriate providers. A face-to-face interview is conducted by the provider, who notifies the team within five days whether the recommended services are adequate. The provider then indicates the services to be offered and their frequency, justifying any refusal to extend recommended services. The team must approve any changes in the client's care plan. Once services are initiated, both a case manager and a case coordinator work to ensure the continued provision of appropriate services.

Standard contracts have been negotiated with a large number of alternative services providers. The contracts include agreement on specific expenditures and cost allocations, a line item budget which the provider cannot exceed, and a system which allows a provider to retain unused funds to expand the program.

Medicus Systems Corporation is evaluating the project under contract to the grantee. Medicus has participated in and reviewed all aspects of the project, including the technical research and the management system. In particular, the evaluation will focus on costs, utilization, health impact, and effectiveness.

Some of the preliminary cost and utilization findings from the first operational year follow. However, analysis of data from subsequent years may change these findings.

- Total Medicaid mean monthly costs for the experimental group are 76 percent higher than for the control group. Medicaid costs exclusive of AHS costs for the experimental group, however, are 9.4 percent less than for the control group. The most significant differences by category of expenditure are for nursing home, inpatient hospital, and physican costs.
- Medicaid nursing home costs are on the average $15.94 a month, 38 percent higher for the control group than for the experimental group.
- Physicians' costs reimbursed by Medicaid are 141 percent higher for the control group than for the experimental group.
- Mean Medicaid inpatient hospital costs for the experimental group are 49 percent higher than for the control group. These cost figures are consistent with the finding that individuals in the experimental group used an average of 5.4 hospital days during the first year of enrollment, compared with clients in the control group who used 4.1 hospital days on the average. This finding may be attributed to the professionals who provide AHS services and recognize the need for hospitalization before it might otherwise be recognized by the client or the family.
- The utilization and service cost figures indicate that 42.6 percent

of the clients have received home delivered services, 14.7 percent have received adult day rehabilitation services, and 2.8 percent have received alternative living services. The mean monthly project service costs of home delivered services per person was $129, adult day rehabilitation, $216, and alternative living services, $212.

The final project report is available from HCFA.

The Georgia State legislature has appropriated funds to expand the AHS program so that it may be adopted state-wide (over a three year period) as part of the State Medicaid plan. Efforts to phase in AHS state-wide began in August 1980. The program is currently working on the transition from a demonstration project to a state-wide program and establishing ongoing linkages with providers and agencies. In addition, the project is auditing providers. Together with the evaluator, AHS is developing a methodology to convert the current financial data base, which is in a charge-based format suitable to a demonstration, to a cost-based format, more suitable to the State Medicaid program.

Monroe County I

The New York State Department of Social Services is conducting a demonstration project under the authority of Section 1115 of the Social Security Act, through the Monroe County Long Term Care Program, Inc. (MCLTCP). Its purpose is to demonstrate alternative approaches to delivering and financing long-term care to the adult disabled and elderly Medicaid population of the county.

The project has developed the Assessment for Community Care Services (ACCESS) model as a centralized unit responsible for all aspects of long-term care for Monroe County residents, 18 years of age or older, who have long-term health care needs and who are eligible for Medicaid benefits. The program will develop and coordinate community services, administer long-term care funds, approve all public payments for institutional and community long-term care services, and collect program data. ACCESS staff assess client needs, assist in planning and obtaining community or institutional services, and monitor the appropriateness of the service. All long-term care services provided under Medicaid in the county must be coordinated with the ACCESS unit for the provider to be reimbursed. Private pay patients may voluntarily use ACCESS services.

ACCESS assessment activity varies based on client location (whether in an acute care facility or in the community). However, actual assessments are all carried out using the Preadmission Assessment Form (PAF) developed by the project to improve upon previous State forms which attempted to document patient condition.

The principal focus of the PAF is to determine the client's capacity for self-care and specific service needs necessary for the patient to remain at home, if possible. Nurses from the County Health Department or the Visiting Nurse Service of Rochester perform the assessments.

Once a patient's needs have been determined, the assessor completes an alternate care plan (ACP) form which provides a detailed home care package identifying required services, personnel, and equipment. On the basis of the ACP, ACCESS determines the cost and practicality of home care for the patient. If the patient and family agree to the service plan, ACCESS initiates services for the client (whether it involves home care or admission to a long-term care facility). As part of its contract with the County Division of Social Services, ACCESS may only approve home services for Medicaid clients who can be assisted in home care for less than 75 percent of the cost of a comparable level of care in a long-term care facility. If costs exceed 75 percent, ACCESS must make a special request to the DSS to allow home services. Non-Medicaid patients (for example, private pay voluntary participants) must arrange for payment of their services on their own, although ACCESS will assist and advise them in these arrangements.

ACCESS tracks its client population with a home review system. Home review visits are made three times a year for Medicaid clients and where necessary and agreed to by non-Medicaid clients. Utilization review forms are routinely shared with ACCESS by three church-sponsored nursing homes and one public facility in the county. These forms determine whether the patient is at the appropriate level of care. If the UR form indicates that a change may be necessary, the Genessee Valley Medical Foundation (which conducts the utilization reviews) transmits the form to ACCESS for review and resolution.

Section 1115 Medicaid waivers permit the project to include the following services: friendly visiting, housing improvement, home maintenance and heavy chore services, housing assistance, transportation, moving assistance, and respite care. Bills for all Medicaid covered (and waived) long-term care services for project clients are submitted to the project by providers. Their claims, based on State Medicaid reimbursement schedules, are reviewed and then forwarded by the project to the State Medicaid office for payment. The project also has the authority to contract with providers for the delivery of certain waived services.

Objectives

The objectives of the project are:

- to provide long-term care services which are appropriate, cost-effective, and acceptable to the client

187

- to provide coordination and continuity of case management for long-term care clients
- to improve long-term care assessment and review procedures
- to collect data about needs, service utilization, and appropriateness of placement on persons requiring long-term care
- to reduce the number of county residents who are in acute hospitals and long-term care institutions
- to reduce the per person rate of increase of Medicaid expenditures for individuals needing long-term care from what it would have been had the project never existed.

Macro Systems, Inc. evaluated the project for three operational years. An evaluation report was published in 1980. In the initial 32 months, ACCESS received 8,862 referrals, 4,766 from hospitals and 4,096 from community sources. The community referrals came from home health agencies (33 percent), clients and/or families (28 percent), long-term care facilities (10 percent), local human services agencies (4 percent), and physicians (5 percent).

The percentage of community Medicaid patients treated at home has increased over the life of the program. During the first year of operation, 88 percent of the Medicaid patients referred from the community were treated at home, but in 1980 (through July), this figure rose to 96 percent. Increases have also been dramatic for non-Medicaid community patients who in 1978 had only 75 percent home resolutions, increasing to 88 percent in 1980. Similarly, more hospital patients have been released to home care since the start of the program. During the first year, 35 percent of the Medicaid patients referred from the hospital were cared for at home. In 1980 (through July), this figure increased to 54 percent. Eighteen percent of non-Medicaid patients were cared for at home in 1978, increasing to 25 percent in 1980.

Medicaid costs for all direct, noninstitutional services for 1,123 skilled-level patients who were assessed at home under the ACCESS system are estimated to be $25.12 a day, or 52 percent of the comparable Medicaid institutional rate (approximately $50 a day). The Medicaid cost for health-related and proprietary home level service packages is also less than half of the comparable institutional rate.

Evaluation findings indicate that home care costs for long-term care patients under the demonstration are from 30 to 50 percent of the county's comparable institutional costs. Skilled nursing services provided in the home through the project were estimated to be $22.22 per day, compared to $50.00 per day for equivalent institutional care. For health-related services (equivalent to ICF care), the costs were $9.29 for home care as compared to $30.00 for institutional care. At the domiciliary care level, the costs were $3.74, compared to $16.00 at the institutional level.

Monroe County II

The delivery model used for the Section 1115 Monroe County Long-Term Care Medicaid project (Monroe County I) will be expanded under the authority of Section 222 of the Social Security Act to include case management and patient assessment services for the county's Medicare population in need of long-term care. This demonstration shares the purpose and goals of the Section 1115 Medicaid project. The addition of this project to the Monroe County Program will enable the county to work toward integrating Medicare and Medicaid long-term care services in the county and to simplify program administration.

In addition to the ACCESS process described for the Monroe County I project, Section 222 Medicare waivers will enable this project to implement a utilization review component, whereby once a client has entered a facility or has been approved for home care, a set review schedule will be used. Medicare-entitled clients will be reviewed in an SNF every 14 days by a utilization review nurse from the Genesee Valley Medical Foundation. Medicare-entitled clients at home will be reviewed by a nurse from a certified home health agency every 28 days. In addition, the Section 222 Medicare waivers will permit ACCESS to certify a client's need for skilled nursing services for up to 14 consecutive days in an SNF and up to 28 days for the provision of home care services, if approved by the client's private physician.

The waived Medicare services under this demonstration include client intake and assessment, noninstitutional SNF services, financial counseling, in-home architectural review, and transportation services. Extended care services will be furnished to participating SNFs if the patient requires daily skilled nursing or other skilled rehabilitation services which can only be provided in an SNF on an inpatient basis. The "post-hospital" Medicare requirements for SNF care and Part A home health care are also waived to implement this project.

This project began operations in 1982.

Delivery of Medical and Social Services to the Homebound Elderly

The New York City Department for the Aging is conducting a three year Medicare demonstration of the delivery of medical and social services to the homebound elderly under Section 222 of the Social Security Act. A separate grant from the Administration on Aging is supporting certain administrative activities and supplemental service delivery costs for the project.

The purpose of the demonstration is to test a community-based methodology which will provide a spectrum of medical and social services, directly and by linkage and coordination, to a home-bound, chronically ill population. Specifically, the project is targeted to persons age 65 and over, entitled to Medicare Part B, who suffer from chronic illness or functional or mental impairment and who are unable to visit a physician without assistance or have no access to medical care.

Four sites will be developed, each serving 100 individuals, with a comparison group of 200 for research purposes. The project's major objectives are three-fold:

- to identify characteristics of this population, needed levels of care, costs of delivering such care, and the effect of care delivery
- to demonstrate the process of coordination and identify mechanisms and strategies to achieve it
- to develop a cost-effective model of coordinated service delivery to be incorporated into the city's system.

A coordinating model has been established to carry out the project. It is composed of separate organizational components, each with specific responsibilities related to coordination and service delivery. These components include a project advisory committee which comprises relevant city departments and four neighborhood-based service delivery sites. The project advisory committee reviews policy, selects sites, and establishes criteria for clients and services. The committee also facilitates agreements between service providers. An interdisciplinary team (nurse and social worker) from the neighborhood-based sites conducts centralized intake, assessment, care planning, reassessment, and monitoring.

Each site has a physician consultant whose responsibilities include:

- participating in selected care planning conferences,
- serving as a consultant to the nurse and social worker on medical management problems of clients,
- making special assessment visits to clients who have no physician in the community and signing off on the care plans developed by the case management team for such clients (wherever a client has a personal physician, he or she will approve the client's care plan), and
- intervening in client situations, on behalf of the assessment team, when current medical care is no longer adequate.

The project has developed the four sites incrementally; two became operational in December 1980, and two more became operational in April 1981. The sites are:

- the Sunset Park Family Health Center (Brooklyn), which is part of Lutheran Medical Center but functions as a freestanding clinic,

- the Community Agency for Senior Citizens, which is sponsored by the Staten Island Home Care Integration Service Coalition and funded under Older Americans Act, Title III B,
- the Jamaica Service Program for Older Adults (Queens), which is a voluntary social service agency providing a broad range of services to the elderly in this borough, including services funded under Title III B of the Older Americans Act, and
- the Comprehensive Family Care Center (Bronx), which is sponsored by the Albert Einstein College of Medicine.

The four sites may provide services directly or contract or arrange for other services in their respective catchment areas.

Services provided through the Medicare waivers are the core around which other community services will be obtained for project clients. These services are homemaker, personal care, transportation and escort, and drugs and biologicals.

The assessment instrument is based primarily on the Georgia Alternative Health Services client assessment interview, together with the New York State DMS-1 Medicaid preadmission instrument.

Long-Term Home Health Care Program—Nursing Home Without Walls

The New York State legislature established the Long-Term Home Health Care Program (LTHHCP), also known as the "Nursing Home Without Walls" Program, effective April 1, 1978. The program provides an alternative to institutionalization for Medicaid clients who meet the medical criteria for skilled nursing facilities (SNFs) or intermediate care facilities (ICFs). A maximum expenditure for home care has been set at 75 percent of the reimbursement rate in a locale for SNF or ICF levels of care for which the client is eligible.

The New York State Department of Social Services received Medicaid waivers in September 1978 under Section 1115 of the Social Security Act to assist in a three year demonstration of the program.

The purpose of the program is to reduce fragmentation in the provision of home care services to the aged and disabled through a single entry system which coordinates and provides these services in (currently) nine sites throughout the State. The single entry system coordinates and provides all of the services. The objectives of the project are to maximize the use of available resources, determine whether various types of providers are differentially successful in providing these services, compare the effectiveness of long-term care programs in different geographical areas, compare the program with traditional home health care provided by certified agencies, and promote cost containment.

191

As illustrated below, each of the nine sites shows a different pattern in development of its patient caseloads.

Sites	Operational Date	Caseload[1]	Capacity
Bronx—Montefiore Hospital	August 1979	54	100
New York City—St. Vincent's Hospital	September 1979	34	80
Queens—Visiting Nurse Service	May 1980	57	75
Brooklyn—Metropolitan Jewish Geriatric Center	May 1979	147	150
Buffalo—24 Rhode Island St. Nursing Home Co., Inc. N.Y.C.	November 1978	38	50
Buffalo—Erie County Department of Health	September 1979	51	100
Syracuse—Visiting Nurse Association of Central New York	March 1979	42	100
Syracuse—Onondaga County Department of Health	March 1979	79	125
Olean—Cattaraugus County Department of Health	April 1979	18	25

---

[1] As of the end of February 1981.

Under LTHHCP, all patients must be eligible for Medicaid and need either SNF or ICF levels of care. For all potential program users, a medical assessment abstract must be completed which produces a predictor score, referred to as the DMS-1 score. The DMS-1 assessment instrument is used in New York State as a tool to determine the appropriate placement of patients in long-term care facilities. When patients are determined to be eligible for the LTHHCP program, an LTHHCP nurse and a caseworker from the local (State) social service district complete a joint, in-home assessment. The caseworker then develops a plan of care and initiates a budget review. This budget review determines whether the total projected costs are within 75 percent of the monthly average Medicaid costs of the going rate for SNF or ICF levels of care for which the client is eligible. A reassessment is conducted every 120 days and a physician reviews patient care needs every 60 days.

The LTHHCP coordinator and caseworker coordinate the services and the case management functions. Professional support must be available to patients through an emergency, on-call system 24 hours a day.

In the initial phases, the State Department of Social Services and Health Systems Management, together with State Senator Lombardi (the author of the LTHHCP legislation), met with local commissioners at each district site to familiarize them with the program and facilitate program implementation. In addition, the State met with hospital discharge planners to make them aware of the program and worked with the local social service districts to train staff and provide technical assistance. However, the project experienced some difficulties in starting. Staff turnover, problems in coordination, and difficulty in obtaining referrals delayed the project. There was also a delay in the enactment of State legislation authorizing financial participation for reimbursement of the seven waived services under the Section 1115 demonstration authority. The implementation guidelines for paying for these waived services became effective in September of 1980. The services are home maintenance, nutrition counseling/educational services, respiratory therapy, respite care, social day care, transportation, congregate meal services, moving assistance, housing improvement services, and medical-social services. For evaluation, the project will also collect primary data on a comparison population for analysis by Abt Associates, Inc. (the HCFA evaluator).

The project has resolved some of its problems by establishing three additional State monitoring staff positions to provide site assistance. Project staff are working with the evaluator to coordinate and develop the data collection strategy. Because there have been delays in the joint assessment process to determine patient eligibility, an "alternative entry procedure" was established, which allows the provider to begin service to the patient immediately based on the provider's initial assessment of the patient. A joint assessment is then conducted with the local social service district.

In the New York City area, where there are four sites, a long-term care task force has been established with participation from the sites and the New York City Human Resources Administration to facilitate communication and coordination of efforts in program implementation.

In addition, the following legislative modifications, passed by the State legislature in June 1980, have facilitated project operations:

• Patient slots have been reallocated among the nine approved sites through a change in the State Hospital Code and legislation authorizing the Commissioner of Health to stipulate the maximum number of persons that LTHHCP may serve.

193

- Passage of a Senate bill will put the 75 percent cap on an annual basis so that if it is reasonably anticipated that average expenditures for a year's time will not exceed the cap, the patient can be admitted to the program.
- The eligibility requirement in the LTHHCP program has been amended to require that the patient be "medically eligible" for placement in a residential health care facility.

The State recently expanded the LTHHCP program to include four additional sites: Jewish Home and Hospital for the Aged, New York City; Visiting Nurse Association of Staten Island; Rockland County Health Department; and Elderly Geriatric Center, Troy, New York.

Multipurpose Senior Services Project (MSSP)

In September 1977, the State enacted AB998, which required the State Health and Welfare Agency to establish state-wide MSSP sites to test single entry access to the health and social services system through case management, care planning, and needs assessment. In October 1979, the State Health and Welfare Agency received a "waiver-only" grant under Section 1115 of the Social Security Act to implement the MSSP demonstration over a four year period. The project began to provide services at some sites in April 1980.

The target population comprises persons 65 and over who are considered at risk of institutionalization and who meet the State eligibility requirements for Medi-Cal (Medicaid). There will be 1,900 participants in the MSSP; 960 will compose the comparison group sample. The sample is being drawn from Medi-Cal eligibles from the community, acute care hospitals, and skilled nursing facilities (SNFs).

The project has received Medicaid waivers to provide certain health-related and social services which are not otherwise provided. These include:

- adult social care
- housing assistance
- in-home support services
- legal services
- non-medical respite care
- non-medical transportation
- meal services
- protective services
- specialized communication
- preventive health care.

During the first operational year, the two most frequently used services across all sites were in-home support services and non-medical transportation.

194

Other services are being provided from existing State funds under Title XIX and XX of the Social Security Act and Title III of the Older Americans Act, as well as the State General Fund. The sites must use these and other available community resources before using waived services.

The demonstration has both comparative and operational objectives. The comparative objectives are to reduce clients' numbers of hospital days, to reduce clients' numbers of SNF days, to reduce total expenditures on social and health services for clients, and to improve or maintain clients' functional abilities. The operational objectives are to estimate the effectiveness of existing services, to compare sites to achieve a more effective mix of long-term care, to estimate optimal expenditures for client care while reducing SNF and hospital patient days, and to eliminate optimal expenditures for client care while improving or maintaining clients' functional abilities.

Individual MSSP sites were required to meet specific State-prescribed criteria before becoming operational. The eight sites are:

- Jewish Family Services, Los Angeles
- East Los Angeles Health Task Force
- Senior Care Action Network, Long Beach
- Mount Zion Hospital and Medical Center, San Francisco
- City of Oakland
- Greater Ukiah Senior Citizens Center
- County of Santa Cruz
- San Diego County Area Agency on Aging.

During the first developmental year, MSSP launched a public relations campaign to inform key State and local officials and agencies about the project. MSSP also conducted comprehensive planning, hired staff, and trained personnel.

The project developed, tested, and finalized a uniform patient assessment instrument. This instrument is in two parts: social assessment and medical assessment. It is administered by a nurse practitioner and a social worker. The instrument is currently being refined further, based on experience at the sites to date.

MSSP has developed the data collection procedures for the participant's information, designed a system to analyze the effectiveness of the program, and designed a computerized management information system (MIS).

During the second year of the project, preliminary reports of Medi-Cal utilization trends, unit costs of services, and the impact of case management hours on client outcomes will become available.

195

Mt. Zion Hospital Long-Term Care Demonstration Design and Development

The Mt. Zion Hospital and Medical Center is conducting a three year Medicare demonstration under Section 222 of the Social Security Act to implement a hospital-based, long-term care services delivery system in a designated service area. This model builds upon components of Mt. Zion's existing geriatric services, including acute care, emergency health services, outpatient services, home care, and information and referral. A consortium of five service providers under the direction of Mt. Zion will cooperate to provide a range of health and social services to the frail elderly in the designated catchment area.

The project is providing centralized intake and case management, including assessment, care planning, and case monitoring. It tests the ability of a consortium of service providers to provide more accessible, appropriate, and cost-effective care.

The project has received waivers to provide certain health-related and social services which are not otherwise provided under Medicare. These include:

- day care services
- homemaker services
- chore services
- home delivered meals
- interpreter services
- respite care
- discharge assistance
- drugs and biologicals
- audiology services, including hearing aids
- optometry services, including eye glasses and contact lenses
- podiatry services, including orthopedic footwear and other supportive devices
- dental care, including prosthodontics
- adaptive and assistive equipment
- transportation of patients by specialty vehicles, cabs, and other private and public means
- case management services
- mental health counseling
- prosthetic and orthotic appliances.

The project uses the Patient Status Assessment instrument, which was used for the Public Health Service Section 222 experiments on adult day health care and homemaker services. This instrument has been expanded to include items which are necessary for care planning and determination of appropriate patient placement. Material from the Monroe County, N.Y. (ACCESS) instrument was used in the revisions. The resulting instrument has been field-tested extensively, further revised, and validated.

The project developed a formal program to train project staff in assessment, care planning, and case management functions. In addition, Mount Zion has established a seminar program to provide project staff, as well as consortium members and other hospital personnel, an opportunity to increase long-term care information. Knowledgeable individuals from the Mount Zion Medical Center and the community are leading the seminars.

The project will have a caseload of 200 experimentals and 100 controls. Its final report will be due in the late summer of 1982.

North San Diego County Long-Term Care Project

This demonstration compares client benefits and costs of care of existing long-term care services and those provided under the project. The project will provide a comprehensive, coordinated system of long-term care for Medicare beneficiaries age 65 and over. The hypothesis to be tested is that a coordinated system of long-term care service delivery for Medicare beneficiaries 65 and over, providing continuity of care with a wide array of in-home, community-based, and institutional resources and stressing client education for self-care and client participation in care plan development, will yield optimal health status and functional independence and help to contain the overall costs of health care.

The project established broad goals: (1) to demonstrate that a Medicare-certified provider of home health services with a range of supplementary in-home support services and an established system of community-wide linkages is an appropriate and cost-effective source of long-term care; (2) to assist the frail elderly, chronically ill, and disabled persons 65 and over to achieve and maintain an optimum level of health, self-care and functional independence in their own homes and cultural environments; and (3) to ensure appropriate and acceptable out-of-home placement only after a thorough exploration of personal and community resources demonstrates that needs cannot be met at home.

The project builds upon existing Medicare-covered, home health services provided by the Allied Home Health Association and the Visiting Nurse Association. Through this delivery model, the project links an existing information and referral network with a centralized single entry system. Project services include professional assessment of client needs, client participation in care plan formulation, and case management. The project contracts with providers for delivery of services.

The project will provide the following services under the Section 222 waiver authority:

197

- adult day care
- home delivered meals
- homemaker services
- escorted transportation
- educational services to enable the patient to follow the physician's instruction for self-care.

Approximately 500 experimental and 250 control participants will be randomly selected for the project.

During the first developmental year, the project revised a patient assessment instrument which has been used by the Allied Home Health Association to include items of broader scope. The instrument provides four levels of information: patient assessment needs, services of existing community providers, services provided by the patient's informal support system, and Medicare-waived services specific to the long-term care project.

The project has trained the initial assessment teams and provided special training for project nurses and social workers in care planning and case management. It has also obtained the commitment of local service providers and referral sources and begun accepting referrals for assessment and case planning.

FIG Waiver Continuum of Care Project for the Elderly

HCFA awarded a grant to the Oregon Department of Human Resources in September 1979 to test the provision of alternative, community-based services to the elderly in a five county area in the southwestern part of the State. This demonstration was funded for the first year of a three year project under the authority of Section 1115 of the Social Security Act. The project has also received a grant from the Administration on Aging to support administration costs and an evaluation component for the project. The HCFA project became operational in January 1980.

The two components of the project—FIG (Flexible Intergovernmental Grant) and the Section 1115 waivers—share the same objective: to serve the elderly more appropriately and contain Medicaid costs. It was expected that each component used separately would affect both problems to some extent; however, use of both of the components together in one of the five counties would ideally maximize the impact on deficiencies in the current system.

The FIG component directly addresses deficiencies in service delivery stemming from uncoordinated, unintegrated service delivery by diverse agencies serving the elderly. It has been designed to address the problems involved with a multiple agency, multiple entry, service delivery system without increasing the available fiscal resources and without initially changing any agency's internal structure. It has the following characteristics:

198

- It depends on a local policy committee (with representatives from all of the agencies which serve the elderly) for local accountability and decision-making.
- It makes available to each agency, for information and referral purposes, a profile of all other agencies which serve the elderly in the local area.
- It uses a common functional assessment tool to assist decision-makers in standardizing placement choices.
- It uses a common data base which returns to each agency an internal report on its own operation and an external report on how that agency fits into the total system.

The waiver component addresses fiscal imbalance in the service system due to Federal funding patterns which encourage Medicaid institutionalization. This is accomplished through the State guaranteeing, as a condition to the waiver, that it will spend no additional Medicaid funds above the projected amount. In fact, no Medicaid funds will be available for alternative services each month until the State can show that it has reduced projected expenditure levels and that 90 percent of the Title XX funds available for these alternatives have been encumbered.

The five sites and their respective research conditions are Josephine County (FIG only), Jackson County (FIG and waiver), Coos/Curry Counties (waiver only), and Douglas County (comparison).

Each site is conducting assessment, care planning, and case management, with follow-up by county personnel. The project is targeted to individuals 65 years or older who are eligible for Medicaid and Title XX benefits and have been assessed as eligible for in-home services instead of nursing home placement.

Certain health-related and social services which are not otherwise provided under Title XIX are provided under waiver authority in the two waiver counties only. These include:

- homemaking and housekeeping services
- chore services
- home delivered meals
- adult foster home services
- adult residential services
- limited transportation services.

The specific objectives of the FIG/waiver project are:

- to overcome fiscal imbalance and service delivery deficiencies in the current Title XIX program,
- to achieve cost containment,
- to provide alternative, community-based service to elderly persons to delay or prevent institutional placement, and

199

- to provide more appropriate in-home health services without increasing current fiscal resources allotted to institutional and in-home Titles XIX and XX program components.

The project's basic patient assessment instrument, which was developed by the State prior to the current demonstration, is the Placement Information Base (PIB). Although shorter than most instruments currently used in demonstration projects, the PIB contains the important items that provide information on which to base a decision to maintain a person in his or her own home. The items are organized to obtain pertinent information regarding an individual's ability to communicate, to ambulate, to manage the living environment, to perform both activities of daily living and instrumental activities, and to handle financial affairs. The instrument is currently being used state-wide for adult services by county agency personnel, by providers (for referrals made to the project), and by project staff. A training program has been developed for all project staff to ensure uniform application of the expanded assessment instrument in the five county area.

Results to Date by County

Josephine County (FIG only)

Since project implementation, nursing home expenditures and caseloads have been well below predicted levels. Community-based care expenditures and caseloads have been consistently higher than the predicted levels mainly due to the FIG component and increased utilization of housekeeper and personal care services, home delivered meals, and residential care facilities (all of which are part of the current Oregon State plan).

Jackson County (FIG and waiver)

Since project implementation, community-based caseloads and expenditures have been considerably above predicted levels. Nursing home caseloads and expenditures have been well below predicted levels.

Coos/Curry Counties (waiver only)

Experience in the first three quarters of the project shows that the nursing home caseload has increased substantially compared to the predicted caseload with or without project intervention. Nursing home expenditures have increased less but are still higher than those predicted with project intervention.

Douglas County (comparison)

Caseloads and expenditures for the nursing home program continue as expected. Both community-based care caseloads and expenditures remain above predicted levels in this county. However, the increase in utilization of community-based services has not significantly affected nursing home growth. The project results in the FIG only and the FIG/waiver counties are similar. Both counties have consistently reduced expenditures of Medicaid funds for nursing home care. The FIG component continues to have significant impact on the long-term care system in both counties. Results in the waiver only and the comparison counties reinforce the tentative conclusion that local agency cooperation and planning are vital in preventing or delaying nursing home placement.

Providing additional financial resources (for example, waivers) without other intervention (as in the FIG component) has not significantly affected nursing home growth in the five counties involved in the project.

The final report was submitted in 1982.

Ancillary Community Care Services

The Florida Department of Health and Rehabilitative Services is conducting a three year, "waiver only" demonstration project under Section 1115 of the Social Security Act, to develop and test ancillary community care services for the chronically impaired elderly.

The purpose of the project is to establish in five Florida counties (Broward, Dade, Duval, Pinellas, and Polk) a model of preventive, maintenance, and restorative health care systems for Medicaid eligibles, who are age 60 or over, non-institutionalized, and functionally impaired. The project's goals include the following: a) to assist persons 60 years of age and older identified as "at risk" of institutionalization to remain in the community by helping them maintain a level of self-sufficiency with health and related services not provided under the State's Medicaid program; b) to conduct a study of individuals receiving ancillary community care services to determine the effectiveness of community-based, socio-medical services; c) to evaluate the organizational structures and costs related to each site, including client impact, staffing, annual budgets, urban/rural orientation, service cost, referral networks, and incidence of undetected health problems.

Each of the five county agencies will be responsible for the development of individual care plans, case management, and contracting for services with local providers. The demonstration project consists of three major components:

- a comprehensive medical-social assessment (CMA) designed to a) provide a comprehensive health examination and a functional assessment and b) collect information about the general health, mental health, physical impairments, availability of social resources, unmet needs, and living conditions of older persons

201

- a case management system
- six ancillary community care (waived) services, including personal care services, specialized home management services, medical therapeutic services, respite services, day treatment services, and medical transportation services.

During the first developmental year of the project, the following tasks were completed:

- Key staff, including the project director, deputy director and data specialist, were recruited and oriented.
- The project developed a protocol manual for implementation.
- The project also developed a training program for the five sites and trained the Duval County personnel. This site will help to orient and train the personnel recruited for the next sites.
- The project initiated working relationships with the State Medicaid program.
- The existing State Medicaid management information system (MMIS) was modified to track all project expenditures, and the project has arranged with Blue Cross to perform a similar service for Medicare services and costs.
- The State Office of Evaluation developed and implemented plans for on-going evaluation of the project.

Community Long-Term Care Project

The South Carolina Department of Social Services is conducting a three year demonstration under Section 1115 of the Social Security Act to test community-based client assessment, services coordination, and provision of alternative services and to develop proposals for permanent modification of the State Medicaid program. The project has also received funds from the Appalachian Regional Commission to pay part of its administration costs. A major goal is to establish a community network of services to help disabled and elderly individuals remain in their communities. The network will have a self-sustaining, community structure without a separate coordinating agency.

Key operational components of the project include community-based client assessment, reassessment, and coordination of services which are alternatives to institutionalization. The population to be served comprises Medicaid-eligible, elderly individuals with functional disability who are at risk of nursing home placement. Two thousand individuals are expected to enroll in the project over the demonstration period (55 percent of caseload from the community; 45 percent from nursing homes). The control group will be random.

The project will provide certain waived health-related and social services which are not otherwise covered under Medicaid. These include homemaker, chore, respite care, alternative housing, home delivered and congregate meals, and adaptive equipment in the home.

The project includes three project sites, located in three different counties (Spartanburg, Union, and Cherokee). Each county site is establishing an advisory committee. The advisory committees will assist the sites in identifying service needs and priorities for new service development.

A major objective of this project is to facilitate cooperation among service providers at the community level. It will coordinate the existing Medicaid, Medicare, and Title XX services for project participants.

The assessment instrument designed for the project was based closely on the instrument developed by the Monroe County, N.Y. ACCESS project. The South Carolina instrument has been revised to meet the unique needs of this primarily rural project. Training has been provided to project staff in the areas of assessment, care planning, and case management.

The project became operational in July 1980 in each of the three counties. Strong support has been provided by the South Carolina State Long-Term Care Council. A Legislative Advisory Committee is providing liaison between the project and the State legislature. In addition, the State has appropriated more money for the project.

Modification of the Texas System of Care for the Elderly: Alternatives for the Institutionalized Aged

The Texas Department of Human Resources (DHR) is conducting a three year "waiver-only" demonstration project under Section 1115 of the Social Security Act. The project will develop and test a comprehensive continuum of care for the aged that is appropriate in terms of quality of care, preferences of recipients, and costs.

This demonstration was initiated as a result of a State legislative mandate to eliminate unnecessary and inappropriate use of nursing home services. The mandate requires DHR to eliminate one of the two Medicaid ICF levels of care (ICF II) and to provide community-based services to patients who can be deinstitutionalized.

As of March 1980, the distinction between ICF II and ICF III was eliminated so that only a single ICF program (in conformance with Federal regulations) now exists below the SNF level. Some of the individuals who were receiving benefits in ICF II are being deinstitutionalized to community-based settings and provided with alternative, health-related services. The remaining individuals will be "grandfathered" into the single ICF program.

The project will assess a 5 percent sample of the 18,000 institutionalized patients in level II ICFs to determine their discharge potential. For those who are deinstitutionalized, the project will develop a care plan and arrange for in-home services through community service providers. In addition, the project will conduct case management, monitoring, and follow-up activities for participants.

The following services will be provided: Medicaid home care benefits, Medicaid personal care benefits, Title XX adult in-home services, and Section 1115 waived community-based, in-home support services.

The objectives of the project are to create a single ICF level of care (by eliminating level II), to increase the availability of alternative care services in communities, to develop a new State assessment instrument that is appropriate for institutional discharge planning, and to ensure appropriate, continuing care for current level II ICF patients.

As of March 1980, the State had terminated all new admissions to level II ICFs. It has revised standards for SNFs and ICFs and established new criteria for ICFs. In addition, the State has developed a plan for monitoring admissions to long-term care facilities.

The project became operational on March 1, 1981.

The State Planning and Evaluation Unit, located within the State Office of Management Services, will conduct an ongoing project evaluation. It will document that the system tests the objectives and evaluates the outcomes of the project.

Medicaid Physician Nursing Home Visitation Project

The primary objective of this project is to determine whether eliminating existing regulations which mandate the frequency and intervals of physician visits to nursing home residents will improve physician involvement in nursing home care, improve the quality of physician-patient interaction, and generally improve the quality of medical care.

The State Department of Social Services plans to contract with the Colorado Foundation for Medical Care to plan and implement the project. The Foundation is the Colorado Professional Standards Review Organization. Currently, the State Department of Social Services, through its Division of Medical Assistance, has a formal relationship with the Foundation.

The project will be carried out in four phases: developmental, pilot, implementation, and evaluation.

During the three year demonstration period, the following activities will receive emphasis:

- development of the research design and demonstration methodology

204

- development of the necessary criteria and standards for the project
- education of physicians and nursing home personnel
- assessment and monitoring of patient care planning efforts and physician performance
- analysis of research results and evaluation of the extent to which the research hypotheses were supported by the data.

Four hypotheses have been identified to prove or disprove the project's primary objective:

(1) A flexible framework of physician-patient encounters for long-term care residents, based on patient need, coupled with physician-patient care planning and supported by a prospecitve planning system in the facility, will change the distribution of patient-physician encounters.
(2) A flexible framework of physician-patient encounters, coupled with patient care planning, will improve quality of patient-physician interaction.
(3) A flexible framework of physician-patient encounters by itself will change the distribution of patient-physician encounters and will not negatively affect the quality of patient care.
(4) The costs of care will continue at the current level in a system where physician-patient encounters occur based on patient need rather than regulation.

The project participants will be divided into three groups: an experimental, a semi-experimental, and a control group. The experimental group will consist of facilities in which existing regulations for physician visitation will be waived. The physician will, instead, develop a patient care plan in which he or she will specify the frequency of physician-patient encounters required by the patients' conditions. The physician will be supported by a system of prospective patient care planning in the facility (that is, facility staff will be trained to operate such a system).

The semi-experimental group will comprise facilities in which existing regulations for physician visitation will be waived. However, there will be no instruction to the physician or the facility with regard to patient care planning.

The control group will consist of facilities which continue to operate under existing regulations and the existing methods for enforcing those regulations.

A total of 9 to 15 long-term care facilities will be selected to participate in this project. Ideally, three to five facilities will be assigned to each of the three study groups.

Data will be collected at specific time frames from each group of participating nursing homes to measure physician involvement in long-term care, physician-patient interaction, quality of care, hospital admission, and costs of care. The monitoring/intervention system will be measured using the management information system of the PSRO.

The research design will be a pre-test and post-test control group design subjected to a six-way analysis related to each of the three treatment groups prior to and during the project.

Four waivers will be granted under the authority of Section 1115 of the Social Security Act to enable the State to implement the project. These are: 1) statewideness to permit the project to be conducted in a sample of experimental facilities in the State; 2) current State and Federal requirements for extended stay review; 3) the visitation schedule, to permit physicians to develop their own schedules according to plans of care based on individual patient needs in ICFs and SNFs; and 4) the requirement for independent Medicare evaluations in SNFs, to permit the State to develop the project research, demonstration, and evaluation methodology in the SNFs.

The project was approved on February 25, 1981. Certain questions about the demonstration and research design require clarification before the project is implemented.

National Long-Term Care Demonstration

Pennsylvania

State Contractor

(DHHS) awarded a contract to the Pennsylvania Department of Public Welfare (DPW) to conduct a demonstration under the National Long-Term Care Demonstration Program. The Channeling Project is located in the DPW Office of Policy, Planning and Evaluation, Bureau of Research, Evaluation and Information Systems. The Office of Policy, Planning and Evaluation is directly responsible to the Secretary of the Department to provide overall direction and coordination for the many program offices within the Department.

The State Departments of Aging and Health helped to develop the proposal and have committed their continued involvement and support toward implementing the project. Before submitting a proposal to the Federal Department of Health and Human Services, the three departments formed an inter-departmental work group and developed a memorandum of understanding which set forth the roles and responsibilities of the group in planning the project. The work group delegated the Department of Public Welfare (DPW) to be the lead agency and recommended that DPW administer the project if it were approved for funding.

206

A long-term care planning group, which includes the original inter-departmental work group, will prepare a State long-term care plan. A working subcommittee, comprising senior staff representatives will assist the planning group. In addition, community-level organizations, consumers, and providers will have input into the planning process.

The Department of Public Welfare is subcontracting with the Philadelphia Corporation for Aging (PCA), a non-profit corporation, to conduct the channeling demonstration. (Philadelphia is the catchment area.)

Channeling Project Organization

The local project is an administratively distinct unit under the PCA's Office of the Assistant Director for Operations. The project director will be assisted by a staff which includes a service management supervisor, two caseworker supervisors, a nurse practitioner, two intake workers, and 12 caseworkers.

Channeling Functions

Outreach/Case Finding: The project will educate agencies about the project and develop relationships with potential referral sources. Referral protocols will be developed along with public information materials.

Screening: Two intake workers, under the direct supervision of the project director, will screen potential participants. As caseloads begin to approach capacity, however, one of the intake workers will be moved to a caseworker position, and a single worker will continue the screening process.

Assessment: Caseworkers with a minimum of a bachelor's degree will assess program participants. These caseworkers will be employed by the PCA and will be supervised by two supervisors with masters' degrees. All assessments will be reviewed by a casework supervisor and the nurse practitioner. When further health care assessment is required, the nurse practitioner may visit the client with the caseworker or recommend an appropriate resource for specialized assessment. Consultant assessment will be arranged through the service management supervisor.

Case Management: Following the assessment and after contacting all client relatives and acquaintances, previous service providers, if any, and/or others who might offer useful information for care planning, a caseworker will develop a care plan for the client. (The above contacts are only made with the client's consent.) The care plan will be reviewed by the worker's supervisor and the nurse practitioner. Then the worker will discuss the care plan with the client, obtain client consent, and initiate service arrangements.

The caseworker will monitor the care plan with service providers, the client and family members, or informal resource networks. The project will develop a process to facilitate feedback from the service provider to the caseworker following the initiation of service.

Monitoring and Reassessment: Caseworkers will monitor the progress of their clients, contacting them at least once each month. They will reassess clients every six months, and determinations will undergo the same review process as the initial assessments. If appropriate, however, clients may be reassessed before six months are up.

Services Audit and Program Review: The Philadelphia Health Management Corporation will audit services and review the program.

Client Caseload: The project expects to serve a caseload of between 720 and 780 clients for which the ratio of clients per worker is expected to range between 60:1 and 65:1.

Texas

Introduction

Through the passage of legislation in 1979, the State has promoted new alternate care services and committed funds to develop community-based programs. In response, the Texas Department of Human Resources, the Governor's Committee on Aging, and other State agencies working in the long-term care network are increasing their efforts to change the delivery system. The Texas Long-Term Care Channeling Demonstration Project, awarded to the Texas Department of Human Resources in 1980, represents an important step in this direction.

Long-Term Care Planning Group

The State long-term care planning group is composed of agency commissioners or lead executives and citizens knowledgeable about long-term care. Two public forums were held in July 1981 in support of the activities of the group. Participants included the 76 State delegates to the White House Conference on Aging, consumers, providers, and policymakers.

Demonstration Site

Houston is the site which will demonstrate channeling. The administering agency is the Texas Research Institute of Mental Sciences Gerontology Center (TRIMS). TRIMS is a research, training, and service facility of the Texas Department of Mental Health and Mental Retardation located in the Texas Medical Center. The project's catchment area includes the Houston central business district and communities to the west, north, and south of the business district. The area includes the incorporated community of Jacinto City. Drawing from this catchment area, TRIMS expects to have a caseload of 370 in the first year.

Project Organization

TRIMS will have 11 staff members. It will directly employ 9 staff members and will subcontract to hire an experienced case manager from Sheltering Arms, a United Way agency, and a case manager from the Houston Department of Human Resources Regional Office.

Since implementation of the project will depend upon interagency collaboration, TRIMS has established a Management Advisory Board and a Channeling Operations Group. The Advisory Board will provide input and review decisions pertaining to the design of service procedures, community relations, public information activities, and interagency agreements. The Operations Group, which will be composed of representatives from the provider agencies serving 50 or more project clients, will convene to review care plans and complex cases.

Channeling Functions

Outreach/Case Finding

The project will conduct case finding and outreach activities to identify a broad spectrum of potential clients, reflecting the diverse population of the catchment area. Referral agreements with community agencies will establish multiple access points to identify potential clients. In addition, the project will establish linkages with police, medical practitioners, and hospitals. Where possible, the referring agency will be encouraged to confer with the site intake specialist directly so that the agency or potential clients who contacted the project directly can be notified of acceptance or rejection from the project without unnecessary delay.

Screening

Because of the importance of the screening function, one staff member will devote his or her total time to screening. This individual will be located at TRIMS Gerontology Center, which will serve as the screening and entry point. As required by the request for proposal, the site screening staff will be administratively separate from the case management staff, with offices in a different location. The intake specialist will receive incoming and in-house referrals of potential clients, gather and record background information on each client using the screening instrument, identify control and experimental clients on a random basis, and link the clients appropriately for information and referral to the project or to other community agencies.

209

Assessment

A case manager or a supervisor on the channeling staff will assess clients. However, in a small percentage of cases, two channeling staff members will assess a particular client. Situations that might warrant this include cases where a married couple is involved, where the client's environment is potentially unsafe, or where specialized consultations are necessary.

Using the prescribed assessment instrument, case managers will conduct at least one home visit or in-person visit to complete the initial assessment. They will also make telephone and face-to-face contacts to obtain more detailed information to complete the assessment. Signed releases of information will be requested to obtain any appropriate written records from sources of medical and/or psychiatric treatment. During weekly supervisory conferences, each case manager will review new assessments with his/her supervisor (nurse or supervising counselor), who is responsible for ensuring uniformity in the assessment procedures.

Case Management

Working with the providers, the case manager will develop a care plan matching available resources with client needs. The client and involved service providers must consent to the plan before it is implemented. With the written consent of the client, a copy of the written care plan will be shared with involved providers of service and discussed with the informal support system so all involved parties understand their respective relationships. The Houston site will ensure that the record forms developed for clients include the eligibility information necessary for the case manager to negotiate public program services.

Monitoring and Reassessment

The responsible case manager will monitor service delivery and changing circumstances of clients. Some cases will require more intensive follow-up, particularly as services are first initiated or are being changed for any particular reasons. Clients with a functioning informal support system will need more routine follow-up. All project clients will be routinely reassessed at least every six months. The timing of individual reassessments will be based on the individual's functional status or significant change in his or her living environment.

Services Audit and Program Review

The Houston channeling staff will cooperate with the Department of Human Resources and the Governor's Committee on Aging to develop standards to evaluate project activities and will assist the Program Review and Evaluation Division in evaluating channeling activities and developing plans for corrective action.

Client Caseload

The proposed, average, annual caseload for the Houston channeling site is 370. Decisions regarding the rate of intake, average annual caseload, and caseload per worker are based on information on the catchment area, anticipated needs of multi-problem channeling clients, and the previous service experience and management data of the proposed channeling agency and the Texas Department of Human Resources. The Houston channeling site will complete approximately 55 comprehensive assessments per month at the beginning of the project and 27 per month once the full caseload is reached. Each of the case managers will have an average caseload of 70 clients, and the supervisors will have a caseload of 45 clients.

Hawaii

State Contractor

The Governor of the State of Hawaii designated the State Department of Social Services and Housing as the lead agency for the National Long-Term Care Demonstration Project. Within the Department, The Public Welfare Division has leadership responsibility for the project. The Public Welfare Division provides two major types of services: 1) income maintenance and economic and medical assistance (including the Title XIX and food stamp programs) and 2) social services programs (including the Title XX and State-funded service programs).

At the State level, the staff includes a project administrator, a planner, and assistance from the Assistant Public Welfare Administrator. The State staff will assist the State Long-Term Care Planning group.

Demonstration Site

The Oahu Branch, Department of Social Services and Housing, located in Honolulu, is responsible for administering and implementing the community-based project. The State has named the program Project Malama. Malama is a Hawaiian word meaning to care for, to keep, to preserve, and to observe. The central channeling unit, or Project Malama, will function as part of the Oahu Branch Administration. The Oahu Branch has units in the catchment area which process applications for money payments, food stamps, and Medicaid, and provide services to recipients.

The project organization will include interdisciplinary teams, a project director, and a project coordinator. The teams will include nurses and social workers. Every effort will be made to have the staff of Project Malama representative of Hawaii's multi-ethnic and multi-lingual population. The project expects to have a caseload of 475.

The interdisciplinary teams will administer the assessment instrument. Specialists from the medical, psychological, and occupational and physical therapy professions will assist in the assessments and participate in case conferences for clients with complex problems. The assessment team will review each client's assessment to identify problems and establish priorities in preparation for developing a care plan. The project recognizes the need to actively involve the client's family and informal support system in the care planning process.

The project coordinator will be primarily responsible for coordinating the assessment. He or she will assign cases to teams, maintain a client flow chart, review cases and completed forms, and approve requests for the use of consultants.

The interdisciplinary teams will monitor and reassess cases. While the teams will reassess clients every six months, reassessments may be conducted more often based on significant changes in a client's functional abilities and living environment.

Services Audit and Program Review

The Medical Care Administration Services of the Department of Social Services and Housing will audit services and review the program.

Client Caseload

A client caseload of 475 is projected by the end of the first year.

Maine

Introduction

DHHS awarded a contract to the Maine Department of Human Services under the National Long-Term Care Channeling Demonstration. The Department is the State's umbrella agency for health and social service programs with responsibility for administering the Title XIX and XX programs of the Social Security Act and Title III of the Older Americans Act.

The Bureau of Maine's Elderly within the State Agency on Aging was designated by the Department of Human Resources as the lead agency for planning and implementation at the State level. The Bureau Director has the overall responsibility for contract management. The State-level project staff consists of a program manager, project officer, research associate, and human services manager.

Background

Because of Maine's commitment to provide a broad mix of community-based health and social services, the Governor convened a Task Force on Long-Term Care for Adults in October of 1979 and appointed key government officials, consumers, interested citizens,

212

legislators, health care providers, and advocacy groups to it. The task force met in subcommittees and working groups to analyze long-term care issues. The report of the task force was published in September 1980. It will be of major significance to the work of the State Long-Term Care Planning Group.

Long Term Care Planning Group

The State has established two distinct (although related) planning groups. The State Long-Term Care Planning Group will consist of Bureau Directors from the Department of Human Services and the Department of Mental Health and Corrections. The composition of the group is consistent with the planning and decision-making structure of the Department and represents a concerted effort to integrate long-range planning for long-term care services into the mainstream of current activities. A second group, which will be directly coordinated with the first, will focus specifically on the operational aspects of the long-term care channeling contract. This group will be chaired by the Director of the Bureau of Maine's Elderly. Members of this group will also include Bureau Directors and representatives of community agencies and other units of State government.

Demonstration Site

The local community demonstration site will be administered under a subcontract with Southern Maine Senior Citizens, Inc., an area agency on aging in Portland. This agency is a voluntary, non-profit group run by a citizen board of directors. The catchment area for the project comprises Cumberland and York counties, which represent an urban, suburban, and rural mix. The case-load will be approximately 500 clients. The anticipated client-case manager ratio will be 60 to 75 cases per individual services coordinator.

Project Organization

The Director and planner of Southern Maine Senior Citizens, Inc., will provide information and support to the site. The site, however, will be managed by a project site director, who will be accountable to the project officer in the Bureau of Maine's Elderly. The site director will be responsible for community education, general public relations, the establishment and monitoring of service linkages with providers, and the supervision of the two community service co-ordinators. These coordinators' responsibilities include participating in the development and implementation of policies and procedures for coordinating service delivery and supervising individual service coordinators. The six service coordinators will represent an interdisciplinary team with backgrounds in nursing, social work, and physical or occupational therapy.

213

Site-level activities will also receive input from a community-based advisory committee, Elders-at-Risk, which represents more than 30 provider and planning agencies, as well as from older persons in the region. The advisory committee will meet on a regular basis to provide community input into the development and operation of the project. The site director will provide staff assistance to the committee.

Channeling Functions

Outreach/Case Finding

The project has identified several community agencies, hospitals, nursing homes, housing authorities, senior citizen centers, and churches as potential sources of referrals. These community representatives will be encouraged to refer potentially eligible clients to agencies that will screen them. In addition, to ensure that the population with French as a first language is familiar with the project, bilingual flyers will be distributed through the referral network and into community social clubs to reach potential clients and their families.

Screening

Designated staff of Southern Maine Senior Citizens, Inc., and intake staff of provider agencies that have signed a memorandum of understanding will screen potential participants. They will exercise special care to inform potential clients about the long-term care demonstration project and the associated requirements for knowledge sharing (about information in records) and to obtain their signed consent if they agree to participate. The screening forms will be sent to the research associate at the Bureau of Maine's Elderly. Once the forms have been reviewed by the research associate, forms of those clients who are determined to be inappropriate for the project will be set aside. The research associate will randomly assign appropriate clients to control and experimental groups. The research associate will notify referral agencies about eligibility determinations. The agencies will then be able to link those clients who will not receive channeling services with the appropriate services in the community.

Assessment

The community service coordinator will assign clients to individual services coordinators for assessment, care planning, and all other aspects of case management. The individual service coordinators will use the standardized assessment instrument to assess channeling clients. Professionals who are not a part of the interdisciplinary team may conduct additional specialized assessments in preparation for care planning.

214

Case Management

Community service coordinators and individual service coordinators will hold case conferences to discuss and review the client's assessment, service needs, and frequency and duration of service provision. The conferences will also focus on the selection of provider agencies, considering the agencies' staffing patterns and types of services delivered.

The individual service coordinators will convene a meeting at which the client and a family member or significant other person are present, as are representatives of one or more provider agencies. Goals will be established and the prescribed services identified. The frequency and duration of these services will be discussed and agreed upon and the expected participation of family members clearly defined. The care plans will be shared with all provider agencies delivering services to the client.

Monitoring and Reassessment

The individual services coordinators will periodically contact clients and involved provider agencies. The agencies will re-evaluate and renegotiate services, depending upon the achievement of goals and changing client functional needs and home environment. Individual services coordinators will conduct formal reassessments every six months.

Services Audit and Program Review

The human services consultant, a full time State staff employee, will audit services and review the program. The consultant will work with the State Title XIX and XX agencies to develop and implement service audit and program review activities that build on, expand, or modify existing review procedures.

Client Caseload

The caseload is expected to be approximately 500 clients. The anticipated client-case manager ratio will be 60 to 75 cases per individual service coordinator.

Kentucky

The Kentucky Department for Human Resources has been awarded a contract to conduct a demonstration under the National Long-Term Care Demonstration Program. This department, an umbrella agency responsible for all human services throughout the State, is mandated by State statutes to develop, implement, regulate, and administer Kentucky's long-term care program. In this regard, the Department delegates long-term care functions to its various bureaus and offices.

The channeling project has a strong commitment from the Secretary for Human Resources for full financial and administrative support. The State project director also serves as the Director of Planning within the Office of the Secretary of the Department for Human Resources, and therefore reports directly to the Secretary. The channeling agency is a special unit of State government made up of staff directly employed by the Bureau for Social Services, Bureau for Social Insurance, and Bureau for Health Services. For the purposes of the demonstration, this unit and its personnel will be directly responsible to the State project director.

The channeling unit will pool the combined resources and experiences of the State service agencies. The Bureaus for Social Services and Health Services have statutory responsibilities for providing social services and health services to the State's citizens. A registered nurse will conduct comprehensive patient assessments. The Bureau for Social Insurance will provide an eligibility worker who will provide the technical expertise necessary for eligibility determinations. A further indication of State commitment is that the Bureau for Social Services is committed to match the $250,000 in services expansion funds which the local site will receive under the demonstration.

Eastern Kentucky, consisting of eight counties, comprises the local demonstration site. These counties are Jackson, Laurel, Clay, Harlan, Leslie, Perry, Knot, and Letcher Counties.

Long-Term Care Planning Group

The State Long-Term Care Planning Group, which consists of 20 members, is made up of key State policymakers and is chaired by the Secretary of the Department for Human Resources. Several subcommittees have been established to work with project and department staff in preparing reports for the planning group. The reports are designed to be the building blocks of the State plan. The planning group is expected to continue as an advisory group to the Secretary for Human Resources and as long-term care advocates beyond the completion of the State long-term care plan.

Local Project

The local project will be administered by a site director who will be directly accountable for the performance of all channeling functions and will be responsible to the State project director. The site director, assistant director, screening staff, and core channeling team will be centrally located for the convenience of the eight counties. A Long-Term Care Advisory Council will be established to assist the local site. This council will consist of service providers, provider agency board members, service recipients, and related sources who represent the geographical areas served. The chair-

216

person of the council will also serve on the State planning group to provide an appropriate link with the State planning effort.

Channeling Functions

Screening

The screening unit, which will be administratively separate from the other functions of the project, will be located at the Frontier Nursing Service in Hyden, Kentucky. Referrals will be received on a toll-free telephone line. The unit will be staffed by social workers with bachelors' degrees who have experience in working with long-term care clients.

The screeners are expected to travel extensively in the early months of the project to identify and cultivate relationships with various agencies, organizations, and other potential referral sources within the catchment area. Once the project begins to accept referrals, screening will be completed mostly by phone. However, in cases where clients have no access to a telephone, a face-to-face interview may be necessary. All referrals will be processed through the screening unit prior to any action by the channeling staff. The screening staff will work with the evaluation and technical assistance contractors who will provide guidance on the use of the screening instrument. Clients can be screened within one working day after referral. The local site director will supervise and monitor the screening.

Assessment

The channeling unit will consist of two components: a core team, including a registered nurse and an eligibility worker (from the Bureau for Social Insurance) and eight county-based caseworkers (one in each county).

Upon receipt of the intake screening document, the caseworker will schedule a face-to-face meeting with the client to discuss the purpose of the project. If the client agrees to participate, he or she will sign a consent form, allowing the caseworker to obtain and share specific information with service provider agencies. The caseworker will complete the standard assessment and any add-on assessment information which is approved by the Department of Health and Human Services. Finally, he or she will interview family members or service provider agencies if appropriate.

When completed, the assessment will be transmitted to the core channeling unit via telecopier. The nurse will review the client assessment for health needs and participate with the caseworker in care planning to ensure consideration of health and social needs. The eligibility worker will review the assessment to determine if the individual is in need of and eligible for public benefit programs. The assistant director will supervise the assessment function.

217

Case Management

The county caseworker will be responsible for case management. However, the core team will provide direct assistance and, in some instances, will be the key broker for specific service needs.

The caseworker, in concert with the client or responsible person, will review the service plan. The parties will negotiate an agreement and, based upon that agreement, the case manager will implement the service plan.

A system of county case conferences will be scheduled when multiple services needs are identified. These conferences will assist the case manager in implementing the plan and will be used consistently throughout the case.

County caseworkers who complete the assessments and manage the cases will be social workers with bachelors' degrees or masters' degrees and community-based experience. Both the channeling assessment and case management functions will be decentralized. Case managers will be located in each county Bureau for Social Services office to be accessible to the target population. To facilitate communications, telecopiers will be used to transmit information to and from caseworkers and the central location.

Reassessment and Monitoring

Monitoring the status of the client and the effectiveness of the care plan will be addressed in detail in a manual of operation. The caseworker and the core channeling team will reassess clients no less than every six months. Criteria will be developed to determine when a client needs to be assessed prior to the six month mandatory interval.

Service Audit and Program Review

The Kentucky Peer Review Organization will audit services and review the program.

Project Implementation Subgroup, composed of representatives from the State's Division for Field Services, will develop a manual of operation which will provide direct assistance to the State and the site director in developing policies and procedures to implement the project.

Caseload

The Kentucky Department for Human Resources expects to serve a caseload of 600 clients through this demonstration project. The anticipated ratio of clients to case managers will be 75:1.

218

Maryland

State Contractor

DHHS awarded a contract to the Maryland Office on Aging to conduct a demonstration under the National Long-Term Care Demonstration Program. A five member, State Long-Term Care Planning Group has been established to serve as the major policymaking group for Maryland's channeling project. In this regard, the Planning Group, which meets monthly, will develop the State long-term care plan.

The Planning Group, chaired by the Director of the Office on Aging, consists of high level policymakers from the Departments of Health and Mental Hygiene, Human Resources, and Budget and Fiscal Planning, and the Governor's office.

A project manager, planner, and community liaison representative compose the staff at the State level. In addition, a State advisory group has been proposed, which would consist of representatives from both private and public agencies throughout the State, as well as consumers.

The Office on Aging is subcontracting with the Baltimore City Commission on Aging and Retirement Education (CARE) to implement the demonstration at the local level. CARE, an umbrella agency, has given the responsibility of administering the project to the Baltimore Area Agency on Aging (AAA), the planning and coordinating arm of CARE. The site location is the city of Baltimore.

Channeling Project Organization

The channeling project director and the assistant director will share administrative functions. The director will be responsible for the overall supervision of the assessment and case management functions. The assistant director will supervise the case finding and screening functions.

The project director will report directly to the director of the area agency.

Channeling unit staff will include four screeners, two nurses, and two social workers. The case management functions, which will be decentralized, will be provided by three agencies under contract to the area agency.

The channeling project will build upon the CARE/AAA existing Coordinated In-Home Services Unit, which currently offers the following services to elderly individuals: intake, screening, and referral to one of the 14 participating health and social services provider agencies.

The Coordinated In-Home Services Unit will become the channeling agency, adding new responsibilities to its current ones. Under the new model, the unit will perform comprehensive assessments

219

using the standard assessment instrument to be designed for the demonstration program.

An existing advisory committee will be expanded to become the channeling agency advisory body. It will be composed of agency directors, provider staff, community leaders, and consumers.

Channeling Functions

Outreach/Case Finding

The area agency will launch an intensive effort to inform the Baltimore community about the channeling project to stimulate appropriate referrals. Such efforts will include meeting with special interest groups, advertising, and informing local decision-makers of the project's progress.

Screening

Intake workers who currently screen potential clients in the existing Coordinated In-Home Services Unit will continue to do so. An additional screener will be added to accommodate channeling referrals.

Assessment

Either a nurse or a social worker will assess clients in their homes. The completed assessment will be reviewed by the opposite member of the nurse/social worker team. If additional consultant expertise is needed, it will be obtained.

Case Management

After the assessment, those individuals accepted for channeling services will be assigned to a case manager. The decentralized case management functions will be provided by one of three agencies: the Baltimore City Department of Social Services (local department of the State agency responsible for Title XX funds), the Visiting Nurse Association (VNA), or the Baltimore Jewish Family and Children's Society. These are well-established professional agencies that together represent social/health and public/private backgrounds.

Case managers will be hired and housed by these three agencies, although administrative accountability of case management staff will be to the channeling director and advisory body. Case managers will be either nurses or social workers and they will serve only channeling clients.

Monitoring and Reassessment

Case managers are expected to continually monitor the services and client response. They will reassess clients at least every six months. Criteria for conducting reassessments prior to the six month required interval include the following:

- The client's needs are multiple, but one or more may be of short duration.
- The client's health is deteriorating.
- The provider agency recommends reassessment and possible revision of the care plan.
- The client's services are altered due to change in his/her situation.

Services Audit and Program Review

The University of Maryland's Department of Epidemiology and Preventive Medicine will audit services and review the program.

Client Caseload

An active caseload of 400 clients will be served through this project. The ratio of clients to case managers will be 40:1.

Florida

State Contractor

The contracting agency for the National Long-Term Care Demonstration Project in Florida is the Department of Health and Rehabilitative Services, within which the Aging and Adult Services Program Office manages the project.

A special channeling team, responsible to the Director of the Aging and Adult Services Program Office, administers the Long-Term Care Demonstration project. The team consists of a director, two professional people, and a staff assistant. It assists the interagency State Long-Term Care Planning Group in formulating a Florida Long-Term Care Plan. It also provides advice, oversight, and supervision to the local channeling site in Miami.

Responsibility for the overall management and for most of the core functions of the local site channeling project is in the hands of the Miami Jewish Home and Hospital for the Aged (MJHHA) at Douglas Gardens.

Channeling Functions

Outreach/Case Finding

Most of the core channeling functions will be centralized in MJHHA. However, MJHHA will often enlist the assistance and cooperation of several community health and social service agencies in carrying out the project. For example, the initial outreach and case finding function is lodged with MJHHA, but this effort will be coordinated among a wide range of community groups and organizations.

221

Screening

The screening process will be delegated to United Community Care, an independent, non-profit agency currently identified by the area agency on aging and Florida's Department of Health and Rehabilitative Services as the lead agency in the State's Community Care for the Elderly Program (CCE). Two specialists will screen applicants.

Assessment, Case Management, Reassessment

The key assessment, case management, and reassessment functions are the responsibility of MJHHA. Two people will administer the comprehensive assessment instrument, and their work will be reviewed by a channeling council composed of senior officials of MJHHA. Eight people, headed by a supervisor, will manage the cases.

Services Audit and Program Review

The Dade-Monroe PSRO, in conjunction with the Stein Gerontological Institute (a component of MJHHA), will audit services and review the program.

Client Caseload

The expected caseload for the Florida channeling project is 400 clients, an average of 50 clients per case manager.

Massachusetts

State Contractor

The contracting agency for the National Long-Term Care Demonstration Project in Massachusetts is the Department of Elder Affairs. This Department is both a cabinet-level secretariat and a State agency responsible for program development, planning, and advocacy on behalf of the State's elderly population. The Department also coordinates various funding resources to provide services to the elderly, including Title III of the Older Americans Act and Title XX of the Social Security Act. To plan and manage the project, the Department is collaborating with the Department of Public Welfare.

In addition to the Department of Elder Affairs and the Department of Public Welfare, there are seven other major departments which play a role in developing, operating, regulating, and/or financing services for the chronically ill and disabled elderly population: Department of Public Health, Department of Mental Health, Department of Social Services, Commission for the Blind, Rehabilitation Commission, Rate-Setting Commission, and the Executive Office of Communities and Development.

The Governor has designated a task force to develop a State long-term care plan. The task force comprises representatives of the State agencies involved in long-term care, the legislative committees, and the various Federal funding sources. Consumer and provider input will be solicited at two public forums which will be held during the planning phase of the project.

Channeling Project Organization

Greater Lynn Senior Services, Inc. (GLSS), will be the subcontractor for site activities. GLSS is a private, non-profit corporation which currently offers a variety of services for persons age 60 and over. It is the area agency on aging (Title III), a home care corporation (Title XX), and a multi-service center offering 14 different services. The agency has established working relationships with the two local hospitals, the home health agency, the nursing homes, the mental health center, and the Councils on Aging. The Department of Public Welfare has established a nursing home preplacement screening program called the case management screening project (CMSP) in the area.

As the subcontracting agency, GLSS will implement an outreach, referral, and screening system to identify channeling clients. GLSS will also employ direct service staff who will provide comprehensive assessment, case management, monitoring, and reassessment of clients. The staff will have direct access to certain services (homemaker, chore, transportation, day care, mental health counseling) and negotiated access to home health, acute health, and housing services.

The above-mentioned preplacement program of the Department of Public Welfare will also play a role in the demonstration project. Through a State-level, interagency agreement with the Department of Elder Affairs, the Department of Public Welfare's CMSP staff will be available to the project to approve or deny levels of care for Medicaid-eligible, channeling clients who may need to enter a long-term care facility. Additionally, the role of the CMSP staff will be expanded to include approval or denial of community-based and in-home services for Medicaid-eligible, channeling clients.

Channeling Functions

Outreach/Case Finding

The overall responsibility for performing the outreach and case finding functions will belong to GLSS, which now has an outreach component of 10 outreach workers and a supervisor. Area health and social service agencies will also perform outreach and case finding. Such agencies include the five Councils on Aging in the GLSS service area, the area agency advisory council, local senior centers, the mental health center, the Visiting Nurse Association, and area hospitals.

Screening

An information and referral/intake specialist from GLSS will screen project applicants. In addition, a CMSP nurse from the Department of Public Welfare will screen Medicaid-eligible clients to determine appropriateness for the channeling project.

Assessment, Case Management, and Reassessment

The key assessment, case management, and reassessment functions will be carried out by seven case managers using a prescribed assessment instrument. Once the assessment is completed, the case manager and supervisor will develop an initial care plan. For Medicaid-eligible channeling clients, the supervisor and case manager will be joined by the CMSP nurse for a review of the assessment and development of the care plan. These same case managers who completed the client assessments will continue on with the client in the case management function.

Services Audit and Program Review

The services audit and program review functions will be performed by an external cost and quality control audit team composed of staff from the Departments of Elder Affairs, Public Welfare, Public Health, and the Rate-Setting Commission.

Client Caseload

The expected client caseload is 450 clients. Seven case managers will serve an average of 65 clients each.

New Jersey

State Contractor

The contracting agency for the National Long-Term Care Demonstration Project in New Jersey is the Department of Human Services. This Department is New Jersey's major umbrella health and social service agency, responsible for Medicaid, public assistance, child welfare, mental health, the mentally retarded, energy assistance, and a host of smaller related programs. Two other programs vital to the contract, Title III of the Older Americans Act and State Health System Planning, are located respectively in the Department of Community Affairs and the Department of Health.

To administer the project, the Department of Human Services has created an Office of Long-Term Care Initiatives, staffed by a senior-level director, two project specialists, and one support specialist.

224

As part of the State-level functions under the project, a 55 member planning group is developing a State Long-Term Care Plan. The members of this body, all appointed by the Governor, are, by design, predominantly policymakers. The public at large may contribute through five public forums, to be held in each of the State's health systems agency (HSA) areas. Leadership of the group is shared by the Department of Human Services with the Departments of Health and of Community Affairs to underscore the interagency cooperation necessary to plan and implement long-term care policy in New Jersey.

Channeling Project Organization

Overall managment of the local site channeling project is the responsibility of the Middlesex County Department of Human Services, operating under subcontract to the New Jersey Department of Human Services. Within the County Department, a distinct Central Administrative Unit will be established to administer the subcontract. This unit will carry out several functions: management, planning, consultation and education, coordination, contract administration, and data collection.

While the County Department of Human Services will exercise management and oversight functions, it will rely on a series of second-tier subcontracts with other local agencies for the performance of core channeling functions, that is, providing help and service to the functionally impaired client.

Channeling Functions

Outreach/Case Finding

As mentioned earlier, various county and community agencies will provide the different channeling services. The tasks of outreach and case finding are assigned to area health and social service agencies, with the channeling project unit in the County Department of Human Services (in particular, the consultation and education specialist) responsible for gearing these efforts to reach isolated and often overlooked clients.

Screening

Screening will probably be performed by the Local Medical Assistance Unit (LMAU) of the New Jersey Division of Medical Assistance and Health Services, the State agency that authorizes, through assessment, the provision of certain health and medical services to persons eligible for the State Medicaid program. The LMAU will provide a separate three or four person unit composed of a social worker, one or two social work aides, and a clerk to perform the screening function for potential channeling clients.

225

Assessment, Case Management, and Reassessment

The Middlesex County Visiting Nurse Association (VNA) will carry out the key assessment, case management, and reassessment functions. A separate unit in the VNA will be established to perform these functions. The assessment instrument will be administered by five social workers and five nurses. These same 10 individuals will also function as case managers—not in teams—being redeployed as necessary to meet intake and caseload requirements. Generally, the individuals who complete the client assessment will *not* assume case management responsibility for the same client. The remainder of the channeling staff at the VNA will consist of a program director, an assessment and case management supervisor, and four clerical workers.

Services Audit and Program Review

Staff of the Central Jersey Health Planning Council will audit services and review the program at appropriate intervals.

Client Caseload

The expected caseload for the New Jersey Channeling Project is 700 to 800 clients. Eight to nine case managers will be serving an average of 90 clients each.

New York

State Contractor

The contracting agency for the National Long-Term Care Demonstration Project in the State of New York is the Office for the Aging, the single State agency that administers programs under the Older Americans Act, in addition to administering several State-funded programs. Two other programs essential to the project, Title XIX (Medicaid) and Title XX, are both located in the Department of Social Services.

There are five other State agencies that provide a wide range of services for the elderly and chronically impaired: the Office of Health Systems Management, the Office of Mental Health, the Office of Mental Retardation and Development Disabilities, the Health Planning Commission, and the Council on Home Care Services.

In addition to the demonstration project, the channeling award to the Office for the Aging includes a long-term care system development component. The State Health Planning Commission, in cooperation with the Office for the Aging, has responsibility for carrying out activities under this component and developing a State long-term care plan.

To carry out system development tasks, an interagency long-term care planning group has been created, composed of the directors

226

or deputy directors of the eight major State agencies involved in long-term care. The Director of the Office for the Aging and the Executive Director of the Health Planning Commission serve as co-chairperson. A major purpose of the planning group is to focus its attention on the delineation and development of interagency efforts to coordinate and manage long-term care resources. Conclusions and recommendations of the planning group will be integrated into New York State's long-term care plan.

The public at large will have an opportunity for input in the development of the plan through at least two public forums to be held during the planning phase of the project.

Channeling Project Organization

The Rensselaer County Department for the Aging will operate the channeling project at the site level. Within the Department for the Aging, the project will become an additional division comparable to the two existing Divisions of Services and Nutrition. This division will focus on solutions to service delivery problems in the long-term care system. The project director will report to the Commissioner of the Department, who in turn reports directly to the County Executive.

The Department, through its existing Division of Services, will screen people who may need long-term care services and will provide uniform assessment and case management for persons appropriate for channeling. The services of all three divisions within the Department will be closely coordinated.

Channeling Functions

Outreach/Case Finding

The tasks of outreach and case finding will be a function of the Division of Services Screening Unit, working with the general community and the existing service delivery network. The Unit will maintain contact with such community resources as churches, fraternal orders, local organizations, neighborhood groups, etc. Formal linkages will be established with a wide range of health care and social service providers and organizations. To encourage community involvement, project staff will undertake media and public education efforts.

Screening

The Division of Services will screen applicants using existing information and referral (I&R) staff throughout the network of six senior service and nutrition centers in the county. The central I&R unit (consisting of the I&R assistant, the program supervisor of I&R services, and the "project alert" staff person) will oversee the screening activities. In addition to conducting screenings, the central unit will serve as the conduit through which the six centers forward their screenings.

Assessment

Seven teams, each consisting of one case manager and one case aide, under the coordination of the senior case manager, will assess clients. Two registered nurses will administer the physical health and Activities of Daily Living (ADL) sections of the assessment instrument. Staff of the County Department of Social Services will be transferred to the channeling project to fill some of the case manager positions.

Case Management

The case management function will also use a team approach, each team consisting of the same case manager and case aide who initially assessed the client. The nurse will serve in a consultative role in case management. Formal procedural linkages will be established between the Department of Social Services Medicaid unit and the case managers. In cases where the client is Medicaid-eligible and the plan of care indicates a cost for home-based services over the average cost of nursing home care, the case will be referred to the Medicaid unit for authorization.

Reassessment and Monitoring

Case managers and case aides will periodically visit the clients' homes to assess their case. Reassessments will be performed at six month intervals by the same teams who performed the assessments.

Services Audit and Program Review

An outside contractor will audit services and review the program at appropriate intervals.

Client Caseload

The expected caseload is 600 clients. Of the seven case managers, four will serve an average of 75 clients in the rural areas, and three will serve 100 clients in the urban areas.

Ohio

State Contractor

The Ohio Commission on Aging, awarded a contract under the National Long-Term Care Demonstration Program, is a cabinet-level commission that advocates the interests of older people and administers social services under the Older Americans Act, as well as administering other State-funded programs.

228

The contractor is primarily responsible for developing a coordinated long-term care plan and policy recommendations, involving all State departments that provide services for the chronically impaired, older person. The State long-term care planning group, sponsored by the Commission on Aging, will develop information about both institutional-based and home/community-based services at the county level, to identify unmet needs and types of services required. The committee will also evaluate coordination among State agencies that plan long-term care services and will develop a strategy for improving the coordination of resources at the State level.

The State does not plan to perform the research and demonstration project itself. The actual demonstration will be carried out in Cuyahoga County. The demonstration is primarily the responsibility of the Western Reserve Area Agency on Aging (WRAAA), under an agreement with the Ohio Commission on Aging.

Channeling Project Organization

In Cuyahoga County, the WRAAA will implement the channeling demonstration. The project has been given the name of "COMPASS." COMPASS will direct all functions except screening of potential clients. Another organization, Senior Information Center, will screen applicants under an agreement with COMPASS.

The area agency's role is to plan for the needs of older people and to provide social services through Older Americans Act funds and the State's own aid to an independent living program in a five county area that includes Cuyahoga County. The area agency is governed by the County Board of Commissioners.

Channeling Functions

COMPASS will have a caseload of 750 clients, the majority of them over age 75. The clients will be moderately to severely limited in activities of daily living and not residing in an institution. Their conditions will require assistance on a regular basis from at least two service providers or informal caregivers for at least six months. These characteristics define the target group.

Outreach/Case Finding

To reach the target group, COMPASS will develop referral procedures with hospital discharge units, private practitioners, social agencies, and the County Welfare Department. Referrals will not be made directly to COMPASS, but to the Senior Information Center. The Center will provide routine information and referrals to people who are not referred to COMPASS.

For research purposes, clients will be randomly assigned to either an experimental group or a control group. The control group

229

does not receive services from COMPASS. As part of the research, the same assessment will be administered to both groups. However, the control group will be assessed by the research team and, if required, will be referred to the Senior Information Center for information and referral

Experimental clients are then referred to COMPASS. A central unit of nursing and social work staff, supervised by a case management coordinator, provides the core channeling functions at COMPASS. The nurse and social worker who assess the client will also develop the client's care plan, arrange for services, monitor the plan, and periodically reassess the client.

Assessment

A total of six social workers will be hired to assess clients. Each will have a caseload of 125 clients. In addition, there will be two registered nurses who will review the assessment and, if needed, conduct a follow-up assessment after consultation with the case management coordinator. One nurse will be assigned to three social workers. Discrepancies between the social work and nursing assessment will be addressed by the case management coordinator. The social workers will also decide whether consultation is needed with other professionals before completing the assessment. Funds are budgeted for consultation.

After assessment, a decision is made regarding whether the client should receive case management. Clients must meet the target group definition stated above. In addition, clients must reside in the catchment area, may not be currently a client of another community care agency, and must require two or more categories of service to maintain independence in the community.

The same assessor is responsible for planning care for a client. He or she will obtain further information from the client and family members during a home visit. The information will include such things as the client's financial matters, what the client is able to do, what personal services or modifications in the home environment are needed to overcome functional limitations in activities of daily living, what tasks family members are willing and able to perform for the client, and where family members need back-up help.

This information will enable the social worker to develop a care plan with the client and family regarding services to be provided by the family and by community agencies and when the client will be reassessed. The nurse will review all care plans.

Case Management

Social workers will manage the cases. COMPASS, the Western Reserve Area Agency on Aging, and the County Welfare Department will enter into agreements with service providers to accept all COMPASS clients referred by the case manager. Implementation of the care plan is the sole responsibility of the case manager.

Implementation of a care plan involves arranging for services and includes these procedures: determining eligibility under Medicare or Medicaid and determining the family's ability to either perform services or help pay for them; referring clients to agencies that are certified to accept third-party payments when the clients are eligible; referring clients to Title III or Title XX funded service agencies if no third-party payee is found; and referring clients whose families are not able to provide the services, who are not eligible for a third-party payee service, and for whom a Title III or Title XX service does not exist to the service expansion fund for payment. Referrals made by COMPASS will be followed-up with a return card system that signifies the agency's acceptance of the referral. Service providers are allowed to alter a care plan only after consulting the case manager and obtaining written agreement from COMPASS.

The case manager is also responsible for monitoring and reassessment. Monitoring involves ensuring that services prescribed and agreed to by an agency or family members are in fact provided. The case manager will correct deficiencies in services provided by families, while the case management coordinator is responsible for resolving routine problems in agency-provided services.

Reassessment and Monitoring

Every six months, the case manager will reassess the client and family (if indicated) using a modified version of the original assessment. All reassessments are to be reviewed by the nurse. Under the following circumstances, reassessment will occur earlier than every six months: acute illness requiring hospitalization, client's or family's dissatisfaction with the care plan, significant improvement or deterioration in the client's ability to perform activities of daily living, or a change in the client's relationship with the family or other caregiver.

Services Audit and Program Review

An external source, under contract with the local channeling agency, will audit services and review the program. The contractor will be selected by a Request for Proposal (RFP). The Ohio Commission on Aging will approve the subcontract.

Client Caseload

COMPASS will have a caseload of 750 clients, the majority of them over age 75.

Medicare/Medicaid Hospice Demonstration

Background

Hospice care in the United States is a relatively recent phenomenon aimed at helping terminally ill patients live with maximum comfort and minimal disruption to routine activity. Hospices emphasize palliative care to control pain and other symptoms of terminal illness. In addition, the hospice concept views the patient and family as a single unit. Many patients are able to remain at home with their families while receiving hospice services. Hospices employ a broad spectrum of professional and voluntary care givers who use a multidisciplinary approach to deliver social, psychological, medical, and spiritual services.

The Medicare and Medicaid programs do not currently recognize hospices as a separate provider category. However, some hospice organizations are participating in these programs within existing provider classifications (for example, hospital, skilled nursing facility, and home health agency). Some hospice services, such as drugs used in the home and bereavement visits to the patient's family, are not reimbursable under Medicare. State Medicaid programs have differing coverage of hospital, nursing home, and home health services, and many States do not cover certain services integral to hospice care.

Project Description

Because the concept is relatively new in this country, HCFA has implemented a hospice demonstration which permits the waiver of certain statutory and regulatory requirements to allow coverage of hospice services provided to Medicare beneficiaries and Medicaid recipients. The demonstration has a twenty-four month, experimental phase during which hospice services will be reimbursed. In addition, there will be a six month wind-down period which will allow coverage to continue for those patients who become participants at the end of the program. The project is likely to provide a basis for considering more flexible approaches to Medicare and Medicaid reimbursement of hospice services. The operational phase of the demonstration began on October 1, 1980.

Twenty-six sites were selected for participation in the HCFA hospice demonstration program. The choice of these 26 was based on the need for evaluation data that would reflect urban and rural differences and variations in hospice provider types. Of the demonstration hospices, 12 are hospital-based, 10 are home health agency-based, and four are freestanding. All 26 organizations are either certified home health agencies (HHAs) or have contractual arrangements with certified HHAs to provide home health services. Some also have the capability of providing inpatient hospice services.

232

There is at least one demonstration site in each of the 10 Department of Health and Human Services regions.

For 24 of these hospices, Medicaid State agencies have also agreed to participate in the project and reimburse for services to Medicaid recipients.

Under the demonstration, the hospices are serving patients who have (1) a life expectancy of six months or less, (2) a primary care giver, such as a relative, friend, or paid attendant who is available to provide simple personal care and emotional support on an around-the-clock basis, and (3) entitlement to Hospital Insurance benefits (Medicare Part A) and Supplementary Medical Insurance benefits (Medicare Part B) and/or eligibility under Medicaid.

Participating hospices may be reimbursed under the demonstration for a number of items and services not currently covered by Medicare and Medicaid. Examples include outpatient prescription drugs, institutional respite and home respite services (primary care giver relief), visits by dieticians and homemakers, supportive and counseling visits to hospice patients during occasional hospital stays, continuous care (by nurses, home health aides, or homemakers) on a shift basis in the home, certain self-help devices, inpatient hospice care, and bereavement services to family members.

The project evaluation is jointly supported by HCFA, the Robert Wood Johnson Foundation, and the John A. Hartford Foundation. HCFA has contracted with Brown University to conduct an independent study of cost, use, and quality of care provided to hospice patients and their families in this project. To more clearly understand the effects of hospice care and of reimbursement for hospice care, HCFA and Brown University will also gather information on other groups of terminally ill patients, including a group of patients served by hospices outside the demonstration and another group of patients served by hospitals and cancer centers which provide conventional medical care.

The evaluation will focus on (1) the types of hospice services provided to terminally ill Medicare and Medicaid beneficiaries and the cost of providing those services; (2) the types of services provided to terminally ill patients by conventional modes of care and the cost of providing those services; (3) the cost of services provided in-home and in inpatient settings by the demonstration hospices and conventional modes; and (4) the adequacy of the care received. HCFA processes all Medicare claims submitted by participating hospices. Medicaid hospice claims from the participating States are either processed by their own fiscal intermediaries or by HCFA. For demonstration services provided to Medicare beneficiaries, HCFA reimburses the hospices on the basis of reasonable cost, subject to retrospective cost reimbursement.

233

HUD/HHS Demonstration Program for
Deinstitutionalization of the Chronically Mentally Ill

The Departments of Housing and Urban Development (HUD) and HHS are jointly funding this demonstration to do the following: (1) integrate the chronically mentally ill into the community and improve the quality of their lives by providing housing linked to supportive and rehabilitative services; (2) provide an environment that protects the privacy and personal dignity of the chronically mentally ill and at the same time offers incentives for them to assume increasing responsibility and control over their own lives; and (3) encourage and assist States in providing housing and comprehensive health/social services for the chronically mentally ill.

For this demonstration, a chronically mentally ill person is defined as "any adult, age 18 or older, with a severe and persistent mental or emotional disorder that seriously limits his or her functional capacities relative to primary aspects of daily living such as personal relations, living arrangements, work, recreation, etc., and whose disability could be improved by more suitable housing conditions." (Alcoholism and drug abuse are not included in this definition.)

The following three categories of individuals may be served:

- chronically mentally ill individuals currently residing in institutions but capable of more independent living
- chronically mentally ill individuals at risk of being reinstitutionalized
- chronically mentally ill individuals with no prior institutionalization who are at risk, but for whom housing linked to services would provide an alternative to institutionalization .

Under this demonstration, the following services are required: case management and program planning, house and milieu management, life skill development, medical and physical health care, and crisis stabilization. Additional services that are recommended but not required are vocational development, education, family relations planning, recreational/avocational activity planning, psychotherapy, and advocacy/legal assistance.

Under the authority of Section 202 of the Housing Act of 1959, as amended by Public Law 86-372, HUD is providing 40 year, direct Federal loans to assist private, non-profit corporations in developing new or substantially rehabilitated housing. Over a three year period, HUD has set aside approximately $69 million in loan reservations for 229 sites in 39 States, including the District of Columbia and Puerto Rico. These sites will house from 3,500 to 4,000 residents. In addition, HUD will provide Section 8 rental assistance for all of the units.

This community-based residential housing (group homes and independent living complexes) will allow chronically mentally ill persons

234

to live more independently in the community. A group home is defined as a small living arrangement for not more than 12 persons with a home-like environment for those who require a planned program of continual supportive services and/or supervision but do not require continual nursing, medical, or psychiatric care. An independent living complex is defined as an arrangement of six to 10 individual apartment units that are supervised by professional or paraprofessional staff living in a separate or adjacent apartment or living off the grounds of the facility. The complex may house no more than 20 individuals with a maximum of two persons per bedroom.

Through a cooperative arrangement with HUD, HHS (HCFA, the National Institute of Mental Health [NIMH], and the Office of the Assistant Secretary for Planning and Evaluation [ASPE]) will ensure that participants in the demonstration receive an appropriate service package and reimbursement for selected services. A steering committee comprising staff from each agency provides review and input into each phase of the program. ASPE has had the HHS coordination role, NIMH provides the guidance, direction, and review of the service component, and HCFA is committed to the approval of Section 1115 waivers to provide Medicaid reimbursement for services that the States are unable to pay for under current funding programs. This reimbursement mechanism is transitional, in that it allows a State time to secure funding for these services and thus fulfill its commitment to HUD. Each site within a State is to be covered by waivers approved for three years.

Up to 26 States are expected to submit Section 1115, waiver-only, grant applications to HCFA. In addition to waiving specific sections of the statutory requirements for the Medicaid State plan, the grants will authorize Federal matching funds for such services as case management, supervision, training in life skills, and transportation. The Minnesota waiver-only grant was approved May 1, 1980 and has provided services at one site. Georgia was approved on April 1, 1981 and will have four sites providing services. Oregon, Vermont, New Jersey, and Tennessee have submitted applications to HCFA and will have sites in operation in 1981. In addition, six more areas (California, Maryland, Washington, D.C., Rhode Island, Maine, and New Hampshire) are preparing Section 1115 applications.

HHS will conduct a four year, cost-benefit evaluation of the demonstration with HCFA as the lead agency. Funding for the evaluation has been committed by NIMH and ASPE. The evaluation design, developed under contract with Urban Systems Research and Engineering, Inc., will be pilot tested in 1981. The schedule of events relating to the evaluation will be determined based on the date on which a sufficient number of sites become operational.

235

Waiver of Prior Hospitalization Requirements for Medicare SNF Coverage

HCFA provided Medicare waivers and contracted with Blue Cross of Oregon and Blue Cross of Massachusetts in 1977 to conduct demonstrations in eliminating the three day prior hospitalization requirement for SNF coverage. The purpose is to determine whether a waiver of the requirement will lower overall costs for both the patient and the Medicare program. In addition, the contractors will determine if the three day requirement ordinarily imposes a burden on Medicare patients who may need SNF care but not hospital care.

The SNF benefit is included in Medicare Part A to provide a lower cost alternative to extended hospitalization. The requirement of a three day hospitalization prior to admission to an SNF is imposed to limit SNF benefits to persons who need continuing care after hospital treatment. The requirement also ensures that medical conditions and needs of Medicare patients admitted to SNFs have been given adequate medical appraisal prior to admission. The Senate Finance Committee recommended that the Secretary of HHS conduct experiments to determine the effects of eliminating or reducing the requirement.

The experimental phase of the projects, which ended in 1980, tested the hypothesis that the hospitalization requirement has resulted in unnecessary hospital stays for Medicare beneficiaries who could effectively use less costly SNF care without hospitalization. The contractors are also studying nursing home utilization and quality of care. Under the projects, approximately 28 facilities in each State have participated in the experimental part of the demonstrations, admitting a total of 970 patients during the first two years. During the experiment, all other criteria involved in the Medicare SNF level of care decisions remained unchanged.

Use of the waiver option in Massachusetts and Oregon was low compared to the HCFA's national estimate of a 25 percent increment in SNF utilization. The Oregon waiver project accounted for 7.4 percent of the Medicare SNF utilization in the 28 participating facilities during the demonstration period; for Massachusetts, it was 11.5 percent. Because some patients involved would have gone to the hospital and then transferred to SNF care afterward, the actual increment in nursing home use to the waiver is somewhat less than these figures. The utilization rates for the two States were 0.38 and 0.23 waiver admissions per bed in Oregon and Massachusetts, respectively; the number of waiver admissions per 1,000 Medicare enrollees was 1.3 in Oregon and 0.7 in Massachusetts. Both States had similar experiences with respect to the length of stay. In Oregon, 79 percent of Medicare covered stays were less than 31 days. In Massachusetts, 69 percent were less than 31 days. The average covered days under the demonstration varied between the two States: 26.6 days for Massachusetts and 20.5 days in Oregon.

The two States differed in sources of admission and patient diagnostic characteristics. In Massachusetts, 70 percent of all waiver admissions were internal transfers from a lower level within the institutions. Direct admissions from home represented another 22 percent, transfers from other nursing homes were 6 percent, and hospital transfers accounted for 2 percent. The composition of admissions differed in Oregon; only transfers from other nursing homes (8 percent) were close to the percentage found in Massachusetts. Home admissions represented 40 percent of all admissions (almost twice the Massachusetts figure), internal transfers constituted 39 percent of admissions (approximately half the rate for Massachusetts), and hospitals were involved in 13 percent of waiver admissions.

Patient diagnostic categories differed for the two States. While fractures and amputations accounted for 27 percent of all admissions in Massachusetts, Oregon patients accounted for only 5 percent of admissions in these categories. This difference can be explained partly by the three chronic rehabilitation hospitals in the Massachusetts demonstration, two of which were entirely rehabilitative in their orientation. There were no facilities of this type in Oregon, which is more typical of the nation. The home admissions in Massachusetts occurred primarily in these rehabilitative facilities (73 percent of all home admissions), and the remaining home admissions were dispersed throughout the free-standing SNFs. Excluding the rehabilitation hospital cases, home admissions accounted for only 6 percent of all admissions. This difference was largely attributable to the better awareness of the demonstration by Oregon physicians and their more favorable attitude toward nursing homes.

The most important aspect of these data is that the numbers of demonstration admissions over the three year experimental period are small in both States—700 in Massachusetts and 648 in Oregon (11.5 percent and 7.4 percent of Medicare SNF utilization in the experimental facilities). These rates raise a key issue for evaluation: Can the same moderate level of use be expected if the program is expanded nationally, or is it a result of either the peculiar environment of each State or the way in which the demonstrations were implemented?

Each demonstration has been explored preliminarily in terms of its environment and special characteristics to identify specific factors that distinguish the two demonstrations and account for the utilization experience that was lower than expected. The low overall utilization could be attributed to the Medicare SNF admission criteria, the physicians' practice patterns, and bed shortages. The major factor that could increase utilization of the Medicare SNF benefit in a non-demonstration setting is a reduction in the strictness

237

of the Medicare SNF criteria themselves or in their enforcement by intermediaries or PSROs. This reduction, however, could affect direct entry and prior hospital stay entry equally.

Finally, not all increases in Medicare SNF utilization might lead to reductions in hospital use. Evaluation interviews suggested that between 35 and 67 percent of the waiver patients probably would have entered a hospital if the waiver option had not been available. Thus, it appears that the waiver option will result in some increases in Medicare SNF costs, but the degree to which these will be offset by reduced hospital stays is not clear and requires further analysis. Analyses will assess the cost of the waiver with respect to Medicare reimbursement for SNF care and will estimate the potential hospital savings to assess the net cost of the waiver of the three day hospitalization stay prior to SNF admission requirement.

HCFA awarded the evaluation contract to Abt Associates in September 1979. The final evaluation report will be available in 1982.

A Social/Health Maintenance Organization Program for Long-Term Care

HCFA awarded a three year planning grant to the University Health Policy Consortium at Brandeis University in 1980 to develop the concept of a S/HMO for long-term care. The S/HMO is a capitation financed delivery approach to meet the needs of the disabled and/or elderly. It addresses two of the most pressing problems in long-term care: the fragmentation of services and the fragmentation of funding sources. The concept promises to integrate health and social services as well as acute care services.

The objectives of the planning grant include the following: (1) to provide technical assistance to several possible demonstration sites; (2) to develop the methodology for estimating utilization rates and for calculating costs and capitation rates; (3) to develop the data system and evaluate plans to ensure maximum test results; (4) to develop criteria for selection of the demonstration sites; and (5) to link the evaluation of S/HMOs to other long-term care demonstrations.

A S/HMO is an approach to the organization of health and social services in which the elderly, including those at high risk of institutionalization, are voluntarily enrolled by a managing provider into an intergrated service system. All basic acute hospital, nursing home, ambulatory medical care, and personal care support services, including homemaker, home health, and chore services, would be provided by or through the S/HMO at a fixed, annual, prepaid, capitation sum. Other offered services would include emergency psychiatric care, meals (home delivered and/or congregate), counseling, transportation, information, and referral. The provider may either employ staff or contract with other providers for the services. In the

238

S/HMO model, financial, programmatic, case decision-making, and management responsibility rest with the provider. The S/HMO provider will share the risk for service expenditures and will act as broker for other needed services which are not covered but which are available from other community providers. Financial risk is defined as absorption of agreed-upon costs which exceed a capitation agreement.

In comparison with other models, the S/HMO integrates health and social services under the direct financial management of the provider at the point of services delivery. The success of conventional HMOs with Medicare contracts and of other managed systems of care (for example, the Triage and Monroe County models) suggests the possibility of expansion to an S/HMO system model.

In the proposed demonstration, the S/HMO will serve persons from a targeted elderly population ranging from the ambulatory, non-impaired aged to those who are extremely impaired. Inclusion of the well-ambulatory permits preventive activities for a population which feeds both hospitals and nursing homes. Early management is expected to result in a delay or reduction in nursing home care. For such a population, survey data indicate that approximately 55 percent are ambulatory and well, 25 percent are ambulatory with modest home care needs, 15 percent are living at home with severe impairments, and 5 percent are very impaired, whether housebound or in nursing homes. While the S/HMO is expected to represent all four groups, the proportion enrolled will depend upon the attractiveness of the program to different groups and the intake procedures established by the S/HMO.

Financing for the S/HMO will flow from some combination of public funds (for example, Medicare, Medicaid, and Title XX), as well as from private payments, deductibles, and potential, private, third-party payers. Reimbursement would be based on prepaid capitation.

The S/HMO will offer incentives to all involved parties. Incentives to the provider organization, for example, include improved cash flow, reduction in the cost of administering third-party billing mechanisms, flexibility in program innovation, financial incentives through negotiated rate ceilings and flexible savings arrangements, greater organizational stability, and growth potential in the long-term care marketplace. Public authorities will gain by harnessing HMO control methodologies to long-term care. The uncontrolled, or diffuse, long-term care costs can be addressed systematically through an integrated financing plan with provider risk-sharing and reduced administrative complexity. Consumers will benefit by having a single-entry access to a wider range of services. These services will be provided in an integrated manner, thus reducing the need and costs of "shopping around." Paperwork usually associated with Medicare will be eliminated.

It is hypothesized that the S/HMO will reduce the number of expensive institutional days for enrollees as well as encouraging significant changes in patterns of use.

Three S/HMO demonstration sites, to be selected, will provide a strong comparative evaluation of different S/HMO modes of organization. They will use common assessment instruments, comparable experiment populations, compatible management information systems, and a common evaluation strategy. The demonstrations will provide answers to questions about cost/benefit effects of an S/HMO, the effects of integrated care on the elderly and on service costs, the administrative feasibility of the S/HMO model compared with the fee-for-service model, and the effects on quality of care.

On Lok Senior Health Services: A Community Care Organization for Dependent Adults

The On Lok Community Care Organization for Dependent Adults (CCODA) is a community-based demonstration providing long-term health and health-related services to functionally disabled elderly in the Chinatown-North Beach area of San Francisco. Participants in CCODA must meet the State's eligibility criteria for 24-hour skilled nursing or intermediate care and be entitled to Medicare. A multidisciplinary team assesses the needs and strengths of each CCODA participant and develops a service plan to meet the individual's needs. The On Lok program delivers all services that are required either by its own staff or providers under contract. Single source reimbursement is provided under HCFA's Title XVIII waiver approval.

The objectives of this demonstration are to develop and operate a centrally-funded and administered community care system, to measure the impact of capitated funding on utilization, quality, and cost of services, to contrast the management efficiencies of the model with those of other systems, and to develop actuarially sound budgeting methods for medical and social needs.

During the first year, On Lok established the outpatient service delivery and reimbursement phase of the demonstration. This entailed reorganizing existing staff and their functions, hiring and orienting additional staff, changing procedures, changing clinical and fiscal record keeping, validating assessment instruments, further developing the research protocol, and establishing data collection and analysis techniques. In addition, the transfer of the participants from the previous On Lok program to the CCODA required extensive time and effort due to the age and ethnic background of the population. The inpatient phase of the project began on February 1, 1980. Inpatient services are provided through negotiated contracts with two hospitals and several skilled nursing facilities in the area. Through the first 20 months of operation, it cost On Lok, on the average, $552 per participant per month to provide all of its out-

240

patient services (day health, transportation, primary medical care, drugs, medical specialty services, home health, etc.). With the onset of inpatient services, an additional $278 per participant per month was spent, bringing the total monthly capitation rate to $830. This rate is below that of On Lok's comparison group of patients ($1,513) and below original On Lok projections ($1,045) for the demonstration. At the end of the second year, the CCODA program had essentially completed its developmental phase and begun normal operations.

The research component of On Lok funded by the Administration on Aging (AoA) has a program-based, policy-oriented perspective to assess the impact of the CCODA program on the quality and cost of long-term care. The research includes process evaluation, which describes and interprets issues and problems in program development and operation. It has also developed and continues to refine a computerized information management system that (1) is used in program operation; (2) monitors information on a regular basis for program administration and development; and (3) establishes a real-world, relevant data base for research analysis. The project has established and maintains a comparison group study, identifying a sample of similar elderly in the traditional long-term care system and tracking them over time, gathering information comparable to that in the information system to assess relative program impact. This study has a sample size of 200. Cost analysis will be a specific area of focus in the coming year. Participant-based predictors of the cost rate (for example, functional level, physical and social characteristics, biographical data, etc.) will be identified, and the proportion of monthly CCODA costs that would be reimbursable under existing programs (Titles XVIII, XIX, XX) will be determined.

HCFA is evaluating the On Lok CCODA through the cross-cutting evaluation of its long-term care demonstrations. This evaluation contract was awarded to Berkeley Planning Associates in September 1980.

Skilled Nursing Pharmacy Services—
Capitated Reimbursement

HCFA awarded a grant in 1979 to the California Department of Health Services to conduct a pilot project on capitated reimbursement of drugs for Medicaid patients in SNFs, under the authority of Section 1115 of the Social Security Act. The objective is to improve the drug regimen of Medicaid SNF patients, which in turn should improve the overall quality of care and reduce costs.

The California State Department of Health Services (DHS) currently administers a program of medical assistance under Title XIX of the Social Security Act. The program provides a broad range of medical services to a beneficiary population that is predominantly linked by category. Medicaid usually pays for these services on a

241

fee-for-service basis. Approximately 2.5 percent, or 67,500, of the nearly three million beneficiaries receive their care in SNFs. Medicaid payment for health care for these beneficiaries is made to the individual providers of service, for example, the SNF, physician, dentist, physical therapist, or pharmacist. To control use of pharmacy services, Medicaid employs a closed formulary, that is, a specific list of covered drugs, with prior authorization required for unlisted agents. In addition, either a *minimum quantity* per prescription (how many times the prescription may be renewed) or a *minimum supply* per prescription (how many pills in a bottle) is required for certain medications unless the prescription represents the initial order or has been previously authorized for a smaller quantity or duration of therapy. Minimum quantities are commonly required of drugs used for chronic medical conditions, and the minimum supply requirement commonly applies to certain drugs dispensed to patients in SNFs. Current costs of pharmacy services for SNF inpatients average approximately $26 per patient per month. To determine whether the current expenditures for drugs for SNF patients in the Medicaid program can be reduced, the California State legislature enacted Assembly Bill 1395. The legislation authorized a pilot project in which pharmacists would be reimbursed on a capitated basis for pharmacy services provided in SNFs.

The project proposes to establish capitation rates for 30 selected SNFs based on 25 pharmacies' experiences with those facilities. The monthly capitation rate will be calculated for each facility and will be paid to the pharmacy in advance for each Medicaid patient it serves. In addition, pharmacists who participate will be granted the authority to approve non-formulary drugs necessary for the treatment of the patients.

Participants will reflect the geographic and bed size distribution of nursing homes in the State. Contracts will be prepared to establish project requirements with the participating pharmacies. A group of pharmacies and SNFs will be selected for comparison. The project will be a three year effort with a one year pre-capitation period for selecting participants, collecting baseline data, determining rates, and developing the evaluation methodology. A one year period of capitation will be followed by analysis and reporting of the results.

Capitation rates will be determined by dividing the prior year's Medicaid expenditures for drugs in the facility by the number of patient months for which the facility was paid by Medicaid. This figure will then be increased by an inflation factor for the year of the demonstration to account for increases in ingredient costs.

Pharmacists will be required to submit an invoice monthly, in advance, listing the names and Medicaid ID numbers of those patients for whom the capitation rates are claimed. In those cases where recipients are reported to the State and are ultimately determined to be ineligible, future capitation payments will be offset. Submittal of a current label or copy of the ID card for the month at issue will satisfy eligibility questions. Participating pharmacists will be required to submit claims forms for data collection but not for payment.

The project will allow the pharmacist to bypass the usual utilization controls of the Medicaid program and to exert his or her professional judgment to a maximum degree, consistent with a high quality of care. Minimum quantity rules, prescription audits, and diagnosis restrictions will all be waived for the patients served under this project.

In those instances when the pharmacist does not feel that a prescribed non-formulary drug is necessary, the service can only be denied by the Medicaid consultant. The State and the pharmacy association both feel that the professional arguments that may be raised against use of any particular medication will probably provide adequate justification for the consultant to support the pharmacist's position. This feature is built in, however, to prevent obvious under-utilization on the part of the pharmacy and to enhance the professional relationship between prescribing physicians and pharmacists.

The State will evaluate any changes in costs and utilization of services which result from the project. An outside contractor will conduct a second evaluation, using a multidisciplinary team of physicians, pharmacists, pharmacologists, and nurses, to evaluate the professional decisions involved in the approval of treatment authorization requests (TARs), as well as the overall quality of care received by the patients.

Capital Investment in Nursing Homes

In August 1980, HCFA awarded the West Virginia Department of Welfare a Section 1115 grant. This allowed waiver of the current methodology for determining capital costs included in the Medicaid reimbursement of SNFs and ICFs. The basic objective of this demonstration is twofold:

- to determine whether the proposed reimbursement system produces satisfactory patient care within the operating cost standards
- to determine whether the proposed system results in lower reimbursement rates when compared with a system of reimbursement based on historical costs for all service factors (for example, a Medicare formula).

There is reason to believe that controlling cost by cost center is preferable to using an aggregate operating cost cap, but the data required to evaluate this hypothesis are not currently available. This project will, therefore, focus upon the investment component and the total reimbursement rate under the following operational assumptions:

- Functional and physical variances from the model facility standard result in operational and nursing services deficiencies, inefficiencies, and diseconomies.
- Quality of care is ensured and verified through review of the monthly long-term care services invoices and quarterly nursing services audits.
- Both the rates of reimbursement and the manner in which they are determined significantly affect investor confidence in the industry and the quality of services provided.

Given these assumptions, West Virginia has implemented two parts of a three component reimbursement system. The *nursing services component* is compensated on the basis of actual nursing services required by and delivered to individual patients. The *operating costs component* is compensated by cost center and facility class. Caps on operating costs will be derived from industry experience within the State. Incentives for efficiency and economy will be introduced through the operating cost component by encouraging costs less than the cost caps, with quality of care assured and verified. As a management incentive, the State will share with the facility any savings when actual costs fall below established caps. That incentive will consist of a percentage of the difference between actual facility cost and the established cost caps, provided that such facilities meet all certification and quality patient care standards.

The *investment component* of the new reimbursement system (which is being implemented under this demonstration) should allow for the reasonable costs of investments in long-term care facilities, including a reasonable return on the investment. A unique aspect of this system is the method for determining the allowance for value of the investment component (land, building, and equipment) of the reimbursement rate.

The standard appraised value (SAV) method establishes the value of the fixed assets as a long-term care center, not only by encouraging functional utility, but also by discouraging features which detract from or do not contribute to that function. The model facility standard is drawn from Federal and State regulations and guidelines and from accepted industry practice. It offsets the fundamental difficulty of the reproduction cost approach by providing a stable base for deriving consistent appraisals of long-term care properties.

First year tasks included the design and implementation of uniform accounting and reporting procedures, definition of the model facility standards, initial appraisals of all facilities, the evaluation

244

of the appraisals, and the establishment of a rate of return. In designing the reimbursement formula, the State intends to base the rate of return on the yield generated by the Federal National Mortgage Association's (FNMA) conventional mortgages. This yield will allow enough flexibility to keep current with the recent volatility in the mortgage market. This different method of reimbursing capital costs will ideally discourage rapid turnover in facility ownership and encourage greater stability. Implementation on a state-wide basis will be effected in 1981. Since this project has just begun, no findings are available.

Incentive Payment Grant—Encouraging Appropriate Care for the Chronically Ill Elderly

Early in 1981, HCFA approved a Section 1115 waiver grant to the Department of Health Services in Sacramento, California. The purposes of this two year grant are to improve appropriateness of care and encourage more efficient use of resources. The project will encourage nursing homes to admit sicker patients who require more care and who might otherwise remain inappropriately hospitalized; thus discouraging unnecessarily high costs for care. It will also improve residents' outcomes through improved quality care facilitated by resident-specific goal setting and care planning. Finally, it will encourage discharge of certain kinds of residents who might be served more appropriately by non-institutional services, thus making room for more severely dependent patients.

The cost of the evaluation and incentive payments will be paid through a contract between the National Center for Health Services Research (NCHSR) and Applied Management Sciences, Inc. The contractor will reimburse participating facilities for data collection and will make incentive payments to deserving facilities under the study protocol. The contractor will pay for all other data collection and data processing, including data supplied by the California Department of Health Services. HCFA and NCHSR will analyze the data and final reports.

Methodology

Thirty-six proprietary nursing homes in the San Diego standard metropolitan statistical area (SMSA), having between 50 and 200 beds, with at least 50 percent normally available to Medi-Cal residents, will participate in the study. Homes will be randomly assigned to treatment or control groups. Approximately 3,472 residents will participate in the demonstration, one-half in the experimental and one-half in the control homes. The demonstration will attempt to encourage long-term care facilities to admit and provide quality care to severely dependent residents and to dis-

245

charge less dependent residents into lower levels of care or to provide continuity of care for discharged residents.

As an incentive, the demonstration will pay nursing homes for admitting severely dependent residents. Participating homes will also receive outcome incentive payments for achieving specified goals in selected patients who require special care to improve or maintain their functional health status. The demonstration will also pay nursing homes for appropriately discharging residents (who must be kept at a lower level of care or in the community for at least three months). No incentives will be paid for residents who should not have been admitted or for those expected to stay for less than 90 days.

Applied Management Sciences will collect the data, and NCHSR will analyze them. Final reports on the demonstration should be available early in 1984.

Survey-by-Exception (SBE)

In July 1980, HCFA awarded a Section 1115, waiver-only, quality assurance grant to the Massachusetts Department of Public Welfare. The purposes of this 18 month project are to reallocate surveyor time so that facilities with the greatest certification compliance problems can receive additional consultation and technical assistance and to improve the quality of care in SNFs and intermediate care facilities (ICFs).

This project tests an experimental survey process in Medicaid and Medicare facilities. The medical review and the independent professional review patient survey will be performed as usual. Massachusetts has developed a facility screening instrument which it will pretest for reliability and validity before using it in the demonstration.

Methodology

The facility survey is a modification of the screening survey developed by the Wisconsin Quality Assurance Project. The design for the demonstration classifies facilities into three groups, based upon their performance on annual surveys for the preceding three years.

The Massachusetts Long-Term Care Information System (LTCIS), a management information system containing the results of all facility surveys since 1976, aggregates survey results at the facility level so they can be compared across facilities. The criteria for facility classification are as follows:

- Screening Survey Group—Compliance scores of 93 or above on annual inspections for three calendar years prior to the inspection date (classified as outstanding)

246

- Abbreviated Survey Group—Compliance scores of 85 to 92 for the past three calendar years (classified as acceptable)
- Full Survey Group—Compliance scores below 85 for the past three calendar years (classified as unacceptable)

The demonstration is planned as a 2X2 experimental design with test facilities in outstanding and acceptable groups assigned randomly to the traditional method of survey and the SBE method. The design calls for 120 of the 160 facilities in two geographic areas, the northwest and southeast sections of the State, to be assigned to the four cells of the design; 60 will be eligible for SBE and 60 will receive the traditional survey.

Hypotheses to be tested include the following:

- Quality of care in the screening and abbreviated survey facilities in the experimental groups will increase or remain constant relative to those in the control group.
- Quality of care will improve in the full survey facilities.
- Time spent on certification visits will decrease in facilities in the abbreviated and screening survey visits.
- Time spent on certification visits will increase or remain constant in the poor performance group.
- The number of interim visits, follow-up visits, and consultation visits, and the time spent on such visits, will increase in each of the three groups.
- Provider attitudes toward the State survey agency will be more favorable in facilities participating in SBE.

The demonstration was initiated October 1, 1980, after pretesting and compliance with conditions attached with the Notice of Grant Award. It will be evaluated by a contractor chosen by HCFA to evaluate all of the survey/certification related demonstrations.

Findings to date include the following:

- SBE decreases the amount of time spent on certification visits.
- Surveyors spend more time on consultation and follow-up visits.
- The number of "trivial" deficiencies declined with SBE.

The final report is expected in the fall of 1983.

New York State's Nursing Home Quality Assurance Program

HCFA awarded the New York State Department of Health a Section 1115 waiver-only grant, effective September 2, 1980. This three year demonstration is part of an overall effort by the State to improve the quality of care provided in residential health care facilities (RHCFs), which include both SNFs and ICFs.

247

Description

The objectives of this project are to simplify and streamline the MR, IPR, and Medicare review process for all RHCFs in New York State. The current system is very cumbersome, particularly when 8,000 reviews are processed per week. The new system will use a screening survey (based upon the screening survey developed for the Wisconsin quality of care project). It will combine a form to be filled out by the facility with a relatively brief form to be filled out by the reviewers when they visit the facility. This latter form would reduce the number of items for the SNF survey from 1,285 to 241 and the ICF requirement from 780 to 223. MR and IPR will be combined into a single process. The first stage will be an outcome-oriented system which will look at Sentinel Health Events (SHEs). These are events representing a potential failure in the care system. Examples include the presence of bedsores, urinary tract infections, and contractures. If the number of these events exceeds a threshold (to be established on the basis of the patient mix and the facility), then the second stage of the proposal will be initiated. In this stage, a more detailed investigation of the process of care for a sample of patients having the untoward events will be undertaken, using specifically designed protocols for each SHE.

The research design assesses three things: (1) the review of 20 percent of the facilities requiring intensive surveys, (2) the validity of the outcome-based screening and the process-based follow up, and (3) the causes of deficiencies in the new process. Finally, it will apply various statistical measures to test the increased efficiency of the new system over the old one.

Hypotheses to be tested include the following:

- The survey emphasis on the structural measures of quality of care will complement the outcomes/process measures of the MR/IPR to more clearly define the causes of lack of facility compliance with State and Federal regulations. Corollaries of this hypothesis are:

  —The deficiencies in the new process will be traced to underlying causes rather than symptoms to a greater extent in the new system than in the old.
  —The plan of correction filed by the facilities will treat underlying causes rather than symptoms to a greater extent in the new system.

- Each SHE is a reliable measure.
- The SHEs will point to areas of poor quality care.
- Different reviewers will reach the same decision as to whether a Stage II review is needed.

248

- Stage II review reliably and efficiently documents poor quality care when compared to the present system.
- The new system will document more problems associated with direct patient care rather than indirect factors related to patient care.

The following has been completed:

1. HCFA attached several conditions to the grant award and these were all satisfactorily met.
2. Two field tests of the SHEs have been completed. They resulted in revisions of the definitions and protocols for measuring the SHEs.
3. A training curriculum for surveyors has been developed anɟ training programs have been evaluated in the State.

The project was implemented in Albany, Buffalo, Rochester, and Syracuse in July 1981 and in White Plains and New York City in October 1981.

HCFA will select an independent evaluator to assess the project.

Nursing Home Quality Assurance Project (QAP)

The Wisconsin Department of Health and Social Services is in the fourth and last year of a Section 1115, waiver-only project to improve the quality of care in nursing homes using an experimental survey and certification methodology. This demonstration is based on the premise that the State should reallocate surveyor time so that more time is spent in nursing homes that are cited as having deficiencies and less time in nursing homes providing good care.

Project Objectives

The primary goal of the project is to improve the quality of care in nursing homes in the demonstration areas using cost-effective techniques which reallocate the State's resources.

To increase the efficiency and effectiveness of the facility review process, QAP does the following:

- uses a screening technique which allows teams to separate homes into three categories: homes performing well, homes with minor problems likely to be resolved with consultation, and homes with one or more serious problems requiring detailed analysis for possible negative action
- omits the full facility survey except where indicated by a history of problems or after using the new facility screening technique
- involves nursing home administrators and rehabilitation specialists in the facility survey to provide a broader base of knowledge for the evaluation

249

- trains survey staff to collect data which will hold up in court when negative action is indicated
- schedules survey visits at less predictable and more frequent intervals to collect more accurate data.

To increase the efficiency and effectiveness of the MR and IPR of patient care, QAP:

- uses a statistical quality control methodology to choose a stratified sample of patients for intensive review, rather than performing a cursory review of all patients currently in the home
- reallocates staff time to comprehensively evaluate the home's system for identifying and meeting patient needs
- omits the full MR and IPR survey except where indicated by a history of patient care problems or after using the new patient sampling technique
- provides feedback to the facility survey by citing deficiencies and documenting cases of poor patient care for court use.

To improve the quality of nursing home care by resolving the problems discovered through the facility survey and patient review, QAP has done the following:

- developed criteria for quickly choosing corrective actions from a list ranked by severity
- added new options to the list of correction/enforcement actions, including consulting with survey team members and contracting for technical assistance
- provided more immediate feedback to homes detailing deficient areas of patient or institutional management, especially for homes evaluated as needing enforcement action.

Since these last three elements are considered essential in any quality assurance system, they are used in both control and experimental sites. The experimental design separates the effect of these changes from those caused by the experimental facility and patient review processes.

Methodology

The Bureau of Quality Compliance, Wisconsin Division of Health, is demonstrating two new approaches to the control of quality in nursing homes. These approaches deviate from traditional State and Federal requirements. The first requirement is that a nursing home be evaluated for compliance with applicable State and Federal regulations at least annually. The second requirement is that every Medicaid nursing home resident be evaluated at least annually for appropriateness of placement and level of care.

Facility Screening

In place of existing requirements for annual surveys of nursing homes, a screening survey to quickly identify problems in critical areas is being tested. Further action, ranging from informal consultation to decertification, is taken on problems found during screening. The time saved through this screening process is used to more rigorously pursue enforcement in homes that are endangering the health of their residents.

Sampling Patient Review

In place of existing requirements for reviewing Medicaid recipients in nursing homes, a scientifically chosen, 10 percent sample is taken of all patients in the home. As in the facility screening, decisions for further action are based on problems found during the careful review of this sample. State surveyor time saved by not examining all patients is devoted to more extensive consultation and enforcement.

In July 1978, during the first phase of the demonstration, Wisconsin studied 122 facilities (SNFs and ICFs) in a rural area using a 2X2 factorial design of the treatments, facility survey, and patient evaluation. The two options for facility "treatment" are the old full survey and the new screening survey; the two options for the patient "treatment" are the old 100 percent medical review and the new patient sampling technique.

In the second phase of the project, Wisconsin added 40 more homes in a large urban area to the demonstration. In half of these nursing homes, the screening survey and patient sampling techniques were used, and in the remaining 20, the old full survey and 100 percent medical review were carried out. In addition, another 20 homes were selected as control homes in the urban area.

Two additional changes were made in the second year which affected the demonstration methodology. First, HCFA approved a waiver of the Life Safety Code so that a screening survey instrument could be used by the engineer/architect. Second, HCFA's Health Standards and Quality Bureau agreed to accept less than the full report for Title XVIII certified facilities, which permitted their inclusion in the demonstration.

In the last phase of the demonstration, 40 additional facilities were added to the sample. These facilities are located in a mixed rural/urban area of the State. The methodology has been slightly changed in the last phase to further eliminate the possibility of surveyor bias. In these areas, separate survey teams have been assigned to each treatment cell. One team uses the screening survey and patient sampling methodology, and the other, the full survey and 100 percent patient sampling.

251

With this last expansion, the demonstration project includes 31,000 residents/patients and 281 (59 percent) of the State's nursing homes.

Findings to date include the following:

- The total time for survey and certification visits using the screening survey and 10 percent sampling of patients for MR/IPR is two days in homes of 100 beds or less, while the traditional methods in homes of the same size require 15 working days.
- The State survey staff and nursing home administrators and staff have positive attitudes about the screening survey and sampling technique.
- The number of nursing home administrators participating in the screening surveys has increased but has not yet reached 100 percent.
- Surveyors are making increased use of the option to switch from the screening survey to the traditional method. The most common reasons cited are a poor survey record, a new administrator, or a new director of nursing.
- Surveyors in the rural districts make more frequent surprise visits than those in the urban areas.
- Surveyors using the new methods spend proportionately more time on facility assessment than when using the traditional method, less time on resident assessment, and only a slightly greater proportion of time on follow-up.
- When the new methods of survey and certification are used, slightly more Class A violations (probability of death or injury to a patient) and slightly fewer Class B (direct threat to health and safety) and Class C (does not threaten health and safety) violations were found.
- Surveyors using the new methods more frequently use a variety of State follow-up actions, that is, consultation, special advisor, and return to follow-up.
- A lower percentage of patients are observed to be at an incorrect level of care using the sampling methodology. However, after reviewing the history of facilities in the study, the QAP findings reflect pre-existing differences in these homes.

HCFA awarded a grant for an independent evaluation of the demonstration to the University of Wisconsin in July 1980. The final report will be submitted in the summer of 1982 and the independent evaluation report should be available shortly thereafter.

References

Analytical Review of the Literature, Mental Disorder and Primary Medical Care, Services D. No. 5, National Institutes of Mental Health, 1974.

252

Archives of General Psychiatry, Volume 35, June 1978.

Budget Issue Paper, "Long Term Care for the Elderly and Disabled," Congressional Budget Office, February 1977.

Budget of the United States Government, Fiscal Year 1981: Appendix, U.S. Government Printing Office, Washington, D.C., 1980.

Callahan, James J. "The Organization of the Long Term Care System and the Potential for a Single Agency Option," Brandeis University Health Policy Consortium, 1979.

Commission on Chronic Illness, "Care of the Long Term Patient—Volume II," Harvard University Press, 1956.

General Accounting Office, "Entering a Nursing Home: Costly Implications for Medicaid and the Elderly," Report to the Congress of the United States, 1979.

LaPorte and Rubin, "Long Term Care," Praeger, 1979.

LaVor, Judith, "Long Term Care: A Challenge to Service Systems," Long Term Care, Praeger, 1979.

National Long Term Care Project: Final Report, University of Chicago Center for the Study of Welfare Policy, August 1980.

Shaughnessy, Peter, "An Evaluation of Swing-Bed Experiments to Provide Long-Term Care in Rural Hospitals—Volume II," Health Care Financing Grants and Contracts Reports, U.S. Government Printing Office, Washington, D.C., 1981.

Sheehan, Daniel M. and James E. Craft, "Final Report of the Study of Placement Needs of Mental Hospital Patients," Texas Department of Mental Health and Mental Retardation, National Institutes of Mental Health, 1974.

Statistical Reports on Older Americans, "Some Prospects for the Future Elderly Population," Administration on Aging, January 1978.

U.S. Bureau of the Census, Current Population Reports, Series P-20, No. 363, "Population Profile of the United States: 1980," U.S. Government Printing Office, Washington, D.C., 1981.

U.S. Bureau of the Census, Current Population Reports, Series P-25, No. 704, "Projections of the Population of the United States: 1977 to 2050," U.S. Government Printing Office, Washington, D.C., 1977.

U.S. Department of Health and Human Services, The Need for Long Term Care Information and Issues: A Chartbook of the Federal Council on the Aging, U.S. Government Printing Office, Washington, D.C., 1981.

U.S. Department of Health and Human Services, Health Care Financing Administration, "National Annual State Medicaid Statistical Report," U.S. Government Printing Office, Washington, D.C., 1981.

Wallack, Stanley, "Services for the Chronically Mentally Ill: The Implications of Financing," Brandeis University Health Policy Consortium, 1979.

Chapter VII

The Alternatives Question

by Hans C. Palmer

Rapid escalation in the costs of nursing home care, social services, and health care have renewed interest in long-term care "alternatives." These cost-based interests have reinforced worries about the quality of life in institutions, worries caused in large measure by revelations of scandalous conditions in many nursing homes. In this chapter we will specify issues associated with differing modes of long-term care (LTC), to present some alternative analytical approaches to assessing the relative effectiveness of different care modes, and raise some key theoretical, methodological, and empirical issues about the quality of alternatives research. The framework developed here will provide a basis on which to assess other modes of LTC.

Most discussions of alternatives in LTC emphasize substitutes for the nursing home, with special emphasis on care in the patient's home. For example, home (health) care (HC) has been projected by many analysts and public figures as *the* alternative pattern of care, one which they assert is more natural, more satisfying to the patients and their families, and, above all, cheaper (Demkovich, 1979).[1] Actually, the term "alternatives" is something of a misnomer and may carry the wrong connotations. Discussions of one or another mode of care as preferable to the nursing home also can pose the analytical issues incorrectly. As was pointed out in Chapter I, analysts and policymakers should consider a spectrum of care modes rather than sets of either-or alternatives. Moreover, the appropriate spectrum is not two-dimensional, in terms of one alternative phasing into another as in the model of "progressive patient care" (a patient moving from more to less institutionalized settings in definite steps). Instead we should be thinking more of a crystal lattice with various modes of care linked to each other in

---

I would like to thank Margaret Stassen for her many helpful suggestions for this chapter.

[1] Careful analysis of the alternatives issue shows that HC may not be the sole solution to the problem of long-term care. The advocates of HC may, however, be accurate in their assertion that many types of dependency are created, rather than relieved, by current provision of long-term care. Their analysis of the pro-institutional biases and policy foibles of present legislation and regulations may also be fairly accurate.

a multi-dimensional framework, sometimes as substitutes, sometimes as complements, sometimes in a progression. In this sense, home care, for example, would not be considered just as an alternative to the nursing home. It could also be a substitute provider of routine services, a low-care complement to high-intensity care in a skilled nursing facility (SNF), and/or a stage in a dependent person's movement in the system of care.

The Range of Care Options

If the objectives of LTC include helping individuals cope with their disabilities, reducing their dependencies on others, and narrowing the gap between their actual and potential functional capabilities, then it is clear that the nursing home is not the only appropriate site of care (GAO, 1979). LTC services (health, social, and income support) can all be provided in the home, adult day care centers, outpatient ambulatory care facilities, and, in cases of great disability and/or lack of major social supports, the nursing home or the acute hospital. This circumstance has led many policymakers and analysts, to say nothing of the patients and their families, to ask: Do we get what we want for the billions in public and private money which go for services provided in nursing homes and acute hospitals? Are there better ways of providing care, better sites for care in which it could be provided more cheaply and with greater satisfaction to those being served? These questions motivate much research in LTC alternatives.

LTC sites differ in the types of care they provide, or they offer the same actual types of care but "package" them differently. For example, physical therapy (PT) can be offered in the home by visiting professionals or can be provided in a hospital or day hospital setting. Of course, some technologies are unique to certain settings; it would be hard to imagine offering certain types of mechanical life support outside an acute general hospital.

Clearly, the sites of care and the services they offer can operate as substitutes or complements in a static sense. In a dynamic sense, they can serve as steps or sequences in a continuum of care which may begin with the home, involve an episode of hospitalization, find the patient in some sort of extended care facility, and end with the patient back at home and with many movements back and forth as in the lattice. For these reasons, it is inadequate to analyze only HC, or any other individual option, merely as a substitute. The following examination of alternatives will accordingly identify sites and services from a number of perspectives to analyze costs and compare cost-effectiveness. Because the nursing home is the dominant form of U.S. institutional LTC provision, absorbing most of the official resources devoted to long-term care, much of what follows will compare the nursing home with other alternatives.

256

Why Have Alternatives?

A major purpose of LTC is to enhance the quality of life for recipients and their families. Presumably, LTC interventions of all types relieve the effects of disease or injury, enhance or maintain functional capacities, and enrich the quality of life. Many advocates of alternatives, however, assert that their favorite options uniformly offer advantages over more institutionalized care, especially that in nursing homes. According to them, patient satisfaction is enhanced, and costs are reduced, because alternatives are cost-effective substitutes for nursing homes and/or hospitals and because they may delay institutional admission.

Although LTC alternatives are not always substitutes for the nursing home, the possibilities of such substitution and the widespread advocacy of non-institutional alternatives force consideration of some crucial questions about purposes, appropriateness, and limits to use from a perspective of substitution (Weissert, 1979). The analysis obviously also has implications beyond substitution.

Considering the purpose of alternatives raises questions about which populations are to be served. Are alternatives to be considered only as substitutes for nursing home care or might they not serve as replacements for other forms of intervention, such as doctors' visits? Are alternatives to be targeted only for the population now defined as eligible for care in SNFs and intermediate care facilities (ICFs), or should other categories of dependency be considered? If alternatives are actually complements to institutional care, which population groups should receive the additional care? Many of the questions relevant to purpose relate, as well, to appropriateness, an issue which touches age groups, medical/functional/psycho-social conditions, etc. As to limits, the most binding are economic, although administrative, bureaucratic, and political obstacles may be as constricting. With respect to costs, the key issue is really that of trade-offs between cost-containment and the desire to have effective programs, where effectiveness is measured in terms of the attainment of outcomes. Costs also impose the need to choose between enhancing quality of life for the limited number of people now being reached by various types of care and the desire to extend care to broader reaches of the community, even on a very modest basis. So also, one form of cost reduction may increase other costs. For example, an alternatives program might enhance quality of care and life at the cost of losing much of the family support now forthcoming because alternatives are limited in number and accessibility. Perhaps the most troubling aspect of cost lies in the substitution of services versus their augmentation, an aspect which surfaces explicitly in some of the cost analyses surveyed in following sections.

257

Questions of costs and trade-offs again raise some of the central issues of appropriateness versus the need to make a cost-effective program actually operative. As Weissert points out (1979), if cost-effective limits are to be imposed, alternatives will be institutional substitutes, and the alternatives must be restricted to those people who would probably otherwise be institutionalized and who would use alternatives if offered.

The cost constraint raises the question of how to determine the probabilities of institutionalization. In general, older, more disabled, and socially isolated people are more likely to be institutionalized, but the mere appearance of these characteristics among certain groups still does not allow predictions about specific individuals. Furthermore, because institutions vary greatly in their services and the attributes of their patient populations (even though the institutions nominally may be of the same type), and because all vulnerable, elderly people are high users of care, predictions for individuals based on group characteristics are very shaky indeed. In actuality, there is no way to protect against the possibility of excluding some people at risk of institutionalization from alternatives, just as there is no way to avoid including some people who are not at risk. These constraints do not preclude trying to sort people into appropriate groups for the offer or non-offer of alternative care. Rather, as in the case of nursing homes, they indicate that much more knowledge is needed about explanatory and predictive factors linking personal characteristics and circumstances to vulnerability to institutionalization and to suitability for alternative care.

Cost Analysis

Because we are dealing with a system of provision that is largely publicly financed, access, quality, and cost are of special importance in connection with alternatives, as they are with nursing homes.

Access in any public system should be provided to all persons defined as eligible for provision. *Quality* should be high enough to ensure that there is no danger to life, that common standards of comfort and decency are maintained, and that there is a reasonable expectation that the services provided will contribute to achieving an intended outcome, such as the elimination of an acute condition, the improvement of function, the custodial maintenance of a patient, etc. *Costs,* in a general sense, should fall within limits set by the political process and by society's resources and should yield most benefit for the amounts expended. (In other words, it should be cost-effective.) For this last reason, cost measurement (and cost-effectiveness or cost benefit analysis) has assumed special importance in most of the studies of different modalities of care.

258

These cost analyses have approached the cost question most often via the cost function. Little effort, so far, has been devoted to the production function for alternatives, probably because of the difficulty of identifying the appropriate outputs. Overall, cost function analysis has emphasized the effects of case-mix (or patient characteristics), outcome and process quality, and facility characteristics. To be sure, not all analyses have considered all of these factors, while others have introduced special factors, for example, focus on care for a closely defined set of illnesses, such as stroke, neoplasms, senility, etc. In general, then, analysis of alternatives has not been as sophisticated as that for the nursing home. The general lack of systematic and careful economic analysis of alternative care settings is particularly striking in the heavily researched area of home care, which has led to an ongoing program at the University of Colorado Health Services Center to assess the cost-effectiveness of nursing homes and home health care agencies.

Cost-Effectiveness and Cost-Benefit

Cost-effectiveness is a familiar analysis to students of government policymaking and policy choices and, increasingly, to the policy-makers themselves. As Doherty and Hicks point out, cost-effective-ness is one of a set of techniques (including operations research, cost-benefit analysis, and cost-effectiveness analysis) which employ engineering concepts and the theory of choice as developed by economists to assist decision-makers in choosing among possible alternatives (Doherty and Hicks, 1975, 1977; Doherty, Segal, and Hicks, 1978). While operations research, as a study, emphasizes the determination of the most technically efficient methods of generat-ing outputs from inputs, cost-benefit and cost-effectiveness analyses introduce notions of economic efficiency into the calculations, so that choices can be framed in terms of alternatives foregone, that is, the opportunity costs of choosing one course of action rather than another. Since policymakers must operate within specified limits of financial and physical resources, verifiable and manageable techniques for making choices offer numerous advantages.

Cost-benefit techniques usually frame both outcomes and costs in terms of money. By calculating the ratios between monetarily stated costs and benefits, especially at the margin (or when a change in levels or direction of efforts is indicated), the policy chooser can compare among programs, selecting the most gain for the resources and efforts expended. Two ingredients are essential: both costs and benefits must be calculable in terms of money or some other common denominator, and the potential programs must bear some realistic relationship to the problem at hand. Because not all benefits may be calculable in money or other discrete terms, and because the

259

nature of the benefits or outcomes may be a conglomerate of many objectives, analysts and policymakers often resort to cost-effectiveness analysis.

Costs and Outcomes

The cost-effective technique does not always require a close specification of objectives in quantifiable terms. Rather, it may involve the specification of desired objectives, sometimes in qualitative terms, which then are to be attained with the least expenditure of resources. Because the objectives merely have to be identified rather than quantified, the cost effectiveness technique is very useful when there are social goals or outcomes not specifiable in economic or monetary terms. This is presumably the case with LTC for the elderly, where many outcomes may not yield an economic payoff (for example, in the sense of restoring someone to a wage-earning job) but rather generate intangible and personal outcomes such as increased independence, improved family feeling, and a better "quality of life" (Grimaldi and Sullivan, 1981). Some of the outcomes of long-term care, however, are more closely quantifiable. For example, changes in functional condition or mental acuity are clearly measurable; yet even in these instances, comparisons or progress may have to be measured in ordinal rather than cardinal terms.

Doherty's and Hicks' model (1975) of the cost-effectiveness method results in a list of seven requirements for a successful analysis:

1) identifying alternative programs and their objectives,
2) constructing models of these programs,
3) establishing outcome and cost models,
4) applying outcome and cost models,
5) arraying the results of the application of these models in outcome/cost ratios,
6) applying decision-making rules subject to program goals, objectives, and constraints, and
7) arraying alternatives in order of preference.

The first and third requirements are the most important, since they capture the essence of the choices to be made. The other questions are mostly process-oriented, although they must be answered to analyze cost-effectiveness.

Specifying Outcomes

Specifying and quantifying desired outcomes for long-term care may be quite difficult.[2] As Doherty and Hicks point out, health and

---

[2] In fact, the degree of such difficulty, stemming partly from the multi-faceted nature of long-term care dependency, has led Sonia Conly to question the appropriateness of cost-effectiveness or cost-benefit analysis

well-being include numerous dimensions of physical, social, and psychological conditions, considerations especially relevant in LTC. This circumstance heightens the need to simplify the outcomes specification and to make it as explicit as possible in operational terms. The specification must be decided prior to investigating the cost-effectiveness of the project(s); otherwise both the data collection and analyses become the subject of quarrels among investigators and skepticism among the audience.

Despite the need for clarity and simplicity in specification, the analyst must avoid trying to gather all of the facets of concern into a single indicator. For that reason, it is necessary to specify a small number of outcome areas, leaving the relative weights to a later stage of the analysis or to those who make policy. In LTC for example, a favorite approach is to specify changes in functional ability (the ability to bathe, dress, feed oneself, etc.), changes in instrumental functional ability (the ability to shop, use a telephone, manage a checkbook, etc.), and changes in psychological status as evidence of outcomes. However, since research from demonstration projects has not shown much improvement in functional abilities as a result of most LTC services, functional outcome measures could probably be supplanted or complemented by other indicators to get a better picture of progress towards outcomes. For example, client or family satisfaction could be useful, especially in connection with less medically-oriented services. One implication of adding satisfaction measures to the set of outcome indicators may be that less costly support services (telephone checking, visiting, etc.) turn out to be more cost-effective in terms of quality-of-life than more costly, medically-oriented services. Of course, who makes the choices for the individual and who decides the weights of various types of outcomes still must be addressed as political questions (Stassen and Holahan, 1981).

One danger of aggregating too many separate outcomes stems from the ordinal results generated by many of the indicators. In many cases, for example, on the Katz scale for assessing the ability to cope with the activities of daily living (ADL), the scores reflect the presence or absence of certain capacities. The Katz system rates clients in terms of six levels of disability, but a score twice as large does not necessarily denote twice as much disability. Rather, it suggests a larger number of categories of incapacity. Nonetheless,

---

for evaluating and making decisions about alternative care modes. (See, "Critical Review of Research on Long-Term Care Alternatives," DHEW, Office of the Assistant Secretary for Planning and Evaluation, June 1977, pp. III-6ff.) Conly offers, instead, a program of analysis which presumably allows consideration of multiple objectives in terms of social costs and indicators of success. In operational terms, however, her approach appears similar to cost-effectiveness analysis but with a stronger social component.

one is tempted to add the scores on various disability measures in search of some composite measure of disability.

In framing any set of outcome measures, one must also avoid a "fallacy of composition," that is, outcomes for individuals may not necessarily be applicable to the groups to which the individual belongs. Given the objectives of social policy, an intervention may be judged more desirable for an individual than for a group, and *vice-versa*. Thus, outcomes do not necessarily have to be specified solely in individual terms. As a result, cost-effectiveness measures based on outcomes may be misleading when assessing group effects. For example, heavy doses of home care may be cost-effective for an individual when compared to nursing home care. When considering groups, however, nursing homes may enjoy some economies of scale or other cost advantages which make them the cost-effective choice. The preferred strategy would then reflect the relative weights given to the satisfaction of the individual versus the group and possibly the relative weights assigned client/family satisfaction versus maintenance of functional ability.

Although the point is emphasized elsewhere, it must be repeated that any specification and measurement of outcomes must be logically, and clearly linked to the interventions being compared.

At a very fundamental conceptual level, we must also recognize that much cost-effectiveness analysis may just be accepting the traditional policy and intervention variables. In LTC, this can involve an analysis based on functional or satisfaction measures of the types just discussed, or it may, at a more elemental level, seek to identify the cheapest manner of providing something simply known as "care." However, if cost-effectiveness is to develop, especially as an alternative to cost-benefit analysis (mainly because of the difficulty of quantifying outcomes in common terms), then it must be sharpened. This may well demand conceiving new types of outcomes, defining new outcomes measures, and developing new methods of measuring outcomes with respect to those newly defined outcomes. Such new outcomes could be linked to increased independence, improved family feeling, and a better quality of life. These conceptual and definitional tasks still remain before us (Stassen and Holahan, 1981).

Many Costs and Services

Costs appear to cause fewer difficulties to the analyst than do benefits, but they still create a number of definition and calculation problems. For example, revenue-based expenditures must be distinguished from the actual costs of producing care. Frequently, policy analysts will focus solely on the expenditures of government revenues; yet, to society, the costs of maintaining a program of support may considerably exceed direct funding allocations from public money (Grimaldi and Sullivan, 1981).

In this vein, Grimaldi and Sullivan (1981) citing the 1977 GAO study on home care, note that informal (largely family) care accounts for more than one-half of care costs at all levels of impairment and for more than 80 percent of care for the extremely impaired. They also question the claims of the Minnesota Age and Opportunity Center (MAOC) of being a cost-effective alternative to nursing homes on the grounds that 1) MAOC only considered governmental outlays and not family costs or rent paid while living in the community, 2) not all medical costs were added in, especially those from sub-sidized inputs, 3) the true value of volunteer costs was understated, and 4) MAOC subtracted both the patients' incomes above $25 per month from nursing home costs (on the grounds that these had to be paid by the patients and thus reduced government budgeted costs) and the patients' contributions to meals-on-wheels provided as part of home care programs (on the same grounds). In both cases, contributions from clients were part of the costs to society, even though not to the government.

Actually, there are many sets of costs associated with supporting an elderly person in the community. Doherty and Hicks (1975) distinguish three sets of care costs which do not always reveal themselves in cost studies. In providing HC, for example, there are the direct costs of providing the health-related services to the patient. Second, there may be health-related costs which are picked up by the patients, families, or friends, and which are not supported by external funding.

Third, there are personal living expenditures for the patient and the family. These are especially important when comparing home care with nursing homes, in which room and board are part of the total cost.

These extraordinary costs can also be viewed from the perspectives of the community, the socio-medical services system, and the family. Again with respect to home care, there may be additional social services and family costs to bring in supports not provided by Medicare and Medicaid. Among the former might be an additional social worker to help a family cope with the presence of a difficult older person; among the latter one might find the foregone earnings of family members who stayed home to care for an elder, or whose productivity was reduced by the caring effort and by associated psychological strain. (See the work of Grad and Sainsbury on home maintenance of mental patients in Britain in this connection.)

Grimaldi and Sullivan (1981) also have cautioned against a costing approach based on too narrow definitions. They assert that analysis must distinguish among total costs, total fixed costs, and total

263

variable costs. Even when these categories are adequately defined analytically, there is a danger that some costs deemed variable might actually be fixed, and *vice-versa*. For example, the cost of salaried personnel paid on a yearly basis might be listed as a variable labor cost. The marginal (additional) care costs of certain types of patients/clients may also differ, yet the analysts may assume that all categories have the same costs. This is particularly a problem when, for example, HC is analyzed as an alternative for patients discharged from nursing homes. In this case, the discharged patients may have actually been cheaper to serve as residents in the nursing home than those who remain, so the saving in discharging the former to HC may be lower than claimed. In like manner, newly eligible patients may be more costly to serve than presently eligible persons, possibly because of start-up costs associated with processing the former.

According to Grimaldi and Sullivan, proper costing analyses must be certain that alternatives characterized as substitutes are not actually complements (and *vice-versa*). Likewise, they assert that correct substitutes must be chosen. For example, the substitute for nursing home care may not be home care but rather intermediate care or domiciliary care of lower intensity. Furthermore, they warn against uncritical use of input costs as proxies for care costs, since inputs may vary in definitions of input units, intensities of input uses, patients actually benefited from use of a given input, and non-comparability of input units.

A Service Packages Model

David Dellinger of Duke University has developed a systemic model for the analysis of costs (1975). It examines the interactions of demanders and suppliers, focusing on the structures within which care is provided and by whom it is financed. (See Figure VII–1.)[3]

If the choice of service site and modality is to be considered as an economic problem, Dellinger argues that proper economic decisions can be made only if the costs of the services provided to the elderly (or any other target group) are compared to the value of those services to the elderly and to the society. (He does not explicitly consider the externalities question, but the flavor of his analysis suggests that it is to be included.) These costs and values will be generated by the combination of service packages and associated technology which will require resources to produce services and the satisfactions they yield. Service packages relate to individuals who require help rather than to particular producers of

---

[3] Outcomes and dependency levels were determined in accordance with the Duke OARS analysis and assessment instrument.

264

FIGURE VII-1
Schematic of Model

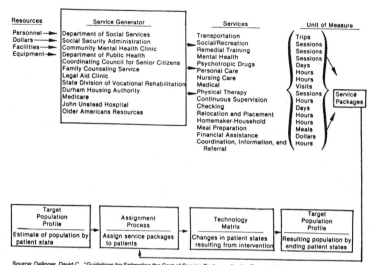

Source: Delinger, David C., "Guidelines for Estimating the Cost of Service Packages for the Chronically Impaired." (Apendixes omitted), Durham, Duke University Graduate School of Business Administration, July 1975, p. 1-3

services (many different producers can provide the same type of service) or to the place of residence of either the producer or client. Balancing value and cost leads to the determination of funding levels for specific types of care and the choice of service outputs within the funding limits.

In view of these considerations, the objectives of cost analysis are to estimate the future costs of service packages yet to be provided, the social opportunity costs of providing specified services in a given manner, the supply function of a capable producer, and the costs in terms of the use of physical resources, which can then be translated into money terms. The last proposition is important because of the distortion which existing institutional factors, especially the payment mechanism, may introduce into the analyses. Overall, those producers and technologies which yield lowest costs to achieve a given level of outcomes should be chosen.

In the Dellinger model, costs of given service packages are a function of the numbers of particular service packages to be produced (for example, nursing care), the nature of the institutions producing them (such as a nursing home or a home health agency), the identity of the particular institution responsible (the XYZ Nursing Home), and the other products of the specified institution (XYZ's home chore services, acute level hospital procedures, etc.). Amounts of output are relevant not only because of effects on total costs, but also because average and marginal costs may be affected by economies of scale in output production and in the use and/or production of inputs. The type of institution is significant because of the effect of a particular organizational structure, while other products of the institution may influence costs as a result of high cost outputs, such as available medical care.

A number of potential problems can create major analytical difficulties. First, the allocation of clients among producing units can alter the organizational structure of producers and thus their cost functions, especially if economies or diseconomies of scale are present. Similarly, producers may contract with specific suppliers of inputs who cannot adjust to sudden increased demands. Some of these suppliers are specialized for certain types of institutions (hospital laundry supply services, for example), even though their products are not unique. This type of problem is especially awkward if new Federal programs create a larger demand for specific types of service packages. Often this circumstance will dictate financial outcomes different from real resource use outcomes, so it is better to assess resource rather than money cost effects, particularly if the reallocations of clients are to be permanent.

The problem of institutional definition also arises. Often large "equivalence classes" or categories of producers must be employed for policy and analytical convenience. For example, Federal reimbursement rules use the SNF/ICF dichotomy to determine level of care (level of service intensity) in cost-related reimbursement formulae. These groupings may be too broad, concealing actual differences in the nature of service packages. In the long run, these differences may be eroded; in the short run, they probably will not. Perhaps the main equivalence class problem arises in connection with private homes as the site of HC. All homes are not the same for these purposes. Indeed, differences in size, amenities, internal arrangements, capacity for stress, and level of family support may account for much of the success or failure of identical HC programs in ministering to similar patients.

Cost analyses of service packages can founder on the familiar problem of joint costing. For example, if there is both a baby and a dependent elder to be cared for, a relative or even a home health service may find that the marginal cost of taking care of one, given the presence of the other, is negligible. The analytical problem of costing for policy purposes in such cases is formidable.

In view of these considerations, Dellinger offers a number of guidelines for conducting costing studies. Where possible, one should develop cost functions, rather than point estimates of costs, since the latter provide little help in predicting the results of changed circumstances. The cost functions, to be of maximum use, must allow for the nature of the service packages to be produced, the numbers actually produced, and the intended levels of output. Market structures are important, since they affect suppliers' behavior, the costs of changing from one type of service package to another, and the availability of inputs. Although such structural influences are important for the behavior of suppliers, real resource costs should be sought if the social opportunity costs are to be accurately assessed. Definitions of equivalence classes must be precise. Simultaneously, differences among those classes must be distinguished from differences in managerial style. One may generate actual differences in costs because of fundamental differences in production functions, etc., yet the cost differentials may be artifacts of personality or organizational history, which change only over time.

Although Dellinger's methodology of analysis is highly abstract and ambitious in its standards, his approach provides some important guidance for the cost analyst who should, in theory, follow the recipe provided or at least try to make some defensible substitutions for the desired types of data which may not exist.

Dellinger emphasized data and methodological issues as he attempted to apply the specified cost analysis to 18 dependent elderly in Durham, North Carolina to assess the private home as a provider of service packages. He initially analyzed the parts of

267

service packages provided from inside and outside the household. Dellinger's definition of household production was anything used in the home which was made or purchased with household resources. He excluded services produced by the dependent person for her/himself and any routine household chores which the household would provide without the presence of the dependent person.

Thus, the provision was that of care or extraordinary personal services which members of households would not routinely provide to each other. The admittedly preliminary findings showed that 10 of the 18 dependent elderly in the survey received household-generated, non-supervisory services; all 10 were supervised by members of their households, who offered this service jointly with other services. The most common services provided by family and friends outside the household were nursing, home chore aid, transportation and checking, but these were only provided in four cases. Very importantly, family and friends outside the household did not provide much help, suggesting that the "relevant other" has to be close by to make much difference. Although Dellinger's data relate to few care recipients, they shed light on sources of service. The experiment also indicates the nature and complexity of the service costing which must take place to develop valid cost analyses.

Secondary and Tertiary Costs

William Pollak, in a study for the Urban Institute (1973), has extended the concepts of relevant costs to explicitly embrace the issues of secondary and tertiary costs, as well as the extraordinary family and community costs just considered. His argument, like those of Doherty *et al*, Grimaldi and Sullivan, and Dellinger, is that cost calculations should include all costs, regardless of how such costs are distributed. Costs to Pollak are a function of family status, level of functional competence, and quality of care provided. Clearly, these factors determine the parameters of the service packages defined by Dellinger. In the specifics of costs, Pollak includes housing, nutrition, supervision, environmental hygiene, personal care, transportation, recreation, medical care, and miscellaneous small or patient-specific items.

Among the more important (and difficult) costing questions are those associated with the attribution for rent or cost of housing space, especially in owner-occupied housing, when considering provision of home care. The key question is how to account for the equivalent of the housing services which a nursing home by its very nature provides. The need to provide shelter, whatever the care site, suggests that some attribution must be made for housing costs, even if there is only a "shadow price" or presumptive basis for costing.

The shadow price question is even more taxing when evaluating the services of volunteers and family members. Although volunteers may provide valuable services through their labor, it might be argued that such labor is socially costless, since volunteers presumably gain utility or satisfaction from their efforts. These utility gains supposedly compensate for any income foregone by not engaging in paid work. On the other hand, if volunteers are used in one setting, they cannot be used in another, so there is an opportunity cost of their services. (After all, there are never as many volunteers as one wants!) In addition, Pollak argues that many volunteer programs contain the germs of much larger programs which may require the services of paid staff (as has happened with, for instance, the American Red Cross). If that change is expected, it is all the more important to use the cost of labor which would have to be paid if volunteers were not available. Otherwise, volunteers are overused or not used rationally.

Pollak applied his costing logic to a number of specific circumstances, among them foster family care and family-provided home care. In the case of foster families, one could assert that the true costs of care are measured by payments to the foster families from the paying source, since foster families presumably balance their gains and costs in deciding to participate. However, the present system of foster care is, in many cases, highly unstable, with elderly people being shunted from one family to another. Therefore, one can reasonably argue that the true cost of a more stable system would be higher than is the present cost. Also, the supply of foster care may only be expandable (in the face, say, of an expansion in major, publicly-financed care programs) at increasing (marginal) cost. This would be especially true if an expanded system drew in increasingly impaired patients. Pollak, in effect, is calling for more research on foster family supply curves for care. The same imperative applies to the supply of volunteer care.

The proper costing of family services might, by contrast, appear quite straightforward. That is, one could impute the costs of family services as the income lost because of staying home to take care of an elderly family member. This simplicity is, however, illusory for two reasons. First, the helping family member may not have been employed, hence not incurring any opportunity costs. Second, there may be some gain to the "relevant other" family member or friend which reduces the loss which may be experienced by foregoing paid labor. Pollak concludes that the proper rate of imputed labor cost in this case would be greater than zero but less than the market wage for the type of labor provided. The level is not clear. Note that in imputing the costs of family care, one must avoid the double counting which would occur if both foregone earnings and the imputed value of family caring activities were added in. If a family

269

member works at home to give care, that work, in a theoretical sense, should be construed as having a cost equivalent to the work income foregone. Alternatively, that effort could be costed at the prices paid to agencies in the community which provide equivalent services. Both, however, cannot be done. The nascent theory of family labor supply, coupled with empirical econometric work, provides the basis for some urgently needed research, particularly if home-based services may be expanded.

Costs and Impairments

One of Pollak's main contributions to the discussion of care costs is his systematic analysis of the relationship between the costs of care and the level of impairment. This issue has been analyzed in connection with nursing home costs where patient characteristics were recognized as an argument in the cost and production functions. In Pollak's models for assessing the costs of alternatives in a cost-effectiveness mode, patient impairment level is joined with (attempted) quality of care in a given care setting to determine cost per client per day. Figure VII-2, which generates a "cost surface," all points corresponding to combinations of impairment and quality, presents his argument. The diagram measures quality on one axis and impairment on the other. For each impairment level, different qualities of care yield differing costs, and *vice-versa*. Note that a different surface can be generated for each different type of care setting. Note also that the cost-effectiveness comparison enters the scene in terms of the specified desired outcomes of any given care regimen. Desired outcomes can thus be explicitly included.

The cost-quality-impairment surfaces can be "sliced" at any point on the quality or impairment axis to show changes in costs for, say, changes in impairment. Pollak shows such a slice (assuming quality constant) as a curve linking cost of care to level of impairment. The cost surfaces of a number of care sites may generate such curves, allowing cost comparisons to be drawn at a given quality level between or among care sites. For a given level of quality (measured as process, outcome, or some weighted combination of both) of care, the costs of caring for patients with differing levels of impairment can be directly compared between care sites. (See Figures VII–3 and VII–4.) The individual curves and the comparisons using curves from two or more care sites have become quite familiar, forming a basis for comparative cost studies. (See the General Accounting Office's analysis of home care services in Cleveland; 1977, 1979. See also Jay Greenberg's 1974 study of Minnesota alternative care sites.) Using Pollak's graphic comparison and following his method of comparing costs based on quality and impairment, one may avoid the pitfalls of relying on single number comparisons, which implicitly hold both of these variables constant

270

FIGURE VII-2
Cost of Care in a Particular Setting

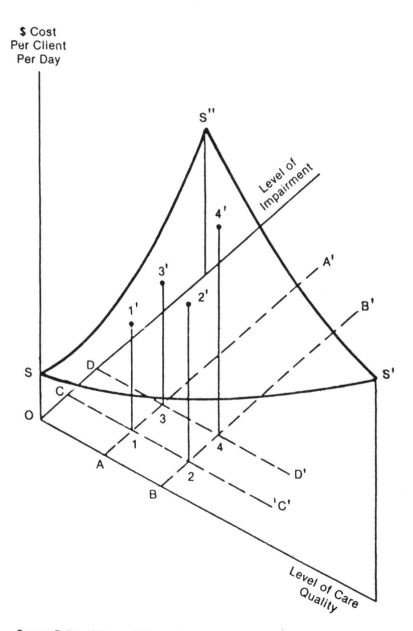

Source: Pollak, William with the assistance of Joanne Helferty, "Costs of Alternative Care Settings for the Elderly," Urban Institute, Working Paper 963–11, March 12, 1973.

FIGURE VII-3
Cost of Home Care

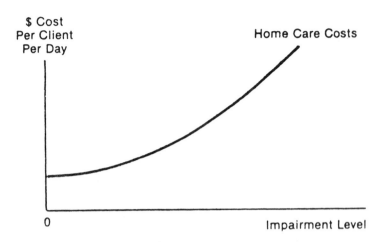

Source: Pollak, William with the assistance of Joanne Helferty, "Costs of Alternative Care Settings for the Elderly," Urban Institute, Working Paper 963-11, March 12, 1973.

FIGURE VII-4
Cost of Home and Nursing Home Care

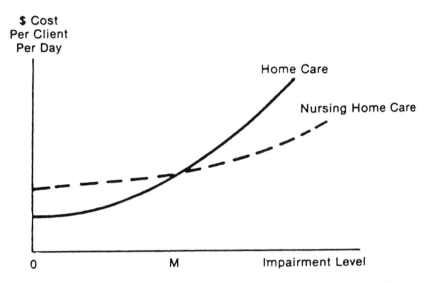

Source: Pollak, William with the assistance of Joanne Helferty, "Costs of Alternative Care Settings for the Elderly," Urban Institute, Working Paper 963-11, March 12, 1973.

FIGURE VII-5
Tabular Display for Cost-Effectiveness Analysis of Day Care, Home Care, and Institutional Care
(Format adapted from Kazanowski)

Program	Number Patients In First Assessment	Effectiveness Criterion						Per Diem Cost ($)		
		IADL		ADL		MSQ	Total	Primary	Secondary	Tertiary
		Number	Ratio	Number	Ratio	Number	Ratio			
Day Care	45	37	.082	40	0.88	38	0.84	27.38	18.60	3.20	5.58
Home Care	78	55	0.70	61	0.78	54	0.69	22.43	14.26	2.05	6.12
Institutional Care	60	45	0.75	42	0.70	31	0.52	26.69	25.12	1.57	0

Number and proportion of patients in first assessment whose function on each scale was maintained or improved in second assessment

Source: Doherty, N. J. G. and Barbara Hicks, "Cost-Effectiveness Analysis and Alternative Health Care Programs for the Elderly," *Health Services Research*, Summer 1977.*

*Reprinted with permission.

274

in the analysis without any justification. Unfortunately, many comparative analyses of home care and nursing home care fail to recognize this difficulty.

A Convenient Method for Showing Cost-Effectiveness

Doherty and Hicks (1977) have offered a form of Kazanowski's tabular display approach (TDA) as an alternative to more mathematical formulations which may confuse readers. The tabular approach allows for simplicity in presentation when more elegant mathematical formulations may be inappropriate because of unsuitable data. Moreover, the tabular method readily permits the evaluation of programs on the basis of criteria that are not easily measured. According to Doherty and Hicks, the TDA can be used ". . . to evaluate performance within a care program or among alternative programs." It also may be used cross-sectionally or longitudinally. Furthermore, the TDA allows analysis of multiple criteria and complex programs. Figure VII–5 shows an example of a TDA on which the multiple criteria are shown as column headings and the different care modalities as row headings. Obviously a number of tabular arrangements are available to researchers. For example, criteria can be arranged in decreasing order of importance, allowing concentration on the more important objectives of the analysis. Again, this display should be set up prior to the formal investigation so that crucial elements can be given most attention in the research.

Lining up programs in the TDA manner presumably will make the particularly weak and strong choices obvious, but it will not necessarily show any one choice as preferable on all bases. Nevertheless, the TDA method narrows the range of choices for the policymaker, who then may assign weights and choose programs. This is important for the dependent elderly in the long-term care system because the choice of effectiveness criteria may be unusually difficult, since many of the relevant concerns cannot be put into operation in very specific terms. Rather, they have to do with maintenance, deterioration, or improvement in functional status. Nonetheless, in the TDA argument, three sets of criteria related to functional capacity and ability to cope in the community were identified and could be used as sources of data. The criteria of choice are ADL (as measured by the Katz scale), the IADL (a measurement of ability to undertake instrumental tasks that allow a person to function), and MSQ (a measure of cognitive ability).

In applying the TDA method, one might begin with a set of initial assessments of patients in various care sites/modalities. These assessments would be later repeated, and the number of patients who have shown maintenance or improvement of function, as measured by the three scales, would be compared with the number of patients at the beginning of the program. Note that this particular

275

use of the TDA is coupled with maintenance or improvement of functional capacity as the desired objective. Other objectives in long-term care might lead to the use of other instruments of assessment and/or other weights being given to the results.

In the example taken from Doherty and Hicks, the data are arranged to show the proportion of patients maintaining or improving functional capacity between two assessments (the effectiveness criterion). *Per diem* cost of patients in the different care modes is also shown, so that analysts and policymakers may view their relative cost-effectiveness based on differing criteria. For example, day care is preferred on the basis of the three effectiveness criteria, but home care is preferred on cost grounds. As noted, the choices will not necessarily be unambiguous, and the policymakers will have to assign their own weights.

To accommodate subgroups within the patient sets, outcomes for each effectiveness criterion (function status in this case) may be subdivided into high, medium, and low. Patients could then be classified by such finer status screens at the beginning and during the progress of the programs and so-called transition matrices calculated. Carried further, the transition process can show numbers and proportions of possible changes in functional status measured on a number of dimensions. (See Figures VII–6 and VII–7 for examples of the transition matrices). If enough patients are available, one can calculate Markov chains to indicate the probabilities of passing from one status set to another in different modalities of care. Also, one may be able to set standards, norms, or expectations for changes in status for differing programs. Additionally, the probable effectiveness of different programs in dealing with patients with different characteristics can be stated.

Despite the mechanical attractiveness of the TDA approach as one method of assessing cost and effectiveness simultaneously, the techniques cannot remove the need to make choices and judgments about preferred criteria and about the combinations of desirable outcomes. For example, one cannot, from the TDA method by itself, decide if a change in functional status for a group of patients from high, medium, and low to high, low, and medium (on ADL, IADL, and MSQ, respectively) represents an improvement or a decline. However, to repeat an earlier point, TDA can simplify the presentation of data on widely disparate outcomes and allow the policymaker to simultaneously compare costs among different programs.

Structural and Institutional Aspects of the Alternatives Question

In addition to the definitional and methodological questions just raised, a number of structural and institutional issues complicate

FIGURE VII-6
Transition Matrix for Patients' Changes on One Program

Function Status at First Assessment	Function Status at Second Assessment				Number Maintained	Number Improved	Effectiveness Ratio[1]
	High	Medium	Low	Dead			
High	15	3	2	0	15	0	0.75
Medium	15	10	5	0	10	5	0.75
Low	1	7	8	4	8	8	0.80

[1]Ratio of number of patients with improved and maintained function to number (29) in each function status group at first assessment

Source: Doherty, N.J.G., Joan Segal, and Barbara Hicks, "Cost Effectiveness and Alternative Health Care Programs for the Elderly," *Health Services Research*, Summer 1977.*

*Reprinted with permission.

FIGURE VII-7

Transition Matrix: Changes of Status on Three Function Criteria

	Assessment II. Criterion Scores					
	(H,H,H)	(H,H,M)	(H,H,L)	(H,M,H)	...	(L,L,L) (dead)
Assessment I Criterion Scores	(H,H,H)					
	(H,H,M)					
	(H,H,L)					
	(H,M,H)					
	⋮					
	(L,L,L)					

Source: Doherty, N.J.G., Joan Segal, and Barbara Hicks, "Cost Effectiveness and Alternative Health Care Programs for the Elderly," *Health Services Research*, Summer 1977.*

*Reprinted with permission.

the analysis of alternatives in long-term care. Most of these issues present themselves in comparisons with the nursing home, which has abundant institutional and structural problems of its own.

Perhaps the most significant difficulty lies in the strong institutional bias of the present pattern of long-term care. This bias has been ascribed by some analysts to the attitude of professionals, especially the MDs, who may believe that their time is more efficiently used in a hospital or other institutional setting. (This would not explain, however, why physicians are allegedly seldom in nursing homes.) It has also been claimed that hospitals may find it more profitable to serve inpatients rather than outpatients in a scheme of outpatient-day care-home care programs. Another alleged source of difficulty is the family, which supposedly has a desire to institutionalize elders. As shown previously, however, this attitude does not exist to the extent usually claimed. Yet another cause of problems has been the shortage of trained professionals to staff the various types of alternative systems.

Some observers suggest that the key reason for the strong growth of the U.S. institutional system of LTC may lie in the rapid increase in the number of elderly persons at risk. While increased numbers may increase the demand for LTC services, they alone do not justify increasing institutionalization. They could possibly be equally well served at home or in less intensely institutional settings than the nursing home. Ultimately, a basic cause of the institutional bias may be found in the method of reimbursement under public financing programs, especially Medicare and Medicaid. Although some of the effects of the programs have been mitigated by Title XX of the Social Security Act, which allows the development of community-based services, and by home care and nutrition programs under Title III of the Older Americans Act, the combination of State discretion under Medicaid and the strong medical bias (the medical model) under Medicare has rendered the development and financing of alternate care systems very difficult. These influences are all the more important since Medicare and Medicaid expenditures for LTC are many times greater than those under Titles XX or III.

Medicare's Medical Orientation

Medicare was conceived mainly as a program to relieve elderly people of the financial burdens of medical and hospital costs. Its primary focus is on acute and institutional care. In fiscal year 1979, Medicare spent almost $30 billion; of this, only $373 million went for nursing home care, whereas almost $22 billion went for hospital care, and $6.4 billion for physicians' services (Gibson, 1980). In fiscal year 1978, out of a total Medicare outlay of almost $24 billion, only $430 million went to home care (HCFA, 1980). Almost one-third of the HC visits were to people living in the Northeast.

279

Under present Medicare regulations, entitlement to home care and other community care services is contingent on a physician's determination of such need on a medical basis pursuant to a care plan established within 14 days after discharge from a hospital. To qualify for 100 visits of home care under Part A (Hospital Insurance), an individual must be homebound and certified by a physician as in need of skilled nursing or physical or speech therapy. Under Part B (Supplementary Medical Insurance), there is no three day requirement, but the medical pre-condition still applies. Beneficiaries must also be homebound and require skilled nursing services, as under Part A. As if to reinforce the strong medical orientation of the Medicare entitlement and the institutional flavor of even the services provided at home, the list of covered HC services is heavily medical: nursing care, physical, speech, or occupational therapy, medical social services under the direction of a physician, part-time services of a home health aide (not a home chore aide), medical supplies (other than drugs and medications), medical appliances, and medical services provided by an intern or a resident-in-training. On the other hand, many services which would be important in a home health or alternatives system are not covered under Medicare: drugs and medicines outside of an SNF or an acute hospital, vision care, including spectacles, dental care, hearing aids, periodic examinations, etc. Lack of these services may drastically hinder the ability of elderly people to function in the community, thus contributing to their apparent need for more intensive nursing care.

The problem of limited covered services is symptomatic of a larger difficulty, that of non-participation in Medicare by many elderly who cannot meet the deductible and copayment requirements. If they cannot participate in the system at all, they obviously cannot gain access to those types of provision for which prior participation is a pre-condition.

Medicaid's Limits on Alternatives

Many poor elderly people who would rely on Medicaid are also caught in the predicament of not being poor enough to qualify as medically needy (or they live in a State like Texas, which has no medically needy program) or they do not have income adequate to pay for the home or other alternative care services they require. GAO (1979) cites an example from Austin, Texas, in which the income necessary to pay for home care services was lower than the median income of elderly in the area.

The low incomes of many elderly and the inability of many of their families to support them provide strong incentives to institutionalization. Specifically, commitment to a nursing home entitles the patient to a wide range of support services, including board, room, and personal care. Alternate care modes, by contrast, carry

280

no such entitlements. If these elderly were to remain in the community, many would not qualify for any type of Medicaid support. Even if Medicaid-provided home or other alternate care benefits became available, the range and frequency of services might be so small that the clients and/or their families could not provide the remainder of support. In some cases, lower income and asset limits are applied to community-based clients than to nursing home residents. In other cases, poor elderly who cannot pay for, say, home care services and who have incomes too high to qualify them for Medicaid home care benefits may enter a nursing home as private patients and then "spend-down" to the qualifying income levels for nursing home Medicaid support. Perhaps one of the greatest ironies of these income and eligibility problems is that, even if a home or other alternate care program is developed for which many nursing home residents might once have been suited, extended nursing home residency incapacitates a person for independent living. Heavy physical dependencies develop, while the vital network of family and friends has been disrupted. In some cases, households have been disbanded, thus requiring the creation of a whole new set of relationships and physical arrangements, frequently an impossibility.

Medicaid's alternative care benefits appear to be broader than those of Medicare. In fiscal year 1979, however, home health services, as an example, only accounted for $264 million, while expenditures for nursing homes came to $8.7 billion.[4] Of the over 358,000 Medicaid HC recipients in fiscal year 1978, over 55 percent lived in New York, which accounted for 77 percent of national Medicaid HC spending. Under Medicaid, home health care, personal care, and adult day care are all options which the States can offer to beneficiaries. Until 1976, however, the States were also empowered to impose Medicare-like restrictions on eligibility, that is, to require a previous hospital stay, etc. Since that year, skilled nursing and previous hospital stays can no longer be required, but recipients of HC, for example, may still have to be homebound to be eligible. Furthermore, home health care (which does not usually cover personal and housekeeping chores) and personal care (which allows for support to help with activities of daily living) have to be prescribed by a physician, as does adult day care (a collection of medical and health-related services provided by clinics to disabled Medicaid beneficiaries). Although HC is a covered benefit in every State or jurisdiction participating in the Medicaid program, only nine States cover personal care services, and only six cover adult day care.

---

[4] Unpublished data from HCFA's Office of Research, Demonstrations, and Statistics

State discretion regarding types of programs also applies to types of services and amounts of utilization which they may choose to cover under Medicaid. Many States have accordingly curtailed amount, duration, and comprehensiveness severely. They also set low reimbursement levels for covered services, an action which has caused some major problems for the provision of nursing home care as well as for home, personal, and adult day care. Reimbursement restrictions (either denials of charges, very low allowances, or both) have forced many home health agencies, for example, to refuse Medicaid patients. In addition, individual States have imposed stringent regulations on providers (often using Medicare standards) and, to the extent permissible under Federal law and regulations, on beneficiaries as well.

Title XX As An Alternative Support

Under the Title XX social services program it would appear that there is leeway to develop and use alternative types of care. Although the range of permitted services is quite broad, the program is subject to a limit on Federal expenditures, ($2.9 billion in fiscal year 1979) limiting State matching funds as well. Title XX programs are means tested and, moreover, are highly skewed to children and AFDC recipients, as well as to recipients of SSI payments. As a result, the elderly often must compete with other client groups for a rather limited pool of resources. This further limits the potential expansion in home care and other alternative service systems under Title XX.

Overall, the combination of medical bias, limited support for service development under Medicaid, and the means testing of certain eligibilities under Medicaid and Title XX may have truncated the development of alternative care systems. The extent to which this is true, however, is a matter more of assertion than of analysis, and more research is required on these issues. Not only must analysis focus on these aspects of regulation and reimbursement, but also on the effect of copayment and deductible provisions.

Fragmentation of Alternative Services

The fragmented provision structure also hinders the development of alternatives. With a few notable exceptions, often the creations of Federally-sponsored demonstration projects, agencies which function well independently are unaware of each others' services and organizationally incapable of any sort of joint support. Because of this lack, a number of demonstration projects (Triage; Monroe County, New York; Wisconsin Community Care Organization; Georgia Alternative Health Care Systems; etc.) have designed programs of assessment, care planning, care management, and services for specific groups of elderly people living in the community. The results of these demonstrations are not conclusive, although pre-

282

liminary data are encouraging, at least in terms of the ability to coordinate service provision. (See Chapter VI.) Congress has also mandated a series of so-called "channeling agency" demonstrations. These are being jointly organized by the Department of Health and Human Services' Assistant Secretary for Planning and Evaluation, the Health Care Financing Administration, and the Administration on Aging. Another type of coordinating agency is the social health maintenance organization (SHMO), proposed by Brandeis University's Heller School, which combines assessment, care planning, service provision, and case monitoring to ensure quality and appropriateness of services (Diamond and Berman, 1979).

A lack of information among elderly clients and their families aggravates the problems created by lack of coordination. Particularly for those elders who may be ill, confused, and frightened, it is often next to impossible to know one's rights and entitlements. It is even more of a problem to know where to go for which services or who to contact for help. Even if services exist in the community, dependent individuals and their families may be unable to combine these resources in the appropriate service packages. As a result, services may go unused or only partially used unless some agency can perform the brokerage function.

The potential user of alternative services is limited by a lack of income, combined with the nature and skewing of the Medicare/Medicaid system. Many elderly people have limited incomes and assets. Consequently, they cannot explore alternatives to the nursing home. SSI and social security benefits, as well as limited pensions, may not permit many elderly to demand alternative services which might support them as effectively as nursing homes. The price reductions (to users) of subsidized institutional care and the relative lack of subsidies for non-institutional LTC services hamper the development of alternatives. Certainly, for those elderly without families or spouses, being poor makes it harder to fend off institutionalization and thus to support the growth and prosperity of alternative care systems.

Specification and Identification Problems

Even if the elderly can gain access to coordinated support systems as proposed by Dellinger, it is still necessary to identify and assess family and client problems and to ensure the quality of the services provided. These issues are discussed elsewhere, but their particular applicability to the alternatives question must be emphasized. Sager (1979), for example, has shown that there is wide disagreement among professionals as to the appropriate amounts and types of care which should be provided to dependent elderly, even though there may be general agreement as to their level of dependence. His findings also show that individual assessors and care planners diverge widely with respect to the care to be provided to specific individuals, although they do ordinally rank the intensity of need for care consistently. Differences in amounts of care appear related to professional discipline (for example, doctors and nurses prescribe more hours of home care in their areas of specialization), more knowledge about patients (which implies more prescribed care), and greater experience as a case consultant (which implies less prescribed care).

The shortage of appropriate screening procedures and the emphasis on medical characteristics by the Professional Standards Review Organizations (PSROs) in conducting LTC reviews may well have led to the waste of resources via inappropriate placements. GAO (1979) claimed that 55 percent of Medicaid and 48 percent of non-Medicaid supported patients had few ADL problems and possibly could have stayed in the community at a lower public cost. At a conceptual level, these issues relate to the problem of specifying outcomes; yet they are administrative issues as well. As part of the lack of coordinated services, there is also a great lack of means to screen the elderly (or other populations at risk) for the presence and prevalence of conditions which create dependency that requires intervention.

Also, there have been few specifications in either a process or outcome sense for measuring the quality or performance of providers of alternative services. This lack also exists in the case of nursing homes, although there the state of the art and the practical means for assessing quality are rapidly developing. (See the discussion of nursing home quality in Chapter IV.) Filling this gap in knowledge and practice is one of the purposes of the recently-funded University of Colorado comparative study of hospital-based and free-standing nursing homes and home health care facilities. At this point, however, quality assurance in home care and other long-term care alternatives remains largely unexplored.

Alternatives Research

Having considered a number of issues and approaches to the alternatives question, it is appropriate to assess the nature of the research about alternatives, particularly in relation to present and potential utilization, effectiveness, and cost. These categories have clear links to the access, quality, and cost issues discussed earlier.

An extended list of the findings on alternative LTC programs will not be provided here, since information on studies can be found in a number of excellent recent research reviews. (See Applied Managment Sciences, 1975; Conly, 1977; Doherty, Segal, and Hicks, 1978; GAO, 1979; and Stassen and Holahan, 1981.) (For examples of cost and outcome findings, see Figures VII–8 and VII–9.) In addition, a

284

FIGURE VII-8
Cost Findings from Alternative Care Programs

Program	Objective	Type of Service	Number of Clients	Year	Estimated Daily Savings per Client (1976 dollars)[b]
Home Care Association Rochester, N.Y.	Reduce length of hospital stays	Home care	458	1973	141
Pre-Planned Post Hospital Home Care, N.Y.,N.Y.	Reduce length of hospital stays	Home care	5,000	1960	82
Blue Cross/Blue Shield of Greater Philadelphia	Reduce length of hospital stays	Home care	3,940	1970	225
Home Care Program St. Luke's Hospital, N.Y.,N.Y.	Reduce length of hospital stays	Home care	25	1971	225
Chelsea Village Program, N.Y.,N.Y.	Reduce length of hospital stays	Home care	222	1973	215
Schenectady Rehabilitation and Day Hospital Schenectady,N.Y.	Reduce length of hospital stays	Day hospital	80	1960	75
Burke Day Hospital White Plains, N.Y.	Prevent institutionalization	Day hospital	79	1975	68
Highland Heights Experiment Fall River, Mass.	Prevent institutionalization	Sheltered housing	91	1971	142
Project Able Multnomah Co., Ore.	Prevent institutionalization	Home care	1,400	1974	13
Personal Care Program Hartford, Conn.	Prevent institutionalization	Home care	202	1974	5 (13) ($5 when compared with intermediate care, $13 when compared with skilled care)
Brightwood Day Care Center Athens, Ga.	Prevent institutionalization	Day care	18	1974	- 6
Center for Creative Living Lexington, Ky.	Prevent institutionalization	Day care	30	1974	none
Mosholu-Montefiore Geriatric Day Care Program, N.Y.,N.Y.	Prevent institutionalization	Day care	90	1974	-11
On Lok Senior Health Services Center San Francisco, Ca.	Prevent institutionalization	Day care	92	1974	2
Health Care by the Day Program Syracuse, N.Y.	Prevent institutionalization	Day care	39	1974	-2
St. Otto's Day Care Program Little Falls, Minn.	Prevent institutionalization	Day care	14	1974	8
San Diego Senior Adult Day Care Program San Diego, Ca.	Prevent institutionalization	Day care	129	1974	4
Tucson Senior Health Improvement Program Tucson, Ariz.	Prevent institutionalization	Day care	390	1974	4
Levindale Hebrew Geriatric Center and Hospital Baltimore, Md.	Prevent institutionalization				
Day-Care Program		Day care	30	1974	10
Community-Care Program		Home care	24	1974	18
Concord Housing		Sheltered housing	28	1974	16

a. For programs above the line, estimated savings were calculated from a comparison of *per diem* program costs with *per diem* hospital costs. For programs below the line, estimated savings were calculated from a comparison of *per diem* program costs with *per diem* nursing home costs.

b. The estimate of daily savings is the difference between institutional and alternative care costs adjusted to 1976 dollars by the medical component of the Consumer Price Index. The semi-private room figure was used to adjust the institutional costs, and the total figure for hospital and professional services was used to recalculate alternative care costs. For programs whose reported costs were averaged over several years, an average of the respective index figures for that period was used ("Medical Care Component," 1977).

Source: Doherty, N. J. G., Joan Segal and Barbara Hicks, "Alternatives to Institutionalization for the Aged: Viability and Cost Effectiveness, *Aged Care & Services Review*, Vol. 1, No. 1, January/February 1978, p. 11."

*Reprinted with permission.

FIGURE VII-9

Outcome Findings from Alternative Care Programs

Program	Outcomes
Home Care Association, Rochester, N.Y.	Hospital stays were reduced by 21 days per patient.
Pre-Planned Post Hospital Home Care, N.Y., N.Y.	Hospital stays were reduced by 22.6 days per patient.
Blue Cross/Blue Shield of Greater Philadelphia	Hospital stays were reduced by 12.9 days per patient.
Home Care Program, St. Luke's Hospital, N.Y., N.Y.	Home Care patients had shorter hospital stays, fewer re-admissions for recurring strokes, and fewer deaths than controls, and were able to remain self-sufficient in the community.
Chelsea Village Program, N.Y., N.Y.	Hospital stays were reduced by 14 days per patient. Ten percent of the patients improved in functional independence, and 52 percent remained stabilized at home.
Schenectady Rehabilitation and Day Hospital, Schenectady, N.Y.	Physical functioning measured by five different scoring methods "showed considerable improvement in a significant percentage of cases."
Burke Day Hospital, White Plains, N.Y.	Physical functioning improved for stroke patients and patients with musculoskeletal disorders.
Highland Heights Experiment, Fall River, Mass.	Experimental group had improved self-rated health, greater satisfaction with housing, more socialization and satisfaction with social contacts than control group. No short-term differences in measures of physical functioning and cognitive and emotional states were reported.
Personal Care Program, Hartford, Conn.	Clients showed improved mental health and life satisfaction; social supports were increased. There were no differences in activities of daily living over time.
Levindale Hebrew Geriatric Center and Hospital, Baltimore, MD. (Day-Care Program, Community-Care Program, and Sheltered Housing	For effectiveness, measured by functioning status, day care ranked first, community care second, sheltered housing third, and institutional care fourth.

Source: Doherty, N. J. G., Joan Segal and Barbara Hicks, "Alternatives to Institutionalization for the Aged: Viability and Cost Effectiveness," *Aged Care and Services Review*, January/February 1978.*

*Reprinted with permission.

recent Medicaid data base search performed for this long-term care study (1980) showed 247 separate articles covering the subjects of home care for the elderly and deinstitutionalization of the elderly, while a recently published bibliography showed well in excess of 325 items on home health care.[5] Thus, our purpose here is to summarize results and judgments about research quality. (See Figures VII–8, 9.)

Much of the summarized research has actually described demonstrations and specially created projects, rather than provided the careful theoretical and empirical assessments demanded by scientific analyses of utilization, effectiveness, and cost. Additionally, there is not always a clear distinction between research to assess the results of existing systems and the evaluation of demonstrations that examine the consequences of changing systems.

Cost questions motivate much of the research on the alternatives. In addition, home care (and, to a lesser extent, day care and congregate housing) has elicited an enthusiastic band of followers, many of whom have been impressed with European experiences. These advocates—some policymakers, some providers, some clinicians, some academics—have provided powerful impetus to establishing and researching alternative care systems. Although these efforts are often mounted to enhance the quality of life of those in the care system or to reduce the costs of providing care, the intensity of the advocacy has contributed to certain problems of research quality and usefulness. Fortunately, the situation since 1975 has changed dramatically, most recently with the establishment in 1979 of the *Home Health Care Services Quarterly,* a scientific journal for the field.

In general, much of the research reviewed in these surveys is positive about desirability and cost-effectiveness of alternatives, but it has been unsymmetrical. Most of the alternatives have been compared with acute hospitals and nursing homes, rather than with each other. Also, the emphasis has been on various forms of home care.

Additionally, outcomes were often unspecified, statistical techniques inappropriate, and surveyed populations were not necessarily candidates for the institutions against which alternatives were compared. These problems are examined in the following discussion.

Assessments of Research Quality

As indicated, much of the alternatives reasearch demonstrates some weakness. The surveys just listed include a number of useful

---

[5] There is much overlap between the data base searches and published bibliographies. See DHEW, Health Resources Administration, *Home Health Care Programs: A Selected Bibliography* (HRA Publication 79-60, Hyattsville, Maryland: July, 1979).

assessments of the quality of research on alternatives. Such assessments are found in AMS (1975), Conly (1977), and Stassen-Holahan report (1981). In addition, a recent review by Grimaldi and Sullivan (1981) for the American Health Care Association and the National Foundation for Long-Term Health Care is very helpful. Many of these reviews considered some of the same research projects.

Grimaldi's and Sullivan's analysis provides a useful introduction to evaluations of alternative care research and offers many comments about the results and methods of the specific studies reviewed, one by TransCentury Corporation, one by the National Center for Health Services Research, and one by the Stanford Research Institute.

The TransCentury study covered 10 adult day care programs funded as demonstration projects under Section 222 of the Social Security Act. On the basis of extensive data on available services, admissions criteria, persons served, staffing patterns, and costs, the study concluded that ADC offered significant cost savings when compared to nursing home care. The total annual cost of ADC per patient in the median facility was between $4,500 and $6,200, depending on weekly attendance rate. (Note that direct ADC costs were augmented by estimated living costs to generate the cited number.) By contrast, nursing home costs were over $7,000 per year.

In commenting on this study, Grimaldi and Sullivan agree that for many misplaced nursing home patients, lower levels of care might be more appropriate. Nevertheless, they note that the study assumed that all nursing home inmates would be kept in such facilities for one year, whereas Medicaid data show that many persons who might have been discharged to ADC may well have been in nursing homes for only half a year. For 1976, they note that Medicaid data show that the average length of stay in an SNF was 189 days, with almost half of the residents staying only six months. In ICFs, by contrast, the median stay was 239 days, with only 31 percent staying for less than six months. Survey data from the 1972–73 and 1977 National Nursing Home Surveys support these data. Overall, ADC (on a four day per week basis) would only be cheaper than nursing home care for patients who would have stayed in a nursing home for 231 days or more. In addition, the Trans-Century study seems to have overstated the average cost of nursing home care, failing to account for cost variations based on geography, affiliation, status (level of care), and size. Moreover, the study failed to allow for the statistical difficulties produced by very few patients in some of the homes. Also, the use of Bureau of Labor Statistics budget standards, based on the estimated low-budget expenditures of an independent older couple, may have led to understatement of the costs of community maintenance for a dependent person with specialized requirements. Perhaps most critical

288

was the study's lack of an analytical linkage between the use of ADC or nursing homes and the health status and functioning levels of patients receiving either type of support. Again, there is the problem of failing to specify desired outcomes and standards for measuring progress.

The Stanford Research Institute (SRI) study attempted to compare nursing home care costs with those in alternate settings using eight alternatives from 28 possibilities. The study matched the alternatives with traditional nursing homes, both sets of facilities having to meet the following criteria: 1) operating for two years or more, 2) deriving at least some revenue from non-Federal sources, 3) having similarities between the demographic and health characteristics of the alternatives and the nursing homes, and 4) having providers willing to participate in the study. On the basis of the characteristics of the clients served in the various settings, SRI concluded that, since 44 percent of the total number of patients in the sample were not dependent, a significant proportion of LTC patients currently in nursing homes could be served in alternative facilities. It determined costs in the comparison settings by allocating fixed and variable costs to types of patients with respect to their health/functional status. Overall, the finding was that the total annual costs per patient were much lower (from 97 percent to 33 percent) for alternate care than for nursing home care, even though the average monthly cost in those alternatives which were institutionally based (that is, satellites of hospitals, nursing homes, etc.) was higher than in nursing homes. Monthly costs in non-institutionally based alternatives were lower than in nursing homes or institutionally based alternatives. In general, SRI claimed that many people in nursing homes could have been treated less expensively elsewhere.

In commenting on the SRI analysis, Grimaldi and Sullivan note that 1) sample sizes were very small, limiting the general applicability of the conclusions; 2) huge cost differences between alternatives and nursing homes (97 percent in the case of one New York alternative) robbed the findings of some credibility (for example, for a very highly technical comprehensive New York facility compared with a modest outpatient clinic attached to a housing project); 3) some costs of the alternates were not included, since certain living expenses were not registered at market prices, such as subsidized housing costs in New York; 4) cost determination based on costs for all patients in the relevant facilities may not have raised the actual costs for the patients surveyed, since the latter may have been more or less representative of the total patient pool; and 5) modes of treatment were, again, not tied to desired outcomes nor to measures of progress.

Grimaldi and Sullivan conclude that there is no basis in the

289

present literature for believing that Federal coverage of alternative services will lower the nation's total LTC bill. Many people, they argue, will not use alternatives as substitutes for nursing home or other institutional care. Thus, cost-effectiveness may not be a relevant basis for judging whether to embark on alternatives programs. Rather, they feel that choices about quality of life for dependent people and their families may be the appropriate bases for deciding whether to initiate such programs.

As Grimaldi and Sullivan note, questions about cost-effectiveness of alternative services are reinforced by two recent studies, one by the Congressional Budget Office (CBO) and the other by the General Accounting Office (GAO).

The CBO analysis (1977) develops four scenarios: one for estimates of care costs under present law, one for estimates under an option expanding alternative services to persons presently covered by Medicare/Medicaid (Option A), and one replacing current programs with a social insurance program entitling all aged and disabled persons to the most cost-effective care for their particular needs (Option B). The fourth option, C, was developed because of the high estimated costs of Option B. Under Option C, Medicare changes would be enacted as under Option A, but, additionally, the Medicaid LTC funds and Title XX social services funds would be combined in a comprehensive LTC grant. The States would receive Federal grants roughly based on the number and proportion of elderly in the State's population, the income levels of the elderly and disabled relative to the cost of living and the cost of LTC services, and the amount of Federal funds currently going to the individual States for LTC purposes. To qualify for these grants, the States would have to establish community LTC centers. The main cost saving of Option C is that it would not be an entitlement program but one that could be limited by Federal and State appropriations.

Estimates of the total and specific costs for institutional care and for non-institutional alternatives under various options are given in Figure VII–10. It is clear that even with no expansion in present entitlements or services, the total LTC bill will rise from about $30 billion in 1979 to as much as $75 billion in 1985. Under present policies, perhaps $30 billion more will be spent on nursing home care and between $1.8 billion and $6.4 billion more on home health services. Under Option A, assuming that supply would expand to meet Federally-financed demand, home health costs could rise to $18 billion, more than twice the maximum possible expansion under present law. Option A removes several present Medicare restrictions on home care, for example, that HC be intermittent, that it not include occupational therapy, and that HC aides must be supervised

FIGURE VII-10

Estimated Cost of Select Long-Term Care Services
Under Three Assumptions, 1979–1985
(billions of dollars)

Program/Service	1979	1980	1985
Present Law			
Total Cost	$28.0 - $31.7	$32.0 - $36.3	$63.7 - $ 74.5
Institutional care	26.0 - 28.9	29.9 - 32.9	59.4 - 64.8
Nursing homes and personal care facilities	19.8	23.0	48.6
Sheltered care facilities[2]	0.4 - 3.1	0.4 - 3.5	0.7 - 6.2
Others[3]	6.0	6.5	9.9
Ambulatory and home care	1.9 - 2.9	2.2 - 3.4	4.3 - 9.8
Home health services	1.4 - 2.2	1.6 - 2.7	3.2 - 8.6
Other services[4]	0.5 - 0.7	0.7 - 0.8	1.0 - 1.3
Option A			
Total Cost	$28.0 - $32.0	$32.6 - $37.1	$66.1 - $ 83.9
Institutional care			
Nursing homes and personal care facilities	26.0 - 28.9	29.9 - 32.9	59.4 - 64.8
Ambulatory and home care	2.0 - 3.1	2.7 - 4.2	6.7 - 19.1
Home health services	1.5 - 2.4	2.0 - 3.4	5.7 - 17.8
Other services	0.5 - 0.7	0.7 - 0.8	1.0 - 1.3
Option B			
Total Cost	$28.5 - $32.5	$33.7 - $40.8	$73.3 - $105.6
Institutional care	26.4 - 29.2	30.8 - 34.2	62.9 - 71.9
Nursing homes and personal care facilities	20.0	23.9	50.1
Sheltered living facilities	0.4 - 3.2	0.4 - 3.8	2.9 - 11.9
Others	6.0	6.5	9.9
Ambulatory and home care	2.1 - 3.3	2.9 - 4.6	10.4 - 33.7
Home health services	1.6 - 2.6	2.2 - 3.8	9.4 - 32.4
Other services	0.5 - 0.7	0.7 - 0.8	1.0 - 1.3

Detail may not add due to rounding.

[1] Excludes administrative cost of insurance and other items.
[2] Includes only persons not capable of independent living.
[3] Long-term hospitals, psychiatric hospitals, homes for physically handicapped, homes for blind and deaf, drug and alcoholism facilities, homes for mentally disturbed, and homes for mentally retarded; first two facilities include only persons not receiving active treatment to diagnose or cure an illness.
[4] Rehabilitation agencies and certain private practitioners.

Source: Taken from Grimaldi, Paul and Toni Sullivan, *Broadening Federal Coverage of Non-Institutional Long-Term Care* (Washington: American Health Care Association, 1981); table based on Congressional Budget Office, *Long-Term Care: Actuarial Cost Estimates*, Tables 3, 6, and 7.*

*Reprinted with permission.

by registered nurses. It also would allow reimbursement, not now permitted, to proprietary HC agencies and to so-called "one-skill" agencies. Medicaid benefits would be expanded to include visits by medical social workers in the HC benefits package. Homemaker services would be available under certain conditions, and physician-certified services would be reimbursed only if needed to diagnose or treat patients or to slow deterioration of health.

Option B might raise total LTC costs to over $100 billion, of which over $50 billion would go to nursing homes, an increase of only $1.5 billion above the level which would hold under present law. Under this option, all aged and disabled people would be entitled to the most economical form of care for their needs. Cost sharing would be required, services being reimbursed only if needed to diagnose or treat, to stabilize or slow deterioration, to maintain or improve capacities to cope with ADL, and/or to postpone institutionalization. Services provided would include HC, nursing home care, and sheltered care. The cost of home health services alone might rise to as much as $32.4 billion. The burdens of cost sharing and/or copayments would be moderated for low income persons/families by linking those payments to family income. Grimaldi notes that official income data for aged persons and families headed by older people suggest that copayments would not be onerous, particularly if they are income-linked. This conclusion varies from that found in a number of other analyses, however. (Option C was not analyzed in the CBO study and so was not considered by Grimaldi and Sullivan.)

The GAO study (1977), undertaken in connection with a larger study of home health care, indicates that the expansion of HC benefits could be very costly, especially if two or more services (or provisions regarding their implementation) are newly offered for the first time. For example, if the requirement that home care include skilled care were eliminated at the same time that home-maker services were added, the costs could reach $2 to $3 billion yearly, rather than the $1.325 billion if home chore services alone were added (Grimaldi and Sullivan, 1981).

The House Ways and Means Committee (1979) reached a similar conclusion about the high costs of adding alternative services in a report to the House Committee on Interstate and Foreign Commerce. The legislative proposals (H.R. 3990 and H.R. 4000) would have eliminated the 100 visit limitation under Parts A and B of Medicare, the requirement for a three day prior hospital stay to qualify for Part A home care benefits, and the $60 deductible for Part B benefits. They would also have added the need for occupational therapy as well as skilled nursing care, physical therapy, or speech therapy to qualify for home care. Both the CBO and the

292

Department of Health and Human Services (DHHS) provided estimates of additional costs of these legislative proposals for 1980–81
and 1985. These agencies put the costs at about $25 million for
1980–81; for 1985, however, CBO's $154 million estimate is almost
double DHHS's $78 million. (The former estimate was adopted by
the committee.) The Senate Finance Committee assessed similar
legislative proposals (H.R. 934), that is, that unlimited home visits be
provided and that the three day hospitalization requirement be removed. Additionally, these proposals would have extended reimbursement for HC provided by ADC centers which are non-profit,
eligible for Title XX funds, and meet certain standards; changed
home health aides to homemaker-home health aides; and expanded
the consumer education program to emphasize maximum independence. Again, the cost estimates (by both CBO and the Senate
Finance Committee) show an $80 to $100 million increase in costs
between 1980 and 1984. While the estimates considered by both
the House and Senate committes are not impressive in comparison
with current spending on nursing homes, they may well augur
more significant cost increases for the future, especially if the
supply of services rises to meet the Federally-financed demand.
Of course, any estimate of cost increases must reflect the effects
of current imponderables: the number of covered persons, the impact of cost-sharing arrangements, and the public's wants for such
services (Grimaldi and Sullivan, 1981).

AMS reviewed eight studies. Three of them are of particular
interest here, since two were among the alternatives demonstrations
surveyed by Doherty et al and since each also dealt with a different
type of alternative, was concerned with differing conditions, and
postulated differing outcomes.

A 1974 study of a home care program for stroke victims alleged
that the home care clients enjoyed shorter hospitalization, fewer
re-admissions for recurring strokes, and fewer deaths than similar
patients who were retained in the hospital in a clinical environment.
Home care patients also received continuous care, could be rein-
stated into their families and the community, and could be provided
for at much lower costs. In its review of the St. Luke's study, however, AMS found that there was no evidence that HC treatments
were of the same nature as hospital care treatments, that the
experimental (HC) patients and the controls (hospital patients) had
not been truly randomly selected (being matched only by age and
sex), that there was no match between experimentals and controls
(who had average hospital stays 10 days longer than the HC group)
for severity of condition, and that there was real danger of bias in the
selection of patients for comparison. Furthermore, there was no
analysis of comparative living arrangements and variations in medi-

293

cal treatments. There was also no specification of a hypothesis to be tested against an alternative. On balance, AMS judged that the St. Luke study claims could not be accepted.

AMS also criticized a 1973 day care hospital study comparing two groups of patients, one which received day care and one which was institutionalized. The study argued that day care recipients exhibited more life satisfaction than institutionalized patients and seemed more involved in family-related social roles. Additionally, the daily costs of day care were $7 per day lower for day care versus institutionalized patients. Inpatients were matched with day care patients on a case-by-case basis, and researchers gathered data by observing patients directly and then interviewing patients and their families. Unfortunately, the AMS review showed that the study did not have any clear hypothesis with respect to social theory or the effect of the services provided. In addition, the study design— so-called *ex post facto*—involved comparing a group of service receivers with non-receivers in terms of outcomes. This method is flawed in that it does not show that the two groups would have been equivalent except for the treatment. Studies of this type suffer from selection effects (that is, recipients self-select in advance) and from mortality effects. In sum, it is impossible to determine that the treatment produced the effects observed. Moreover, although there was some attempt to match the patients, there is no assurance that the matched variables were the relevant ones or that patients matched on other variables. Furthermore, there is some question as to the populations to which the results can be applied because of the nature of the matching. Cost results were also suspect because there was inadequate information as to their derivation. Perhaps most troublesome was the lack of any logical, theoretical, or empirical specification of causal relationships between treatments and outcomes. AMS concluded that the study findings actually only suggest areas for future research.

The third AMS-reviewed study was of a sheltered housing program for the physically impaired. This study examined the impact of residential environments on health and/or well-being of physically impaired adults. The experimental group was project residents. The control group was nonresidents who had applied for residency. The program provided health care for residents, while community dwellers had to find care on their own. Individuals in the two groups were matched on the bases of theoretically important variables and clinical and professional judgments. Outcome areas were health status, housing conditions, degree of social isolation, and cognitive and emotional states. The key question was whether residents were better off than their community counterparts at the end of the nine month study period. The study claimed better health

294

results for residents but no differences otherwise. Again, AMS found this study lacking in a number of important respects. There were no specific hypotheses stated, and the measures of health and social isolation were very crude, no reliability or validity data being provided for the scales used. The matching techniques, while intuitively appealing, were beset by data and methodological problems, possibly subverting randomness and statistical validity. Moreover, no information was presented on the factor, cluster, and discriminant analyses employed to perform the matches. In general, the data were also lacking in cross-validation from other populations and may have not been gathered in an objective fashion because of the varying backgrounds of the collectors. A major problem was the lack of information on the health care assistance received, and other experiences of the non-residents. The study also failed to present any data on cost-benefit analyses or on efficiency of the residential provision.

Both the Grimaldi-Sullivan and AMS judgments about the quality of alternatives research studies are echoed in the Stassen-Holahan review cited earlier, which focused most of its methodological critique on the community care projects. Again, the literature surveyed is faulted for its lack of true experimental design, its failure to examine truly comparable experimental and control groups, its failure to recognize that community care users were frequently less disabled than their institutionalized counterparts, its failure to establish true comparability between areas and groups in the analyses, and its casualness with respect to analytical and statistical techniques. Only the Georgia Alternative Health Services Program study received high marks on methodological grounds among the community care reports surveyed.

In their recent review of research on community-wide coordinated care programs, adult day health care services, and in-home services, Stassen and Holahan examined a number of claims made by researchers who assessed the programs in question, and we may take this work as a good example of the surveys cited. Overall, they found that in the case of community-wide programs, the evidence of substitutability for institutional care was very limited. Although lower Medicaid expenditures were reported by programs such as the Georgia Alternatives project, the Monroe County project, and the Wisconsin Community Care Organization, other programs (Triage, for example) reported higher costs for clients than for those who did not receive such services. Furthermore, many of the research findings were equivocal because of lack of comparability among experimental and control groups, because of failure to control for differences in availability of institutions and services among areas, and because of statistical and technical problems. Simliarly, although first results showed lower program costs for the community-based system, many studies failed to count all relevant costs and did not allow for either an add-on of additional clients beyond the numbers served before the projects were undertaken or the possibility that the deinstitutionalized might just be making way for others who had hitherto not been able to find a nursing home bed. With respect to outcomes, both the studies themselves and the Stassen-Holahan review found that there were no clear results for mortality rates or functional improvement. One finding did stand out clearly: satisfaction levels tended to be higher for patients and families with regimes of community-based care than with institutionalization.

Overall Judgments

Grimaldi and Sullivan determined that most of the alternatives research was methodologically weak and inconclusive on the questions of utilization, effectiveness, and cost (or cost-effectiveness). In the first place, comparability among the different evaluative and research studies was hard to establish because of variations in time for measuring outcomes and in definitions and measurements of costs, and because of use of different assessment instruments. Also, most studies and programs were very small in scope (geographically and populationally), being confined to single sites with a special focus on the northeastern States. Clearly, some agreement on definitions, conventions, time frames, and desired outcomes must develop before comparisons can be made and uniform conclusions can emerge.

In addition to general methodological complaints, AMS in its review cites a list of weaknesses specific to the eight studies it evaluated which may well apply generally to studies in the field. Among these weaknesses are a lack of adequate samples from defined universes of patients, indiscriminate use of statistical tests, the omission of much data on conditions, outcomes, and costs, inconsistent specification of outcomes/variables, lack of direct analysis of service impact on treatment groups, a short time frame which precludes longitudinal analysis, and too much involvement of researchers with the patients. This last probably accounts for much of the lack of random selection and the failure to use random clinical trial methods in the "classic" experimental mode.

As Conly points out (1977), most research on alternatives suffers from conceptual weaknesses at a very fundamental level. Many efforts were not constructed according to consistent theoretical models or with clearly identifiable hypotheses. If models were used, they focused on one or a few aspects of the problem or of a service package, a clear weakness when the essence of the problem may lie in the interaction of many forces and factors, as is true in LTC. Much research does not clearly identify the population at risk

296

or the characteristics which such populations might display. Specification of relevant personal and population characteristics is rare; moreover, these attributes are not often couched in readily measurable, operational terms. Desired or expected outcomes frequently are not stated, and models linking outcomes to services are not presented.

Research and demonstrations often suffered from weaknesses in both internal and external validity. Internally, the data may have been flawed and/or inappropriately collected, thus destroying credibility. Externally, unwarranted generalizations were often made based on limited data or a too narrowly defined set of phenomena. Clients were seldom randomly assigned to experimental or control groups, which, moreover, frequently were not really comparable or completely identified. Control groups sometimes received the same service packages as experimental groups, and sometimes it was hard to determine if both groups did not get additional or different services from sources outside the project. Also, samples were too small and/or periods too short for any changes to make a difference. Exogenous factors, such as changes in client eligibility or the willingness or ability of families to cope were not specified. In those studies dealing with costs, total social costs (especially costs of living, costs to clients' families, and secondary or tertiary costs) were usually not fully considered, documented, or specified. Even direct costs, presumably readily identifiable and quantifiable, were sometimes not offered without error. Because of hospital costing conventions, costs per day are often the unit of measure, when costs per episode, or per case, might have been more suitable.

At a theoretical level, both the results of these reviews and a cursory consideration of project descriptions and of some recent journal articles reveal a definite lack of models about user behavior and provider (producer) responses to market, regulatory, and reimbursement stimuli. In part, this shortcoming reflects the scant attention paid to the alternatives question by social science researchers interested in modeling user and provider behavior in LTC. Consequently, the research is difficult to use as the basis for systematic analysis of behavior and for policy guidance. This problem relates to a difficulty discussed earlier, the lack of coordination among the research, demonstration, and evaluation efforts, whether on the part of research analysts or those responsible for planning governmental efforts and funding. Especially troubling is the lack of evaluation components in the design of demonstrations and in the research reports about such efforts.

Recommended Methods for Alternatives Research

To protect against these weaknesses, Sonia Conly (1977) has proposed a series of recommendations about the necessary conduct of research and demonstrations on alternatives. Her lists (Figures VII–11 and VII–12) stress precision of research questions, definiteness of research design, unambiguous specification of outcomes, models linking services to outcomes, clear specifications of costs, and measures for monitoring validity in terms of the integrity of the research project and of the general applicability of research findings.

Demonstrations Research

Despite this litany of research weakness (and hence of lack of usability), a number of recent demonstrations have generated some interesting findings about the problems of service integration, assessment, care planning, case management, and service provision. According to a GAO review (1979), these demonstrations indicate a need for gatekeeping, that is, the identification of potential and actual vulnerables to determine whether they can be maintained in the community or must be placed in a nursing home. Three projects—the Virginia Preadmission Screening Program, the Monroe County (NY) ACCESS project, and the New York Long Term Home Health Care Program—focused on this issue. The Virginia program requires all candidates for Medicaid-supported nursing home placement to be surveyed by a screening committee (an MD, nurse, and social worker) which must authorize placement on the basis of the client's medical and social support needs. The ACCESS program, which included private pay patients (64 percent of the total assessed), found that 54 percent of the clients determined to need nursing home care could actually be maintained in the community.

Another need identified by these demonstrations is for comprehensive needs assessment to establish individuals' requirements for nursing home care, specify the types and quantities of service required, and determine the impact of LTC services on health, ADL capability, longevity, morale, and risk of institutionalization. Such needs assessment also tries to total the costs of providing home or alternate services to elderly people with various levels of impairment. These projects, which used waivers under Section 1115 to pay for their programs, also appear to show the need for central coordinating mechanisms, especially important in filling gaps in available services in the community. Also, single funding mechanisms apparently are central to the successful functioning of comprehensive programs. This latter is particularly important in view of the manifold services and the numerous payment sources which may overlap in providing services, have differing eligibility rules, set divergent cost and reimbursement limits, etc. The Federal-State-local-volunteer linkages are especially troublesome and must be handled by some central coordinating agency. Last, the demonstrations show that some form of cost control is needed, both on

298

FIGURE VII-11
Guidelines for Proposals and Reports

It is crucial that the research proposal demonstrate Investigator knowledge of both the subject matter area and research design. Adherence to the following guidelines for research proposals would eliminate many studies with little chance of success.

1. Research proposals should demonstrate Investigator knowledge of related research.
2. The proposal should contain a clear specification of the hypothesis to be tested.·
3. The proposal should contain a simple clear specification of the research design.
4. For evaluation studies, the criteria by which treatment success is to be judged must be specified.
5. For evaluation studies, the Investigator should calculate the ability of the research design to detect significant differences with the proposed sample size using plausible assumptions regarding true treatment effect.
6. For evaluation studies, the Investigator must demonstrate that different treatments will be observed or that base time data on comparable untreated population are accessible.
7. The Investigator should show how the cooperation of program administrators will be obtained.
8. The Investigator must demonstrate ability to satisfactorily manage variables other than the treatment variables. This includes a requirement that the Investigator be able to show that variables used to demonstrate comparability of comparison experimental groups are important in outcome and the extent of importance.

Source: Conly, Sonia, "Critical Review of Research on Long-Term Care Alternatives," ASPE, June 1977

FIGURE VII-12
Suggested Guidelines For Research Reports

The following is a set of suggested guidelines for research reports. These guidelines represent the minimum requirements for research reporting that will enable a reader to determine the conclusions of a research study and evaluate the soundness of these conclusions.

1. Interim and final reports should be prefaced with a concise statement of the hypotheses tested, the treatment observed, and the essential elements of experimental design—including sample size, selection of experimental and control group members and management on non-treatment variables.

2. Related research should be reported.

3. Alternative explanations for observed results should be considered.

4. Conflicting and inconclusive results should be included in the report.

5. The treatment should be described as it was applied and any deviations from the original design noted. Changes in treatment during the course of the experiment should be reported and possible effects of the change in treatment noted and analyzed.

6. Sufficient data should be presented to allow the reader to judge the validity of conclusions.

7. The report should document the importance of variables used to demonstrate similarity of comparison and experimental groups. When non-probabilistic selection of experimental and comparison groups is made, the investigator should demonstrate that the possibility of systematic biases was investigated and managed.

8. Distributions of outcome variables as well as means should be reported for both the experimental and comparison groups.

Source: Conly, Sonia, "Critical Review of Research on Long-Term Care Alternatives", ASPE, June 1977

nursing home expense and on the provision of alternative service packages.

Stassen and Holahan also offer a set of research imperatives of both a methodological and substantive nature stemming from their review. They call for further work on the links between levels of costs and impairment. They also recommend development of the concept of full-costing (including community costs) and consideration of full costs in any future cost comparisons. On a related subject, they warn of the reality of high start-up costs for any community care or other alternatives program and, again, warn that these may bias results against alternative systems and must be factored into any costing exercise. Because of the possibility that community-based care systems may make nursing home beds available for people who had not been able to find space in nursing homes before the alternatives were initiated, they recommend further research on the question of total community use of nursing homes and other institutions across all groups in the population. Since budgetary allocations may be limited and costs constrained for all types of LTC, they also advocate more intensive studies of targeting services to specific elements of the population on the basis of type and intensity of service needs. Admitting that this type of targeting is politically difficult, they note that it is essential if cost-effectiveness is to be achieved in reducing institutionalization. Of course, if the goal of LTC service programs is to serve all frail elderly in the community, targeting may not be urgent. However, even this objective usually is constrained by costs, and some targeting is still a necessity. In terms of outcomes, they perceive a need for further analysis of the effects of various care modes on the patients' mental conditions, their capacity for self-maintenance, and their life satisfaction. On a related topic, they urge more analysis of the determinants of family satisfaction. These last research imperatives obviously relate to the call for some reorientation toward personal satisfaction and away from purely functional indicators.

We do not intend to examine the results of these and other demonstrations in detail. Such an examination has already been undertaken in Chapter VI. Rather, the purpose here is to show that, notwithstanding certain methodological flaws (and there may be some, since the final reports on the 1115 demonstrations were not submitted by spring of 1981), carefully designed and implemented demonstrations can generate some useful results.

A Policy and Analytical Program

An article by John Noble and Ray Conley raises some key policy and analytical issues (Noble and Conley, forthcoming). Their analysis begins with a set of questions about Federal responsibility and about the nature of settings-services needed to cater to broad categories of dependent people, especially the elderly and the mentally troubled. At the Federal level, they turn to the issues of the amount of public responsibility which the Federal government should assume, the possibilities of added Federal responsibility in an age of budget limits, the practicability of creating adequate service systems in the face of great fragmentation, and the possibility of countering the medical bias in care at the policy level. With respect to the nature of care, their questions turn on issues of efficiency versus insufficiency and/or bad care, on problems of locating dependent people in care settings, and on the nature of care which should be provided to various categories of patients/clients.

Answers to these sorts of questions clearly require data, most of which are unavailable. In the context of domiciliary care (the initial focus of their article), Noble and Conley assert some key data needs, relevant to the whole LTC field: How many people can be appropriately deinstitutionalized? When will it cost more to maintain a person in a domiciliary care facility (DCF) than in a mental hospital? How many people would never have been institutionalized in the first place had adequate community services been available and provided? Although these are DCF-connected questions, Noble and Conley recognize that answers can only be provided in a more general framework, one that looks at the totality of dependency and at the demand and supply issues related to beds and places in all types of services and settings. These last questions, of course, cannot be addressed without an analysis of the individual States' Medicaid and social services policies as they affect the supply of and demand for places and beds. Given the present lack of data, the above questions clearly lead to a research program with far-reaching implications.

Medicaid policy is also a subject of major reform proposals. Concerned that the social services share of the total Federal welfare allocation may shrink from 14 percent in 1976 to 5 percent in 1985, Noble and Conley suggested that Medicaid expenditures in any State be "capped" on the basis of changes in the cost of living. Such caps might reduce State outlays, as well as Federal matching grants. The resultant "savings" in Federal expenditures might then be added to Title XX and other limited programs to enrich the social services (and therefore, presumably, the alternative LTC component) allocations under Title XX and the Older Americans Act, Title III. Since these titles carry a higher percentage Federal match than Medicaid, the States might be more willing to embrace less institutional LTC alternatives than at present. Of course, as Noble and Conley recognize, we need much more research on the costs and effects of alternative programs and on the impacts of differing

302

incentives systems on users, providers, and State and local governments. Indeed, all of the suggested programs require further research in many areas.

Overall (and this is relevant to all of the considerations and issues of nursing homes and alternates—substitutes and complements), what is needed in long-term care is a set of "cost of condition" analyses. At the social level, we need to determine the direct and indirect costs of catering to various service needs at different quality and availability levels. These latter would be framed in terms of current policy pronouncements about desired outcomes for the dependent population. The cost of conditions analysis could be couched in terms of cost-benefit or cost-effectiveness, although on the grounds of practicality, Noble and Conley prefer an assessment based on program planning budgeting systems (PPBS) approaches. In any event, any evaluation of care systems requires consideration of meaningful care alternatives for the groups in question, a comparison of services/settings for the same group, a consideration of what is an appropriate site of institutional and community care for people with various disabilities (to avoid placing highly dependent people in inadequate care settings), and the development of accurate data systems about disabilities, users, providers, and State actions. We might also add that such a comprehensive view also demands an analysis of the effects of reimbursement formulae and levels.

References

Applied Management Sciences, Inc., "Evaluation of Personal Care Organizations and Other In-Home Alternatives to Nursing Home Care for the Elderly and Long-Term Disabled, Interim Report No. 2 (Revised), prepared for DHEW, Office of the Assistant Secretary for Planning and Evaluation, April 30, 1975 (Springfield, VA: U.S. Department of Commerce, National Technical Information Service, No. PB-256-011).

Conly, Sonia, "Critical Review of Research on Long-Term Care Alternatives," DHEW, Office of the Assistant Secretary for Planning and Evaluation, June 1977 (Project Share, A National Clearinghouse for Improving Management of Human Services, No. SRH-2153).

Dellinger, David C., "Guidelines for Estimating the Cost of Service Packages for the Chronically Impaired," GSBA Paper No. 146 (Durham, N.C., Duke University Graduate School of Business Administration, July 1975).

Demkovich, Linda E., "In Treating the Problems of the Elderly, There May Be No Place Like Home," *National Journal*, December 22, 1979, pp. 2154-2158.

Diamond, Larry and David Berman, "The Social/Health Maintenance Organization: A Single Entry, Prepaid, Long-Term Care Delivery System," Brandeis University *et al*, Health Policy Consortium Discussion Paper 16c, September, 1979.

Doherty, Neville, Joan Segal, and Barbara Hicks, "Alternatives to Institutionalization for the Aged: Viability and Cost-Effectiveness," *Aged Care and Services Review*, January/February 1978, pp. 2-16.

Doherty, Neville, and Barbara Hicks, "Cost-Effectiveness Analysis and Alternative Health Care Programs for the Elderly," *Health Services Research*, Summer 1977, pp. 190-203.

Doherty, Neville J.G. and Barbara C. Hicks, "The Use of Cost-Effectiveness Analysis in Geriatric Day Care," *The Gerontologist*, October 1975, pp. 412-417.

Gibson, Robert M., "National Health Expenditures, 1979," *Health Care Financing Review*, Summer 1980.

Grad de Alarcon, Jacqueline and Peter Sainsbury, "The Psychiatrist and the Geriatric Patient, The Effects of Community Care on the Family of the Geriatric Patient," *Journal of Geriatric Psychiatry*, Fall 1970.

Greenberg, Jay, "A Planning Study of Services to Non-Institutionalized Older Persons in Minnesota," Parts 1 and 2 (Minneapolis, Governor's Citizens Council on Aging, 1974).

Grimaldi, Paul and Toni Sullivan, *Broadening Federal Coverage of Non-institutional Long Term Care* (Washington, D.C., American Health Care Association and National Foundation for Long-Term Health Care, 1981).

Pollak, William (with the assistance of Joanne Hilferty), "Costs of Alternative Care Settings for the Elderly," Urban Institute Working Paper 963-11, Washington, D.C., March 12, 1973.

Sager, Alan, *Learning the Home Care Needs of the Elderly: Patient, Family, and Professional Views of an Alternative to Institutionalization*, Levinson Policy Institute, Brandeis University. Final Report to the Administration on Aging, AoA Grant No. 90-A-1026, November 20, 1979.

Stassen, Margaret and John Holahan, "Long-Term Care Demonstration Projects: A Review of Recent Evaluations" (Washington, D.C.: The Urban Institute, Working Paper No. 1227-2, February, 1981).

United States Comptroller General, General Accounting Office, *Entering a Nursing Home—Costly Implications for Medicaid and the Elderly*, PAD-80-12 (Washington, D.C., U.S. Government Printing Office, November 26, 1979).

United States Comptroller General, General Accounting Office, *Home Health —The Need for a National Policy to Better Provide for the Elderly* (Washington, D.C., U.S. Government Printing Office, December 30, 1977).

United States Comptroller General, General Accounting Office, *The Well-Being of Older People in Cleveland, Ohio* (Washington, D.C., U.S. Government Printing Office, April 19, 1977).

United States Congress, Congressional Budget Office, *Long-Term Care for the Elderly and Disabled*, Washington, D.C., Government Printing Office, February 1977 (Reprinted August 1977).

United States Congress, Congressional Budget Office, *Long-Term Care: Actuarial Cost Estimates*, A CBO Technical Analysis Paper, Washington, D.C.: Government Printing Office, August 1977.

United States, Department of Health, Education, and Welfare, Health Resources Administration, *Home Health Care Programs: A Selected Bibliography* (HRA Publication 79-60; Hyattsville, Maryland: July 1979).

304

United States Department of Health and Human Services, Health Care Financing Administration, *Health Care Financing Notes, Medicare: Use of Home Health Services, 1978* (Washington, D.C., HCFA Pub. No. 03025, June 1980).

Weissert, William G. "Rationales for Public Health Insurance Coverage of Geriatric Day Care: Issues, Opinions, and Impacts," *Journal of Health Politics, Policy, and Law*, Winter 1979, pp. 555-567.

Chapter VIII

The Family Support System of the Elderly

by Judith Sangl

Introduction

Cost comparisons indicate that family care at home is less expensive than an institution for all but the most severely impaired elderly (Comptroller General, 1977). Consequently the role of the family in providing care to the frail elderly has become of special interest to policymakers in view of escalating long-term care expenditures. Family support is also of concern because demographic projections show a great expansion of the elderly population, especially the "old-old" (75 years or older) who are most likely to need care. This expansion is occurring simultaneously with family transformations which are likely to weaken family capacity for caregiving.

Research concerning family support of the elderly comes from a variety of sources:

- Nationally representative household surveys such as the 1976 Survey of Income and Education, the Health Interview Survey (NCHS, 1972), and the 1974 National Council on the Aging Survey (Louis Harris and Associates, 1975), special national 1962 and 1975 surveys of the population 65 and older (Shanas, 1977), and special reports of the U.S. Bureau of the Census (for example, Current Population Reports). These studies include data on health status, living arrangements, family composition, and mutual aid patterns, including assistance during illness.
- Surveys of institutionalized elderly such as the 1977 National Nursing Home Survey and the 1976 Survey of Institutionalized Persons. These surveys provide data on prior living arrangements, reasons for institutionalization, and family involvement.
- Surveys of elderly residents in the community, such as the General Accounting Office study of the elderly in Cleveland (1977), the study of inner city elderly in New York City (Cantor, 1975), and the study of six special groups of elderly in Chicago (Bild and Havighurst, 1976). These surveys contain information on service needs, living arrangements, health status, and family and other social supports.
- Studies of the natural support systems and family caregiving, such as Brody *et al* (1979), Hawkins and Jacobson (1980), Johnson (1979), and York and Calsyn (1977), that give information

307

about the elder's functional level, the caregiving situation, and the extent of assistance from different types of caregivers. This category includes studies examining the effects of caring for the chronically ill elderly, such as Adams et al (1979), Davis (1978), Fengler and Goodrich (1979), and Zarit et al (1980). In addition, some studies have investigated the effects of different programs on family caregiving to the elderly, such as Gross-Andrews and Zimmer (1977), Horowitz (1978), and Rathbone-McCuan (1976).

None of the information obtained from these sources alone provides a complete picture of the family support system of the elderly. Those that are nationally representative are generally limited in scope and detail, while those with a wealth of information have very small sample sizes and are limited in general applicability. Most studies are cross-sectional rather than longitudinal and are primarily descriptive. Consequently, they cannot capture the dynamic processes involved in family caregiving or provide explanations.

Numerous studies have confirmed the viability of family support of the elderly even for the frail and dependent elderly, but commonly held misconceptions about the position of the elderly in the family network remain. These include the following ideas:

- Geographic mobility in our society has caused children to live far from their parents.
- Elderly parents are isolated and rarely see their children or other relatives.
- With the rise of alternative sources of care and long-term care institutions, families rarely provide care to the elderly. Therefore, many of the elderly are in institutions.

All of these misconceptions can be dispelled for the majority of the elderly. Even though there is a great deal of geographic mobility and much emphasis on the nuclear family, kin dispersion has been exaggerated, and most elderly are not isolated and neglected (Treas, 1977). The family of the aged should be viewed as a "kinship system—a network of mutual supports among individual households of persons related by blood and marriage. This network extends not only across households but also across generations of related kin" (Shanas, 1979). Despite the growth of alternative sources of care, the family is still the primary caregiver for the chronically ill and disabled elderly, and no more than 5 percent of the elderly reside in institutions at any given time (Shanas, 1979).

This chapter presents selected research findings from the sources just outlined on the family support system of the elderly and its role in providing long-term care services. It focuses on the following questions:

308

- Who are the caregivers?
- What kinds of assistance do they provide?
- What is the impact of providing such care?
- What can be done to help sustain such family care of the elderly?
- Would formal assistance supplement or supplant this informal caregiving?

Elements of the Family Support System

To understand the family support system of the elderly, we must examine the basic elements of family composition, living arrangements, residential proximity, and interaction and mutual aid patterns. Much of the information here is based on two national probability sample surveys of the non-institutionalized population age 65 and over; one survey was conducted in 1962, and the second one in 1975 (Shanas, 1977).

Family Composition

An examination of the family structure of the elderly provides a sense of what kin resources are available for support. This family composition reflects demographic trends, such as increased life expectancy, differential longevity for men and women.

The number and sex of children is important when examining potential resources available to the elderly. Theoretically and ideally, if there are more children, the responsibilities can be shared without being particularly burdensome on any one child. Research indicates, though, that one child will usually assume primary responsibility (Johnson, 1979). In fact, it has been noted that current economic incentives encourage this. An adult child may claim a tax exemption if he has furnished more than half of a parent's income, and this would assure a parent of social security survivor benefits if the child dies. No tax advantage would accrue to any children sharing equally (Schorr, 1980).

Sex of a child is important, since daughters traditionally take a more active role in caring for parents than do sons. Marital status of children also makes a difference, since married children are more likely to establish mutual help patterns. However, all of these important variables have changed. There has been a trend toward smaller family size, and consequently there are more older persons with only one child. The proportion of elderly people with daughters and the number of married children has also decreased. Eighty percent of the elderly have at least one living child. Of those with children, 90 percent have grandchildren, and 40 percent have great-grandchildren (Shanas, 1977).

At least 50 percent of the elderly are married and living with a spouse. Slightly more than one-third are widowed, and another 6 percent were previously married but are now divorced or separated. Only 5 percent of the elderly were never married. The elderly, both male and female, under age 75 are more likely to be married than those over 75. But regardless of age, men are more likely to be married than widowed and the opposite is true for women, except for those under 69. (Shanas, 1977).

The majority (75 percent) of the elderly are members of multi-generational families due to increased longevity and the shortened time span between the generations. Since women live longer, they are more likely than men to be part of a four generation family.

Most of the elderly (80 percent) have at least one living sibling. Those who are 75 years or older are from families who had an average of five children and with increased longevity, many siblings are still alive (Shanas, 1980). There appears to be a tendency to renew relationships with siblings in old age. Siblings may become a major social resource, especially for those without a spouse or children. Only a small percentage of the elderly (3 percent) are without a spouse, children, or siblings. However, even these elderly are not entirely without family resources and may substitute collateral kin (cousins, nieces, and nephews) and even friends and neighbors to some degree for lack of primary supports.

Simple frequency counts of kin can only suggest potential for caregiving. The concept of functioning kin delineates "merely having a potential support element and having one that is involved in a sufficiently steady and on-going relationship to make meaningful social support a possibility" (Cantor, 1978). For example, a functional spouse is defined as one with whom a person lives. A functional child or sibling is one with whom a person lives or whom the elderly person sees at least monthly or speaks to by phone weekly. Although this concept reduces the number of kin resources, it yields a more realistic estimate. If this definition is applied to the results of the Shanas survey, 75 percent of the elderly have "functional" children and one-third have "functional" siblings (Shanas, 1980).

It is important to point out that there is a major difference in family status between the elderly in the community and those in institutions. Only 14 percent of the institutionalized elderly are married, compared with slightly more than 50 percent of all elderly. There are about three times as high a proportion of persons who had never married as in the elderly population in the community and almost twice as high a proportion of widowed persons. About 50 percent of the institutionalized elderly are childless, while 80 percent in the community have at least one surviving child. Even those institutionalized who have children are more likely to have only one child instead of two or more. Since the median age of the elderly in institutions (82 years) is nine years greater than the median age of all elderly (Brody, 1979), the elderly in institutions are likely to have children who are approaching old age themselves and have less capacity for caregiving. It has been asserted that a "lively, responsible spouse is the surest safeguard against ending up in a nursing home" (Community Service Society, 1980). Also, another study has shown that each additional child reduces one's chances of being institutionalized in old age (Brody, 1979).

Living Arrangements

The overwhelming majority of the elderly reside in the community; as mentioned earlier, only 5 percent of the elderly are in institutions at any one time. Living arrangements among the elderly reflect their preference for independent living whenever possible as well as their kin's desire for privacy. Sharing a household is not a life pattern for most elderly but generally a response to extreme circumstances such as lack of the financial resources or the good health necessary to maintain independent living (Brookdale Center on Aging, 1979). Living arrangements vary by marital status, age, and sex. For those who are married, the most common living arrangement is living in a household with spouse only—about 84 percent (Shanas, 1977). Another 10 percent maintain a household with unmarried children, and the remainder share their households with someone other than their children. These figures reflect an increase from an earlier survey of a greater proportion of intact families in the post-parental and retirement years (Shanas, 1977).

The proportion of unmarried (includes those separated, divorced, widowed, or never married) elderly living alone has increased substantially. According to the survey by Shanas (1977), the proportion increased from half in 1962 to about two-thirds in 1975. This increase in independent living arrangements was more marked for women (46 to 67 percent) than for men (52 to 65 percent) between the two national surveys. Those living with children decreased from 14 to 7 percent. Overall, for women this decrease was from 22 to 11 percent, while for men it was from 17 to 6 percent. Some of the factors that may account for this change are (1) improved health of the elderly, (2) improved financial situation, and (3) greater societal acceptance of living alone as a lifestyle, especially for women (Shanas, 1977). The proportion living with siblings and other relatives has remained the same, about 13 percent. There are some differences depending on sex and age. In both surveys, women were more likely than men to live with unmarried children. This was especially true for very old women, 80 years and over (31 percent) as compared with men the same age (19 percent). In fact, unmarried men in this age group were more likely than women to live with persons other than children (25 versus 10 percent).

311

Living arrangements also differed for those who never married and those who are widowed and divorced. The most common arrangement for both of these groups was to live alone. The second most common arrangement for the never married was to live with siblings, and for the previously married, it was to live with a child. This demonstrates how "family substitution" operates—previously married elderly substitute their children for lack of spouses, and the never married substitute siblings for lack of spouses or children.

About 4 percent of the 65 and over population had at least one parent alive (primarily their mothers), and less than 1 percent had both parents alive. This proportion in the population will increase in the future, due to the greater longevity of the elderly. It is an interesting group to examine since these individuals are balancing demands from their parents with those of adult children and grandchildren when their energy and resources may be declining (Shanas, 1977). In this group, about 50 percent of the parents of the elderly are living with their adult children, about 25 percent were in institutions and the remaining 25 percent were residing in the community independently either alone or with spouse (Shanas, 1977).

Functional ability is also a factor in the living arrangements for both the married and unmarried elderly. Those who have more difficulties with activities of daily living are more likely to live with their children or other relatives than those with less difficulty. Despite the difference in living situation between persons with high and low incapacity, there were potentially alarming changes in the living arrangements of those with high incapacity between the two surveys. More incapacitated elderly were living alone in 1975 (34 percent) than in 1962 (25 percent) and fewer were living with children in 1975 (21 percent) than in 1962 (28 percent).

Living arrangements also differ to some degree by income level and racial/ethnic groups. Previous research has shown that multigenerational living arrangements are more common in particular groups. Shared living arrangements are a very likely response to the financial as well as health needs of an elderly parent for lower-income families and living together has been termed a "lifeboat response" (Schorr, 1980).

Blacks are more likely than whites to compose multigenerational families sharing the same household. This is evidenced by the 40 percent of black families headed by a woman 65 years or older and the 22 percent of elderly black two-parent families containing children under 18 years of age, compared to 10 percent of white families headed by aged females and 4 percent of white, elderly, two-parent families (Bureau of Census, 1977). Black families are more likely to take younger family members into their households than to be taken into households of younger family members. However,

312

white families are just as likely as black families to take in an elderly family member (Hill, 1978).

Hispanic elderly are still often members of extended families, especially in rural areas. Census Bureau data indicate that only 18 percent of the Hispanic elderly 55 years and over live alone or with non-relatives, compared with 24 percent of the total U.S. population 55 years and over (Torres-Gil and Negm, 1980).

Residential Propinquity and Interaction with Family

Even though more elderly now maintain their own households, there still is frequent contact with kin, and their residences are usually located close by. The situation where the elderly and their adult children maintain separate but close residences has been characterized as "intimacy at a distance" (Rosenmayr, 1968).

Despite geographic mobility, studies have shown that about 85 percent of the elderly live less than an hour away from at least one of their children, with 50 percent reporting that their children are within a half hour distance, and a third saying that they live within 10 minutes of at least one child (Shanas, 1979; Cantor, 1975).

Residential proximity data are supplemented by research findings on frequency of interaction. In general, there is a great deal of visiting, telephoning, and other contact between older people and their families. Adult children are the relatives most often seen. Shanas' latest survey (1977) revealed that about three-fourths of the elderly had seen at least one of their children within the past week and about half had seen their children during the past day. Only about 10 percent had not seen a child for more than a month, and this percentage had remained constant between the time of the two surveys.

Frequency of interaction did not differ significantly by place of residence or socioeconomic class. Rural samples of elderly, though they have fewer relatives nearby than their urban counterparts because of migration, do not show significantly different visiting patterns. There is less frequent kin interaction but the same proportionate frequency (Troll, 1971). Middle class children may live farther than lower class children from their parents, but there does not seem to be a difference in visiting frequency (Brookdale Center on Aging, 1979).

The age of the elderly person influences the frequency of seeing a child, with those 80 years or older more likely to have seen a child in the past day at the time of the interview (Shanas, 1977). This may be explained by a greater dependency on their children to meet their daily needs. "Weekly contact which apparently exists between the elderly and their children is more often for purposes of visiting and mutual exchange, while daily contact, when it is reported,

313

is often related to meeting some of the needs of the parent generation" (Shanas, 1977).

Siblings and other relatives are an important part of the kin network for older people. This has been referred to as an "hourglass effect" in which there are many contacts with siblings and other relatives in youth, shrinking in young adulthood and middle age and then expanding in later life (Shanas, 1979). At least a third of the survey population reported having seen a brother or sister in the past week, with women more likely than men to have seen a sibling. There was also a higher proportion of never married elderly, about 70 percent (both men and women) who reported having seen a sibling in the past week. Again, siblings appeared to substitute for the lack of children or spouses for those who were never married.

Other relatives are also included in the family network. About 30 percent of the elderly reported seeing some other relative in the previous week. More distant relatives substitute for lack of siblings or children. It should be noted that not much is known about the quality of the interactions or their nature—whether the visits are "brief or lengthy, friendly and warm, or acrimonious and hostile . . . whether it is a visit or an actual help or giving of services" (Shanas, 1980). We only know that the elderly see their children and other relatives and some exchange takes place.

Mutual Aid Pattern

There is a two way flow of emotional and material support between the elderly and their family members. The large majority of these relationships are balanced, reciprocal exchanges. According to Shanas' 1975 survey, about 71 percent of the elderly help their children or grandchildren, and 46 percent help their great-grandchildren. They generally gave gifts, cared for their grandchildren and great-grandchildren, and helped around the house, with women doing housework and men doing household repairs. On the other hand, about two-thirds of the elderly reported receiving help from their children, with more women than men receiving such help (72 versus 62 percent). A small proportion of adult children (about 3 percent) gave money to the elderly on a regular basis, but occasional money gifts were more frequent (14 percent).

In fact, there is increasing acceptance that government should assume the responsibility of financial support for the aged, primarily through social security (Schorr, 1980); Louis Harris and Associates, 1975; Seelbach, 1977; Cantor, 1980). But financial help can take forms other than cash contributions, such as sharing a home. Studies show a difference in help patterns between working class and middle class. The working class will usually exchange direct services since members are located nearby or share a household,

314

while the middle class will exchange money and serviceable gifts since members live farther apart (Schorr, 1980; Troll, 1981). Schorr has summarized this mutual aid pattern in the following manner:

What children and their parents give one another has little connection with law or compulsion. Cash payment, the only contribution that can be compelled, is now a minor part of the pattern. Helping each other by doing chores, visiting and showing concern—things that cannot be compelled—make up the dominant pattern. . . . In the end, whether from affection or simple acceptance of responsibility, many adult children do what they can. Reciprocity, spontaneity, complexity and (not legal but somehow personal) responsibility—these are the salient qualities of filial relationships.

Lastly, as age increased, the percentage of elderly giving help to the children generally decreased, and they reported receiving greater help from their children.

The Family as a Caregiver of the Elderly

The living arrangements of older persons, their proximity to family members outside the household, and their interaction frequency and exchange of services just described show how the kinship system is functioning as a social support for the majority of the elderly. The question remains, however, how the family support system functions when the health status of the older person deteriorates and dependency results. It is widely believed that long-term care institutions and other human service agencies have replaced the family in providing care to the impaired elderly (Shanas, 1979). However, the proportion of old people that are bedfast and housebound in the community is almost twice the proportion of old people in institutions of all kinds. This ratio of greatly and severely impaired in the community to those in institutions has not changed much since the introduction of Medicare and Medicaid (Shanas, 1979). If those elderly are added to the total who have trouble moving about on their own outside the house (becoming 17 percent of the aged population), the ratio of elderly living in the community with some assistance to that of the institutionalized population (5 percent) is more than three to one.

In addition, research has estimated that the family, and not the professionals or agencies, provides most of the care to the chronically limited elderly. The Health Interview Survey, a national survey investigating health-related home care, found that 62 percent of the medically-related and personal care[1] to persons 65 years and over

---

[1] Medically-related care was defined as bandage changing, injections, and other medical treatment *exclusive* of direct physican care. Personal care was defined as assistance with moving about, dressing, bathing, and eating.

was given by family members, and almost half of the care had been provided for a period of one to five years (National Center for Health Statistics, 1972). The figure would have been higher if other services that relate to disability and that are generally provided by relatives, such as meal preparation, household maintenance and so on, had been included (Brody, 1978). The 1977 GAO study in Cleveland indicated that 56 percent of those surveyed were receiving personal care services from family and friends, and 87 percent reported that they could rely on their family for help if they needed it. Cantor and Johnson (1978) found that 60 percent of the elderly were cared for by family members when sick for less than a week. This figure increased to 70 percent when the sickness lasted between one to two weeks. Another study by Cantor (1975) found that about two-thirds of the elderly received help from their children when ill and received help in chores of daily living.

The nursing home is appropriate for some of the elderly, and it is not reasonable to expect that all elderly should remain in the community. Even for those elderly who are institutionalized, however, the family plays an important role by visiting regularly and volunteering at some homes. It has been reported that residents who had more visitors received better care (Dobrof, 1977; Tobin and Kulys, 1979).

Theoretical Interpretation of Caregiving Patterns

Several groups compose the support system of the elderly (kin, friends, neighbors, and formal organizations), and it is important to know to which group the elderly turn for assistance and why. Two main theories have been advanced to describe this process: (1) the task-specific model and (2) the hierarchical-compensatory model.

In the first model, as postulated by Litwak in his theory of shared functions (Cantor, 1979), support is ordered by the nature of the task and the characteristics of the caregiver. According to this theory, kin are the most appropriate for tasks that require long-term involvement and intimacy. Neighbors would perform those tasks that require speed of response, knowledge and proximity to the living situation. Friends would be able to handle matters relating to peer group status and similarity of experience, such as sharing social activities. Christiansen (1980) has argued that though this division of labor is very plausible, it does not match the fact that most elderly depend more on family members for many of the tasks which the other groups are expected to perform. He believes that the "usefulness of the theory would seem to grow as family resources become thin, and others substitute or compensate for the family."

The task-specific model, in addition to distinguishing functions of the various groups within the informal system, also distinguishes

316

between functions of formal and informal support systems. The elderly would call upon any group within the informal support system when the nature of the task is non-technical and unpredictable, such as assisting in shopping and responding to minor emergencies. Formal organizations would become involved if the level of technical skills or knowledge required is high and assistance can be given in a uniform and predictable manner.

The hierarchical-compensatory model states that support is ordered "according to the primacy of the relationship of the support given to the elderly recipient rather than to the nature of the task. In cases in which the initially preferred element is absent, other groups act in a compensatory manner as replacements" (Cantor, 1979). The model postulates an order of preference for support: kin are the most preferred, followed by friends and neighbors, and finally, formal organizations. Cantor investigated older people's preferences for support agents for different types of tasks to validate this model. Kin, particularly children, were chosen as the most appropriate helping source, regardless of task. In line with the compensatory portion of the model, support functions were shared by other relatives, friends, neighbors, and even, in some instances, formal organizations, as a child was located farther from the aged parents. Those elderly without children chose friends and neighbors, followed either by other relatives or no one. Dono *et al* (1979) point out that preferences for support groups may not indicate which group actually provides the assistance when necessary.

Johnson (1979) takes an intermediate position. Based on her research of caregiving helping patterns, she states that ". . . if one exhausts all intimate kinship resources to the point one must reach out to distant relations for help, the type of care differs greatly and rarely centers on day-to-day care of physical needs as well as social and emotional needs. Neither friends nor relatives of second or third degree can substitute for a spouse or an offspring in the extensiveness of care nor its quality."

Types of Caregivers of the Elderly

Cantor and Johnson (1978) classify caregivers of the elderly into three major categories according to the relationship of the caregiver to the care receiver: kin, close friends, and neighbors. Kin can be further subdivided into spouse and child (the nuclear family), with siblings and other relatives composing the distant family network. These categories can be further inventoried by type of caregiving arrangement (whether it is within or between households) and the type of care provided (instrumental or affective).

Even though the previous review of kin resources, reduced by the concept of functioning kin, indicated a pool of relatives available,

317

research has shown that "primary" responsibility is usually assumed by one person (Johnson, 1979). In general, the spouse is the most likely caregiver, particularly for men who are more likely to be married (Shanas, 1977). "Men take over traditionally female tasks as necessary, women find the strength to turn and lift bedfast husbands. Husbands or wives of the elderly bedfast persons, themselves elderly, are rarely able to manage the care of a spouse without outside help." The spouse as the primary caregiver meets societal norms. Spouses are expected to, and do, provide home care for their partners for as long as possible (Johnson, 1979). This commitment is reflected in the extreme impairment level of the relatively few married persons who are institutionalized (DeVita, 1979). Adult children either in or outside the household were reported as the second main source of help, with many reporting assistance from paid helpers, indicating that they also require outside help (Shanas, 1979). Adult children usually provide care to the unmarried elderly. If there are no off-spring available, brothers, sisters, or other relatives (nieces, neph-ews) may provide assistance.

Friends and neighbors also form part of the social support net-work of the elderly. Dono (1979) determined the importance of peers by showing that widows are more likely to be looked after by other widows, at least where they maintain their own residence. However, relationships with friends and neighbors do not entirely compensate for lack of relationships with spouse and children (Cantor, 1980).

For all categories of caregivers but spouse, the sex is predomi-nantly female. In the study by Cantor (1980), women composed 75 percent of children caregivers, 86 percent of the other relative caregivers, and 92 percent of the friend/neighbor caregivers. Males (excluding husbands) are usually primary caregivers by default, when the family network is all male or they are the only ones avail-able (Brookdale Center on Aging, 1979). If a son is a primary care-giver, his spouse is likely to be very involved in the caregiving process. On the other hand, daughters who are primary caregivers tend to protect their husbands from sharing any responsibility (Horowitz, 1978). Female predominance may be due to greater life expectancy and sex-role differences. The one exception is the category of spouse caregivers where the sex ratio is approximately equal (Cantor, 1980; Soldo and Sharma, 1980). Sex of caregiver is also related to nature of task. There is usually a clear division of labor, with women primarily performing domestic tasks such as cooking and cleaning and males performing tasks such as making repairs in the house (Hawkins and Jacobson, 1980).

Types and Extent of Assistance

The types of assistance provided by family and other informal caregivers of the elderly may be classified into instrumental and

318

affective tasks. Affective assistance provides emotional supports and fulfills socialization needs. It includes activities such as visiting, talking, giving advice, and watching television together. Such emotional support is highly valued by the elderly; in fact, the elderly tend to deem it more important than other assistance (Seelbach and Sauer, 1977). Emotional support can be provided by friends and neighbors. Support from these groups occurs especially for elderly women who are more likely than men to socialize outside the family network (Seelbach, 1979). Although friends and neighbors provide companionship and an outlet for tension, the preference of the elderly remains for family members to provide all types of support, even emotional (Cantor, 1979). Distant relatives do not appear to have much of a role in fulfilling an elderly person's social needs unless a strong bond of affection already existed (Johnson, 1979). It is shown that the more distant the relationship becomes, the more the type of caregiving provided differs from that provided by a spouse or an adult child. The person more likely serves as an "intermediary between the elderly patient and the health care bureaucracy and their major responsibility involves arranging for hired help" (Johnson, 1980). In other words, the assistance is real but lacks intimacy.

Instrumental assistance focuses on particular tasks such as personal care activities, medical management, or transportation and household assistance. A study by York and Calsyn (1977) about families of nursing home patients indicates that the family is very involved in providing assistance to an elderly person before placement in a nursing home. The percentage of families providing regular help is as follows: shopping (72 percent), laundry, medical affairs, and heavy cleaning (69 percent), cooking (58 percent), bathing (32 percent), dressing (21 percent), and using the toilet (12 percent). Although for the entire sample, personal care assistance was less reported than other tasks, about 30 percent of the families took the aged person into their homes before nursing home placement; it is likely that personal care assistance was greater for that portion of the sample.

A study by Cantor (1980) showed a substantial difference in the extent of instrumental assistance as measured by 10 activities among the various types of caregivers. The spouse was the most involved, with a mean number of seven tasks performed, followed by adult children (mean of 5.4) and other relatives (mean of 2.7). Spouses were more likely to be involved in all activities, while children and other relatives were less involved in personal care and assistance with medication. In addition, other relatives were less likely to help with housework. Friends and neighbors were the least involved group. Friends and neighbors may be useful in short-term, crisis situations, but chronic care which requires daily monitoring and nursing care falls primarily within the family realm (Cantor, 1980).

319

The caregiving responsibilities of the family members range from weekly visits to shared housing arrangements. The majority of the caregivers provide care by running frequent errands, providing transportation, and making telephone calls. Cantor (1980) reported a range from one hour to all of the time (84 hours per week) for both affective and instrumental assistance. For the most part, 20 to 30 hours were spent on both types. From the time perspective of the caregiver, it would appear that there was no real distinction between affective and instrumental assistance; both were equally important and time consuming. For about 40 percent of children caring for elderly parents in the same household, Newman (1976) found that they spent the equivalent of a full-time job in caregiving activities.

As the needs of the parents grow, the families generally respond with an increased commitment such as providing constant care or sharing a household. In general, the amount of assistance provided is directly related to health status (Seelbach, 1977) and to the age of the older person and low income (Cantor, 1975). Movement into a relative's home is usually seen as an alternative to moving into an institution, and that living arrangement was often reported prior to institutionalization: 30 percent in the study by York and Calsyn (1977), 54 percent in the study by Miller and Harris (1965), and 45 percent by Townsend (1965). This is buttressed by the fact that there are about twice as many elderly living in multigenerational households—9 percent—than in institutions—5 percent—with more of those 75 years and older living in such arrangements, indicating a relationship to disability (Mindel, 1979). Families view institutionalization as the last resort only after all possible alternatives have been explored (Brody, 1979).

Researchers have argued that with the proliferation of organized programs serving the elderly, a new role for the family has emerged: that of mediator between the institutional bureauracy and the older person. The family can ". . . be a buffer for elderly persons in the latter's dealing with bureaucracies; examine the service options provided by organizations; effect entry of the elderly person into the program of bureaucratic organizations and facilitate the continuity of the relationship of the aged member with the bureaucracy" (Shanas and Sussman, 1977).

Caregiving Impact of the Support System

Although benefits are derived from caregiving, studies have also documented various problems experienced by family members caring for aged relatives. Newman's study of three-generation households in the United States revealed benefits as well as costs when a parent was in the household of an adult child. The benefits included affection, enjoyment, contribution to the household through housework or child care, and relief that the parent was being cared

320

for properly. The majority reported that there had been no changes in the household's routine, but 40 percent reported increased strain and changes in the family (Lebowitz, 1978). These changes included low morale, interruption of domestic routines and social and leisure activities, financial costs, and ill health.

A study by Grad and Sainsbury (1966) indicated that about 75 percent of families with mentally ill elderly reported facing some burden, with 40 percent reporting it as a severe burden. It indicated that the elderly who are mentally ill impose the most severe burden on their families (Lebowitz, 1978). In a study of geriatric day care patients, about half of the families experienced some degree of strain (Rathbone-McCluan, 1976), but it was emotional more than financial. Cantor's study (1980) indicated that spouses were more likely than children or other relatives to experience financial strain, but it was still secondary to the physical or emotional strain. Indirect financial costs, or opportunity costs due to loss of earnings when a caregiver does not enter or not remain in the labor force, may be incurred. Opportunity costs are more likely to affect younger adult children or other relatives who are mostly female, particularly single parents who are most likely to work out of economic necessity, than spouse caregivers who are elderly themselves and not in the labor force.

Direct financial costs to families caring for the elderly are relieved in several ways. Third-party reimbursement, such as Medicare and Medicaid, reduces a large proportion of expenditures for insured items; food stamps for qualifying individuals reduce household expenditures; the elderly person's own income from social security and other pensions reduces direct financial costs incurred by caregivers.

The social and psychological impact of care is expressed by the caregivers in many ways: feelings of worry, burden, frustration, and being "tied down." Caregivers most frequently complain of social isolation due to interruption of friendship patterns and impairment of their mobility (Fengler and Goodrich, 1979). This is accentuated by the fact that usually only one person assumes the primary caregiver role instead of an optimal situation of shared family support which would not overly tax one individual (Johnson, 1979).

Role stress may occur for a spouse in adjusting to a dependent relationship where a mutually interdependent one previously existed, causing anger, frustration, and resentment. Adult children who assume the caregiving role may be confused or angry about the role reversal of the parent-child relationship (Horowitz, 1978).

Conflicting obligations also result in strain. Responsibilities to parents may take precedence over responsibilities to spouse, children, or others because the former is seen as the more pressing need. However, this is usually felt to be a forced choice. Filial duties have a marked impact on the marital and family relations of an adult

321

child. The spouse and offspring may "feel neglected, deprived, bitter, jealous, or resentful, depending on how they view the caregiver's activities. This, in turn, might produce disagreement and turmoil in the marital and parent-child relationships" (Seelbach, 1978).

Women are particularly vulnerable to role strain since they are the principal caregivers to the aged. They have been characterized as "women in the middle," often being in middle age and in the middle generation. They are also in the middle by being subject to "multiple, and often competing, demands of their roles as workers, spouses, filial caregivers, parents, and even grandparents. In addition, they may be in the middle by experiencing conflict due to changing social values, especially the value of women doing out-of-home work *vis-a-vis* the traditional value that care of the elderly is their responsibility" (Brody, 1979).

Women's increased participation in the labor force will have an unknown impact on the caregiving situation in the family. Whether it will lead to a redistribution of responsibilities among the family members or will be an added burden on women and cause more role strain remains to be seen. Reports indicate that sharing of household chores or increased help in families where the women works, however, have not been significant, even with the large rise in female employment. A similar outcome might occur with caregiving obligation (Treas, 1977). Analysis of Survey of Income and Education (SIE) data by Soldo and Sharma (1980) gives evidence that families in which the wife works and no other adult women are present in the house are more likely to purchase care for the elderly than households in which the wife does not work or where there is another woman present.

It is possible that health status of the caregiver may also be affected. Klein *et al* (1968) report that physical and emotional symptoms increase among spouses during caregiving. A study by Myllyluoma and Soldo (1980) on intrahousehold caregiving based on analysis of SIE data indicates that among elderly couples living by themselves, over 5 percent of the caregivers also required a moderate to high level of assistance. This suggests the potential vulnerability of the caregiver, when he or she, too, is elderly and may require assistance, especially as duration of caregiving increases. In a study of effects of caregiving on responsible family members (Adams *et al,* 1979), one-third of the persons reported that their health was affected by their elder's illness. Twice as many of those persons living with the elder reported health problems, compared to those who were not.

Strained affective relationships are another negative consequence of caregiving. For instance, before extensive caregiving begins, the aged parent more likely labels a child as the person to whom he or she feels closest; this is not true afterwards (Tobin and Kulys, 1980).

322

The prevalent notion of family responsibility compels many to care for their elderly parents, regardless of the nature of their past relationships. It seems that a child responds to a parent in need, and "if anything, care is given in spite of, not because of, the past relationship" (Horowitz, 1978).

A history of reciprocity and an affective interaction were associated with the ability to assume and accept the caretaking role with relatively less tension (Horowitz, 1978). Lack of such a positive history was associated with tension related to caregiving. Providing care because one feels obligated could lead to anger and frustration, which in turn might result in ineffective caregiving and, possibly, abuse. One study investigating abuse of the elderly by caregivers found evidence of a rate of abuse of almost 10 percent (Tobin and Kulys, 1980).

Two factors that mitigate the strain of caregiving impact are a perceived support from other family members and a gradual, not sudden, increase in the needs of the older person. Both factors permit an easier adaptation to the caregiving role (Horowitz, 1978).

Sustaining Family Caregiving of the Elderly

Although different caregivers have different tolerance thresholds, family caregiving cannot continue indefinitely in many cases, considering the stresses that families experience in caring for the elderly. Institutional placement more often stems from exhaustion of family resources and excessive burden on family members than a change in the older person's health status (Kraus et al, 1976). In a study comparing institutionalized and community samples of older persons and their families, the family's self-reported ability to provide care as long as needed emerged as the major distinguishing variable (Smyer, 1980).

Much of the literature on family care of the elderly calls for establishing service and/or economic incentives to sustain caregiving. Sussman (1977) states that "the family network is a vast reservoir of energy which can be appropriately harnessed if it is given sufficient resources so that it does not deplete its own stock and that its members have reasonable hopes to meet their expectations for maintenance, a quality of life or achievement."

Studies to date have focused particularly on the role of service provision in assisting the family. In a study of geriatric day care patients, the families admitted that the programs helped reduce family tension, alleviated the burden of care, and prevented further emotional dependence on them. Families indicated that the day care arrangement represented a "last ditch" effort to maintain the older person in the community (Rathbone-McCuan, 1976). Horo-

323

witz (1978) found that when caregivers were provided with services, primarily homemaker, housekeeper, and/or companion-aide, two major benefits were identified: (1) freedom to engage in other activities because more time was available, and (2) freedom from the emotional pressure of having primary responsibility for the parent's well-being. Where the caregiver resented the role reversal of the parent-child relationship, the introduction of an outside source improved the affective quality of the relationship. Gross-Andrews and Zimmer (1977) also reported that family caregivers reported alleviation of stress or of disruption in their lives in emotional, physical, social, and financial terms when provided with up to four services: companion aide, personal care worker, homemaker/home attendant, and housekeeper. Provision of such services would leave the caregiver more time and energy to satisfy the emotional needs of the elderly (Dunlop, 1980).

While these studies suggest that provision of services can reduce the stress on the caregiver, it is still unclear whether provision of services to the family will prevent or delay institutionalization. If one assumes that social services and programs, by providing instrumental assistance, will permit the caregiver to attend to the elderly's emotional needs (Seelbach and Sauer, 1977) and that such emotional support can be crucial in prevention or delaying deterioration in physical functioning (Dunlop, 1980), institutionalization may also be delayed or prevented. For example, in Sager's 1978 study of hospital patients who were to be discharged to nursing homes, the discharge planner believed that three-fourths of the families would have been willing to maintain the patient at home if outside support services were provided. Similarly, in a study by Eggert et al (1977) of elderly disabled patients discharged from the hospital, family willingness to care for the patients and ability to absorb home care costs were the strongest predictors of whether the older person went home or to an institution. This willingness, however, appeared to significantly erode over time when the burden was not shared by supplementary social services. For example, where formal home care and social services were not readily available, 70 percent of the patients' families had provided care for them at home after the first hospitalization, but only 38 percent were willing to give such care after the second hospitalization (Eggert et al, 1977). Although the studies just cited indicate prevention or delay of institutionalization, the Section 222 demonstrations, which studied the effect of provision of homemaker services, did not show any difference in nursing home rates between the control and experimental groups (Weissert et al, 1979).

Several types of economic incentives have been proposed to sustain family caregiving. These include suggestions for direct cash subsidies, tax relief, and low cost loans. Treas (1977) argues that "families who overcome the many obstacles to home care of the aged would seem to warrant direct payments as surely as do strangers providing less personalized services."

Sussman (1976) has proposed offering economic and service incentives to families for care of the aged, under a contractual arrangement that would be for a given time period. The incentives, he argues, would reduce the economic liabilities of caregiving and thereby permit the family to concentrate on providing affective assistance. Schorr (1980) believes that such a proposal would create a bureaucratic nightmare and, in the long run, subvert filial attachments and responsibility. As he points out, "Why would one help a parent for nothing if it seemed that everyone else was being paid? If, in fact, Congress says one should be paid?" Certainly some assessment or goalkeeping procedure would have to be created "unless the government is to pay 80 percent of the home care now being provided free by families."

Another proposal calls for some type of attendance/disability allowance for persons who require care in the home. Currently, the Veterans Administration does provide an allowance to low income, aged veterans who need regular aid and attendance. Schorr (1980) cites suggestions that the United States provide an attendance allowance to everyone who is 75 years old or more without a demonstration of need. A variant of this would provide fewer benefits at age 65 and more at 75 and 85. The government would deal with it as an income strategy and administer it with relative efficiency and simplicity. Other proposals base payment on proven medical need. Some would pay whether home help is purchased or provided by the family, or not provided at all, at the discretion of the beneficiary (Schorr, 1980). Some would provide vouchers to eligible clients with the value based on level of disability and income (DHHS, 1981). These vouchers would be used with formal service providers.

California is an example which uses the former model. Qualified individuals receive a flat sum of money to purchase whatever mix and level of support services they desire from any source, including family. In fact, family members have become the major provider of homemaker, home management, and chores services under Title XX (Callahan et al, 1979). This system permits a large degree of individual choice, but there has been much abuse. Other States limit payments to distant relatives.

Cost is the major disadvantage of these proposals since they are "likely to substitute monetary exchange for what is currently an unpaid, informal care arrangement for many" (DHHS, 1981).

A review by Gibson (1980) discusses how European nations are currently providing such payments and reports that there is a wide variation in the qualifying conditions and benefit levels of the allowances. Some programs pay the elderly disabled person directly to permit consumer choice; some pay the relative directly for pro-

325

viding home care. In England, both the elderly disabled person and his/her caregiving relative can receive an allowance. The impact of these payments has not been systematically evaluated, and it is unclear to what extent, if any, they serve as incentives to family care of the elderly. Some of the payments are so low that they may not be incentives. Others are quite substantial, though still not considered equivalent to a regular wage. So there would still be opportunity costs involved for a caregiver who took care of a chronically ill relative instead of entering or remaining in the work force. England and Sweden provide other benefits which may partially remedy this problem. For example, pension credits are given to persons who leave the work force to care for an elderly or disabled relative.

Tax proposals most frequently mentioned are:

- Income tax deductions to family members for providing care to dependent older members which would be similar to deductions of payments for child care expenses to family members
- specific tax write-offs for expenses incurred in connection with caretaking functions of aging parents
- property tax waivers with some proportional formula for dwelling usage given to the dependent elderly who live with family members (Lowy, 1980).

Such proposals would do more to encourage sharing the burden among several family members than the current requirement of providing more than half of the support to claim an elderly person as a dependent.

Provision of low cost loans to the family for renovating or building an addition to a house to provide suitable space for a disabled older relative is another suggestion. Several other countries, such as Japan, Sweden, England and Australia, provide such assistance to encourage multigenerational living (Gibson, 1980).

An attitude survey by Sussman (1977) provides some insights into what incentives might be preferred by families providing care to the elderly. Individuals were asked to rank service incentives and financial incentives separately. The service incentives were medical care, visiting, social centers, information centers, meals-on-wheels, or home aide services. More than two-thirds chose medical care as the most preferred service incentive. The financial incentive choices were monthly checks, tax deductions, low cost loans, food stamps, rental allowances, or property tax deductions. Of these, two-thirds of the respondents preferred monthly checks. When the financial options were ranked against the service options, 47 percent selected monthly checks as their first choice, versus 22 percent who chose the medical care option first (Sussman, 1977). However, for many of those individuals who cared for or had an older person living with them some time previously, service incentives were preferred over economic ones. It indicates that while the families certainly recognize the benefits of a regular monthly check, "their actual experience with a chronically ill elderly relative indicates a greater need and appreciation for those supports which will make their lives less harried" (Sussman, 1979).

The study also indicated, however, that not all families respond to incentives. About 19 percent of the families interviewed reported that they would not take an elderly relative into their home under any circumstances. Sussman (1979) states that "incentives may just facilitate the process for those already committed and do little to change the minds of refusers."

One conclusion of the study was that demographic variables do not play an important role in explaining willingness of a person to care for an elderly person. Situational variables were more correlated with willingness. These include such things as crowding in the house, perception of spouse's or children's amenability to the idea, presence of relatives who live nearby and could help, favorable attitudes toward the elderly, and previous positive experiences with the elderly (Sussman, 1979).

This is an important finding, for public policy can be formulated to alter these situational variables and thereby increases the family's willingness to provide and continue caregiving of the elderly. Demographic variables are not so amenable. However, as with any attitude survey, attitude cannot guarantee actual behavior.

Policy Issues and Recommendations

The family has an important role in the caregiving of the elderly, being the major provider of care. While policymakers appreciate the usefulness of family ties and seek to maximize the contributions of the family, they must also realize the family's limitations. One costly consequence of excessive burden on the family is assumed to be premature institutionalization of the elderly, although this is difficult to measure.

The issue then becomes what can be done to sustain family caregiving of the elderly. The service and economic incentives just discussed could be universally available and open-ended but realistically, some screening mechanism to target those most in need would be necessary to prevent excessive costs. To develop economically feasible policies, the appropriate forms of family support and who should be supported have to be determined.

However, if the overriding issue is one of minimizing costs (which is usually assumed to be reduction in institutionalization), policy dictates concentrating provision of services or other incentives on those impaired elderly without family supports. "Consequently, those dependent elderly receiving informal care from kin, who may be undergoing severe stress, would tend to be excluded. In this way,

327

the goal of relieving stress on informal care-givers would be for-feited" (Dunlop, 1980). A study in England (Moroney, 1976) found that "services that can be used to support families that are caring for their impaired elderly members are deployed from such families to individuals where there is no viable support." It is assumed that "if resources are not made available . . . , the probability is that the family will still be able to manage, at least for a time. Relatively little is made available to families until they reach the breaking point." The same situation has occurred in Israel, "where if an old person lives with a child or relative, he is informally cut off from the scarce resources of the visiting homemaker or health aide" (Shanas and Sussman, 1977). With limited resources, such competing goals will continue to be a problem.

Limited resources make it essential to provide those services which are the most beneficial. Dunlop (1980) states that "policy-makers need to know the relative value of each type of home-based service and service package." Respite care appears to be a service valued highly by family caregivers. This type of service would alle-viate one of the major problems experienced by caregivers across all socioeconomic groups—restricted mobility (Danis, 1978). It would relieve demands on caregivers and allow them necessary time for themselves, their husbands, wives, and children. The Section 222 demonstration project indicates that a combination of homemaker and day care service might be better than a homemaker package alone (Weissert et al, 1979). Such a service package, however, is likely to have tremendous costs.

More viable alternatives should be developed between the two extremes of institutional care or shared household—generally the only two options that adult children and other relatives consider when extended care is necessary (Robinson and Thurnher, 1979). Service provision has to be adaptable to the needs of particular groups of caregivers, such as spouses who experience tremendous burden in providing constant care but are expected to persevere in accordance with the marital role. For such a group, routine nine-to-five services may be inadequate, and services with more flexible schedules may be required. Linkage to formal services can be facili-tated to ease the family tasks, with more coordination between the formal system and the family network and a division of services that are appropriate for each as expressed by Litwak (1966) in his theory of shared functions. Maximizing the efficiency of both these systems in serving the elderly is admittedly a delicate balancing act. At present there is little information about the best collaboration be-tween the two. Certain suggestions concerning the role of formal organizations were mentioned by caregivers in a study by Hawkins and Jacobson (1980). These suggestions included recognizing the caregiver's assistance, facilitating a support network of other care-

328

givers, counseling and advising caregivers undergoing stress, providing information about services of formal agencies and how to receive them, providing technical assistance in caring for the older person, and providing services on a temporary basis to relieve the caregiver, such as housekeeping and cooking. Certainly, policymakers need to view the elderly in the context of the family network and not as individuals. To that end, the needs of the caregivers should be considered, as well as the needs of the primary client group, the elderly. In fact, the family should be considered the base upon which the services of the formal system for the elderly build, and not the reverse, as is commonly assumed (Hawkins and Jacobson, 1980). Formal service providers, however, have expressed concern about legal and administrative implications of such cooperation with informal caregivers. One concern is the organization's legal liability if it should become the primary facilitator for an informal care-giving arrangement and if the informal caregivers subsequently, for any reason, caused injury to the aged (Hawkins and Jacobson, 1980).

Eggert (1977) questions whether family capacity might be sustained if complemented with particular services. He poses the problem that "if families become accustomed to the availability of supplementary assistance, is there any reason for them not to progressively transfer the burden of care so that over time, social provision displaces present family capacity?"

One national study concluded that:

The services do not undermine self-help, because they are concentrated overwhelmingly among those who have neither the capacities nor the resources to undertake the relevant functions alone. Nor, broadly speaking, do the services conflict with the interests of the family as a social institution, because either they tend to reach people who lack a family or whose family resources are slender or they provide specialized services the family is not equipped or qualified to undertake (Townsend, 1968).

However, because of limited availability of home-based supportive services and other natural limitations on demand, such as the perceived welfare connection of such services (Dunlop, 1980), this question of services possibly substituting for family care rather than supplementing it cannot be addressed fully. It would be difficult to predict the behavior of families if there were expanded public funding of home-based services, especially if the welfare connotation were removed (DHHS, 1981). Very little information is available on this issue. In a study of a program which offered four types of services (companion aide, personal care worker, homemaker/home attendant, and housekeeping), family requests for services were

329

found to be close to what agency staff recommended, and many were extremely modest (Gross-Andrew and Zimmer, 1977).

Current programs and policies need to be reviewed to determine if there is any negative effect on the family support system. Supplemental Security Income (SSI) and food stamp program provisions in particular penalize families caring for the elderly, or if the elderly person and family members share a household, since family resources are counted toward the aged person's income. SSI payments are reduced and food-stamp eligibility may be denied in such situations. These provisions disproportionately affect lower income and minority families who are more likely to share households. However, such provisions may not always act as a disincentive if there is little choice in sharing a household.

Policymakers must remain alert to changing demographics and family situations in developing programs. Such trends include: (1) changes in family composition (for example, more single parents, fewer children, more multigenerational families, and so on), (2) labor market shifts with a greater number of women in the work force, and (3) increased longevity yielding more and older elderly and increasingly older caregivers.

Agenda for Future Research

The introduction to this chapter mentioned the limitations of available research on family support of the elderly. These included insufficient detail, limited general applicability, and the cross-sectional, descriptive nature of studies. Additional research is needed to extend and validate existing studies. Such research should focus on formulating and testing hypotheses and should preferably be longitudinal.

Needed research in this area can be grouped into several major categories:

- more detail of the processes of the natural support system of the elderly, including research on decision-making
- more research on what types of programs or services would best support the family caregiving system
- more research of the costs and benefits of the family caregiving system.

There have been many descriptive studies about types of contributions that family members provide to their elderly relatives, whether well or impaired. More research is needed to determine the conditions and circumstances under which members of varied family networks at different life cycle stages are willing to care for the elderly. This is critical since what constitutes a family today is not particularly homogeneous and will be less so in the future. It is estimated that only 37 percent of families are nuclear (husband, wife, and children), another 11 percent are nuclear dyad (no children), and 11 percent are reconstituted nuclear (remarried husband or wife with children). The remainder are single parent families, extended families, other single adults and experimental forms (Sussman, 1976). Thus, more studies of family forms that differ from the mode are needed since it is predicted that these forms will exist in greater numbers in the future. Since the birth rate is dropping, there will be more elderly who are childless or have only one child. The situation of the childless elderly should be examined—how and with whom helping relationships are established. This may provide information on how family surrogates are developed and how well they compensate for kin.

Other family situations which should be investigated because of their growing numbers are single parent families, dual career families, and four and five generational families where there are aged parents and grandparents to care for because of the increased life span and shorter generation span. More exploration of other than parent-child relationships, such as those with siblings and more distant kin, is needed. Another aspect to be examined is the situation in which more elderly are living with non-relatives in either communal or cohabitation arrangements. In addition, a basic understanding is required of the decision process by which the elderly seek help or the family members and other persons offer care.

Researchers have called for demonstrations which would relate types of family networks, stage of life cycle and lifestyle with respect to specific incentives, the physical and mental status of the elderly person, the attitudes and perceptions of the elderly person and his/her relatives and the physical and social capabilities of relatives and household. Such demonstrations would also provide social and economic cost/benefit estimates for different types of family home care arrangements.

There have been methodological problems with cost comparisons, especially with regard to family contributions. Carefully designed research is needed to know the quality and scope of organized services that substitute for a specific configuration of family contributions. This would then enable assignment of a dollar value to family contributions, particularly opportunity costs involved in caregiving.

References

Adams, Mary, Mary Ann Caston, and Benjamin Davis, "A Neglected Dimension in Home Care of Elderly Disabled Persons: Effect on Responsible Family Members." Paper presented at the Annual Gerontological Society Meeting, Washington, D.C., November, 1979.

Bengtson, Vern and Kristen Falde Smith, "Positive Consequences of Institutionalization: Solidarity between Elderly Parents and Their Middle-Aged Children," *The Gerontologist,* 19 (Issue 5, 1979): 438–447.

Bild, Bernice and Robert Havighurst, "Senior Citizens in Great Cities: The Case of Chicago," *The Gerontologist,* 16 (Issue 1, Part II, February 1976): 3–88.

Brody, Elaine, "Woman's Changing Roles, The Aged Family and Long Term Care of Older People," *National Journal* (October 27, 1979): 1828–1833.

Brody, Elaine, Testimony presented to the U.S. House of Representatives, Select Committee on Aging, November 24, 1980.

Brody, Elaine, "The Aging of the Family," *The Annals of the American Academy of Political and Social Science* 438 (July 1978): 13–27.

Brody, Elaine, Linda Davis, Mark Fulcomer, and Pauline Johnson, "Women's Changing Roles and Help to the Elderly: A Three-Generational Perspective," Research paper supported by AoA Grant No. 90–A–1277, 1979.

Brody, Stanley, Walter Poulshock, and Carla Masciocchi. "The Family Caring Unit: A Major Consideration in the Long-Term Support System," *The Gerontologist* 18 (Issue 6, December 1978): 556–561.

Brookdale Center on Aging of Hunter College, Proposal entitled "The Role of Families in Providing Long-Term Care to the Frail and Chronically Ill Elderly in the Community," funded by Health Care Financing Administration, Grant No. 18–P–97541, 1980.

Bureau of the Census, *Current Population Reports,* "Household and Family Characteristics, March 1976," Series P–20, No. 311, 1977.

Callahan, James Jr., Lawrence Diamond, Janet Giele, and Robert Morris. "Responsibility of Families for Their Severely Disabled Elders," Background paper prepared by the University Health Policy Consortium under HCFA Grant No. 18–P–97038, July 1979.

Cantor, Marjorie, "Life Space and the Social Support System of the Inner City Elderly of New York"—Part I *The Gerontologist,* 15 (Issue 1, February 1975): 23–27.

Cantor, Marjorie, "Caring for the Frail Elderly: Impact on Family, Friends and Neighbors." Paper presented at Annual Gerontological Society Meeting, San Diego, November 1980.

Cantor, Marjorie, "Neighbors and Friends: An Overlooked Resource in the Informal Support System." *Research on Aging* 1 (No. 4, December 1979): 434–463.

Cantor, Marjorie and Jeffrey Johnson, "The Informal Support System of the 'Familyless' Elderly—Who Takes Over?" Paper presented at Annual Gerontological Society Meeting, Dallas, November 1978.

Christiansen, Andrew, "Family Care of the Elderly: A Report on the Literature." Working Paper No. 1, Series CPR–MD–80. Prepared under AoA Grant No. 90–AR–2124, 1980.

Community Service Society, Proposal entitled "Impact of Home Services on Functionally Disabled Adults," funded by Health Care Financing Administration, Grant No. 18P–97462, 1980.

Comptroller General of the United States, General Accounting Office, *The Well-Being of Older People in Cleveland, Ohio,* Washington, D.C.: U.S. Government Printing Office, April 19, 1977. HRD–77–70.

Danis, B. G., "Stress in Individuals Caring for Ill Elderly Relatives," Paper presented at the Gerontological Society Meeting, Dallas, Texas, 1978.

DeVita, Carol, "Sociodemographic Differences Among the Institutionalized Elderly by Kin Availability," Working Paper No. 6, Series CPR–MD–79, Paper prepared for AoA Grant No. 90–A–1681, March 1979.

DeVita, Carol, "The Older Institutionalized Population: A Sociodemographic Profile," Working Paper No. 5, Series CPR–MD–79, Paper prepared for AoA Grant No. 90–A–1681, March 1979.

Dobrof, Rose and Eugene Litwak, *Maintenance of Family Ties of Long-Term Care Patients: Theory and Guide to Practice*, Washington, D.C.: U.S. Government Printing Office, 1977.

Dono, John *et al*, "Primary Groups in Old Age: Structure and Function," *Research on Aging* 1 (No. 4, December 1979): 403–433.

Dunlop, Burton, "Expanded Home-Based Care for the Impaired Elderly: Solution or Pipe Dream?" *American Journal of Public Health* 70 (Issue 5, May 1980): 514–519.

Eggert, Gerald *et al*, "Caring for the Patient with Long-Term Disability," *Geriatrics* 32 (Issue 10, October 1977): 102–114.

Fengler, Alfred and Nancy Goodrich, "Wives of Elderly Disabled Men: The Hidden Patients," *The Gerontologist* 19 (Issue 2, April 1979).

Gibson, Mary, "Support for Families of the Elderly in Other Industrialized Nations," Background paper for International Federation on Aging, October 1980.

Giele, Janet, "A Review of Selected Data Sources of the Family's Role in Long-Term Care," Paper prepared by the University Health Policy Consortium under HCFA Grant No. 18–970381, July 1979.

Grad, J. and Sainsbury, P., "Evaluating the Community Psychiatric Service in Chicester: Results," *Milbank Memorial Fund Quarterly* 44 (Part 2, 1966): 246–278.

Greenberg, Jan, "Intergenerational Family Exchanges: Toward a Conceptual Framework," Paper presented at the Annual Gerontological Meeting, November, 1978.

Gross-Andrews, S. and Anna Zimmer, "Incentives to Families Caring for Disabled Elderly: Research and Demonstration Project to Strengthen the National Supports System," Paper presented at the Annual Gerontological Meeting, November, 1977.

Guttman, David *et al, Informal and Formal Support Systems and their Effect on the Lives of the Elderly in Selected Ethnic Groups,* Final Report to the Administration on Aging, AoA Grant No. 90–A–1007, January 1979.

Hawkins, Brian and Solomon Jacobson, "The Role of Caregivers in the Black Community," Executive Summary prepared for AoA Grant No. 90–A–1375, 1980.

Hill, Robert, "A Demographic Profile of the Black Elderly," *Aging* Nos. 287-288 (September-October 1978): 2–9.

Horowitz, Amy, "Families Who Care: A Study of Natural Support Systems of the Elderly," Paper presented at the Annual Scientific Meeting of the Gerontological Society, November 1978.

Horowitz, Amy and Lois Shindelman, "The Impact of Caring for an Elderly Relative," Paper presented at the Annual Gerontological Society Meeting in San Diego, November 1980.

Horowitz, Amy and Lois Shindelman, "Social and Economic Incentives for Family Caregivers," Paper presented at the Annual Gerontological Society Meeting in San Diego, November 1980.

Johnson, Colleen, "Impediments to Family Supports to Dependent Elderly: An Analysis of the Primary Caregivers," Paper presented at the Annual Gerontological Society Meeting, Washington, D.C., November 1979.

Kane, Robert and Rosalie Kane, "Care of the Aged: Old Problems in Need of New Solutions," in Abelson (ed) *Health Care: Regulation, Economics, Ethics, Practice*, Washington, D.C.: American Association for the Advancement of Science, 1978.

Kraus, A., R. Spasoff, E. Beattie, D. Holden, J. Lawson, S. Rodenberg, and G. Woodcock, "Elderly Applicants to Long Term Care Institutions," *Journal of the American Geriatrics Society* 24 (1976): 165–172.

Lebowitz, Barry, "Old Age and Family Functioning," *Journal of Gerontological Social Work* 2 (Winter 1978): 111–118.

Litwak, Eugene, "A Balance Theory Between Bureaucratic Organizations and Community Primary Groups," *Administrative Service Quarterly*, Vol. 11, 1966, pp. 31–58.

Louis Harris and Associates, *The Myth and Reality of Aging in America*, Washington, D.C.: National Council on Aging, 1975.

Lowy, Louis, "Families: Aging and Changing," Testimony to the Select Committee on Aging, U.S. House of Representatives, Hearing on November 24, 1980, in San Diego, California.

Maddox, J., "Families as Context and Resource in Chronic Illness," in *Issues in Long Term Care*, edited by Sylvia Sherwood, New York: Halsted Press, 1975, pp. 317–347.

Miller, M. and A. Harris, "Social Factors and Family Contacts in a Nursing Home Population," *Journal of American Geriatrics Society* 13 (1965): 845–851.

Mindel, Charles, "Multigenerational Family Households: Recent Trends and Implications for the Future," *The Gerontologist* 19 (Issue 5, 1979): 456–463.

Moroney, Robert M., *The Family and the State: Considerations for Social Policy*, New York: Longman Group Limited, 1976.

Myllyluoma, Jaana and Beth Soldo, "Family Caregivers to the Elderly: Who Are They?" Paper presented at the Annual Meeting of the Gerontological Society in San Diego, November 1980.

National Center for Health Statistics, *Home Care for Persons 55 and Over*, Vital and Health Statistics, Series 10, DHEW Publication No. (HSM) 72–1062, 1972.

National Retired Teachers Association, American Association of Retired Persons and Wakefield Washington Associates, "Family Support Systems and the Aging: A Policy Report," Paper prepared for the White House Conference on Families, 1980.

O'Brien, John and Donna Wagner, "Help Seeking by the Frail Elderly: Problems in Network Analysis," *The Gerontologist* 20 (Issue 1, Feb. 1980): 78–83.

Rathbone-McCuan, Eloise, "Geriatric Day Care: A Family Perspective," *The Gerontologist* 16 (Issue 6, December 1976): 517–521.

Robinson, Betsy and Majda Thumber, "Taking Care of Aged Parents: A Family Cycle Transition," *The Gerontologist* 19 (Issue 6, 1979): 586–593.

Rosenmayr, Leopold, "Family Relations of the Elderly," *Journal of Marriage and the Family* 30 (Issue 4, November 1968): 672–680.

Sager, Alan, "Learning the Home Care Needs of the Elderly: Patient, Family, and Professional Views of an Alternative to Institutionalization," Final Report to Administration on Aging, AoA Grant No. 90–A–1026, November 20, 1978.

Schorr, Alvin, "Thy Father and Thy Mother . . ." SSA Publication No. 13–11953, July 1980.

Seelbach, Wayne, "Gender Differences in Expectations for Filial Responsibility," *The Gerontologist* 33 (Issue 5, October 1977) Part I, 421–425.

Seelbach, Wayne and William Sauer, "Filial Responsibility Expectations and Morale Among Aged Parents," *The Gerontologist* 17 (Issue 6, December 1977): 492–499.

Shanas, Ethel, "Social Myth as Hypothesis: The Case of Family Relations of Old People," *The Gerontologist* 19 (Issue 1, Feb. 1979): 3–9.

Shanas, Ethel, "The Family as a Social Support System in Old Age," *The Gerontologist* 19 (Issue 2, April 1979): 169–174.

Shanas, Ethel, *National Survey of the Aged*, Final Report to the Administration on Aging, AoA Grant No. 90–A–369, 1977.

Shanas, Ethel, "Older People and Their Families: The New Pioneers," *Journal of Marriage and the Family* 42 (Issue 1, February 1980): 9–15.

Shanas, Ethel and Marvin Sussman, "Family and Bureaucracy: Comparative Analyses and Problematics" in *Family, Bureaucracy and the Elderly* edited by E. Shanas and M. Sussman, Durham, N.C.: Duke University Press, 1977: 215–225.

Soldo, Beth and Mahesh Sharma, "Families Who Purchase vs. Families Who Provide Care Services to Elderly Relatives," Paper presented at Annual Gerontological Society Meeting, San Diego, November 1980.

Smyer, Michael, "The Differential Usage of Services by Impaired Elderly," *Journal of Gerontology* 35 (Issue 2, March 1980): 249–255.

Sussman, Marvin, *Incentives and Family Environments for the Elderly*, Final Report to Administration on Aging, AoA Grant No. 90–A–316, February 1977.

Sussman, Marvin, *Social and Economic Supports and Family Environments for the Elderly*, Final Report to the Administration on Aging, AoA Grant No. 90–A–316(03), January 1979.

Sussman, Marvin, "The Family Life of Old People," in *Handbook of Aging and the Social Sciences*, edited by Robert Binstock and Ethel Shanas, New York: Van Nostrand, 1976.

Tobin, Sheldon and Regina Kulys, "The Family and Services," in Carl Eisdorfer, ed., *Annual Review of Gerontology and Geriatrics* (New York: Springer Publishing Company, 1980: 370–399.

Torres-Gil, Fernando and Mona Negm, "Policy Issues Concerning the Hispanic Elderly," *Aging* Nos. 305–306 (March-April 1980): 2–5.

Townsend, P., "The Effects of Family Structure on the Likelihood of Admission to an Institution in Old Age: The Application of a General Theory" in E. Shanas and G. Streib, *Social Structure and the Family*, Englewood Cliffs, N.J.: Prentice Hall, 1965.

Townsend, P., "Welfare Services and the Family" in Shanas, E. *et al, Older People in Three Industrial Societies*, New York: Atherton Press, 1968.

Treas, Judith, "Family Support Systems for the Aged: Some Social and Demographic Considerations," *The Gerontologist* 17 (Issue 6, December 1977): 486–491.

Troll, Lillian, "The Family of Later Life: A Decade Review," *Journal of Marriage and the Family* 33 (Issue 2, May 1971): 263–290.

U.S. Department of Health and Human Services, Health Care Financing Administration, "Long-Term Care: Background and Future Directions," Discussion Paper HCFA 81–20047, January 1981.

U.S. House of Representatives, "Future Directions for Aging Policy: A Human Service Model," report by the Subcommittee on Aging, 96th Congress, 2nd Session, May 1980.

Weissert, W., T. Wan, and B. Livieratos, Effects and Costs of Day Care and Homemaker Services for the Chronically Ill: A Randomized Experiment, Executive Summary, Hyattsville, Md.: National Center for Health Services Research, DHEW, January 1979.

York, Jonathan and Robert Calsyn, "Family Involvement in Nursing Homes," *The Gerontologist* 17 (Issue 6, December 1977): 500-505.

Zarit, Steven, Karen Reever, and Julie Bach-Peterson, "Relatives of the Imparied Elderly: Correlates of Feelings of Burden," *The Gerontologist* 20 (Issue 6, December 1980): 649–655.

Chapter IX

Home Care

by Hans C. Palmer

Introduction

Home care is one of the most frequently advocated forms of alternative provision of long-term care (LTC). To many, home is the "natural" place for care; to others, home is obviously a cost-effective site for LTC, which is considered to consist mainly of hotel services. In this chapter, we define home care (HC), suggest some classifications for HC, place it in the spectrum of alternatives discussed in the alternatives chapter, and assess some of the analytical literature on home care. Among the analytical issues to be considered are cost-effectiveness of HC versus the nursing home, the choice of proper assessment indicators, appropriate and equitable service allocation, the role of the family, and an alternative payment mechanism to evoke more voluntary assistance with HC. We will discuss a number of recent HC studies and evaluations in relation to these issues. The chapter concludes with presentation of a new model of client placement and suitability for HC developed by Thomas Willemain.

Actually, as is true of other modes in the LTC spectrum, the terms "home care" and "home health care" refer to a number of combinations of services, although the home (the client's or the family's) is usually the site of care. For this analysis, the term home care (HC) will be used, and "health" and other modifiers will be introduced where needed. Within the home care structure, current opinion recognizes as strong a psychological and social focus as a medical one, although the intensity of medical services may be heavy. Another expected characteristic is the significant involvement of available family and friends of the client.

In one sense, home care may be viewed as pre-institutional (reducing length of stay by preparing the patient for hospitalization) or post-institutional, as in the famous "after care" programs of some New York and Boston hospitals designed to reduce the cost of acute care episodes. It may also be designed to substitute continuously for either hospital or nursing home care. Home care may form part of a spectrum of care for a particular patient, complementing adult day care and other service programs. In a broader planning sense, HC can be part of a large pattern of offerings whose utilization

I wish to thank Judith Feder, John Holahan, Alan Sager, and William Scanlon for helpful comments on this chapter.

depends on eligibility, medical, functional, and psychological criteria, and other indicators of appropriateness.

One helpful way of studying HC, given its heterogeneity, is through the three-or four-part classification scheme suggested by Callender, LaVor, and a number of health care groups. Specifically, they have identified *intense* HC as a largely medical provision featuring extensive use of physicians, RNs and LPNs in a home setting into which some high technology apparatus may have been introduced. The essential purpose of intense level care is to shorten hospital stays (Callender and LaVor, 1975). At the other end of the spectrum are two care sets, *maintenance* and *personal*. (These are combined in a *basic* category by Callender and LaVor.) At this level, the purpose is to maintain people adequately in their homes ". . . at effective levels of health and function over long periods of time or permanently without recourse to more concentrated care or to institutionalization" (Calender and LaVor, 1975). *Intermediate* level of care is largely an undefined category, although usually it includes some medical provision and nursing care along with some of the maintenance aspects of basic care. Intermediate care usually has a shorter duration than basic care. Its objectives are often mixed, including the prevention of hospitalization and the prevention and deferral of institutionalization.

Still another way of looking at HC is by length of stay. Some HC is essentially short-stay, augmenting acute hospital care. Other HC is long-stay and is aimed at continuing home maintenance of disabled and/or dependent people. Many hospital-based HC programs are of the former type; much of the concern with HC as an alternative for the dependent elderly (mainly candidates for nursing homes) focuses on the latter.

These classification schemes may permit the more precise analysis of HC as a set of alternatives in terms of access, quality, and cost for each of the various categories identified. They also may permit locating HC more precisely in a total spectrum of care as a substitute or a complement and assessing the effects of regulation and reimbursement on the use and supply of care. This is important, since many of the weaknesses noted in existing HC cost-effectiveness research stem from the lack of precise definitions. These considerations, of course, all parallel those found in the other chapters on alternatives.

Home Care in the United States

Home care, at least that provided from other than household resources, is not so widely used in this country as in Europe, where there are many mixes of home health care, home-provided special therapies, and home chore aid. In January 1981, there were 2,908 Medicare/Medicaid-certified providers covering users. (See Chapter V for details on HC utilization, eligibility, etc.) Official data indicate that in 1979 about $1.1 billion was spent on HC through Federally supported programs (Medicare, Medicaid, Title XX, OAA Titles III-B and C). (More recent estimates put the figures much higher, however.) Currently there are no hard data on the amount of private HC expenditures. Karen Rak, publisher of Home Health Line, stated (1982) that privately paid HC costs came to about $2.3 billion for 1980.

In the 20th century, both hospital and nursing home development have seemed to make the home an unusual site for care, at least in the minds of many policymakers and much of the public. Actually, the home remains the site of much care, most often being replaced only when high technology interventions, heavy nursing care requirements, or the method of finance have dictated a shift in patterns of (largely acute) care. Also, the desire of physicians to concentrate patients in their offices and/or in hospitals to economize on professional time has led to the abandonment of house calls in most areas and thus reduced the ability of the home to maintain an adequate support system, or so it has been assumed. However, as the need for care (because of demographic changes) and the perception of that need have shifted increasingly toward LTC, with its requirements for continuing personal and functional support, and away from high technology interventions, using the home as a care site has become more attractive. This attractiveness is, of course, enhanced by the increasing cost of institutional LTC, especially that provided in the nursing home.

HC in the United States may well have been a part of the outreach of many charitable institutions and of some hospitals for some time. In a more formal sense, however, provision and financing for HC emerged in the early part of the 20th century, notably in the program of the Metropolitan Life Insurance Company, which was seeking to improve conditions for the acutely ill and for newborn babies and their mothers. The goal of Metropolitan's programs was to improve the company's claims experience by reducing mortality, preventing disease, cutting hospital stays, and, in general, promoting good health (Rawlinson, 1974). The Metropolitan system, initiated in 1909, continued for 44 years, was affiliated with 850 visiting nurse associations, employed 700 nurses at a time in over 400 sites, and existed in 7,500 towns in the United States and Canada. Total visits during the life of the program amounted to 107,500,000, provided to 20,150,000 policy-holders at a cost of $115,700,000. In some circumstances, Metropolitan helped support local providers; in others, its own staff had to be used because of low standards and/or unavailable providers. The Metropolitan experience is useful for present circumstances because it encountered many of the same problems of distribution and provision adequacy presumably plaguing the current HC

339

situation. The peak utilization year was 1931, when 770,000 policy-holders were given care at home. By 1950, the number had fallen to 330,000. Service was discontinued at the end of 1952 (Rawlinson, 1974).

Paralleling the development of the Metropolitan system was the increased importance of the visiting nurse associations (VNAs) and the corps of public health nurses. These organizations were initially strongest in New England, offering help to the "sick poor." VNAs tended to expand in the east with a medical, adult care focus, while in the west, the emphasis was on the public health nurses and the care of children and mothers. HC entered its modern phase during World War II, when the physician shortage and an increased aware-ness of European experiences stimulated the expansion of home services administered by nurses. These factors were reinforced by the experiments with organized pre- and post-hospital care at home at such places as Montefiore Hospital in New York. HC, like adult day care, clearly originated in the community through local govern-ment and private sector initiatives (Callender and La Vor, 1975).

The Federal Government and Home Care

Federal involvement (aside from that of the Veterans Administra-tion) with HC really began with the Kerr-Mills legislation, under which medical provision for the elderly was linked to Old Age Assistance. This law allowed payment for home health aides who, in addition to providing nursing service, were permitted to perform light housekeeping in the patients' rooms and/or near the sickbed. In effect, this law divided health care from housekeeping, which may have clarified matters for reimbursement purposes but which also introduced a false distinction into a pattern of continuous provision (Trager, 1972; Ricker-Smith and Trager, 1976).

Medicare and Medicaid, in the minds of HC advocates, appeared not only to bring a new era in finance of health care for the elderly and indigent but also to open the door to the implementation of alternative strategies, especially HC. Actual regulations and the laws themselves soon moderated these expectations. In the first place, Medicare definitions of HC, as noted earlier, proved to be very "medical" in their orientation. Reimbursable in-house services under Part A were almost exclusively skilled nursing or medical, provided subject to a care plan devised by a physician and supervised by an RN, LPN, or licensed vocational nurse (LVN). Under Part B, no prior hospitalization was required, but the patients had to be housebound and needing care as prescribed by a physician.

Under Medicaid, it would appear that HC of many types could be provided; yet the program is means-tested and subject to the eligibility definitions and budget limits of the States. Furthermore,

340

intermediaries handling Medicaid reimbursement tend to apply Medicare standards, thus reducing the range of available options. (Oklahoma's personal service options and New York's home care programs are notable exceptions.) Both Title XX of the Social Security Act and Title III of the Older Americans Act may appear to expand HC coverage, but in both instances the limits on program expenditure by the States have limited the application of broad-spectrum programs.

In 1967, new regulations narrowed the Medicare reimbursement definitions even more. Not only did patients have to be housebound and medically dependent, but they also had to be unable to use their lower extremities. Home health aides were virtually restricted to bedside care. The 1969 regulations restricted reimbursable services even more tightly: the actual "laying on of hands" in a nursing sense was needed. Not surprisingly, estimated HC benefit payments (according to HCFA actuaries' calculations) under Medicare showed a pattern of increase from fiscal year 1967 ($21 million) to 1970 ($89 million), followed by a decline to 1972 ($70 million). In fiscal year 1978, they stood at $521 million (HCFA unpublished data, 1981). Under Medicaid, HC payments amounted to $70 million in fiscal year 1975 and $210 million in fiscal year 1978 (DHEW, 1975; HCFA, unpublished data, 1981).[1]

The Analytics of Home Care

As indicated earlier, home care has been the subject of extensive research and publication, some of which we will review. Much of this research has been motivated by the desire to demonstrate the superior cost-effectiveness of HC, as well as its putative benefits to the quality of life of clients and/or their families. Unfortunately, much of the HC research suffers from weaknesses common to most analyses of alternatives (discussed in Chapter VII): poor problem specification, lack of models linking services to outcomes, inability to ensure the comparability of client groups, failure to consider secondary, tertiary, and family costs, etc. It should be acknowledged, however, that much of this literature, while plagued with analytical difficulties, offers valuable data about the nature of clients served, services provided, and costs of programs. Also, descriptive studies are helpful in spotting organizational and program weaknesses.

Cost-Effectiveness Questions in HC

As indicated, much of the analysis of home care has been stimulated in part by the belief that HC is more cost-effective than institutional care. Additionally, many of the partisans of HC and of alterna-

---

[1] Considerable data on HC are available from Karen Rak's *Home Health Line's Decade Report, 1980* (Washington, D.C.: 1980). This publication also contains an extensive legislative history and analysis.

tives generally have felt the need to prove their case as they sought resources for the programs they believed were superior to institutionalization. Cost-benefit and cost-effectiveness analyses have, however, been difficult to undertake. While much of the following discussion might apply to studies of other non-institutional LTC modes, many of the criticisms surveyed relate to HC evaluations; thus it is appropriate to include them here.

Judith LaVor, in an afterword to the previously cited Callender-LaVor study of HC, has succinctly stated two of the key practical and methodological problems hampering useful analysis of cost-effectiveness. First, she noted that data are often not comparable among programs or their components; second, she pointed out that HC and institutional data are often not presented in comparable terms. For example, hospital and other institutional data are expressed in *per diem* terms, while HC data appear in per visit or per service unit terms and may reflect only health or health-related items, not personal care or housekeeping.

Despite these limits, however, LaVor asserted that HC is an economically and socially cost-effective system compared with institutionalization, although she admitted that there was no detailed empirical evidence for that proposition. In the first place, she noted that, in 1975, Medicare/Medicaid expenditures for HC were minuscule compared with costs of institutionalization. A doubling of HC funds, even in 1981, would constitute a minor addition to overall public LTC spending. Furthermore, citing the Social Security Administration's actuary, she suggested that expanded HC would be offset by reductions in hospital and skilled nursing facility (SNF) costs. Crucial here is the presumed inverse relationship between HC and institutional use. Lack of a system of community care, however, deprives us of the possibility to test these data. Note also that the possible filling of nursing home beds vacated by HC clients is not considered by LaVor in her statement about reduced SNF and acute hospital care costs.

LaVor quite rightly recognized that a critical determinant of HC cost-effectiveness is the type of care: intensive, intermediate, and/or basic. In general, she believed that intensive HC is cost-effective compared with hospital care. Intermediate HC (provided as a substitute for SNF or ICF care) may involve episodes of skilled care of shorter duration than in the intensive situation. Because of this periodic skilled service requirement, intermediate HC may not be as cost-effective *vis-a-vis* nursing home care as is intensive HC compared with acute hospital care. On the other hand, intermediate level HC is not required daily, whereas nursing home services are; therefore, the comparison may be more attractive over the course of a year.

342

LaVor acknowledged that basic level HC generates major problems in analyzing cost-effectiveness. This level aims at maintaining ability to perform activities of daily living (ADL) or slowing its deterioration and involves custodial services as well as a modicum of medical provision. Because of the uncertainty of the care mix, cost-effectiveness comparisons may have to be made on a case-by-case basis. Such analyses could reveal that basic care is not cost-effective, but it may be highly desirable from the perspectives of patient/family contentment and quality of life.

Overall, LaVor argued that expanded systems of HC provision may initially increase outlays from the public purse. Present residents of institutions are not likely to be removed in large numbers. Rather, the gains may accrue from keeping many present and future vulnerable people out of institutions by offering them the opportunity to remain in their homes.

John Craig presented a highly useful summary in the Callender-LaVor report of some of the key methodological problems raised by cost analyses in home health care and in the studies assessing HC costs. His review provides some perspective on the LaVor arguments and on the general assertion that HC not only enhances the quality of life but also is cost-effective compared with institutionalization. In his review of various HC cost studies, he noted that in-depth studies were rare as of 1975, that raw program data were not available at that time, and that many studies were not primarily aimed at comparing cost-effectiveness. (The studies Craig reviewed are shown in Figure IX-1, taken from the Callender-LaVor report.)

Craig grouped the studies into three broad categories: (1) reports on specific hospital-based agencies, community home health agencies, or home health departments of major insurance companies (these studies appear to provide most of the bases for assertions about the cost-effectiveness of HC); (2) descriptions of particular HC or alternative services demonstration projects which had not (in 1975) generated much cost data (see Chapter VI, which summarizes many of these demonstrations); and (3) in-depth analyses of data from particular home health agencies or groups of agencies, potential sources of many fruitful conclusions about HC and HC costs. Unfortunately, the latter studies, especially the methodologically good ones, were (are) scarce.

As Craig recognized, evaluations of HC cost studies are hampered by three major obstacles. In the first place, home health and home care programs differ widely in their objectives. Some are designed to substitute for acute hospital care, others are designed as SNF or intermediate care facility (ICF) substitutes, and yet others are aimed at improving the condition of frail elderly at home. Obviously, costs of one type of project can not be compared with other types of

FIGURE IX-1

PROGRAM/PROJECT	Date of Program	Hospital Based	Community Based HHA	Acute Care Orientation	Chronic Care Orientation	HMO Bases	Summary of Reports Available	Cost Information Supplied	Cost-Effectiveness Statements Made	Cost Anaylsis Attempted	Demonstration Project	In Planning Stages Only	Patient Characteristics Given	*Cases (C) Patients (P)	
Blue Cross of Greater Philadelphia	1962-70	X					X	X	X				X	2,495,267c	
Associated Hospital Services of New York	1960-	X		X			X	X	X				X	5,000C	
Rochester Home Care Association	1970		X	X			X	X				X	X	1,554C	
New Jersey Homemaker - Home Health Aide Service	1970		X	X								X	X	9,380P	
San Franciscan Home Health Services	1957-66	X	X										X	3,024P	
Benjamin Rose Hospital (Cleveland) Home Care Project	1966-67				X			X					X	100C	
Kaiser Permanente Experience	1966-68*			X	X		X	X	X	X			X	420C	
Saint Luke's Hospital (Denver) Home Nursing Care Project	1969	X		X	X		X	X		X			X	100P	
Nassau County (New York) Department of Health Home Care Project					X										
Alternate Care Arrangements Project-Caledonia Home Health Care Agency	1969-70	X			X		X	X			X		X	17P	Cost data expected
Community Care Organizations, Wisconsin			X		X		X	X			X	X	X		
Home Care Corporation, Massachusetts			X	X							X	X	X		
Home Care Pilot Project - Coordinating Vendor Agencies - NYC	1973-74		X				X				X		X	200C	
Lincoln-Lancaster County Areawide Model Project on Aging - Nebraska	1972		X								X	X	X	200P	*Cost data expected
Minneapolis Age and Opportunity Center	1970	X		X			X				X		X		*Cost data perhaps could be generated
Personal Care Program, Community Life Assn. of Greater Hartford	1974		X		X		X				X		X	300P	
Project Independence, Maine	196		X		X		X				X	X	X	10,000P	
Triage - Connecticut Department of Aging	1974		X		X		X	X			X	X	X	1,000P	*Cost data expected
Michigan Blue Cross Coordinated Home Care Program	1963-70	X		X	X		X						X	10,000C	
Health and Hospitals Corporation's Home Care Programs, NYC	1970-71	X	X	X	X		X	X					X	2,242P	
New York SMA Home Health Services Study	1969	X	X	X	X						X	X		275P	
Minnesota - Minneapolis Home Health Service	1972-73		X	X								X		47C	
St. Luke's Hospital Home Care, Stroke Patients, NYC	1971	X			X						X		X	50P	

Source: Taken from Craig, John. "Cost Issues in Home Health Care." Part IV, Marie Callender and Judith LaVor. "Home Health Care: Development, Problems, and Potential." U.S. DHEW ASPE. April 1975 (Mimeo), p. 49

344

programs. Yet, as noted, much of the claimed cost advantage for HC derives from studies of acute care substitutes. Valid cost-effectiveness analyses must therefore define program objectives and carefully define the range of the comparison.

A second difficulty arises because most studies fail to acknowledge key health, demographic, social, and economic attributes of the populations from which project clients might be drawn. Again, studies of affluent, family-supported, dependent elderly may have little relevance to the poor and the isolated. Also, studies of urban HC programs may have little relevance to rural areas.

Third, administrative arrangements differed widely among the projects studied. Obviously, such differences affect project effectiveness and program costs. Unless some means of controlling for such administrative variation can be found, comparisons among programs and between HC and institutional costs will be almost meaningless. This realization has evoked suggestions for research on programs with similar administrative structures, such as channeling agency demonstrations.

In Craig's methodological discussion, he (like LaVor) first singled out data problems in HC cost analyses, for example, the need to define a common costing unit for HC service and for institutional provision and the need to include all elements of HC costs, including food, housing, transportation, and administration.

Craig also found fault with the actual comparison of costs in many studies. He noted that in many cases, a health professional (physician, nurse, etc.) will review a set of files chosen at random (with no control for differing population characteristics, etc.) to determine number of hospital or institutional days saved, the costs of those days, the costs of HC provided, and the difference between the last two magnitudes. This procedure is flawed by the subjectivity of the analyst and the widely fluctuating estimates of HC and hospital need. Such divergences of opinion could lead to widely different estimates of cost savings. For example, in a study of Philadelphia area HC programs, a downward shift of 30 percent in the number of estimated hospital days saved could have reduced estimated cost savings by over $1 million (from $1.3 million to $261,000).

At a macro level, Craig noted that most cost comparisons assume that HC is a substitute for institutional care. At a program-specific level, especially in connection with small, hospital-based HC programs providing after-care, this assumption may be warranted. However, if broad-based, large-scale programs featuring broad entitlements were introduced, newly defined clients and newly provided services may well add significantly to the total LTC cost burden. This problem of complementarity versus substitutability has already been noted in the chapter on alternatives and in the discussion of the research of Weissert and others.

345

Having praised the Minnesota studies of Jay Greenberg (discussed subsequently), Craig then discussed means of obtaining data for making judgments about cost-effectiveness and the desirability of initiating HC programs. He found that large scale simulation methods are weak because of the relative insignificance of HC provision in the total health service structure, because of inconsistencies and weaknesses in available cost data, and because of the paucity of analytical tools powerful enough to control for variations in program objectives, program benefits, and program administration. Alternatively, one might experiment by enlarging the HC system (by expanding Medicare/Medicaid financing) essentially to "see what happens." This approach, while appearing truly experimental, faces high administrative start up costs (thus leading to charges of waste) and the need to promise to continue support of the service. Failure to make good on such promises would be hard on dependent clients and problematical for politicians who would probably rather not initiate expanded programs anyway. On the other hand, large scale expansions may be necessary to generate enough data on changes in utilization patterns, complete costing of services, etc. Complexities at the macro level may, in short, demand expansions of benefits if macro consequences are to be understood.

On balance, Craig appeared to favor carefully designed experiments which avoid the perils of simulation and the potentially huge increases in costs associated with program expansions. His guidelines for these experiments follow those of Conly (discussed in Chapter VII): a large enough number of settings, adequate controls for demographic and economic population characteristics, accurate and standard costing procedures, standardization of program benefit definitions, and clarity of specification for program objectives and outcomes. Experimentation has risks—an adequate number of experiments may prove as costly as major HC program expansions, macro issues may still be uncertain, and good experimentation may take more time than the political process will allow. In any event, arguments by Craig and others undoubtedly contributed to the expansions of experiments and demonstrations discussed in Chapter VI.

In a 1979 analysis of patient, family, and professional views of alternatives to institutionalization, Sager also discussed the weaknesses of much HC and other alternatives cost research. His review (part of a large study of HC, discussed shortly) provides a useful summation of the many methodological and data problems running through the research on alternatives. He identifies four commonly employed methods of comparing costs: (1) comparing costs of new HC services with those of the institutional days believed to have been saved; (2) costing the HC services which would be needed to maintain otherwise "inappropriately institutionalized" dependent people at home; (3) costing the HC and institutional care of groups

346

of patients who are retrospectively matched on a number of personal, medical, functional, and psychosocial characteristics; and (4) conducting a truly prospective random clinical trial (RCT).

Each of these methods has major problems. The first, comparing costs of new HC services with those of existing institutional services, suffers from lack of evidence about reductions in nursing home costs stemming from the introduction of new HC. Beds emptied may be quickly filled, and it is not clear whether the new HC thus represents added LTC services and/or whether the new nursing home occupants really needed to be institutionalized. Additionally, this type of study does not adequately consider questions of the actual amounts of services needed by patients, the long-term versus short-term need for HC service, the relative disability of continuing and deinstitutionalized nursing home patients, the actual need for all HC services provided, and the complete sets of relevant patient/client characteristics.

The second study method suffers mainly from a lack of definition as to what constitutes "inappropriate" institutionalization. The third, matching, suffers from an inability to define all relevant characteristics to be matched and from an inability to make comparisons across broad groups of highly dissimilar people. The RCT method, while attractive from a control perspective and useful in testing certain drugs and surgical procedures, suffers from both the need for very large sample sizes, especially when outcomes are expectedly small and/or occur over a long time, and from certain ethical hazard problems. In LTC, particularly, it may be hard to identify accepted treatments for the problems at hand, to identify true alternatives for whatever treatments or regimes are in vogue, and to accumulate evidence for the superiority of alternatives. In short, the requirements for an RCT usually cannot be met in long-term care because of the essential system nature of the LTC requirement and the inability to specify outcomes. Perhaps most troubling for the RCT method as applied to long-term care is the need to secure informed consent from the subjects of the experiment. Since it is difficult to offer clear statements of the risks and benefits of alternative modes in LTC, and since many of the potential subjects are not fully capable of providing informed consent, the RCT method presently holds little promise.

Because of the limits noted by Sager in the four methods, another approach is suggested. Essentially, this new method involves directly costing institutional services for a specified group of nursing home patients, all of whom would actually become institutionalized. Before entering the homes, however, these people would be completely assessed physically, medically, functionally, and psychologically. On the basis of these assessments, a group of health/social services professionals would design home care plans for these

347

clients. The costs of the "typical" plans could then be compared with those of institutional care. This method, Sager claims, allows use of the patient/client sample as its own control and, furthermore, by using many professionals' judgments, eliminates many of the problems of defining "inappropriateness" of institutionalization and appropriateness of various HC service packages. Also, by seeking consistency among care plans and assessments, Sager claims that both horizontal (same assessments imply same care) and vertical (more disabled get more care) equity can be achieved. (We will consider the results of the Sager analysis in the various sections on costing and other HC analytical problems.)

Hospital-Linked Studies

Among the more successful of the traditional studies of HC have been those of the hospital-based, (usually) short-term services, such as those provided by Montefiore Hospital in New York City, the Chelsea-St. Vincent's Hospital program in New York, and the Massachusetts General Hospital in Boston. These studies dealt for the most part with patients whose suitability for hospital care was not a matter of doubt, so comparability was never much of an issue. Furthermore, the therapeutic links between intervention and outcomes were often clearly clinically established.

Some cost savings claims were impressive. Findings at Montefiore through 1974 indicated significant cost reductions in connection with acute episodes. For example, they showed home care costs of $10 per day (excluding the value of caregivers' time) versus $175 per day for a hospital stay. The $175 figure reflected average daily hospital charges, not necessarily marginal costs, so the comparison is not quite symmetrical.

Chelsea-St. Vincent's claimed total savings of $150,000 per year for HC for community-based patients with HC compared to episodic hospital bed utilization and $340,000 for HC yearly over nursing home placement for 70 patients.

The Boston program, aimed at post-hospital episodes for chronically ill patients, sought to save money and increase life satisfaction by substituting home care for SNF and/or hospital care. The program was initially motivated by the long waiting lists for SNF beds for patients no longer needing acute care and by the resultant queues for acute care beds because patients could not be moved out of the hospital. Another powerful stimulus was the Massachusetts Medicaid ruling that denied reimbursement for administratively necessary days, that is, acute bed occupancy forced upon the patient (and the hospital) by the lack of SNF space. An average cost savings of almost $31 per day or $900 per month per patient was claimed. Over three years, $34,000 per patient was saved (Rossman, 1974; Brickner et al, 1975; Tolkoff-Rubin et al, 1976).

348

The impressiveness of these cost savings must, however, be modified by two considerations. First, some studies showed that hospital-based after-care programs were even more cost-effective than home care, largely because of reduced transportation costs, concentration of specialists' efforts, and economies of scale available at a single care site. Second, in many cases where hospital beds were freed by SNF-eligible patients receiving HC, the actual spending on acute care rose as new patients occupied those beds.

Gerson and Hughes (1976), using Canadian hospital and short stay HC data, have shown that even the more complete and successful comparative studies of HC versus hospital care have really not dealt with all the relevant categories of service or cost. They argue that most studies do not compare costs for equivalent levels of care or for patients with comparable conditions. They also make the previously mentioned point that the relevant comparisons are those between costs per care episode rather than costs per day, the latter a favored calculation because of the ready availability of data gathered according to hospital accounting conventions. Acknowledging the difficulty of establishing complete comparability among patients, they nonetheless claim that their method of calculating and comparing costs shows few savings for HC over hospital care unless additional beds would have to be constructed for those patients otherwise cared for at home. It should be noted that Gerson and Hughes' costs included physician and surgeon fees, in-hospital laundry, housekeeping, and food expenses, homemaker costs, physical therapy costs, home nursing costs, and transportation costs. Secondary, tertiary, and family costs were not calculated, however; hence the total social cost comparison could not be made (Gerson and Hughes, 1976). Nonetheless, their article shows that even the comparisons for direct costs of services cannot be based on time alone, but must incorporate patient condition, quality of care, and length of stay. The amount of attention these authors paid to the problems of patient comparability in two care modes also is notable.

Cost Analysis in the Sager Study

Sager (1979) directly compared actual nursing home and hypothetical HC costs for the 50 patients in the Massachusetts sample. Note that this comparison was explicitly between two types of long-term care. The former costs were determined straightforwardly on the basis of actual expenditures, while the latter were established based on the prescriptions of the 18 different professionals who assessed and prescribed for the patients in the sample. In the analysis of nursing home costs as correlated with patient characteristics, Sager noted that many of the conventionally assumed variables (marital status, number of medical diagnoses, measure of functional ability, etc.) exerted measurable but statistically insignificant influences on nursing home costs. Only anticipated discharge site, determined by hospital discharge planners as SNF or ICF level, was positively and significantly linked to costs. Similarly, a multiple regression analysis of the effects of patient characteristics on costs again showed that discharge site was the most important influence on costs, although being married (negative), number of disabling conditions (positive), and number of medical conditions (positive) were of some influence. Together these factors explained about 57 percent of the variation in nursing home costs.

Since the HC packages were prescribed by professionals based on client characteristics, it is not surprising that such attributes were directly related to costs. What is surprising is that nursing home costs were so much less related to characteristics. Evidently, institutional costs reflect location and age of nursing home rather than patient condition, at least in the Sager study. In the analyses of nursing home costs summarized in Chapter XIX, the impacts of patient condition and care quality were very difficult to trace, while reimbursement systems, location, and other facility characteristics were often linked to costs.

Aggregate HC costs were calculated in three ways: (1) taking the mean of the hours prescribed by each of the 18 care planners, (2) taking the mean of the median prescription for each patient by each professional, and (3) taking the mean across 50 patients of the 33rd percentile of HC costs for each patient. Taking these various estimates of typical HC costs for paid services, to which was added a Bureau of Labor Statistics estimate for costs of living at home in the Boston area (with family = $50 per week, alone = $76 per week), yielded weekly mean costs of $574 (method 1), $513 (method 2), and $395 (method 3). Sager did not include opportunity cost of family time nor many of the secondary and tertiary cost items discussed in Chapter VII, such as possible extra social worker time, home modifications, etc. The mean number of paid hours of service was 84.3. This high figure, as well as the high figure for mean total number of hours (paid and unpaid) needed, did not imply very high service costs, since so much of the time was unpaid and since much of the paid time was that provided by low-skill, low-wage workers.

Similar correlation analysis of the same 16 patient characteristics examined in connection with nursing home costs showed that five were significantly related to HC costs: number of persons with whom the patient resided before hospitalization (negative), better psychosocial status (negative), better anticipated functional ability score (negative), percentage of nursing services used in hospital (positive), and amount of decline in functional ability (positive). (Functional ability was measured with the Barthel score, as discussed subsequently.) Anticipated discharge site exerted only a small and insignificant influence. Interestingly, the Sager analysis showed a significant divergence among care prescribers in estimated costs of HC. Most agreement, however, was found among prescribers in connection with older patients with marked decline in functional ability, need for many nursing services, and more recent episodes of illness.

A comparison of weekly HC with nursing home costs shows that the latter ($373) were, on average, lower than the former (method 1: $574). Nevertheless, Sager argues that for many institutionalized patients, HC would be cheaper than the nursing home because of their less than average need for HC services or because of their higher than average need for nursing home services. Among the 45 patients for whom complete data could be assembled, between eight and 14 could be cared for more cheaply at home than in an institution. The number depended on which method of costing HC was used. If administratively necessary days (ANDs) were included in nursing home costs (to accommodate patients in hospitals because nursing home beds could not be found), then HC was cheaper for an even larger number. For individual patients, the savings derived from their being diverted to HC ranged from 11 percent to almost 26 percent of LTC costs. System savings, however, cannot be so readily calculated because of changes in numbers and characteristics of patients being served in the two settings. Clearly, freeing nursing home beds through HC placements would be relevant here. Reduced aggregate system LTC costs might only be produced if beds freed by expanded HC services were closed. If they are filled by more dependent patients, and/or if the number of LTC service recipients rises, then system costs very likely would rise.

Sager also points out that if nine patients were diverted to HC because their HC costs were lower than institutional costs (as determined by method 2), $1,889 per week could be saved. If this money were used to subsidize other patients for whom institutional care was only marginally costlier, an additional 15 patients could be served with HC. If the total of LTC funds is fixed, and/or if home placement is considered desirable on other than just costs grounds, this added diversion represents an added plus for HC.

Patients for whom HC was cheaper than institutional care were primarily those living with others, those less likely to be married, those whose families were willing to have them at home, those with higher anticipated functional scores, those taking more medications while in the hospital, and those requiring fewer nursing services in the hospital. Perhaps most significant was that most of these patients for whom HC would have been cheaper were discharged to SNFs or rehabilitation hospitals. What emerges from this catalogue of attributes is two groups for whom HC may be cheaper than nursing home care. One is a modestly disabled group with few care requirements; the other is a heavily impaired group with heavy care demands which can be more cheaply met at home. (See Figure IX-2, taken

FIGURE IX-2

One View of Home and Institutional Care Costs

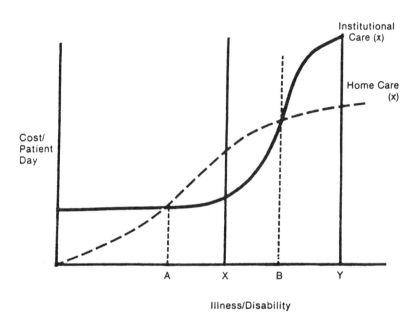

Source: Taken from Sager, Alan, *Learning the Home Care Needs of the Elderly: Patient, Family, and Professional Views Of An Alternative to Institutionalization* (Waltham, Mass.: Brandeis University, Levinson Policy Institute, November 20, 1979), p. 252

from Sager.) This finding runs counter to some conventional wisdom that light care cases are the only ones for whom HC is cheaper. It is, however, buttressed in the Sager analysis by the finding that if we take the difference between HC costs and institutional costs and correlate that difference with various patients' characteristics, we will find that smaller cost differences are related both to higher functional capacity (on the one hand) and to anticipated discharge to a heavy nursing care or rehabilitation facility on the other. In other words, both the more and the less disabled will have HC costs which are lower in relation to nursing home costs than will the moderately disabled. (Interestingly, Skinner and Yett found that the moderately disabled were also more costly among nursing home patients, as did Birnbaum *et al.*) A similar finding and argument appears in the second Minnesota study and in Willemain's analysis, both of which are discussed subsequently. Sager notes that his study is too small to support drastic changes in HC policy and in the diversion of heavy care patients to HC, but the data suggest that further analysis of this type of function-cost relationship should be undertaken to consider some redirection of HC policies.

Other Key Aspects of HC Analysis

Problems other than cost analysis are as relevant to HC as to other types of LTC services. Among these problems and issues are those related to client characteristics and need for service, equity in service provision, family-service agency cooperation, and mobilization of family and volunteer support. Family roles in LTC were discussed extensively in Chapter VIII and will only be touched on here.

Client Characteristics and the Need for Service

Many studies and analyses have assumed that any candidate for LTC was also a candidate for HC or some other care alternative. Recent debates over enlarging HC and other alternatives have, however, forced a sharper focus on suitability for particular forms of LTC provision, particularly as outcome definition and measurement have also become more clearly defined. Recent work by Fortinsky, Granger, and Seltzer (1981) has shown that functional diagnostic instruments are valuable in helping to target HC to candidates for whom it is particularly suitable.

Their analysis begins with the assumption that functional incapacity, rather than medically defined illness, is the key determinant of the need for LTC in general and for HC in particular. (This argument parallels those of Katz and others.) Functional incapacity, alone, however, is not enough to explain HC need; rather the availability of family, certain psychosocial characteristics, and a given level of economic resources must also be considered in establishing suitability. Because of the presumed interaction among physical functioning and other environmental and psychosocial characteristics, Fortinsky and his colleagues analyzed a group of 89 clients receiving "basic care" services from the Visiting Nurse Association of Providence, Rhode Island during February, 1978. The sample was predominantly female (74) and had a mean age of 73 years with 20 of its members 85 and older. Measurement instruments used in the sample included the Barthel Index, which measures a person's ability to function independently in performing activities of daily living. The ESCROW profile, a measure of environment (stability of housing, etc.), social supports (personal contacts versus formal agency supports), clusters of family members, resources (mainly financial), outlook (ability to make decisions), and work or school situation was employed as a measure of social and economic support. Psychosocial characteristics were measured by the Brief Psychiatric Rating Scale (BPRS) which assessed anxiety, depression, somatic concern, emotional withdrawal, disorientation, hostility, uncooperativeness, and conceptual disorganization.

In addition, the researchers compiled a list of essential tasks and identified the performer of the task (patient, family member or friend, VNA home health aide, or nurse from the VNA). Performance of the tasks was coded 4 for patient, 3 for family, 2 for home health aide, and 1 for nurse. The scores for the 72 tasks were then matched against client characteristics as shown by the Barthel, ESCROW, and BPRS values. In this manner, the researchers could observe relationships among hypothesized measures of patient need and level of support required for the patients.

Results of the analysis suggest that most of the clients were not highly functionally dependent, since the mean Barthel score was about 75 (high scores indicate more independence), individual scores ranging from 0 to 100. The mean group ESCROW score of almost 16, however, indicated that the group showed much need for social and economic support. Barthel scores were also used to establish relationships between needs and services provided. In the first place, there was a strong linkage between scores and ability to perform tasks. Notably there was a break at a score of 60: below that level, individuals were able to perform no more than 10 tasks independently. A second analysis focused on the individual tasks and showed that the Barthel score was strongly associated with the capacity to perform most personal care tasks, especially feeding, grooming, dressing, toileting, and transferring—key indicators of personal care need. Additionally, the scores were linked to light housekeeping, cooking, and meal service, that is, those instrumental tasks most closely related to ADL in the home. By contrast with the sharp diagnoses shown by the Barthel scores, the ESCROW scores could not indicate any specific needs for VNA agency services, probably because the ESCROW measure is not sufficiently refined.

The Fortinsky et al analysis was extended to include interactions among the various indicators of need in relation to tasks and to service provision. The techniques employed (mainly correlations between the various indicators of need) suggested that functional impairment as measured by Barthel score was associated with the presence of psychological problems and increased age. In addition, among the ESCROW indicators, the only significant relationships were those between environment and social supports, that is, people who live in poor housing need more social supports. A multivariate analysis, employing stepwise linear regression also showed that Barthel score was significantly related to age, depression/emotional withdrawal, and disorientation/conceptual disorganization.

Overall, Fortinsky et al concluded that the modified Barthel index can serve as a screening or targeting device for potential users of HC services. A care providing agency or a channeling agency could then determine the level of care required and the amount of time to be provided on an individual client basis. In addition, the researchers believe that explicitly linking requirements to functional condition may be valuable in educating physicians who must, under Medicare (and in some States, Medicaid), be responsible for prescribing HC services. Greater education of physicians may be especially important in a time of constrained LTC resources. The linkage of functional and psychosocial problems shown so clearly in this analysis also has important implications in relieving family tensions and providing services appropriate to psychosocial need.

Areas identified as requiring more assessment attention and additional research were the role of family support networks in determining care needs and the evaluation of the effects of particular interventions in changing functional capacities. Again, outcomes in relation to interventions are critical.

Appropriate and Equitable Provision of Services

Although techniques such as those of Fortinsky et al may allow better targeting of services to clients on an individual basis, there may still remain problems of equity and appropriateness in the distribution of services. Two recent studies—the cited Sager study and another by Boyd et al—of the distribution of HC services have assessed the equity and appropriateness of new patterns of professional assignment of services (Sager, 1979; Boyd et al, 1980; Boyd et al, 1981). These studies were stimulated by perceptions of inequities in service provision, that is, people with identical dependencies were not getting the same amounts of service, and people with higher levels of dependency were not necessarily getting larger amounts of service. In addition, the issue of who should determine

355

use and allocation of HC resources has come to the forefront of much LTC discussion. The latter question is of special importance for the Sager study.

Sager's point of departure for his analysis was the recognition that the cost and cost-effectiveness analysis of HC or any other LTC mode depends, in part, on the identity and function of those who allocate services for individual patients. That realization raises the question of who should make the allocation decisions: patients, family, or professionals? There are strong pressures to expand the realm of consumer sovereignty in LTC provision because of the key role of families in LTC and because the technical requirements of LTC services are relatively low. Consequently, Sager argues that if families, patients, and professionals do not significantly disagree on the allocation of services, the locus of decision-making may not be an issue. On the other hand, if there is major disagreement, the appropriate decision-maker(s) will be the one(s) making the most equitable, efficient, and effective choices. Since efficiency and effectiveness are not concrete in LTC, equity will have to be the measure. Overall, if there are no differences, we may as well use the judgment of professionals, since they may have a useful margin of additional knowledge over that held by patients and families. With that perspective, Sager considers the possibility and meaning of disagreements among professionals. He hypothesizes that consistency within the deciding group indicates that equity is being achieved.

Using the Patient Appraisal and Care Evaluation (PACE) instrument, 50 Massachusetts patients about to be released from acute care hospitals to nursing homes were assessed in terms of functional, medical, and emotional well-being. With these data, 18 different health and social service professionals each developed an HC service package for each client. The care packages were designed to ensure that each patient could live at home in a "safe, adequate, and dignified" manner. The professionals were divided into two groups: 15 discharge planners, MDs, and home health agency planners and three others, each directly concerned with the individual patient's hospital care—his/her MD, hospital discharge planner, and floor nurse.

Professional, family, and patient views were then compared. The views of all three groups about the amount of weekly episodes of help required were remarkably similar. Families and professionals both wanted more episodes per week than did patients (130 versus 118), while professionals assigned a higher percentage of paid help, 71 percent, than did either of the other two. Families assigned least paid help, 55 percent; patients wanted 64 percent. With respect to the specific types of services assigned, all three groups roughly agreed on the amounts of each type to be allocated: personal care, housekeeping, nursing, and medical-therapeutic. Major differences emerged in the balances assigned to paid and unpaid care. In personal care, family willingness and ability to provide appeared greater than expected by professionals and patients. In nursing care, families and patients expected more family support than did professionals.

It appears from the Sager analysis that the three groups roughly agreed on the appropriate amount of different types of care which should be provided to the average patient. To determine who might be better able to design HC plans which are valid for individual patients, Sager suggested testing for vertical equity, that is, do care allocators assign more service to the more disabled? He also argued that high levels of consistency among raters would signal a high level of prescription validity.

Using a Barthel scale of functional ability, Sager found that all three groups again similarly linked number of needed episodes of care per week directly to clients' level of disability. Professionals tended to be most linear in their assignments; families, the least. With the aid of multiple regression analysis, Sager also found that professionals consistently used only a small number of characteristics as indicators to assign care to patients in accordance with need. Despite possibilities of disagreement stemming from definitional problems (for example, the meanings of safe, adequate, and dignified), the different interpretations of the PACE data, differences in prognoses, and divergent opinions about providers, professionals displayed remarkable agreement about HC needs.

MDs, discharge planners, and home health agency planners agreed at the aggregate level. Agreement was less impressive about amounts of services needed in the four separate service categories, decreasing even more when specific types of service were considered. The weakest consistency was shown by individual professionals' estimates of individual patients' needs for specific services. Professionals did not agree among themselves about total prescribed hours and amounts of particular types of service. In fact, professionals clustered across roles and training. Another finding was that the more experienced professional, in general, assigned fewer service hours in total than did the less experienced. On the other hand, professionals having more information about specific patients prescribed more help for them than for patients about whom they knew less.

Sager believes it important that professionals were consistent over time with respect to the service needs of specific patients. (The simple correlation between total amounts of service assigned by the same professional to the same patient at two different periods, three to six months apart, was 0.91.) More experienced professionals were more consistent, as were those who prescribed for more dependent patients. Large disagreements among professionals as to amount and types of care to be assigned were accompanied by less con-

357

sistency over time. Further analysis of the data also showed that professionals agreed about which patients needed more or less care, but they may have disagreed about the actual number of hours needed to sustain individuals at home. (This finding parallels those of McCaffree *et al* in connection with professional assessments of nursing home patients.) Overall, professionals tend to be consistent with their own views of patient need over time and across patients.

In view of the agreements and disagreements among professionals, one is still left with the question of whether professionals should enjoy more, less, or the same amount of control over the allocation of HC services to individual patients. Sager argues that his analysis shows no dramatic evidence to support supremacy in the HC allocation decision by any one of the three groups. While professionals may be able to devise vertically equitable care plans with some degree of reliability, family- and patient-devised plans tended to cost less. In light of these trade-offs, Sager suggests some means for balancing influences, for example, allowing families more weight in areas in which professional agreement is less certain, such as allocating household services. This procedure could be developed, for example, by setting an absolute ceiling on the amount of household help to be allowed any patient, with families and patients distributing that total among various services as they see fit.

Another important finding of the Sager study was that fears of uncontrollable increases in spending brought about by irresponsible family and patient use of HC services are not justified, since families and patients desired less expensive plans than did the professionals. This finding suggests that the locus of care planning—whether controlled by patients, families, or professionals—should be selected to enhance patient well-being, since spending is not likely to go out of control. Better understanding of outcomes and of intervention-outcome linkages is crucial.

Despite this argument, Sager believes that because of legislators' and administrators' biases, most care planning decisions will probably have to be left with professionals. Greater participation by families and patients is indicated, however, and means to bring that involvement about should be made a basis for experimentation. Additionally, society must consider the safety and adequacy implications of allowing families and patients to choose lower allocations of publicly-supported HC services to be able to keep dependent elderly people at home.

Another study focusing on the equity issue was recently conducted at the School of Social Work at the University of California, Berkeley (Boyd *et al*, 1980; Boyd *et al*, 1981). This study was motivated by the perceived inequalities among the HC service allocations made by different social workers to seemingly similar clients in counties around the San Francisco Bay Area under California's

358

In-Home Support Services (IHSS) Program. California underwrote a three-year study and demonstration because of perceptions that HC services were inequitably distributed.

Boyd, Pruger, and Clark, researchers on the project, argued that if social workers all adhered to the same standards in making service awards, both vertical and horizontal equity would be ensured. The system chosen to achieve similarity of standards was based on so-called "worker judgment averaging," a technique made possible by the use of interactive computer facilities. Essentially, the technique involved using the computer to gather information both on client characteristics and on the service awards made to clients with particular sets of characteristics. By feeding data to the computer, social workers would reveal their individual explicit and implicit decision rules. These rules would then be grouped to reveal typical rules across the whole body of service allocations, initially in the individual service offices. As more data were gathered, the typical rules would become more faithful to typical decision-making among all social workers within and across the various counties. Individual workers, seeing the rules used by their peers, would strive to bring their own practices into line with modal behaviors, and more consistent (hence more equitable) allocations would be made. Over the first year of the project, consistency in linking awards to needs increased markedly from 60 percent to 79 percent.

Data manipulation would also identify the variables central to the social workers' decisions. On the basis of dependency data shown by five-point ratings in each of 10 functional areas (meal preparation, eating, bathing, etc.) plus two sets of binary ratings (laundry and special functioning), multiple regression analyses indicated the weights assigned to different characteristics by different social workers. Also, the goodness of fit of the model to social worker decisions could be determined by means of the R^2 value, thus indicating how much confidence could be placed in the inferred model as a mirror of allocators' actual decision rules. Unfortunately, the system suffers from multicollinearity (interaction among independent variables) which leads to unstable coefficients or indicators of the influences of particular client characteristics. For this and other reasons, a multiplicative, interactive model was chosen over a linear one.

As developed, the model of social worker award behavior permits continual monitoring of individual worker actions. It also presumably allows for continuing improvement of assessments and sharpening of guidelines, both of which lead to greater consistency among awards and, presumably, to greater equity.

Despite its impressive achievements over the first year, the system and the model revealed some major problems. Social worker use of the system was hampered first by technical barriers, most prominently disbelief in the credibility of the model's technical aspects,

359

the need to provide computer predictions to the social workers before the latter actually made their awards, the initial tendency of the computer to predict only aggregate hours of service, and the lack of continual evaluation of worker performance provided both to workers and to supervisors. Process barriers included workers' tendencies to make up their minds about awards in advance, workers' lack of concern with equity in their decision-making, lags in the entry of data into the system (especially in smaller offices without their own computers), and the dead weight of tradition.

Researchers posed questions about social workers' using the model to justify service awards to protesting clients. However, since the system had not really been used as an information source by most workers at the time the first year's report, the answer seemed negative to the researchers. Another question dealt with the social workers' use of the system to nudge service awards upward. Since each worker's awards would be compared to the standards of the group, the researchers believed this game could not be played for very long. Another possibility was that workers might adjust awards to predictions to avoid adverse performance ratings. Perhaps some 20 percent of workers were doing so, possibly giving rise to much inequity. To the extent that workers came to understand the model and realize that their actions might result in inequities, Boyd and his colleagues believed that the problem would be corrected. In addition, supervisors would have to recognize the legitimacy of workers' diverging from computer predictions in making awards. These requirements could only be met through education, a time-consuming process.

Another major area of concern was that of worker norms, of which two categories influence equity: those rules used by workers in determining awards based on need and the extent to which all workers adhere to the common rules. Distributional equity, it is argued, depends on a common set of rules and adherence to them.

Another category of norms has nothing to do with equity. One of these has to do with worker burdens: 71 percent of all cases were reviewed in the first year, but only 22 percent of the awards were changed, suggesting that workers wished to avoid clashes with supervisors or clients, to avoid finding new or additional providers, and to avoid additional paperwork which changed awards demand. The other non-equity related norm had to do with the need to find providers. In some instances, scarcity of providers stimulated workers to increase awards to make it worthwhile for providers to respond.

Overall, Boyd et al claimed success for the computer assisted project. Over the course of the first year, all field offices raised the goodness of fit of their individual models (as shown by increased R^2s). Causes of this improvement were alleged to be a better model, clearer guidelines, and the greater receptivity of social workers to the system and to the computer.

Performance during the second year of the project reaffirmed the researchers' optimism in the system's ability to enhance equity and efficiency. Among the achievements of the second year were continual increases in goodness of fit between client characteristics and service awards (the R^2s went up in almost every office). In addition, Boyd et al concluded that, because of increased efficiency in data processing and interpretation, the computer itself was a powerful influence in attaining greater equity and efficiency. Furthermore, workers seemed to use the system more routinely, guidelines for assessment and service awards had been improved, and workers were participating more fully in designing new methods. The biggest frustration was the continuing lack of direct participation and involvement by the State's IHSS bureau.

While the Sager and Boyd projects offer some impressive evidence about the process of award decision-making, and while the Sager effort presents some critical patient condition and cost evidence, some methodological issues remain. Most importantly, it is not clear that consistency in making awards necessarily implies vertical and horizontal equity. Equality may be ensured across clients with similar impairments, and the amount of service awarded may be a direct function of level of impairment, but equality may not ensure equity unless an independent argument can be framed to that effect. Moreover, providing more service to more disabled people may not meet their needs unless there is an established relation between the intervention and the purpose of intervening in the first place. Cardinal as well as ordinal differences are important. These considerations again summon up the problems of outcomes and reasonable links between services and outcomes. Efficiency and effectiveness, in short, must be directly involved in the analysis, no matter how difficult that may be, since equity cannot be ensured without them.

HC and the Role of the Family

As shown in Chapter VIII and in many studies, the family is a crucial element in the provision of LTC services, especially HC. These matters are extensively discussed in Chapter VIII, but it is appropriate here to raise the issue of public policy in support of the family's caring role.

Francis Caro, in a paper for the Community Service Society of New York (1980), argues that public support systems could significantly alleviate the burdens borne by families in providing for their elders, and in so doing, could sustain the family in making even further efforts. As it is, family burdens may be exacerbated by tax policies which allow deductions for paid care but none for family care. Similarly, Medicaid and Medicare provision both favor institutionalization over home care which, if provided in modest amounts, might allow a family to maintain a dependent elder at home. So also, inadequate coverage for home care locks many family members into a heavy care environment from which employment stimuli and privacy are removed and in which the caregiver's mental health may suffer.

In a similar vein, Amy Horowitz (1978) notes that family capacity to maintain dependent people at home can be significantly enhanced by HC seed money programs which allow time for new activities, release of emotional pressure, and relief of guilt. Coordination of HC leads to better quality of all care by relieving some pressures on the family caregivers and possibly prolonging the ability of the family to provide care. Certainly the experience of the British with holiday relief beds suggests that prolonging family ability costs relatively little (Griffiths and Cosin, 1976). Even if more formal HC may be needed because of demographic changes which leave fewer younger caregivers at home, the role of the family is crucial enough for us to seek ways to ensure that it can be sustained.

A Voucher System to Ensure Care

Because of rising LTC costs, a potential shortage of HC workers, and dangers of eroding HC quality, Drob et al (1980) have suggested a voucher or marker system under which volunteer care providers could ensure themselves of care in the future. Noting that an expansion of HC financing seems unlikely in the near future and that many able-bodied people may wish to provide some form of HC service, they propose a system in which people of similar backgrounds who know each other and who enjoy elements of mutuality and responsibility can join together to ensure care for themselves.

Essentially, volunteers would, to use the authors' words, be able to "stockpile their good deeds" through accumulating markers representing the amount of care they had contributed for the benefit of another. These saved results of volunteering could be spent at will by the caregivers and/or their families when they need care. To ensure provision of care to those at the end of the line, guarantor agencies would have to ensure that care could be paid for. Such agencies could accumulate guarantee funds and be responsible for the initial organization of the system. Ideally, churches, unions, and other similar "propinquity groups" would be guarantor agencies, since they already have committee structures, some degree of organization centralization, and usually a fair degree of longevity. Volunteer workers presumably would be more humane, especially with members of their own groups, and bureaucratic problems could be minimized. Presumably some coordination would be needed among volunteers, home health agencies, and social service providers.

362

Certain key problems must be recognized despite the many attractive features of the proposal. A major difficulty lies in preventing overuse of the system by those who first get care without previously having been volunteers. This problem is similar to that encountered when social insurance schemes are initially established. A related question is how many markers should initial users be given, and how should they be valued? Other practical questions concern the actual operation of the system: How does the agency protect against continuing overuse? When are markers earned? Would markers be initiated by the guarantor agency? What should the size of the guarantee fund be? Should there be a limit to the number of markers issued? What types of services are covered? Can markers be inherited?

Although this proposal is only tentative and may be impractical, the central idea opens up the possibility of using volunteers at the same time that constraints on the availability of HC resources are clearly in evidence.

Comprehensive Analytical Studies of Home Care

In addition to the Sager study, a number of comprehensive research efforts have analyzed various programs of HC from differing viewpoints. These studies offer a number of perspectives on patient conditions, effects of interventions, and comparative costs of HC and nursing home care. They also demonstrate methodological strengths and weaknesses of the types discussed in this chapter.

Veterans Administration Programs

The only programs of Federally-provided HC are those of the Veterans Administration. Known as hospital based home care (HBHC) programs, these were initially funded in fiscal year 1972 under legislation which expanded the definition of VA outpatient care to allow the VA Administrator to provide such home health services appropriate to the "effective and economical treatment" of veterans' disabilities (Veterans Administration, 1980). HBHC programs are similar to those of the British National Health Service, since they involve direct provisions of home services rather than payment for those services. Provision includes nursing care, physical, occupational, and speech therapy, medical-social services, dietetic consultation, home health aide services, drugs, medical appliances, and home adaptation. The range of provision is very wide.

In early 1980, there were 30 HBHC teams, each with an average of 9.25 personnel. Each team was expected to provide 350 visits per month.

A recent assessment of these VA programs, pursuant to a mandate from Senator William Proxmire, examined their effectiveness in terms of cost and outcomes. The study period was October 1 through

December 31, 1979. The time span of the study was too short to effectively analyze cost-effectiveness. The VA report thus described the program and focused on costs (Veterans Administration, 1980).

Despite its inability to assess program effectiveness, the VA set forth the bases for such an assessment. It identified five general outcomes:

- discharge when program goals have been achieved
- discharge to a less intensive level of care, usually to outpatient care, when maximum improvement in HBHC has been achieved
- discharge through death in the home
- long-term maintenance of current health status
- deterioration with the need for more intensive care, usually in a hospital or nursing home.

Recognizing that cost-effectiveness cannot be identified by comparing average daily cost of care in the home with average daily cost of care in an institution (because of the need to quantify family and patient contributions to HC), the VA nonetheless listed five major issues in any cost-effectiveness exercise:

- determination of the need for HBHC
- program descriptions including types of patients, services provided, and the costs of providing professional care
- measurement of outcomes of care relative to HBHC services provided
- comparison of patient care outcomes among different HBHC programs
- comparison of patient care outcomes between HBHC and alternative treatment settings.

Although the agency recognized the difficulties of undertaking cost-effectiveness studies, it clearly understood the implications of the type of analysis which would be required to perform a comprehensive examination of its program.

In examining the 10 sites (out of 30) in its sample, the VA focused on patient morbidity characteristics, patient disability levels, services provided, and specific problems encountered by care providers and family members. As of October 1, 1979, the 10 sites served 516 patients. An additional 260 were added to the program over the study period, while 289 were discharged. It should be noted at the outset that the VA population crucially differed from most LTC groups in the country, in that, of the patients receiving HBHC during the study period, 98 percent were male. The average age was also only 68 years. The group was thus more male and younger than most LTC recipients nationwide.

Most HC recipients were relatively poor (average monthly income only $700 per month), lived with others, and had been referred by a

364

local VA facility (79 percent). The typical client had an average of five conditions. The most common conditions were heart disease, cancer, and stroke. The levels of disability were about evenly divided among severe, moderately severe, and moderate (about 27–32 percent each). Mild levels of disability only accounted for about 10 percent of all patients.

The average number of medications per patient was 7.5; the average number of prosthetics and durable equipment was 3 per patient. The 10 study sites made 10,500 visits in the three-month study period, for an average of four visits per patient per month. Most visits (36 percent) were made by registered nurses.

The most common problem encountered by the professional providers was coping with stress of the family caregiver. Often the caregiver was old and in poor health. In general, the problems confronted reflected the difficulties tied to chronic, debilitating conditions. This finding parallels much anecdotal evidence about limits on HC created by the problems of the aging family as it seeks to cope with debilitated elderly at home.

Although the VA, in this study, did not directly compare cost-effectiveness between HBHC and nursing homes (or other LTC institutions), it did attempt to directly derive costs for the services provided. However, no imputation was made for family costs. Costs were divided into direct (provider time, services and procedures, medications, etc.), indirect (VA Medical Center overhead cost percentage imputed to costs of the HBHC program), and total costs, or the sum of direct and indirect costs. Direct costs were calculated on a per unit basis, that is, per patient or per visit, by determining the amount of services and time used per unit. Indirect costs were applied on a formulaic basis. When all costs had been added, they showed that cancer was the most expensive (per day and per visit) condition to treat in the HBHC program, although on a cost-per-visit basis, diabetes and organic heart disease were close behind ($69 versus $68 per visit). Costs per patient day for the program ranged from $13 to $17. As expected, average costs rose directly with disability levels, although mildly disabled patients were more costly than moderately/severely disabled on the basis of average cost per visit.

One of the more interesting aspects of the VA study was its review of other research, some of which is considered elsewhere in this chapter. Overall, the VA concluded that most of these other studies were not satisfactory from the standpoint of comparing costs among care modalities while controlling for patient disabilities. The studies also seemed to show that the costs of caring for patients increase as disability increases. If disability is great enough, home care may be more costly than institutional care. Even so, these studies did not provide for suitable control groups; they did not appropriately

365

allocate HC and institutional costs (especially with respect to indirect costs); they did not provide a comparision based on common units of measure (for example, HC costs usually are expressed in costs per case, hospital costs in average daily cost per patient.)

The VA study provides a beginning for a longitudinal study of one of the few comprehensive direct provision HC systems in the United States. Its cost figures can be compared with those of other HC schemes, and its attempt to control for both diagnosis and disability levels offers some useful bases for comparison with services to patients in other care modes. The VA effort, however, needs to be generalized by including some imputations for family and community costs. Also, because most VA clients are male, the results are not as generally applicable. Nevertheless, they may be significant as more of the LTC population becomes male, at least in absolute numbers. It is to be hoped that changes in patient condition will be monitored as the VA study continues.

Weissert's Home Care Studies

Among recent important studies of Section 222-financed homemaker (as distinguished from home health) services is that of Weissert, presented in connection with his adult day care (ADC) analysis, discussed earlier (Weissert, 1978; Weissert et al, 1978, 1980). His research does not compare cost-effectiveness between or among alternatives, but rather compares the HC outcomes between two groups of clients, one receiving HC, the other, a control.

Although analytical comments on the Weissert ADC analysis apply as well to the homemaker and combined homemaker-ADC study, the HC conclusions are illuminating with respect to patient characteristics and costs. The HC studies covered 630 clients, one-half in the experimental group, the other half in the control group.

Homemakers were used 368 hours per year on average. Among specified users, 41 percent were visited twice a week; 26 percent, once a week, and only 2 percent four times per week. Among those who survived the year, the figure was 430 visits per year. Most heavy users were trauma sufferers; cancer victims were least common. Older, female, white patients and patients living with others were heavier users than younger, male, and black patients or patients living alone. One interesting finding was the wide range of utilization across the various sites: from 30 to 611 hours per year and from 27 visits of one hour each per year to 116 visits of five hours each. A number of explanations for these differences were offered, including divergence of professional need assessments and care prescriptions, the various types of provider organizations, and patients' attitudes toward HC use. Clearly, these institutional and professional aspects of provision must be considered in any analyses of HC and, indeed, in any form of provision before uniform statements can be

366

made about the outcomes and costs (or cost-effectiveness) of any program. In a sense, organization and institutions must thus be a variable for policy and scientific research.

Analysis of the data showed the same results. The rate of institutionalization was not appreciably different for the HC users than for the non-users. For the over-74 females living alone and suffering from cancer or circulatory diseases, there were slightly fewer SNF days than for the controls who received no HC. On the other hand, the controls had fewer days of hospitalization. There was small difference for rates of admission to SNFs (16 percent of the experimental group, 18 percent of the controls) and little divergence in length of stay once admitted to an SNF (23 and 24 days, respectively). As with the ADC users, Weissert found that a very small proportion of HC users or non-users appeared destined for the nursing home. Also, both groups had high rates of hospitalization and comparable stays (24 days versus 22 days). Again, these findings may suggest that HC serves as an additional service rather than a substitute for many services for large numbers of the LTC-dependent population. A larger proportion of HC users improved physical functioning, especially among the older clients.

When those who died in the course of the study are taken out of the analysis, users still did better in terms of functioning, but the differences were not statistically significant. As with the ADC analysis, improvement in ADL with home care showed some lagged effects, that is, improvements often appeared in the quarter after the services were received, but, again, the differences were not statistically significant. On the other hand, intensity of HC use was associated with improvement in ADL functioning on a lagged basis; however, if clients who died are excluded from the figures, differences in ADL functioning associated with intensity of HC use disappear. One interesting finding was that HC use was associated with increased probability of survival.

Average hourly costs of HC services were $7.61; total annual cost was $2,290 for the study year. HC users, overall, cost $3,432 more than non-users annually, a difference of 60 percent. Given the lack of any real measured outcome differences between the experimental and control groups, such cost differences suggest that an HC program might have to be justified on grounds other than cost. In light of the Weissert study, final judgment on this question must be reserved until other research is completed. This is especially pertinent, since Weissert's analysis of a small California group receiving both ADC and HC again showed no significantly different outcomes on grounds other than death rates, contentment, and psychological well-being, as well as showing a much higher (38 percent) annual cost for users than for non-users. Of course, the improvement in contentment and psychological well-being may be as important from society's perspective as cost-saving.

Weissert and his colleagues also considered HC from a multivariate perspective (Wan et al, 1978). They also examined their data sets of users and non-users, experimental groups and controls (those not selected to receive HC in the experiment) in the same manner as for the ADC groups. Essentially they examined users and non-users and experimental and control groups with "contaminated" cases included (Weissert et al, 1980). (Their previous bivariate and multivariate analyses had excluded contaminated cases). Again, use of home-maker services was associated with reduced mortality. Weissert speculates that this reduction may have little to do with HC as such. Rather, alert homemaker aides may have spotted conditions which required help in time for their patients/clients to be taken to the hospital. This conclusion would seem to be consistent with the finding that male users living with others and/or severely dependent users had higher levels of hospital use than did non-users. Also, members of the experimental groups had consistently higher levels of hospital use than did members of the control groups. Otherwise, there seemed to be no effect of homemaker services on institution-alization or physical functioning. As with ADC, the majority of homemaker users and controls did not use nursing homes during the study year. Again, the questions arise of suitability of HC for nursing home prone patients and the add-on of services.

Greenberg's Minnesota Studies

As noted in Chapter VII, Jay Greenberg (1974) at the University of Minnesota has developed a study of the comparative cost of nursing home and home care, following and enriching the Pollak models. The methodological part of the study begins by discussing the four parts of the comparative costing problem: (1) determination of the direct costs of home care, (2) determination of the direct costs of the nursing home, (3) development of effectiveness measures and cost comparison calculations, and (4) estimation of the indirect and systematic effects of any changes in policy and/or the structure of provision. In dealing with all of these costing issues, Greenberg assumes that producers (providers) operate efficiently, that is, they produce each level of output in the most technically and eco-nomically efficient manner.

Assuming that the key issue in a comparative cost analysis for home care is the total social cost of keeping someone out of an institution, Greenberg tackles the direct costing question in terms of client and agency characteristics. He defines home care (non-institutional) costs as does Pollak, in total social terms, because the costs of a non-institutional environment are those of reproducing the services provided by an institutional environment in another setting. As we will show, his definition of social cost is somewhat more restricted than that developed in Chapter VII. In all of his analysis, he also argues that quality is part of the outcome of provision, that is, it is the level of care to which the system and the providers aspire. This contrasts with much other cost analysis which makes quality one of the "inputs" or characteristics of the inputs.

To Greenberg, the most prominent patient attributes are their physical, psychological, emotional, and social circumstances. These can be displayed as linked to cost of care of a given quality per unit time, although the actual shape of the relationship must be a matter of empirical finding. (See Figure IX–3.)

Given patient impairment, cost can also be hypothesized as systematically related to family ability (willingness) to cope. Again, the relation can be pictorially displayed. (See Figure IX–4.) In this case, the willingness to cope can only reduce costs by so much, however, since beyond a certain point (X in the figure), care requirements may be beyond a family's ability to make much of a difference. Similarly, the cost-impairment relationship can be framed in terms of family ability to help by means of two curves, one showing the cost-impairment link without help, and one with (Figure IX–5). It seems intuitively correct that costs will be lower for each level of impairment with more family support. Note that in all of these comparisons, the output is care of a given quality level. By making this assumption, Greenberg eliminates a troublesome problem, the quality issue; however, this issue must be addressed.

Acknowledging that the literature had (by 1974) not generated any theoretical models of HC or other alternatives, Greenberg asserted that a comparative cost analysis must recognize the possibility of high cost and low cost providers, the implications of economies of scale (in, for example, comparing families with agency providers), and the role of geography in influencing input prices. He also noted that, despite many claims on behalf of so-called "integrated," multi-service firms, no one has shown them to be cost-effective in LTC; yet their presence or absence may exert significant influences on cost and must be considered in any cost analyses.

To Greenberg, direct costing of nursing homes is a much more modest affair (at least in Minnesota) since their cost data are matters of public record and they have thoroughly analyzed the data. In effect, he argues for taking nursing home data at face value. As shown in Chapter XIX, that assumption may be a bit risky. In making comparisons of this type, moreover, it must be remembered that observed costs of nursing homes may be functions of reimbursement policies.

Having laid out the basics of cost structures, Greenberg turns to the explicit comparisons he wishes to make. His contention is that

FIGURE IX-3
The Cost-Impairment Linkage

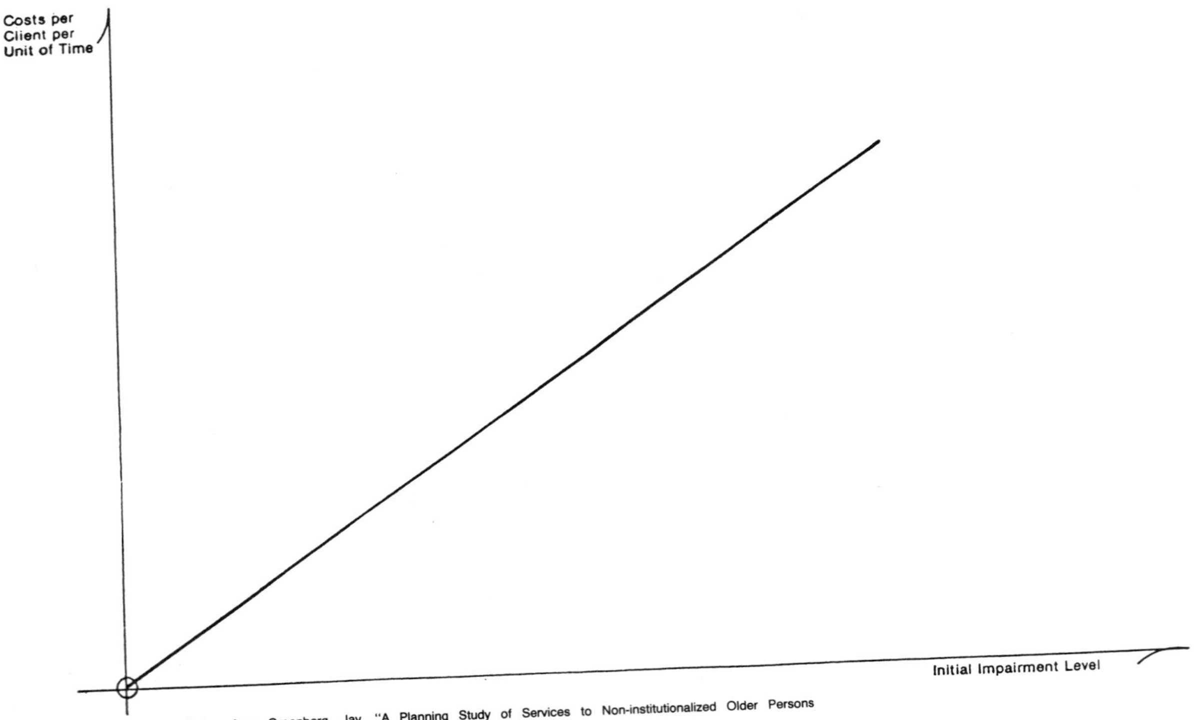

Costs per
Client per
Unit of Time

Initial Impairment Level

Source: Taken from Greenberg, Jay, "A Planning Study of Services to Non-institutionalized Older Persons in Minnesota," p. 4

370

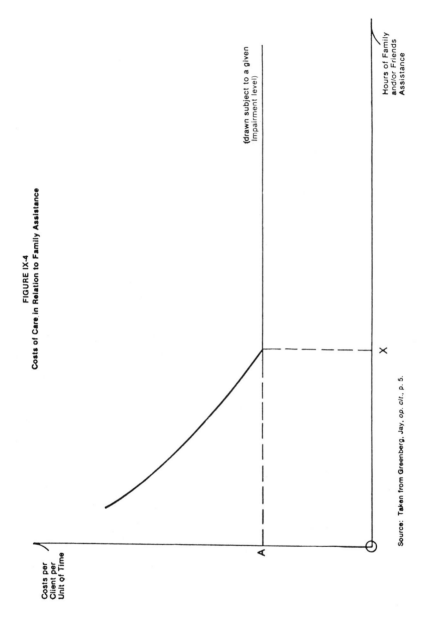

FIGURE IX-4
Costs of Care in Relation to Family Assistance

Costs per
Client per
Unit of Time

(drawn subject to a given
Impairment level)

Hours of Family
and/or Friends
Assistance

Source: Taken from Greenberg, Jay, *op. cit.*, p. 5.

371

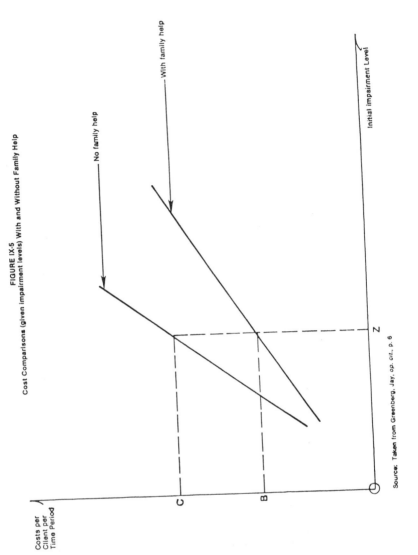

FIGURE IX-5
Cost Comparisons (given impairment levels) With and Without Family Help

No family help

With family help

Initial impairment Level

Costs per
Client per
Time Period

C

B

Z

Source: Taken from Greenberg, Jay, *op. cit.*, p. 6

372

analysis of cost-effectiveness is the most appropriate, since simple costing studies beg the questions of effectiveness, while technical cost-benefit analysis requires specification of benefits in monetary terms, something often impossible to achieve. In making the cost-effectiveness comparisons, it must be remembered that the level of effectiveness or quality must be common to both modalities to be compared and that quality level must be held constant across levels of impairment. Otherwise, assertions about relative cost-effectiveness will be meaningless. If those requirements are satisfied, then finding Pollak's "break-even" point, that point at which costs of care in two modalities are equal, is feasible. In technically framing the investigations, it would be preferable to randomly sort potential patients between care programs, but politically this may be impossible. Also, effectiveness levels should be specified in advance, but, again, one may have to settle for some highly subjective statements. To the extent, however, that professional judgments can meaningfully and operationally define outcomes, these should be developed in advance of an experiment/cost comparison to ensure that both modalities are really producing the same thing. Also, as Weissert points out (1981), the alternative should have some benefit for the users.

The specific comparative cost analysis performed by Greenberg involved using a "typical" agency, that is, one with a case-mix (in disability terms) representative of all agencies in the relevant area, in his case Minnesota. Using a global disability scale, shown in Figure IX–6, he compared HC and nursing home costs by disability levels. Food and housing were included in his total costs of HC, but he excluded the labor of volunteers and families.

As expected, Greenberg's cost comparisons show that, for lower levels of disability, HC is cheaper than nursing home care, but that for those patients who need complete help with personal care (Disability Level IV), nursing home care is cheaper. Living with someone else reduced HC costs substantially, though this advantage is more apparent at lower disability levels than at higher ones. For the former, living alone almost doubles costs, while for the latter, the spreading of fixed costs (mostly housing) in a service package that includes much disability-related nursing care yields few advantages over living with someone else. The role of nursing care appears very important in determining cost, even for the same level of disability, possibly because home chore or personal care is so much cheaper and may suffice for some patients with modest levels of disability (Level II).

On the basis of his cost comparisons for the early 1970s, Greenberg claims that for 300 people, it would be necessary to spend between $104,000 and $109,000 monthly to offer a home service package to elderly dependent patients. On a cost-effectiveness

373

FIGURE IX-6
Global Disability Scale Used in the
Greenberg Minnesota Study

Rating of one: This individual would be medically stable and mentally alert. He would be able to ambulate with little or no human assistance, (although mechanical assistance such as a walker may be necessary). For the most part, he would need help with food preparation, shopping or cleaning or laundry.

Rating of two: This individual would be medically stable with no more than minimal amount of mental disability. He would need minimal assistance with personal care such as tub bathing or shampooing and would also require assistance in non-personal care as in category one.

Rating of three: This individual would be medically stable but may need limited rehabilitation services. He would have difficulty in ambulation, and require moderate assistance with bathing, dressing, or toileting.

Rating of four: This individual would be medically stable or changing in a predictable way (e.g. declining or terminal); may be moderately confused, need complete help with personal care and/or at least one person to help with ambulation.

Source: Taken from Greenberg, *op. cit.,* p. 24f

basis, given the highest level of disability which could be served at home, HC would have saved almost $392,000 per year over nursing home costs for an estimated 1,490 skilled nursing patients. These cost comparisons must, however, be modified by an understanding of the structural implications of substituting HC for nursing home care. In the first place, it must be possible to supply the resources which an expanded HC system might require. This aspect of system dynamics has not been adequately researched, either with respect to staffing and capital requirements or with respect to users' (including social service agencies') demand responses to a new supply of a new type of service. Also, it must be recognized that patients change and that costs may consequently shift. Finally, there is the systemic question of the effects of removing the lighter case loads from the nursing homes which may increase their costs at the same time that HC cost savings are overstated. These marginal cost effects must be included as offsets to the savings from HC. Additionally, there may be a heavier or lighter case load in the acute hospital.

The Minnesota Home Care-Nursing Home Comparison Study

Another major study of clients, services, and costs in nursing homes and home care settings was completed at the University of Minnesota (Anderson, Patten, and Greenberg, 1980). This effort directly compared personal, social, and health characteristics of nursing home and HC clients. It also considered the characteristics of major sub-groups in both sets of service receivers and the degree of overlap between them. The study also examined the amounts and types of service provided, the relation between service use and patient characteristics, the relative well-being of clients receiving HC and nursing home care, and the public income transfers received by both groups. The comparative cost analysis was an important component. Although a cost-benefit or cost-effectiveness analysis was implied, none was explicitly undertaken because there were no specifications of outcome objectives or achievements.

In the study, approximately 550 clients of seven HC agencies were compared with approximately 450 residents of 11 nursing homes, all residing in three Minnesota counties around the Twin Cities. Data were gathered by interview and by consultation of service and cost records. Initial data were obtained in February 1978 with a follow-up nine months later. These data showed HC clients were more likely to be female, unmarried or widowed, and living alone than Minnesotans in general. Average age was 76; most were white. Nursing home residents, by contrast, were older (average age 82), more likely to be female, less likely to be married, and less likely to come from a blue-collar family. Thirty to 34 percent of both groups had no living children; 55 percent of HC clients lived alone versus 52 percent of

375

the nursing home residents before institutionalization. Nursing home residents had been receiving services for about two years longer than HC recipients. Previous hospitalization was not more likely to be related to being in a nursing home or receiving HC. HC receivers were divided into those receiving nursing care only; nursing, home health, and homemaker services; and homemaker services only. Nursing home residents were divided into SNF and ICF clients.

In considering receipt of services and costs, the functional, mental, and medical characteristics are presumably of crucial significance. HC clients were somewhat incapacitated according to indicators of ADL capacity and instrumental ADL (IADL) capacity (ability to use telephone, checkbook, etc.), although they were less so than the nursing home residents. A major finding running through the analysis was that ICF residents were less incapacitated than the total HC group. ICF residents were more like homemaker HC recipients, while the SNF group was more like the nursing/home health aide/home-maker/HC service receivers. Both nursing home groups were more impaired in mental functioning as measured by the Mental Status Quotient (MSQ) than any of the HC sub-groups. Without the MSQ ratings, 22 percent of the nursing home residents had the same characteristics as the HC groups. Mental status, however, seems to be a major discriminator between the two groups. It should be noted that much mental difficulty diagnosed as dementia may actually be reversible depression; hence mental status circumstances must be analyzed with extraordinary care in any such comparison.

In terms of mobility, nursing home residents were more impaired than HC receivers, but the total HC group was less mobile than the ICF sub-group. With respect to ADL functioning, nursing home clients were worse off than HC clients, but again the ICF sub-group was less impaired than the total HC group. For all clients, bathing, dressing, incontinence, and locomotion were the most troublesome; eating, bed mobility, and moving from one place to another were less so. Similar results were shown for IADL. Two-fifths of nursing home residents versus one-fifth of HC receivers were moderately/severely incapacitated in IADL. The most troubling IADL areas linked to ADL problems were doing housework, going grocery shopping, doing laundry, and going places out of usual walking distance.

Overall health status was rated with respect to dependency and ability to live alone. On both counts, the nursing home groups were more impaired than the HC recipients: 47 percent versus 37 percent dependent and 67 percent versus 40 percent needing supervision to live alone.

Services received were organized into the following major categories: case management, mental health, personal care, home-making/housekeeping, and nursing. HC clients used fewer of all services than nursing home residents, although the highest 20 per-

376

cent of HC service users took most HC services and accounted for higher percentages of service use within their group than did either the SNF or ICF residents. Not surprisingly, HC users received much informal care (largely provided by families): ten times as much informal as formal nursing and personal care services and three times as much informal as formal housekeeping services. Most informal care was provided by spouses, many of them old themselves, a circumstance which evokes important questions about replacements when caregivers are incapacitated.

Higher percentages of HC users received more emergency room care and dental care than did nursing home clients, raising some interesting questions about the role of ER care as a part of LTC provision. Total service use (formal plus informal) was greater among nursing home users than HC users, but ICF clients received only 60 percent as much personal care and about the same amount of nursing care monthly as did HC users.

Only a few client characteristics appeared to be the prime determinants of amount and type of service used. Physical functioning was the sole attribute significantly related to the receipt of each provided service among HC recipients. Overall, the level of physical functioning was a better predictor of the quantity of services received. Among medical diagnoses, only cerebro-vascular accidents (CVA or stroke) was a good service use predictor and then only for personal and nursing care in nursing homes. Despite claims for the ability to tailor HC services to the needs of clients, these data show that nursing homes did a better job of meeting needs than did HC, since models of service provision in nursing homes were better explainers of the observed variations in service use than were models for HC. Evidently, more research is needed on how services are allocated and how they should be allocated in HC.

A particular focus of the Minnesota study was the question of costs. Home care was seen to be cheaper in costs of formal services, but if the implicit costs of personal care and nursing care (valued at the wage rates for those functions) were added in, HC use of those services was seen as more expensive than use in nursing homes. Overall formal costs for HC came to about $80 per month; SNF costs were over $950, and ICF costs were almost $675.

Formal plus informal nursing in HC came to almost $127 versus $86 for SNFs and $32 for ICFs; personal care formal costs plus informal costs came to $251, $152, and $36, respectively. Note that these cost comparisons only count service costs. (No allowance is made for housing, food, extraordinary social services, or family opportunity costs.) The excess of formal-plus-informal personal and nursing services costs over nursing home costs may be considered a proxy for the burdens borne by families for users of HC. If so, then that magnitude may give some notion of the outer limit of the amount

377

of burden which might be relieved by public policy. In addition, if formal HC services are to be expanded, say by public funds, then the cost increases may be a function of the level of ADL incapacity among the older population and of the amount of informal care which families are now providing.

In any comparison of care modes, the relative effectiveness of either form of intervention should be analyzed. Specifically, LTC is aimed at maintaining, reversing, or delaying deterioration and allowing a maximum possible quality of life. In the Minnesota study, such outcome comparisons could not be made directly. Rather a number of indicators were used as proxies. In the first place, it was found that after one year, only 50 percent of the original HC users were still receiving services; 8 percent had died, 8 percent had gone into nursing homes, and 12 percent were receiving services from other than the original sources. Among the nursing home groups, 17 percent had died, and 80 percent were still receiving services. Over a nine-month comparison period, there were no appreciable differences within the HC group with respect to changes in functional and other disability scores. In three out of four indicators of well-being (social contacts, satisfaction with services, and satisfaction with living arrangements) HC showed some marginal advantages over nursing home care, which enjoyed an advantage only in overall life satisfaction. The study concluded that the two groups, HC and nursing home, showed no significant differences in well-being. Although the data did not warrant any large-scale inferences about the expansion of HC, the researchers reasoned that if HC and nursing home care produced essentially the same results in objective well-being, HC shouldl be expanded because it is preferred by most patients and most professionals.

This conclusion takes on added weight when we recognize that HC recipients gain less from public income transfers than do residents of nursing homes. On the basis of social security, SSI, Medicare, and Medicaid cash and in-kind transfers, HC clients received $439, compared to $861 per month for nursing home clients, a difference of $422. If Title XX allocations are added to HC benefit packages, the difference drops to $252 per month. It thus appears that horizontal equity is not achieved in the allocation of services and income transfers between HC and nursing home service recipients. Even if functional incapacity is accounted for, the differences between the two groups do not substantially change. Only for the very impaired HC clients are the benefits comparable to those received by nursing home clients.

The GAO Cleveland Studies

One of the most important consequences of the Pollak-Greenberg type of "break-even" analysis was a series of studies by the General

Accounting Office on the questions of death, well-being, HC, and institutionalization among the elderly in Cleveland, Ohio. The GAO-Cleveland studies were based on the interviews and assessments of over 1,600 people over 65 years of age in Cleveland, and on the analysis of the effect of a number of Federally-assisted programs on their health and well-being.[2]

The December 1977 study focused on the linkages among impairments, living arrangements, and costs of home care versus care in institutions. Five sets of patient characteristics were also considered in connection with impairment and costs: (1) social circumstances, (2) economic level, (3) mental condition, (4) physical condition, and (5) level of ADL functioning. Average usage rates of services were calculated for impairment level, and costs were assigned on the basis of the actual costs of provision from agencies and of imputed costs of family support at the same rate as agency costs. Again, there was no attempt to develop total social costs, that is, Doherty's secondary costs, or a full spectrum of family opportunity costs.

Among the major findings of the December 1977 GAO study were the following:

- Sixty percent of the extremely impaired live in the community, not in institutions.
- Families and friends contribute more to the costs of long-term care than do agencies.
- Home care costs are greater than institutional care costs for the greatly or extremely impaired.
- Eighty-seven percent of the institutionalized population is greatly or extremely impaired, versus only 14 percent of those in the community.
- Families and friends contribute about 50 percent of the costs of care at all levels of impairment and about 70 percent of the costs of care of the most impaired living in the community.
- Institutional care is cheaper than HC for only 10 percent of the impaired population.

The methodological emphasis of this study was the search for the break-even point between the costs of HC and those of nursing home care. In the GAO study, social security and SSI payments were defined as offsets (that is, they reduced costs) against nursing home care but as add-ons for HC. Physician costs were excluded in both cases. Total HC costs ranged from $63 per month for the least impaired to $845 per month for the most impaired. The family and friends' share rose from 59 percent of the total for the least impaired to 80 percent for the most. The break-even point was found in the

---

2 The parent study is GAO, April 19, 1977. Also see GAO, December 30, 1977 and September 20, 1979.

penultimate level of impairment, for which HC costs were $407 per month, of which the family was estimated to pay $287 and public agencies, $120. Overall, 37 percent of the extremely impaired were in institutions.

Notice that the question of quality of care was not explicitly addressed, nor was the impact of living arrangements linked to the cost findings. On the latter issue, it was pointed out that few institutionalized people had a spouse or lived with their children at the time of admission in the year-long survey period. Of the 217 greatly or extremely impaired who were maintained in the community over the year, 29 percent were married, and an additional 25 percent lived with their children. GAO concluded that the most likely candidates for institutionalization were the 31 percent of the greatly or extremely impaired who lived alone; 76 percent would enter institutions. These account for only 5 percent of the non-institutionalized persons 65 and over, but 66 percent of the institutionalized are from this group.

Two major policy recommendations resulted from these findings. First, Congress was encouraged to proceed with training programs under welfare reform to create 200,000 public service jobs for welfare recipients to help the sick elderly in their homes. Second, the jobs should focus on helping the sick elderly who live alone and have no family support.

On the basis of its analysis, GAO concluded that the cost of major proposals for restructuring HC benefits under Medicare and Medicaid would not add significantly to Federal costs, except for the elimination of the skilled care requirement under Parts A and B of Medicare, which might add $1.3 billion yearly. Removing the limits on numbers of visits and the prior hospitalization requirement would add only $12.5 million each yearly. Purging the homel ound requirement would generate only $92.5 million in new costs, while adding homemaker/chore services to the list of required services under Medicaid would account for only $75 million.

The Willemain Model

Although the GAO study appears to have addressed the central issues of family circumstance and dependency in connection with cost comparisons between home and institutional care, its methodology and recommendations have been challenged in a paper by Thomas Willemain (1980). Willemain's critique starts with the method of costing for establishing the break-even point. For example, he points out that social and recreational provisions are omitted from family costing by GAO but included in the costs of agency services. A total social cost perspective should include both. Also, family nursing and extraordinary chore services are quoted at the agency rate, ignoring agency economies of scale (thus possibly inflating family costs) and side-stepping the family quality advantages (thus deflating family contributions); there is no reason to assume that these factors cancel out. He also points out that both HC agency and nursing home costs are set at the Ohio or Cleveland averages, although service costs are a function of client impairment levels in both types of care. In fact, this is one of the major analytical and empirical questions now at issue. Willemain also notes that there is no reason for the asymmetrical treatment of social security and SSI payments with respect to HC (added to costs) and nursing homes (deducted). Additionally, he finds no justification for omitting physician costs from either cost calculation, since even the Medicaid regulations (1974) required more doctor visits for patients in ICFs (7.5 yearly) and SNFs (12.9 yearly) than for elderly in the community (6–7). These criticisms on the costing side, most of which appear justified, evoke considerable caution in using the GAO cost comparisons as bases for policy or as sources of data.

The major Willemain criticism, however, and one which leads to some important new analytical and policy perspectives, concerns GAO's conclusions about risk of institutionalization. Noting that the merging of the Duke/Durham and Cleveland data sets to link impairment, institutionalization, and living arrangements is suspect because of lack of comparative information on nursing home bed supply, Willemain points out that living alone is not identical to living in isolation. Therefore, it may not be valid to assume that high impairment level and living alone together raise the risk of institutionalization, unless additional analysis of these factors separately, and then together, definitely show this to be the case. On statistical grounds as well, the small number of persons institutionalized during the study year does not warrant inferences about living/impairment state and institutionalization. Lastly, Willemain questions the merging of the two highest impairment rates as a single impairment measure because the extremely impaired have significantly higher service needs.

These criticisms greatly weaken the base for the GAO recommendation about creating jobs to provide service to the sick elderly living alone. Certainly, the assumption that families will withdraw their support if their dependent elderly get additional public support must be independently tested as a basis for such a policy recommendation. A longitudinal study might be the best approach to this type of analysis, but even with existing cross-sectional data, one should be able to determine if, within each type of living arrangement and at each level of impairment, increased public support is correlated with decreased (or the same or even increased) levels of private (family) support. As a matter of fact, the GAO data appear to indicate that private support increased much more rapidly with level of impairment than did public support. Willemain concludes that if the objective of increasing HC resources is to maximize the number of nursing home admissions saved per unit of HC resources, the best way to do this may not be to focus on the patient group with the greatest risk of admission (the highly impaired living alone) but rather on some other group. This observation leads him to develop a model to select potential clients of an HC system, one which presumably avoids a trap which caught the GAO analysis: the fact that the GAO model linked impairment, family support, and public HC with the break-even point analysis but failed to consider public and family HC supply or nursing home bed supply in linking impairment and institutionalization. In the accompanying diagram (Figure IX-7), the GAO's links to institutionalization are made without considering the level of HC supply or nursing home bed supply, so the system is indeterminate.

Assuming that the goal of HC and LTC policy is to prevent institutionalization, one should target HC services to those individuals for whom there is the greatest probability of remaining in the community. The corresponding model is based on the assumption that everyone faces a risk of institutionalization, R, positively related to level of impairment, I, and negatively related to availability of HC, H. Thus,

$$R = R (I, H) \tag{1}$$

The probability that an individual with risk $= R$ will be in the community in one year can be denoted as $P(R) = \exp(-R)$ since it can be shown that a constant risk of institutionalization is exponentially related to such a probability. The object of a policy of targeting HC is to maximize the value of P, that is, the change (presumably positive) in the probability of keeping someone in the community. If the inverse relationship between R and P,

$$P(R) = \exp(-R) \tag{2}$$

is plotted on a graph, a unit reduction in R for a high-risk individual will produce a smaller improvement in P than will a unit reduction in risk for a low-risk individual. (See Figure IX-8.) On the face of it, this graphical result appears to run counter to the GAO recommendations.

To return to the mainstream of the argument, R can be changed by I or H (availability of HC), and P can be changed by changing R. A reduction in R will produce an increase in P, the chance of staying in the community. Thus, for a given R,

$$\Delta P = \exp [-(R + \Delta R)] - \exp (R), \text{ which becomes} \tag{3}$$

$$\Delta P \approx \exp (-R) \Delta R \text{ for small } \Delta R \tag{4}$$

The change in risk, ΔR, will depend on the increase in HC, ΔH, which, on the grounds of diminishing returns or scale economies,

382

FIGURE IX-7
Conceptual Model Linking Home Care to Institutionalization

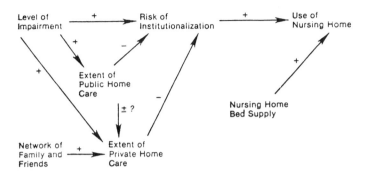

Source: Taken from Willemain, Thomas, "Beyond the GAO Cleveland Study: Client Selection for Home Care Services," p. 13

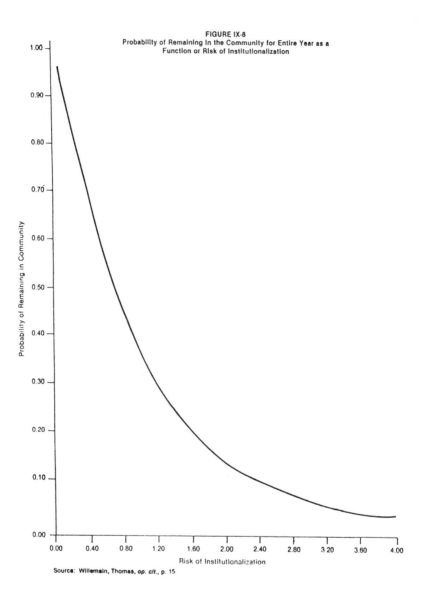

FIGURE IX-8
Probability of Remaining in the Community for Entire Year as a
Function or Risk of Institutionalization

Source: Willemain, Thomas, *op. cit.*, p. 15

384

may depend on the pro level of HC. Of course, since R is a joint function of I and H, the level of impairment is crucial also, and the elasticity of R with respect to I must be considered.

Given the links between P and R, it is now necessary to consider the nature of the risk function, R. Willemain, working from the previous discussions on the effectiveness of HC, argues that the risk function should show that risk increases with impairment, that risk decreases with HC, that R should reflect either economies or diseconomies of scale or some threshold effect (there may be a necessary minimum amount of supply for HC to be effective), and that the elasticity of effect with respect to impairment may moderate the impact of HC on R. Such a function might look like this:

$$R = I(1 + a^I H^b)^{-1} \qquad (5)$$

I and H reflect client characteristics; a and b pertain to the effectiveness of HC.

The parameter, a, shows the effects of impairment, such that if $0 < a < 1$, HC has a greater impact on the less impaired. If $a > 1$, the more impaired will benefit more from HC. Production processes are reflected in b, such that if $0 < b < 1$, there are decreasing returns to scale. If $b > 1$, there may be a threshold effect, increasing as b increases. Figure IX–9 shows this property.

This formulation permits the linking of the change in the probability of remaining in the community to the change in HC via the determination of R. The expression for change in probability, given the introduction of new HC, is

$$\Delta P_{new} = I \exp(-I) a^I (\Delta H)^b \qquad (6)$$

Maximizing this expression with respect to the level of impairment, I, produces

$$I^* = (1 - \log_e a)^{-1} \qquad (7)$$

as the level of impairment yielding the highest value of ΔP_{new}. This expression indicates that the effect of HC crucially depends on the elasticity of response with respect to impairment, denoted by I. Note that a client may be too much or too little impaired for efficient targeting. Willemain, however, believes it unlikely that a home care agency's pool of possible clients would contain many individuals too impaired to be selected. The implication of these manipulations is that patients should be selected on the basis of their impairment level's response to the use of HC.

For clients already receiving services, ("old" clients),

$$\Delta P_{old} = I a^I b H^{b-1} (1 + a^I H^b)^{-2} \exp[(-I)(1 + a^I H^b)^{-1}] \Delta_H \qquad (8)$$

Again, the best targeting is on the client's impairment level, I^*, and current HC level, H^*, which maximize the value of equation (8).

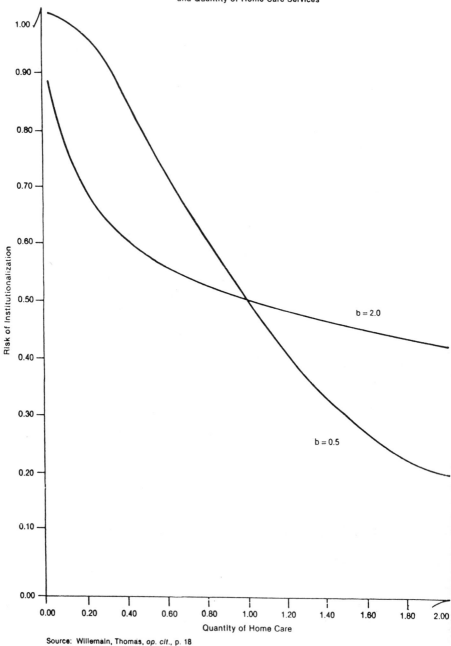

FIGURE IX-9
Hypothesized Forms of Relationship Between Risk of Institutionalization
and Quantity of Home Care Services

Source: Willemain, Thomas, *op. cit.*, p. 18

Again, the values of parameters a and b are crucial. This formulation appears to provide important guidance on the choice of individuals to receive increases in HC. Specifically, clients should be chosen on the basis of the links between impairment level and responsiveness to services. Also, the nature of the returns to scale in the production process must be considered, particularly if there is a question of increasing services to old patients or starting services for new patients.

Obviously, this approach is in its initial phases. Empirical work is needed to determine values for a and b, at the same time that the most appropriate form for R must be found. Equation (5) merely represents a convenient form which Willemain asserted. In addition, as Willemain emphasizes, choosing a most appropriate candidate for services is not the same as choosing a most appropriate group, often the crux of policy debate.

Although this analysis does not necessarily support the proposition that those most at risk of institutionalization are the most suitable targets for an HC program, other factors may make the highest risk group the most politically attractive. Among these are the number of clients in each disability or risk group who must share increases in support, the elasticity of family provision with respect to public HC provision, and the political strength of groups with differing impairment levels. In light of these considerations, a smaller group with a better base of political support may appear more able to produce politically-preferred (in the sense of more closely attuned to public preferences) sets of clients. (They may not, however, correspond with professional assessments of "need" in the community.) In any event, as Willemain points out, the fact that the more impaired tend to have higher ratios of family support to public support than do the less impaired may make them an attractive target. They may also accommodate policymakers' desires to avoid funding seemingly limitless amounts of care for mildly-impaired groups ("maid service" for the frail). The major problem in targeting so closely may lie in equity considerations, especially if a number of similarly impaired groups differ mainly in the amount of political clout they can muster.

Willemain's analysis clearly leads to the realization, implicit in much of what has been discussed before, that much research is needed on alternative policies and procedures for targeting existing and/or increased HC benefits. This research demands strong analytical work on the costs, effects, outcomes, and politics of serving existing and new groups of clients.

References

Anderson, Nancy N., Sharon K. Patten, Jay N. Greenberg, *Summary, A Comparison of Home Care and Nursing Home Care for Older Persons in Minnesota,* Volume III (Minneapolis: University of Minnesota, Hubert H. Humphrey Institute of Public Affairs and Center for Health Services Research, June 1980, for Minnesota Board on Aging and U.S. DHHS, Administration on Aging under Grant No. 90–A–682).

Boyd, Lawrence, Robert Pruger, Maureen Clark, *et al,* "In Home Support Services, Equity and Efficiency Project, First Year Report" (Berkeley: University of California, School of Social Welfare, January 1980, under Dept. of Social Services, State of California, Contract No. 38831).

Boyd, Lawrence, Robert Pruger, Maureen Clark, Martin Chase, *et al,* "In Home Support Services, Equity and Efficiency Project, Second Year Report, 11/1/79–10/31/80" (Berkeley: University of California, School of Social Welfare, January 1980, under Dept. of Social Services, State of California, Contract No. 38831).

Brickner, Philip W., Sister Teresita Duque, Arthur Kaufman, Michael Sarg, Jeffrey A. Jahre, Susan Maturlo, and James F. Janeski, "The Homebound Aged, A Medically Unreached Group," *Annals of Internal Medicine,* January 1975, pp. 1–6.

Brickner, Philip W., James F. Janeski, Gloria Rich, Sister Teresita Duque, Laura Starita, Richard LaRocco, Thomas Flannery, and Steven Werlin, "Home Maintenance for the Homebound Aged: A Pilot Program in New York City," *The Gerontologist,* February 1976, pp. 25–29.

Callender, Marie and Judith LaVor, "Home Health Care: Development, Problems and Potential," U.S. DHEW, Office of Social Services and Development, Assistant Secretary for Planning and Evaluation, April 1975 (mimeo).

Caro, Francis G., "Objectives in Long Term Care" (New York, Institute for Social Welfare Research, Community Service Society, January 1980, mimeo).

Drob, Judah, Alan Sager, Stephen C. Sunderland and M. Virginia Davis, "Mutual Self Help Over Time: Can It Aid the Elderly?" (Washington, D.C.: 3238 Chestnut Street, N.W., February 1980, mimeo).

Fortinsky, Richard H., Carl V. Granger, and Gary B. Seltzer, "The Use of Functional Assessment in Understanding Home Care Needs," *Medical Care,* May 1981, pp. 489–497.

Gerson, Lowell W. and Owen P. Hughes, "A Comparative Study of the Economics of Home Care," *International Journal of Health Services,* Vol. 6, No. 4, 1976, pp. 543–555.

Greenberg, Jay, "A Planning Study of Services to Non-Institutionalized Older Persons in Minnesota," Parts 1 and 2 (Minneapolis: Governor's Citizens Council on Aging, 1974; mimeo).

Griffiths, R.A. and L.Z. Cosin, "The Floating Bed," *The Lancet,* March 27, 1976, pp. 684f.

Horowitz, Amy, "Families Who Care: A Study of Natural Support Systems of the Elderly," paper presented at Gerontological Society, 31st Annual Scientific Meeting, Dallas, Texas, November 1978 (New York: Community Service Society, n.d.).

Rak, Karen, *Home Health Line: Decade Report, 1980* (Washington, D.C.: Home Health Line, 1980).

Rawlinson, Helen L., "Existing and Potential Roles of Third-Party Payors in the Development, Expansion, and Effective Utilization of Home Health

388

Care Services," report prepared in compliance with Order No. PLD–90242–73, October 22, 1973 (mimeo).

Ricker-Smith, Katherine and Brahna Trager, "In-Home Health Service in California: Some Lessons for National Health Insurance," *Medical Care,* March 1978, pp. 173–189.

Rossman, Isadore, "The After Care Project: A Viable Alternative to Home Care," *Medical Care,* June 1974, pp. 534–540.

Sager, Alan, "Decision-making for Home Care: An Overview of Study Goals and Methods" (Waltham, Mass: Brandeis University, Levinson Policy Institute, April 1980 under AoA Grant 90–A–1679 (01)(02)).

Sager, Alan, *Learning the Home Care Needs of the Elderly: Patient, Family, and Professional Views Of An Alternative to Institutionalization* (Waltham, Mass., Brandeis University, Levinson Policy Institute, November 20, 1979 under AoA Grant No. 90–A–1026 (01)(02)).

Tolkoff-Rubin, Nina E., Susan L. Fisher, Joanne T. O'Brien, and Robert J. Rubin, "Coordinated Home Care: The Massachusetts General Hospital Experience," *Medical Care,* June 1976, pp. 453–464.

Trager, Brahna, *Homemaker/Home Health Aide Services in the United States* (Washington: U.S. Government Printing Office, June 1973).

United States Comptroller General, General Accounting Office, *Conditions of Older People: National Information System Needed,* HRD–79–95 (Washington, D.C., September 20, 1979).

United States Comptroller General, General Accounting Office, *Entering A Nursing Home—Costly Implications for Medicaid and the Elderly,* PAD–80–12 (Washington, D.C., November 26, 1979).

United States Comptroller General, General Accounting Office, *Home Health Care Benefits Under Medicare and Medicaid* (Washington, D.C., July 9, 1974).

United States Comptroller General, General Accounting Office, *Home Health: The Need for a Better Policy to Provide for the Elderly* (Washington, D.C., December 30, 1977).

United States Comptroller General, General Accounting Office, *Home Health Care Services—Tighter Fiscal Controls Needed,* HRD–79–17 (Washington, D.C., May 15, 1979).

United States Comptroller General, General Accounting Office, *Identifying Boarding Homes Housing the Needy, Aged, Blind, and Disabled: A Major Step Toward Resolving a National Problem* (Washington, D.C., GAO, HRD 80–17, November 19, 1979).

United States Comptroller General, General Accounting Office, *The Well-Being of Older People in Cleveland, Ohio* (Washington, D.C., April 19, 1977).

United States Department of Health, Education, and Welfare, OPPS, *State Tables 1975, Medicaid: Recipients, Payments, and Services,* NCSS Report B–4 and B–4 Supplement.

United States Senate, Special Committee on Aging, *Nursing Home Care in the United States: Failure in Public Policy,* Supporting Paper No. 7, "The Role of Nursing Homes in Caring for Discharged Mental Patients (And the Birth of a For-Profit Boarding Home Industry), Washington, D.C.: March 1976.

United States Veterans Administration, Dept. of Medicine and Surgery,

"Services and Costs of the VA Hospital Based Home Care Program" (Washington, D.C., Veterans Administration, February 1980, mimeo).

Wan, Thomas T.H., William G. Weissert, and Barbara B. Livieratos, "Determinants of Outcomes of Care in Two Geriatric Service Modalities: An Experimental Study," paper delivered at the November 1978 meeting of the Gerontological Society.

Weissert, William G., "Toward a Continuum of Care for the Elderly: A Note of Caution," *Public Policy*, Summer 1981, forthcoming.

Weissert, William G., Thomas T.H. Wan, Barbara B. Livieratos, and Julius Pellegrino, "Cost Effectiveness of Homemaker Services for the Chronically Ill, *Inquiry*, Fall 1980, pp. 230–243.

Weissert, William G., "Costs of Adult Day Care: A Comparison to Nursing Homes," *Inquiry*, March 1978, pp. 10–19.

Weissert, William G., Thomas T.H. Wan, Barbara B. Livieratos, and Sidney Katz, "Effects and Costs of Day-Care Services for the Chronically Ill," *Medical Care*, June 1980, pp. 567–584.

Weissert, William G., Thomas T.H. Wan, and Barbara B. Livieratos, *Effects and Costs of Day Care and Homemaker Services for the Chronically Ill, A Randomized Experiment*, DHEW (DHS) 79–3258 (Hyattsville, Maryland: National Center for Health Services Research, February 1980).

Willemain, Thomas R., "Beyond the GAO Cleveland Study: Client Selection for Home Care Services," Discussion Paper DP–23, Brandeis University, University Health Policy Consortium, January 1980.

Chapter X

The Significance of Housing as a Resource

by Steven G. Thomas

This chapter analyzes the significance of housing as a resource of long-term care. It begins with a review of how and under what conditions the elderly are housed and then summarizes the major housing problems of the dependent elderly. It continues with an examination of the housing policy objectives and programs initiated by the Federal government to assist the elderly. Finally, the government's housing efforts are evaluated according to how well the programs serve the chronically ill or functionally disabled older person. Complementing this final evaluation are recommendations for improving the range and quality of housing options for the frail and impaired elderly.

Overview

How are the Elderly Housed?

"Housing is a major variable physically, socially, and psychologically, in the lives of older people. It is an integral part of the trinity that perks up one's quality of living, the other two being sufficient income and good health" (U.S. Senate, Special Committee on Aging, 1980).

To fully appreciate the significance of housing and its relationship to long-term care, we must first review the characteristics of the chronically impaired elderly. This overview is a useful introduction to a more detailed analysis of how housing may affect the life of a dependent or frail elderly person.

Several national surveys have attempted to estimate the size and physical condition of the dependent elderly population. In 1975, the *National Survey of the Aged* (Shanas, 1977) reported that the proportion of non-institutionalized elderly who were bedfast and housebound at home was greater than the proportion of older persons in institutions of all kinds: 10 out of every 100 older persons surveyed were bedfast or homebound. Fourteen percent of the non-institutionalized sample group were restricted in their mobility. (Restricted mobility was defined as bedfast, housebound, or experiencing difficulty in going outdoors.)

In 1976, a National Center for Health Statistics survey found that 45 percent of all elderly were limited in their activities due to chronic conditions. A Congressional Budget Office (CBO) report in 1977 estimated that between 11.8 percent and 16.8 percent of the elderly population was functionally disabled.

Finally, it is important to review the results from a 1976 housing survey conducted by the U.S. Department of Housing and Urban Development (HUD, 1979) to gain a perspective on how the elderly are housed. The major flaw in this survey is that the data do not describe how all of the nation's elderly are housed. HUD only surveys households (one or more people living together) which are "headed" by people 65 or older. The data do not account for the elderly men and women living in households headed by someone younger than 65. Nor do they include the elderly who reside in nursing homes, hospitals, or various types of group quarters. The implications of these incomplete data and the need for more extensive research will be discussed later.

Nonetheless, this product contains, to quote HUD, "the most complete and detailed housing data available." These results provide a framework within which a more comprehensive understanding of the specific housing needs and characteristics of the dependent elderly can be developed in the future.

Total Households and Ownership

- 14.8 million households (20 percent of all households) are headed by a person 65 years or older.
- 10.9 million heads of households, out of the 14.8 million (71 percent of elderly households), own their homes; ownership is highest for couples (83 percent) and lowest for men living alone (52 percent).

Types of Housing

- 4.1 million (28 percent of elderly households) live in structures that have two or more housing units (for example, multi-family dwellings).
- 729,000 (5 percent of elderly households) live in mobile homes.
- 76,000 (less than 1 percent of elderly households) live in hotels or rooming houses.

Household Composition

- 6.7 million households (45 percent of all elderly households) consist of two people headed by a male 65 years or older.
- 465,000 households (3 percent of the elderly households) consist of families where the wife is absent.
- 1.4 million (9 percent of the elderly households) consist of families where the husband is absent.
- 1.4 million (10 percent of the elderly households) consist of men living alone.
- 4.9 million (33 per cent of all elderly households) are composed of women living alone.

392

Location

- 63 percent of all elderly households reside in Standard Metropolitan Statistical Areas (SMSAs), and they are concentrated primarily within inner cities.
- 37 percent live in non-SMSA areas.

As will be shown, these characteristics relate intimately to the satisfaction of an older person's needs and requirements for some form of long-term care. Moreover, the results from these and future surveys are essential to guide the planning and operation of quality long-term care housing programs.

The Ideal: Appropriate and Adequate Housing

Housing conditions and services can have a dramatic impact on an older person's ability to cope with a chronic illness or disability. Consequently, the impaired or dependent elderly are vulnerable to the housing environment in which they must live. The most common housing problems experienced by a chronically disabled, elderly person are the result of an inadequate or inappropriate setting.

"Adequate" housing means that the structure and other physical characteristics of a dwelling are conducive to a healthy lifestyle. Some of the common defects found within an inadequate housing unit are a faulty heating unit, a broken-down or incomplete plumbing system, and structural flaws resulting from lack of repair and maintenance. These and other inadequate housing conditions may worsen the dependent status of a chronically disabled, elderly person. Furthermore, flawed physical conditions may actually create dependency and thus a need for institutional long-term care.

"Appropriateness" refers to the level of support services provided (if any) and the size, design, and location of the housing unit. For example, most elderly are homeowners, but the size and architectural features of some homes prevent chronically disabled, older people from managing and maintaining their residences properly. Or an elderly person may be living in a nursing home receiving skilled nursing care when his or her level of impairment and mental capacity would permit a more independent setting.

Whatever the setting (private home, boarding home, nursing home, etc.), the crucial factor is whether the nature of the dwelling and the services offered (if any) are appropriate for the level of care required by a dependent, elderly person. Every functionally limited, older person needs a certain combination of housing and services. The difficult policy and program task is to provide appropriate levels of housing and/or services to match the diverse needs of a dependent population.

Although difficult to separate, the terms adequate and appropriate must be distinguished. Long-term care theory and policy must be concerned with the physical adequacy of a dwelling as well as the appropriateness of the setting. Unless a sensitive understanding is developed and maintained, every long-term care housing strategy will be misdirected.

Major Housing Problems Confronting the Dependent Elderly

Limited Income

Income status usually determines whether dependent older people are able to locate, maintain, or continue living in adequate and appropriate housing. The HUD housing survey found that, compared with other age groups, the average elderly person must pay a larger proportion of his or her income for housing. More importantly, "The need for adequate income is perhaps the most critical problem confronting the aging population of the United States . . . older persons' economic insecurity is a problem that permeates all other dimensions of existence" (Binstock, 1979).

The functionally disabled elderly are especially vulnerable to the relationship between income and housing. Many dependent older people must endure larger health care costs than the average elderly person because of chronic ailments. Also, some of the chronically disabled require a unique combination of housing and services. Such a setting is usually more expensive than a normal rental or housing unit on the market.

This brief review examines the income status of all the elderly. Unfortunately, there are no data which describe the economic status of dependent older people. Yet, this overview illustrates the crucial interdependence between older people's incomes and the quality of their living environments.

Housing costs absorb a disproportionate amount of an older person's income, and in 1979 an elderly person's income was (on the average) 50 percent less than that of a non-elderly person. In 1978, the median annual income for families headed by a person 65 years or older (8.5 million families) was $10,141. This is about 52 percent of the median income for families with younger household heads. The 7.6 million older persons who were either living alone or with non-relatives in 1978 had a median income of $4,303, compared with $8,530 for the similar group under 65 (U.S. Senate, Special Commitee on Aging, 1980).

Moreover, elderly low income is often at the poverty level. In 1978, 3.2 million elderly, or 14 percent of the 65 plus population, were poor according to the poverty definition. In comparison, 24.5 million persons of all ages (11.4 percent of the total population) were below this poverty threshold. However, the person who developed that index, Mollie Orshansky, has recently revamped it to reflect current conditions. The estimates are that 8.7 million elderly, or 36 percent of the aged, are currently living below the revised poverty line (Binstock, 1979).

A complete review of the income status of the elderly must recognize the important role assets play in supplementing an older person's income. Assets accounted for 18 percent of the aggregate income for all elderly (those 65 or older) in 1976. In the same year, 56 percent of all the elderly received a median income of $870 from assets. By far the most valuable, non-liquid asset for most elderly is equity in their homes. Home ownership can provide both direct and indirect income benefits. Since most elderly have their mortgages paid off, they are able to live in a rent-free dwelling. Cash can be generated by renting a portion of the home, selling the home, or borrowing against its appraised value. Income can also be generated through income tax deductions for property taxes and mortgage interest payments.

For some of these home equity assets to be taken advantage of, the house must be sold and replaced by less expensive, suitable quarters. Many elderly people, however, have a psychological attachment to their homes which, in terms of health and well-being, may outweigh its cash value. Also, the major portion of an elderly homeowner's assets are in a form that is difficult to use.

The Absence of a Housing Continuum

Another housing problem experienced by the chronically ill or disabled elderly is the absence of a variety of appropriate housing environments. Within the current housing market, the dependent elderly usually confront two housing options: one, a totally independent unit which must be maintained by the renter or owner or two, an institutional setting. The alternatives are very limited or nonexistent for the frail or chronically disabled older person who requires a combination of adequate housing within an appropriate setting or facility.

Since the "housing continuum" concept is playing an increasingly important role as a guide for future elderly housing policy, it is useful to review several formulations of this ideal.

At the 1971 White House Conference on Aging, delegates called for a national statement of goals on the provision of a spectrum of housing for the elderly. Included in this spectrum were:

- long-term care facilities for the sick,
- facilities with limited medical care and food and homemaker services for those who needed continual supervision and assistance,
- congregate housing with food and personal services for those who require some assistance but who only need routine medical care, and

- housing for independent living with recreational and program activities provided.

More recently, HUD officials have recognized the need for a spectrum of facilities, but they say that such a concept has not materialized because of the conflicting perceptions held by HUD and the Department of Health and Human Services (HHS). As a result, the housing and personal needs of the elderly person tend to be provided in a rigid, uncoordinated manner. HUD uses an "aging spectrum" to show how the two agencies view the needs of the elderly differently. (See Figures X-1 and X-2.) At the "younger" end of the spectrum (60 to 70) a person's housing needs are primary, and HUD is attempting to provide the necessary assistance. HHS, however, (according to HUD) begins with medical and social assumptions which usually result in the provision of institutional and/or acute medical care. Finally, in the middle of this spectrum lies a gap where the social, personal, and housing needs of the elderly, especially the dependent elderly, are unmet by any type of institution. Ideally, to minimize this gap, housing solutions must incorporate social service assumptions rather than medical assumptions. This includes congregate housing and dining, group residential facilities, and homemaker and personal care services.

From HHS' perspective, the Health Care Financing Administration's (HCFA's) Task Force on Long-Term Care has also developed an ideal range, or continuum, of settings for long-term care. In this Department's view, the setting in which long-term care services might be delivered is among the most important issues in long-term care policy. Aside from developing a setting which is most beneficial to the needs of the individual, the following issues must also be considered:

- cost-effectiveness of service delivery in alternative settings,
- mechanisms for quality assurance appropriate for various settings,
- alternative uses of personnel in the different settings, and
- evaluation of the real range of alternatives available at a particular time in a particular place, and the cost of those alternatives.

Functioning Within a Private Home

HUD's 1976 survey found that the rate of physical deficiencies or inadequate conditions for housing for the elderly was comparable to that of the total household population. However, even though 90 percent of housing for the elderly was deemed adequate, 47 percent of all elderly households lived in housing built before 1940, and almost 60 percent of the older households lived in structures built before 1950. In comparison, 30 percent of the younger households

396

FIGURE X-1
Different Agency Perceptions:
HUD vs. HHS

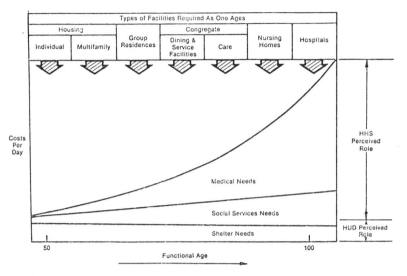

Source: Morton Leeds
Congregate Services Division
Department of Housing and Urban Development (1980)

397

FIGURE X-2
Changing Needs with Increasing
Age and Disability

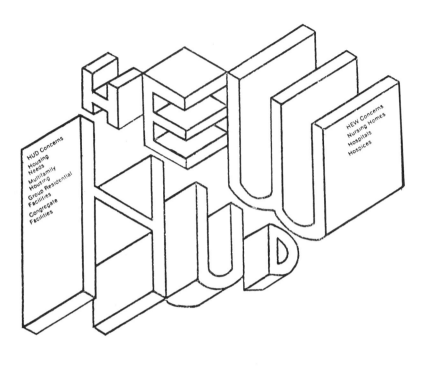

Increasing Age and Disability ▶

Source: U.S. Department of Urban Development, *Challenge,* Vol. X, No. 8, August 1979

lived in units built before 1940, and 40 percent lived in housing built before 1950.

These statistics are significant because the age of a housing unit can create a variety of problems for a dependent older person. An Urban Institute report (Lee, 1980) found that the rate of housing inadequacy increases substantially with the age of the structure. Consequently, since many elderly households live in older units, it is likely that they will experience a variety of maintenance and repair problems. And yet, for some elderly with chronic disabilities and/or modest income, their ability to contend with maintenance and care-taking chores is limited.

In addition, a large number of elderly homeowners may be "over-housed." (Overhousing is a condition of having an excess or inappro-priate amount of living space.) As family members mature and leave their homes, parents may find that they have more space than they desire. This situation of having excess room often requires extra housekeeping and maintenance work. Over time, the older person's ability, physically and financially, to preserve an adequate living environment diminishes. For the functionally disabled elderly it is especially difficult to cope with a chronic condition within an in-appropriate setting. Architectural features such as stairs may impair the ability of dependent, older people to live and manage in their own homes.

Limited Availability of Rental Housing

For those dependent elderly who are unable to adequately main-tain their own homes, the practical solution may be to move into a smaller rental unit. According to the Bureau of Census, however, in 1979 the vacancy rate for rental housing dropped to its lowest point in recorded history. By March 1979, the rate had dropped to 4.8 per-cent nationwide for average-size dwellings (U.S. Senate, Special Committee on Aging, 1980). The higher costs of construction, con-version, and abandonment of buildings have contributed to the scarcity of rental units.

Within this tight rental market, the functionally disabled older per-son is hard-pressed to find appropriate, affordable units. Many frail or chronically ill elderly people are unable to compete with younger persons because of their limited mobility and income. Furthermore, an extremely low occupancy rate hinders the development of alter-native housing settings, because the construction industry turns to more lucrative housing ventures.

The Poor Condition of Small Community and Rural Housing

The housing problems experienced by the chronically impaired rural elderly are potentially more severe than what an older person in an urban area may confront. Thirty-eight percent (8.4 million) of all elderly persons reside in non-SMSA areas (U.S. Senate, Special Committee on Aging, 1980). In 1979, the greatest incidence of poverty among the aged was in rural areas. Also, 60 percent of the nation's substandard housing is located in rural America, with about 25 percent of these units occupied by an older individual (U.S. Senate, Special Committee on Aging, 1980). Finally, more than 50 percent of the rural elderly live in homes that were built prior to 1915.

For the chronically ill and immobile, these features of rural housing and rural life can be very frustrating. Very old homes in need of repair and with too much space, a scarce supply of appropriate, alternative housing settings, and the isolated lifestyle of rural living can have a devastating effect on the well-being of a dependent older person. As policymakers consider developing a spectrum of housing, it is essential that they be sensitive to the special circumstances of the dependent rural elderly.

Deficient and Misleading Housing Terminology

The development of alternative long-term care settings has been stifled by the confusing and misconstrued terms used to define various housing/care arrangements. "Conceivably, in different states, the terms nursing home, proprietary home, foster home, or senior residential facility could be defined differently . . . Varying terminology may be used to describe similar facilities, and the same terminology may be used to describe varying facilities" (Kerschner and Cote, 1979). This poorly defined classification system of housing creates a number of problems for the chronically impaired elderly.

First, the amount of income assistance that a dependent elderly person may receive is partly determined by the classification of his or her housing/care facility. Stipulations concerning housing arrangements are incorporated into the eligibility requirements of the Supplemental Security Income program. Furthermore, the distribution of Medicare and Medicaid funds is contingent on the type of setting in which the long-term care is provided. For example, income eligibility levels under Medicaid may be higher if a person is in a nursing home than in his or her own home, receiving home health care.

Secondly, a confusing array of housing terms makes it difficult for a dependent person to search for and select a suitable dwelling. Without a uniform classification of housing types and settings, many frail and impaired older people must expend precious amounts of physical and emotional energy locating an appropriate unit. Until housing concepts are accurately reflected in standard terms, the chronically disabled elderly will continue to struggle with locating and choosing an adequate and appropriate setting.

400

Finally, the lack of a coherent and detailed housing terminology leads to ineffective and unresponsive long-term care policy. Without a clear set of terms, officials are unable to develop the precise understanding which is needed to debate and formulate future policy initiatives. Also, the policy-making arena requires more quality research concerning the housing needs of the dependent elderly. (This need for more research will be discussed in more detail later in this chapter.) But for the research to have any value, a standard criterion for housing settings must be adopted so that comparability across studies can be enhanced.

The Federal Perspective

The public sector, especially the Federal government, has become an important provider of housing for the functionally disabled elderly. Through a variety of direct subsidies and loan programs, the government has been able to influence the type and amount of housing supplied. In addition, other Federal program efforts, such as income maintenance, play a critical role in determining an impaired elderly person's ability to acquire both adequate and appropriate housing. Because of the government's prominent role, it is necessary to review federal housing initiatives and determine the effect of these government programs on the development of alternative housing/service arrangements.

The Most Significant Federal Housing Programs for the Elderly

Six programs will be examined to determine how they reflect the government's understanding of the housing problems confronting the dependent elderly. Also, the Federal policy objectives for housing the elderly, as exhibited through current program efforts, will be reviewed. Lastly, these six housing programs will be evaluated according to how well they reflect a Federal appreciation for the relationship between elderly housing and long-term care requirements. The first four programs to be examined are significant because they have funded the greatest proportion of Federally-subsidized elderly living units. The final two programs are important because they represent the government's most significant attempt to provide for the special housing needs of the chronically impaired elderly.

(1) Low-Income Public Housing—Section 3, Section 4, Title II
529,000 elderly units (as of June 30, 1978)

The elderly have been eligible for low-income public housing since its initiation under the U.S. Housing Act of 1937. Among the major problems with public housing is that most prospective residents must wait several years for an available unit. Also, the construction of public housing specifically designed for the elderly was not authorized until 1965. Consequently, much of the public housing is structurally inadequate for frail or chronically ill older persons. In addition, public housing agencies are faced with increasing numbers of the elderly who, as they age, become more frail or impaired. Usually public units are not appropriate for occupants who can only maintain semi-independent living. Recently, HUD has been attempting to coordinate its efforts with other agencies so that support services can be provided to the chronically ill or disabled elderly. With the introduction of the Congregate Housing Services Program, a small number of public housing facilities will begin to provide meals and personal care.

(2) Low-Income Rental Assistance Section 8, Housing and Community Development Act of 1977, as Amended

Existing units—199,718 (as of April 30, 1979)
New units—251,034 (as of April 30, 1979)
Rehabilitated units—28,253 (as of April 30, 1979)
Total number of elderly units—478,465

Ideally, the Section 8 program (by providing rental assistance to residents) encourages the construction of new units, the substantial rehabilitation of units, and access to existing dwellings. Under the Section 8 program, no family may pay more than 25 percent of its income for rent. The eligibility requirements have been expanded to include two or more unrelated elderly living together, or one or more individuals living with a person who needs their care and support.

There are, however, several major problems with the Section 8 program. One, only a limited number of Section 8 units are available. Two, most units cannot accommodate the frail or chronically ill older person. And three, only a small proportion of the Section 8 units are included in the Congregation Housing Services Program.

(3) Direct Loans for Housing for the Elderly and Handicapped— Section 202 of the Housing Act of 1959

110,239 elderly units (as of April 30, 1979)

Under Section 202, Federal loans to private, non-profit sponsors are provided to develop new or substantially rehabilitated housing for the elderly or physically handicapped. The program is mandated to have all sponsors classified as private, non-profit organizations, and it provides construction loans that cover 100 percent of the project costs. Over half of the program sponsors have been religious institutions, with the remaining half composed of union, community-based, and cooperative organizations. There are two periods of Section 202 history: The "old" program, which existed from 1959 to 1968, and the "new" program, from 1974 to the present.

402

Along with the living units, Section 202 projects are required to provide a variety of necessary services for elderly occupants. HUD's own evaluation of Section 202 housing projects revealed that the program had produced highly sought-after housing projects, that the projects were sponsored by capable, non-profit organizations, and that the resources were provided at a cost which compares favorably with other elderly housing programs (U.S. House of Representatives, Select Committee on Aging, 1979). Most Section 202 projects have extremely low turnover rates and long waiting lists. Many officials who are familiar with the Federal housing initiatives feel that Section 202 is HUD's most successful program. Much of this success is attributed to the commitment, accountability, and quality of the non-profit sponsors.

As with all Federal housing programs, the availability of 202 units is limited. Some blame the two or more years it takes HUD to approve 202 projects. There simply is not enough loan money to fund all eligible 202 applicants. Another issue is that tenants in 202 projects have traditionally been white, middle-income, elderly females. Under the "old" 202 program, only 7 percent of all residents were minorities. Although there are no income limitations, most 202 projects are now linked to Section 8 subsidies, and a greater effort is being made to fund minority projects. Because of the low turnover rates of their aging tenants, 202 projects are experiencing an increasing need to provide specialized services. The Congregate Housing Services Program was created, in part, to make Section 202 housing more responsive to the service and care needs of the frail and aging elderly residents.

(4) Mortgage Insurance for Housing for the Elderly—
Section 231

65,979 elderly units (as of fiscal year 1979)

Section 231 is HUD's principal program for assisting the elderly who live in unsubsidized rental housing. This program insures lenders against any losses on mortgages used to build or rehabilitate rental accommodations for older persons. The intent of Section 231 is to insure loans for rental units which would help to improve the ability of an elderly or handicapped person to live independently. However, the provision of supportive and personal care services is not a component of this program.

(5) Nursing Home and Intermediate Care Facilities—
Section 232

141,289 elderly units (as of December 1978)

About 10 percent of all nursing homes are financed through this guaranteed/insured loan program for the construction and improvement of nursing homes and related facilities.

403

Funding this type of elderly "housing" has become a controversial initiative. Many argue that nursing home assistance reflects the instituitional bias which underlies most Federal programs for the dependent or chonically impaired elderly. Moreover, some claim that there may be an oversupply of institutional beds because of the emphasis on Federal subsidies. Yet more analysts are claiming that there is a nursing home bed shortage. Whatever the arguments, it is clear that the Federal government directs most of its housing money for the dependent elderly into institutions. And there is evidence which shows that some elderly may be institutionalized unnecessarily because no other housing options exist.

(6) Congregate Housing Service Program—Title IV of the 1978 Housing Act

Potentially 1,600 elderly units

The Congregate Housing Services Program is designed to encourage the development of a housing continuum which relates directly to the realities of the aging process. Under this Act, public housing agencies and Section 202 borrowers may receive funds to provide meals and other supportive services to eligible project residents. These services are meant to help elderly occupants live independently, preventing their premature or unnecessary institutionalization. The basic service component, however, is the food program: all the other services, such as personal assistance, household chores, and transportation, are optional. Overall, the program ties support services to housing to guarantee a long-term funding source, provide an incentive for the construction of congregate facilities, and fill the gap in the housing spectrum.

Ten million dollars were appropriated in both fiscal years 1979 and 1980 to fund congregate projects. Out of each year's allocation, HUD retained $1 million for inflation allowances and other adjustments and is distributing the remaining $9 million over a three-year, contract period. Funds will be split between public housing agencies (50 percent) and Section 202 projects (50 percent). Within this division, approximately 80 percent of the money will go to existing projects and 20 percent will support new construction. HUD estimates that the elderly will receive about 85 percent of the total funds, with the non-elderly handicapped receiving the remaining 15 percent.

Housing for the Functionally Impaired Elderly and the Government's Interpretation of the Problem

The housing programs outlined above address, from the Federal government's perspective, the major housing problems confronting all elderly. First, there is only a limited supply of adequate living units for those elderly who can live independently. Second, because most of the elderly are living on very limited or fixed incomes, they need rental assistance and homeownership subsidies. Third, some elderly, due to functional disabilities and insufficient support from families or friends, are unable to live independently; therefore, intermediate care and skilled nursing home facilities are required.

What is significant, however, is that the objectives and perspectives embodied in these Federal programs are quite different from the views expressed in current government documents. In contrast to the actual programs, the Federal housing literature presents a more comprehensive and detailed understanding of the housing problems experienced by elderly persons. Accordingly, Federal officials have outlined on paper a series of elderly housing objectives which (if they were properly implemented) would produce a more complete spectrum of housing alternatives.

There are numerous examples of this discrepancy between Federal objectives for housing the elderly and actual program efforts. For instance, on paper the Congregate Housing Services Program is the most important housing policy innovation in recent years. This new legislation recognizes the need to implement a housing/services continuum; it is sensitive to the relationship between housing and long-term care, and it realizes the necessity for interagency coordination. Moreover, the Congregate Housing Program was expected to help prevent the premature or unnecessary institutionalization of the dependent elderly. In its present form, however, the project will have little impact on the development of congregate care facilities. Until the program receives more financial, political, and administrative support, congregate housing will continue to be a concept for the future.

As a second example, most Federal officials agree that a well-planned, consolidated delivery system is needed to produce a successful program of dependent elderly housing/services. One of the major objectives behind the congregate housing legislation was to coordinate the Federal programs serving the chronically impaired and to avoid a duplication of services. Although the potential exists, an effective system of interagency cooperation has not developed.

The current focus of Medicare and Medicaid funding is another illustration of how the government has failed to implement what it considers important policy objectives. Critics argue that the unnecessary and costly use of institutional care has been encouraged because these programs offer limited funding for alternative housing options. HCFA's Long-Term Care Task Force reported that long-term care services currently provided in non-institutional settings are minimally supported by public money and, to a large extent, are subsidized by private sources. In contrast, institution-based services are substantially financed by public expenditures. Fifty-three percent of the total nursing home bill is underwritten by public programs; 90 percent of all public dollars earmarked for long-term care is spent on nursing home care (U.S. Department of Health and Human Services, 1980).

Both Congress and Administration officials are beginning to realize that this institutional bias within the health care financing programs is stifling the development of non-institutional settings, including appropriate housing, for the chronically impaired. Nonetheless, major changes in Medicare and Medicaid legislation which might reduce the institutional bias have not been enacted.

Finally, two programs deserve mention because they, too, were created to address some of the housing problems of older people. Yet once again, these programs are an example of how Federal efforts have produced very minimal results. Many elderly homeowners, especially the functionally disabled, experience difficulties in maintaining or repairing their homes. Given the number of elderly homeowners, and the disproportionate age of their homes, it is ironic that the Federal loan program for housing rehabilitation (Section 312, Housing Act of 1964, as amended), provides what one HUD official called an "insignificant amount of funds." Furthermore, most older people are not anxious to use credit and assume a debt. In short, the 312 program, due to limited funds and poor program design, is not a valuable source of housing assistance for the elderly, despite its housing rehabilitation focus.

The second necessary, but minimal, housing effort is directed by the Farmers Home Administration. As was mentioned earlier, many of the rural elderly live in very old homes which, combined with various aspects of rural life, can be debilitating for a frail older person. Rural housing loans under Section 504 provide funds to qualified low-income applicants to make basic repairs to improve the health and safety conditions of a home. Section 502 provides loans for the building, purchase, or rehabilitation of modest homes.

Once again, limited funding and the nature of the Section 502 and 504 programs stifle their effectiveness. In fiscal year 1980, $24 million was available for 504 loans, and $3.08 billion for 502. But most of the money is dispersed through loans which discourage elderly participation. Moreover, neither of the programs has been designed to meet the long-term care requirements of a dependent older person.

This brief review of some very important, but relatively ineffective, Federal housing programs serves two purposes. One, it illustrates how officials can experience tremendous difficulties as they attempt to translate policy objectives into actual programs. If major, innovative housing legislation is to be enacted, planners of long-term care for the elderly must learn how to maneuver housing program objectives through a very competitive policy arena. More important, these insignificant efforts show that the government is becoming concerned and more aware of the housing requirements of the

406

dependent elderly. Granted, a more substantial commitment is necessary, but many Federal officials appear willing to establish a more complete spectrum of housing facilities.

Federal Objectives for Housing the Dependent Elderly

As this review shows, the range and focus of the Federal housing initiatives for the dependent elderly are very narrow. At the program level, Federal officials have been insensitive to the limited availability of appropriate housing arrangements for the chronically impaired elderly who do not require an institutional setting. Overall, Federal housing initiatives have addressed the need for adequate units, but these policies have failed to recognize the demand for appropriate settings. And yet, an appropriate setting is a vital component of long term care for an impaired older person.

Recently however, the government has begun to recognize that most publicly-supported housing units are inappropriate settings for the functionally disabled. But, within the total realm of housing programs for all the elderly, there are few initiatives which demonstrate any Federal intentions to encourage the development of a spectrum of housing settings. Moreover, all the housing objectives which address the needs of the dependent elderly reflect the government's limited understanding of housing and its relationship to long-term care. Most of the objectives concerning housing for the chronically impaired are expressed in vague generalities; no real, substantive policy goals are suggested.

Aside from subsidizing the building of nursing homes, the government is beginning to support a small number of housing alternatives which provide for the long-term care needs of a chronically impaired older person (for example, the Congregate Housing Services Program). Also, in theory at least, Federal officials now recognize the need for a spectrum of housing and care. Along with a desire to ensure a suitable array of long-term care services, the Government is very anxious to develop alternative care settings to offset the tremendous costs of institutional care. With political and financial pressures demanding a more efficient system, it is both expedient and wise for the government to encourage the creation of a more complete range of housing settings.

Long-Term Care Analysis and Recommendations

In the analysis that follows, several recommendations will be introduced which are just as essential as the most encompassing reform proposal. Housing advocates for the functionally disabled are certainly aware of the issues which will be discussed. But quite often the significance of these particular reforms is downplayed within the housing policy arena. Because of the pressures and the

407

nature of the legislative process, it is extremely difficult to maintain a complete perspective on the many important factors related both to housing and long-term care. The specific reforms outlined below are needed to implement and support the development of a spectrum of housing care settings.

1) A coordinated, systematic approach for planning, and delivering housing services to the dependent elderly must be established.

The planners and providers of housing for the chronically impaired must develop a more comprehensive perspective concerning the relationships between housing and the provision of long-term care services. They must review and appreciate the entire social environment; housing must be seen as a social service which must be linked with income, social services, and health care programs.

Part of the current problem lies with HUD and its "engineering" approach to planning housing services. As an agency, HUD has opposed the Congregate Housing Services Program from the beginning, because (said one HUD official) "We are engineers, not social service providers." Settings for the functionally disabled can no longer be viewed just as shelter, but must, as well, be recognized as a service(s) center.

This sensitive and comprehensive approach for the planning and provision of housing can only be achieved within a coordinated, well-managed delivery system. Presently, however, the Federal government has no systematic method for developing and guiding its housing programs for the elderly, especially those needing long-term support. As one HUD official wrote, ". . . there is no longer any point of focus in HUD for elderly concerns . . . only on special occasions . . . have the experts in assistance to the elderly been required to collaborate on anything like a systematic basis for any period of time" (Leeds, 1979). According to Rep. Claude Pepper, there are at least 11 programs administered by three different agencies within HUD that directly affect the elderly (U.S. House of Representatives, 1979).

The Congregate Housing Services Program is a victim of this unorganized effort to provide housing to the elderly. Administratively, most doubt that the necessary cooperation between HUD and HHS will develop fully. In fact, some officials believe that congregate housing, subsidized by the government, will cost more than institutional care because of redundant and uncoordinated administrative efforts.

Consolidating all elderly programs and coordinating among agencies are essential to create a spectrum of adequate and appropriate housing programs. Before this ideal can be realized however, some

408

fundamental organizational and administrative reforms must be initiated.

2) Housing maintenance programs must also be concerned with providing appropriate housing.

All elderly, independent and functionally-disabled alike, require adequate housing. Current maintenance programs, however, do not address the issue of appropriate housing for the chronically impaired elderly. Physical improvements to an older person's home, such as roof repairs or weatherization, are important, but, because of a chronic condition, the person may require a completely different, more appropriate housing setting.

Yet, the focus and intent of housing maintenance programs could be expanded to finance home modifications. Along with addressing the problem of inadequate housing, these programs could eliminate structural barriers from the homes of frail and physically impaired older people. Such efforts would improve the appropriateness of a dependent person's housing environment and may delay the need for a more institutional setting. Overall, the focus of government housing maintenance programs must be altered to include a concern for providing an appropriate living environment.

3) The institutional bias contained within the income maintenance and health care financing programs must be eliminated.

The Medicare, Medicaid, and income maintenance programs have been blamed for stifling the development of alternative housing/care facilities. In general, these programs will only provide maximum benefits if the recipient is either able to live independently or requires intense medical care. Medicaid and Medicare eligibility and reimbursement policies create financial incentives to use nursing homes rather than community-based long-term care services. This is because both programs provide slight coverage for care provided in the home or in other non-medical facilities. Program expenditures reflect this emphasis on institutional care: 41 percent of all Medicaid funds went to cover nursing home costs in 1978. In the same year 1 percent of other total expenditures were used to fund community-based, long-term care services (General Accounting Office, 1979).

For the most part, this institutional bias is the product of a narrow perspective held by policymakers. As the Social Security and Supplemental Security Income programs evolved over time, officials failed to recognize the varied long-term care requirements of the dependent elderly. As a result, stipulations within these programs (for example, Section 1616(e) of the Social Security Act and the long-term care provisions of Title XVIII and Title XIX) are so

409

stringent that providers have only had an incentive to supply a limited range of housing facilities. The fundamental assumptions behind these current policies must be altered so that a greater variety and less expensive array of housing arrangements can be subsidized. Specifically, officials must realize that the chronically impaired require funds for various levels of care within different settings.

4) Housing programs for the chronically impaired must be sensitive to the needs and characteristics of future residents.

A scarce supply of funds combined with the need for appropriate housing settings requires a long-range, comprehensive planning technique. Currently, the government expends most of its housing planning energy on altering or patching up the flaws in present policy. The nature and tradition of our policymaking process requires immediate and incremental reforms. Federal officials however, must also use existing tools and knowledge to provide a variety of housing arrangements that will "remain vital and appropriate over time" (Newcomer, 1976).

In the words of Robert Newcomer, "If decisions for the future are made in relation only to today's needs, priorities, and resources, without consideration of likely future events or population preferences, the buildings and environments produced will probably constitute serious handicaps as the future unfolds. It is essential that flexibility be programmed into plans and service systems, while incorporating as much as can be known of future contingencies" (Newcomer, 1976).

5) The crucial relationship between the quality of a housing setting and an older person's income status must be recognized.

At present, housing policy for the chronically impaired is being formulated within a vacuum; planners have not realized the need to synchronize and coordinate Federal housing initiatives with the broad array of income, health care financing and tax programs. Programs other than housing must be evaluated for their economic impact so that the dependent elderly can be assured an adequate and appropriate housing environment.

Equally important, but often overlooked, is the prominent role which assets and taxes play in determining an older persons level of income (Baer, 1976).

. . . a very important subsidy program to the older (homeowner), is that established through special provisions in the Federal income tax. The value of the income derived from net housing services is not declared as income by the owner occupant; that is, there is no declaration of imputed rent. The homeowner of any

410

age can also deduct that portion of his mortgage that goes toward interest and the amount of his yearly property taxes. The amount of subsidy derived from just the homeowner income tax deductions was $1.7 billion for all elderly homeowners in 1970. In contrast to these homeowner tax benefits, there are no explicit federal income tax provisions for renters.

Overall, the effectiveness of new housing initiatives will be directly influenced by how well officials are able to complement their programs with adequate income maintenance and tax programs.

6) More pertinent research concerning the housing and long-term care requirements of the chronically impaired is required.

"By far the most visible mechanism for feedback and input to the policy planning and design process of housing for the elderly has been research" (Newcomer, 1976). And yet, even though a considerable amount of literature has been published, very little has been written on the relationship between long-term care and the housing requirements of the dependent elderly. The list for suggested research is extensive; however, there are some fundamental studies, suggested below, which should receive immediate priority.

The size and characteristics of the chronically impaired elderly population need to be measured and studied more thoroughly. Several studies which attempt to generate this information were cited earlier in the chapter. Yet, as William Pollak (1976) has written, ". . . accurate information about the size of different population groupings is rare, and planners and policymakers have no choice but to use figures whose measuring is unclear" (Pollak, 1976).

In addition, housing planners must know more about the specific housing problems confronted by the dependent elderly. Officials require information that would improve their understanding of how inadequate and/or inappropriate housing conditions aggravate or create a need for long-term care services. But as Lawton has stated, "Data do not exist that would tell us the extent to which housing and other environmental problems compound this group's vulnerability" (Lawton, 1978). Regardless of these limitations, a better perspective on how the housing setting interacts with the dependent lifestyle of a chronically impaired older person is essential.

An attempt must be made to measure the potential utilization for each type of housing setting contained within the long-term care housing spectrum. Furthermore, this research must be supplemented by studies which indicate how many dependent elderly are currently housed under inadequate or inappropriate conditions. Data from both types of studies are important because (when used with current utilization numbers) they can help to identify gaps in the present housing system and enrich our understanding of utilization patterns

411

(Pollak, 1976a). Moreover, the most efficient and effective distribution of limited program funds is dependent upon knowing how many and what type of housing units are required.

Pollak (1976a) presents a good overview of the research needs in this policy area and offers various suggestions for improving future utilization studies. He also cites two prominent studies that examine the optional and actual placement of functionally impaired elderly persons in different parts of upstate New York: *An Areawide Examination of Nursing Home Use, Misuse, and Nonuse* (Davis and Gibbon, 1971) and *Health Care of the Aged Study* (Hill, 1968). These and other similar research efforts could serve as useful models for formulating more extensive and thorough utilization studies.

The merits of this type of research are obvious, but Pollak identifies several pitfalls which make it difficult to project housing utilization levels. One, nobody knows how one housing service will be substituted for another arrangement, once the various settings are developed. And since there is a limited range of housing types, there is no real program experience on which utilization forecasts can be based.

Policymakers must also have information about the costs of providing long-term care services to the dependent elderly in a variety of settings. In general, there is a need for more complete and comprehensive research that accounts for all the elements which influence the cost of providing long-term care in alternative facilities. Currently, assertions about costs are plentiful, but accurate data concerning the total costs of different housing arrangements are scarce. Pollak (1976b) has stated, "The real social cost of providing care for an elderly person in particular settings will depend critically on (1) the clients' functional impairments (2) the family status of the individual and (3) the quality of the care provided."

Because of individual differences in impairment levels, family status, and quality of care required, the cost of providing care in each of the different settings will vary a great deal. Researchers must be sensitive to these individual characteristics and formulate their results accordingly. In the end, cost comparisons between settings will not be fixed, since the real cost will depend upon the health and family status of the individual. This also means that no one setting will be least expensive for every dependent older person.

The interdependence between income and housing must be analyzed. Throughout this chapter, the importance of a dependent older person's income status has been emphasized. Yet, there is little research to clarify the influence of income on a dependent elderly person's housing. More information is needed concerning the effects of Social Security, SSI, pensions, and assets on a dependent older person's ability to live appropriately. In addition, the

412

significance of a person's home as equity is obvious, but the potential advantages and problems in using this asset need to be examined. The value of quality research as a guide for producing new and innovative housing initiatives is apparent. However, unless these studies are properly managed and coordinated, the usefulness of the results will be minimal. Furthermore, these research efforts must be a practical aid to policymakers as they strive to develop more effective housing programs for the dependent elderly.

Although research is essential, the focus of a study is dependent upon the type of housing program being evaluated. Specifically, the potential use of alternative settings cannot be based on projected estimates of unmet needs (Pollak, 1976a). Utilization of different housing settings will be determined in part by how many and what type of units will be supplied by the Federal government. Policymakers must provide researchers with a clear set of possible program goals and objectives to provide the necessary direction to housing research.

References

Baer, William C., "Federal Housing Programs for the Elderly," in M. Powell Lawton et al, eds., Community Planning For An Aging Society (Strouds-burg, Pa.: Dowden, Hutchinson, and Ross, Inc., 1976).

Binstock, Robert H., "A Policy Agenda On Aging for the 1980's," National Journal Issues Book: Aging Agenda for the Eighties, (Washington: The National Journal, 1979).

Brody, Stanley J., "The Thirty-to-One Paradox: Health Needs and Medical Solutions," National Journal Issues Book: Aging Agenda for the Eighties (Washington: The National Journal, 1979).

General Accounting Office, Entering a Nursing Home—Costly Implications for Medicaid and The Elderly (Washington: U.S. Government Printing Office, November, 1979), GAO Report.

Kerschner, Paul A. and Meredith Cote, "Deficiencies in Terminology: The Effect on Public Policy," in AAHA, Long Term Care of the Aging A Socially Responsible Approach, (Washington: American Association of Homes for the Aging, 1979).

Lawton, M. Powell, "The Housing Problems of Community-Resident Elderly," HUD Occasional Paper #1, 1978.

Lee, Olson and Neil Mayer, The Effectiveness of Federal Home Repair and Improvement Programs in Meeting Elderly Homeowner Needs (Washington: The Urban Institute, April 1980).

Leeds, Morton, "Housing: Serving the Aged," in U.S. Department of Housing and Urban Development, Challenge, Vol. X, No. 8, August 1979.

Newcomer, Robert J., "Meeting the Housing Needs of Older People," in M. Powell Lawton et al, eds., Community Planning for an Aging Society (Stroudsburg, Pa.: Dowden, Hutchinson, and Ross, Inc., 1976).

Pollak, William, "Utilization of Alternative Care Settings by the Elderly" in M. Powell Lawton et al, eds., Community Planning For an Aging Society (Stroudsburg, Pa.: Dowden, Hutchinson, and Ross, Inc., 1976), 1976a.

Pollak, William, "Costs of Alternative Care Settings for the Elderly," in

413

M. Powell Lawton *et al,* eds., *Community Planning For an Aging Society* Stroudsburg, Pa.: Dowden, Hutchinson and Ross, Inc., 1976), 1976b.

Shanas, Ethel, *National Survey of the Aged 1975,* Final Report to the Administration on Aging, AoA Grant #90–A–369, 1977, processed.

U.S. Department of Health and Human Services, Health Care Financing Administration, Long-Term Care Task Force, *Report on Long-Term Care,* June 1980, processed.

U.S. Department of Housing and Urban Development, *How Well Are We Housed,? The Elderly,* (Washington: U.S. Government Printing Office, 1979).

U.S. House of Representatives, Select Committee on Aging, *Oversight Hearings on Section 202 Housing for the Elderly and Handicapped* (Washington: U.S. Government Printing Office, April 10 and 27, 1979).

U.S. House of Representatives, Select Committee on Aging, *Teamwork in Delivery of Federal Programs to the Elderly* (Washington: U.S. Government Printing Office, October 24, 1979).

U.S. Senate, Special Committee on Aging, *Developments in Aging, 1979,* Part 1 (Washington: U.S. Government Printing Office, 1980).

414

Chapter XI

Adult Day Care

by Hans C. Palmer

Among the most commonly proposed long-term care alternatives to the nursing home are those gathered under the umbrella of adult day care (ADC).[1] Actually, ADC is not an "alternative" but usually part of a spectrum of care. It is not a simply defined category of provision, nor is it simply a substitute for other components of health care.

ADC in some analyses and policy discussions refers to a set of medical, nursing, physical therapy, occupational therapy, and other specialized procedures. It often includes podiatry, personal hygiene, nutrition, meals, eye examinations, hearing examinations, and personal-social services of various types. In some cases, social and recreational activities may be included, and the mix of health and social services will often indicate the emphasis of a particular ADC program. ADC is provided in an institutional setting to which the patients are transported. They do not, however, require 24-hour nursing care, hence they can live at home or in some other residential or sheltered care facility. Most patients are presumed to be functionally disabled in varying degrees and to need assistance with some of the activities of daily living (ADL). Most commonly, referral is from a physician, a hospital discharge planning program, or the social services system. Note that ADC may include all or some of the listed services.

Other services and ADC may co-exist in combined programs of care. For example, home health and homemaker services often jointly support dependent elderly in comprehensive programs of community care. Alternatively, ADC may complement some form of formal residential care (for example, domiciliary care), especially if care from the family is unavailable. In yet another form, ADC can provide a wide spectrum of support to someone who may be an outpatient for highly specialized service at an acute general hospital. Note also that ADC is distinguished from outpatient care in that the former generally includes transportation to the care site. Addition-

I wish to thank Margaret Stassen for her helpful suggestions for this chapter.

[1] A good discussion of ADC is found in Trager, Brahna, "Adult Day Health Care—A Conference Report," Arlington, Virginia, September, 1977, and Tucson, Arizona, September, 1978, Grant No. 1 R13 HS 10580–01, NCHSR, OASH, May 1979.

415

ally, outpatient care usually emphasizes medical procedures and makes no assumptions about the level of ADL capabilities on the part of the patients.

It should be stressed, however, that no uniform definition or measure of ADC exists at present.

Amounts and Supports of ADC

Europe is much more familiar with ADC than is the United States. Many British geriatricians (John Brocklehurst, Lionel Cosin, Bernard Isaacs, etc.) have installed ADC services as central organizational components in their maintenance programs. Such programs and services are readily accepted parts of the long-term care offerings of the British National Health Service, at least in those areas where there is a clinician with an interest in long-term community care. In the United States, major initiatives for the development of ADC came from the community, not from Federal or State agencies or funding services.

In 1980, there were about 617 ADC programs in 46 States. Their average daily census (1980) was about 13,500. This figure does not represent the same patients all five days of the week, since average weekly attendance ranges from one to five times. The majority attend two to three times per week, implying some need for service on non-ADC days.[2] The number of sites has grown rapidly, from 200 in 1977 to 300 in 1978, and to 600 in 1979.

Sources of support for ADC vary greatly. Overall, few public financial support programs directly reimburse for total ADC programs. Rather, there is provision for specific services, such as nursing, physical and occupational therapy, medical social work, etc. For example, in two-thirds of the States, Medicaid pays for certain specified services, varying among jurisdictions. Medicare covers all usage of certain specified services, regardless of site provision, as long as the services are prescribed by a physician and/or meet other regulations. In addition, under Title III of the Older Americans Act, administered by the Administration on Aging (AoA), some States support ADC-type services. For most programs, the amounts spent on ADC in total is unknown. Under Medicare/Medicaid, for example, it is not possible to trace the ADC connection of many of the covered services. Under Title III, AoA cannot separate ADC services from other types of social services. Title XX data do, however, permit the breakout of ADC support, and these show an annual intended expenditure of $42.6 million in fiscal

---

[2] This information comes from a personal communication with Edith Robbins, HCFA. If the primary emphasis of ADC is medical, it is sometimes referred to as adult day health care or ADHC.

416

year 1979 (Kilgore and Salmon, 1979). This includes some child day care and care for adults under 65.

In addition to the major Federal and State programs cited earlier, other support for ADC comes from voluntary agencies (for example, United Way), philanthropic groups, local governments, and some Federally-funded demonstrations conducted under Medicare waivers. Some health insurance carriers cover ADC, and out-of-pocket fees also are assessed, often on an income-linked, sliding scale. At present, there is no way to determine the amount spent by these various sources on ADC, partly because of the integration of ADC-related services with other types of health care. Knowledgeable observers suggest, however, that possibly 50 percent of the costs of some ADC programs are being paid out-of-pocket. Obviously, such fragmentation in funding support contributes to fragmentation of programs, leading to confusion among users and providers and lessening the beneficial results which ADC might have.

Types of ADC Services

ADC services are sometimes grouped into various "models," such as restorative, maintenance, and social. The *restorative* model presumably has an intensive health care focus, emphasizing constant monitoring, one-on-one therapy, and psycho-social (as well as medical) services. Discharge is usually to a less intensive care site or program after 3½ to four months. *Maintenance* programs are of longer duration, but they also emphasize individual care plans with periodic reassessments with much less intense monitoring, and often with group therapies. *Social* programs, though often directed by a registered nurse, are much more activity-oriented than health-oriented, offering services to lonely, old clients in a protected environment and, at times, arranging for therapies outside the ADC care site. Some social ADC programs strive to keep clients in the community as long as possible by keeping them in contact with their environment (Trager, 1979). Some ADC facilities offer joint levels of care, but most stress one of the listed types of programs.

Weissert (1976) also has provided a useful classification for analyzing ADC systems. Model I focuses heavily on rehabilitation and emphasizes medical provision. Model II has a more social orientation, often approaching the British Day Centre in its wide ranging provision of social and recreational services and in its focus on enhancing the social life of the patients. Model II also may be presumed to cater mainly to patients whose needs are for maintenance; Model I focuses more on therapeutic treatment of diseases. Of course, these distinctions are a bit arbitrary as are the services supposedly found in each. Nonetheless, this typology—much like

417

the previously discussed three-level model—provides some useful axes for comparison among programs. Also, it may facilitate comparison between ADC and other care modes.

It should be noted that the sorting of ADC into "models" of care has been criticized by a number of ADC specialists as being more suited to reimbursement formulae than to the needs of patients (Trager, 1979). Furthermore, these categories cannot capture all of the variations in service configuration. Despite such objections, these classification schemes may be useful starting points for analysis.

Major appropriate client groups for ADC appear to be the severely developmentally disabled over 21, victims of cerebro-vascular accidents (CVAs) and trauma, and the elderly who cannot cope with ADL. In general, as with all other aspects of long-term care, functional disability, coupled with weak social support systems, makes people logical candidates for ADC. In identifying possible clients, patient medical condition, the severity of that condition, and the lack of a suitable support structure all combine to form the profile of need. In light of these determinants of need, enthusiasm for emphasizing so-called preventive efforts of ADC without an educated awareness of the need to set goals, consider the feasibility of restorative programs, and note the other subtle effects that produce surprising outcomes can lead to major disappointments. So also, mental health issues are central to the establishment, analysis, and success of any ADC program, as they are for any type of long-term care, since mental health problems (especially among the elderly) often accompany medical problems and since clients with socio-medical difficulties can disrupt any ADC organization and program. During episodes of mental illness, ADC may not be of any use to them.

The services required in successful ADC programs are very complex. In most cases, health services or, at least, supervision are necessary. Nursing care is often a key element. In addition, most ADC should include nutrition programs, both to provide good meals and to counsel clients on how to eat and prepare food. Information and referral services are essential in coping with complicated socio-medical problems, as are the efforts of client assessors, care planners, counselors, and others who can assist with integrating patients into (or back into) the community. These activities might, to varying degrees, also be found in other care modalities, but the community interaction of ADC programs and their express purpose of keeping clients in the community, while offering socio-economic assistance, renders some of the services all the more critical.

Somewhat unexpectedly, providing transportation in ADC has generated much controversy. On the one hand, there are those who argue that transportation services are crucial for outreach to the community to bring in many clients who otherwise could not come

418

in. Others argue that the ADC centers should not provide too much transport, since family involvement and contributions are crucial to the success of any ADC program. Both sides, however, agree that transportation should emphasize the use of multi-purpose equipment. A key problem with transport, of course, is its cost, which can often reach 50 percent of program expenditures.

In providing service, proper space is central to success. Not only must space be adequate, but also access to needed services and supports must be guaranteed, for example, the rehabilitation facilities of an acute general hospital. In some cases, these facilities suggest a tied relationship to a hospital or other high-level care facility; in others, the ADC site should probably be free-standing. Within the ADC site, the need to incorporate a number of services puts a premium on the close interactions of specialists in a number of disciplines, who must be able to assume other roles and shift emphases in mounting a team effort, another crucial aspect of successful ADC services.

Access and Quality in ADC

As with all types of care, access, quality, and cost are central to any consideration of ADC. A fragmented funding situation, coupled with a lack of program initiative in the public sector, probably has reduced access to existing ADC services and precluded the development of new ADC facilities and programs. Extensive research, however, is needed to determine the actual and potential need and possible utilization of ADC, to identify the effects of the reimbursement systems under various public funding programs, and to assess the consequences of open entitlement to ADC for all disabled in the community without a means test. Costs and implications of such open access must be considered and investigated, especially with respect to the cost-effectiveness of ADC *vis-a-vis* other care modes.

Among the more important access-related questions are those associated with the organization of ADC facilities and their relationships to each other. Currently, there are at least three modes of organization: *individual* (freestanding or hospital-based), *satellites* around a central planning and logistical support office, and *networks* composed of ADC centers as parts of an integrated long-term care structure. Satellites usually are more general types of facilities than those in a network, in which there is more specialization according to service and client group. Some analysts argue that the network system, emphasizing team concepts and more socio-medical models of care, is capable of greater consistency and, thus, can acquire greater public acceptability (Trager, 1979). This issue also demands further research.

419

Quality in ADC programs can be viewed (again in common with other aspects of social and health care) in terms of input measures, process, and outcomes (or outputs). As yet, ADC quality issues have not been sufficiently analyzed, nor have general standards been set. It seems clear, however, that input quality standards relate to staff number and type, the definition of program and staff goals, the development of team capabilities, and a good data system. High process quality demands comprehensive assessment, periodic re-evaluation, proper case management, and support by and of the home environment. Good output quality requires identification of changing functional status, measures of re-integration into the community, and means of enhancing the self-perception of individuals. In all three cases, the quality indicators pertain to all facets of care, but, again, the lack of general standards and the high community profile of ADC demand special attention to the integration of all aspects of quality. Research is urgently needed in all these areas.

Specific State ADC Programs

Massachusetts

A number of individual State ADC programs have been analyzed by administrators in the States concerned. Among these have been ADC projects in Massachusetts and California. Neither one specifies desired outcomes, assesses the vulnerability of the client population to institutionalization, provides much evidence of the comparability of experimental and control groups, or develops evidence that the services provided and the clients served were actually comparable between ADC and other types of care with which comparisons were made. Nonetheless, these descriptions offer a rich set of institutional facts and provide insights on the type of research designs which would enable us to use their data and their institutional backgrounds to best advantage. They also contain some analytical insights.

Massachusetts has one of the most extensive programs in ADC. Beginning with six sites in 1975 (using Section 222 authorizations), the State's Medicaid authorities have increased the number of sites to 45, serving 807 clients as of August 1979.[3] The experiments were undertaken because of the increasing public attention to a wider variety of service options, the Federal initiatives under the 1972 Social Security Act amendments, and the belief among policymakers that fiscal probity and a better quality of life for the chronically sick (and their families) were progressively harder to attain

---

[3] Masschusetts' ADC programs are discussed in Klapfish (1979, 1980).

through institutionalization. The objectives of the Massachusetts ADC program are to provide alternatives to institutionalization or to delay it; to provide respite for families who may have to manage heavy nursing care responsibilities at home or who, in desperation, may have to turn to institutionalization; and to provide cost-effective care options to policymakers and to vulnerable populations. Outreach, both in case-findings and educating the public about ADC, is deemed a crucial part of the Massachusetts effort.

Initially, the Massachusetts Adult Day Health Program was to be organized on the three-part (restorative, maintenance, and social) model, but very quickly the State authorities realized that their own approach, based on six desired outcomes (to restore health, provide therapeutic recreation and services, provide social services and counseling, provide personal care, assist with adequate nutrition, and provide necessary transport) was more suitable. Accordingly, sites were chosen and standards were set with these outcomes in mind.

Eligibility for the ADC program is determined by one or more of the following characteristics: the client's need for medical and/or nursing services; the possible usefulness of rehabilitative and/or emotional support services in facilitating the client's return as a functioning member to the community; a high risk of nursing home placement for the client; the possibility that the client, presently in a nursing home, could, with ADC, return to the community; the client's being chronically ill and unable to survive without constant supervision. More generally, patients are eligible if they are candidates for a Massachusetts Level III nursing home, that is, they require 24-hour supervision (not necessarily nursing care). Private pay and Medicaid patients can attend.

ADC sites are open eight hours a day, five days a week. Participants are supposed to spend six hours a day at the center (exclusive of transport). A minimum of a two-person staff is required; otherwise there must be one staff professional for no more than six patients. An RN must be present for four hours a day, and all sites must be barrier free for wheelchair-bound and other handicapped patients.

Clients for the Massachusetts program are admitted after a three-week regimen of visits, interviews, and assessments by a multidisciplinary team. Data from the activities in fiscal year 1978 showed 336 new admissions, 52 percent of whom came from health related facilities (hospitals, SNFs, ICFs etc.), 22 percent from community organizations (home care providers, social workers, etc.), and 14 percent from self- or family referral. Increasing success, as well as visibility, for the program was claimed because, in fiscal year 1978, a larger number of referrals had come from hospital discharge planners, now more familiar with ADC than they had been a year

421

earlier. This claim suggests that a critical minimum familiarization period must occur before an ADC program gains legitimacy among those health care professionals whose involvement is essential in generating an adequate clientele and in making ADC a viable long-term care alternative.

Data from 1978 also showed that many clients had mulitple medical problems although most suffered from hypertension (26 percent), arthritis (17 percent), diabetes (19 percent), CVA (18 percent), and chronic brain syndrome (7 percent). Most frequently, clients were disabled in one or more of the following categories: mobility, walking, bathing, climbing stairs, dressing, feeding themselves, toileting, and wheeling in a chair. About 5 percent were incontinent. More than 50 percent were disabled in four out of the eight areas—a disabled population, indeed! Between 1977 and 1978, the vulnerability of ADC clients in ambulation, dressing, and bathing increased slightly; in wheeling, it rose dramatically. The former increases may have arisen because of greater visibility of the ADC programs, the latter because of the newly-imposed, barrier-free requirement. Such changes suggest that ADC planners must be aware of the possibilities of dynamic changes in their actual and potential client groups, changes which may derive from the regulatory and informational, as well as the clinical, environments. Not surprisingly, large proportions of the clients were over age 60 (79 percent; 46 percent over age 75) and female (65 percent). On the other hand, 40 percent lived alone (and the number was rising), a bit puzzling since a number of studies show that families appear central to the success of regimes of care alternative to the nursing home. Perhaps ADC staffs were giving special assistance to these people with their daily routines. An alternative explanation might be that these single people were less disabled and required less assistance with ADL. They may also have had strong social supports in the community, such as a child living nearby or an outreach group at a church. Their incomes and sources of support for ADC (for example, private pay, Medicaid) may also be of interest.

On admission to the program, ADC clients were receiving a number of services other than ADC, home health care (15 percent of the clients) and home chore aid (21 percent) being the most common. Also, 19 percent received physical therapy, 13 percent, occupational therapy, and 7 percent, speech therapy. ADC, home health care, and home chore services combined were provided to 8 percent of the clients. Given the position of ADC as one among a set of possible alternatives, such combinations are to be expected. So also, in light of the large proportion of Massachusetts ADC recipients who live alone, the use of home chore aids is expectable. Overall, in terms of medical and functional difficulties and services received,

422

ADC clients were a very dependent group. How many more such dependents there were in the community is unknown.

During fiscal year 1978, 37 percent of the 106 ADC clients who were discharged went to institutions, although some of these might have remained in the community with ADC had stronger family and social supports been available. Although 42 percent were discharged to the community, a large share of that proportion did not leave because they were "cured." Rather, many of them were fearful of parts of the programs, often because of anxieties about traveling in winter. Others were mentally ill and disruptive to the other clients. Still others had transportation difficulties. A small fraction left because they could not afford the fees and/or because their Medicaid eligibility had run out under State regulations.

Among the clients discharged to the community, 40 percent were referred to home health agencies, 10 percent to mental health clinics, and 5 percent to congregate housing. Two points emerge from these considerations of community discharges: one, that regulations may determine outcomes different from those suggested by patient condition and two, that ADC fits into a set, or spectrum, of alternatives, appropriate or necessary in a dynamic pattern of needs.

The Massachusetts ADC program seems to meet a need among Medicaid eligible clients, since 69 percent of participants were in that category. The daily service capacity of the system was 400 places, and, on the average, clients attended 2.3 times per week (though the program assumed a figure of 2.7 times per week). Average absences amounted to 2/5 of the day per week, suggesting that absenteeism may constitute a significant element in program costs, since staff and other costs are based on assumptions about care actually programed for client groups. If the centers operated at 100 percent of capacity, program costs per client came to $13.16 per day; at 80 percent, they amounted to $16.46. Staff allocations absorbed 74 percent of total costs; overhead and other program costs (independent of staff) accounted for the rest. Transport costs were estimated at $4 to $5 per round trip per person, most clients traveling in ADC vehicles or other community vehicles.

Based on these figures and assessments of clients' satisfaction (and provider perceptions), the Massachusetts authorities claimed that their ADC program was cost-effective. While it is true that the average daily program costs were far below those of a nursing home, there were no data on the total social costs of the program, nor was there any information given comparing services provided and service quality between ADC and other care modes. Similarly, there was no comparison of the effectiveness of ADC and other care modes in serving similar populations. Moreover, the numbers

423

served are quite small in comparison to the total long-term care clientele, so that the efficacy of ADC in dealing with the mass of long-term care vulnerability in Massachusetts has yet to be demonstrated. As indicated earlier, these omissions are shared with many other analyses of alternatives. Nevertheless, the Massachusetts reports are instructive for their insights about client characteristics, the role of transport, the technical possibility of maintaining highly disabled people in an ADC-supported environment, and the need for a multi-faceted approach to ADC. In the Massachusetts analyses, furthermore, the dynamic element and the impact of regulations and other institutional barriers emerge very clearly. So also, the complementarity of ADC with other forms of care and its potential as an "add-on" to other long-term care provision is definitely shown.

California

Some of the California reports are particularly interesting because they focus on changes in the conditions of the ADC clients and because they are concerned with comparative costs. Most of the latter appear as a result of discussions between the California Department of Finance and the State's Health and Welfare Agency (California Health and Welfare Agency, 1979).

In general, the California reports on a series of Section 1115 demonstrations assert that ADC is more satisfactory than nursing home care on the grounds of convenience, personal response, and quality of life. The most startling outcome of the California ADC programs was the claim that 70 to 79 percent of the ADC clients were *eligible* for SNF/ICF care and yet were maintained in the community. (Note that they may not have used such care.) Overall, the ADC clients were highly disabled: 20 percent were disabled in five or more ADL categories; 71 percent were disabled in one or more. In general, the clients of the various State-supported Section 1115 projects were helped in regaining continence of bladder and bowels (90 percent), losing their aphasia (50 percent), and regaining the ability to dress themselves (40 percent). There were also improvements for diabetics, who were able to administer their own insulin, for insomniacs, and for those suffering from depression. Families were also helped in their abilities to cope with stress and to accept their relatives' disabilities.

On the cost side, the California officials claimed that the chronically sick not in ADC programs were significantly more expensive (in terms of State revenue allocations) than were ADC clients. In the case of the San Diego experimental (ADC) and control (non-ADC) groups, 75 percent of the latter's costs stemmed from hospital and ICF usage, presumably unnecessary for the ADC clients. Put in other terms, it was claimed that, by contrast with non-ADC users, ADC users experienced large cost savings for combined hospital

424

and nursing home care, hospital care alone, and nursing home care alone. Overall, the total cost of services provided by MediCal (California's Medicaid program), SSI, and home care (used by 14 percent of the San Diego and 33 percent of the Sacramento ADC clients) was $396.51 per month, well below that of nursing home provision.

As with the Massachusetts reports, those from California are rich in institutional detail, but they provide modest information on assessing costs and effectiveness. For example, although experimental and control groups were presumably analyzed, no data were presented on the dimensions of comparability. Did these groups really have the same characteristics? What were the outcomes for those patients not in ADC programs? What would have happened to the ADC clients if they had had no ADC programs? With respect to costs, no contrasts were offered between the costs of the same services in differing modalities. In addition, the State health administrators rejected the inclusion of family and other secondary and tertiary costs on the grounds that they were already included in the SSI payments. (It should be noted that the California Department of Finance had included family costs.)

General Analyses of ADC

In general, ADC has not been as thoroughly analyzed as has home care (though much institutional data does exist), yet the work of Kiernat and Weissert offers some insights into both the substantive issues and the problems inherent in assessing ADC or any other alternative care mode.[4]

Kiernat's survey in the early 1970s of ADC programs found only 15 which met the conventional and Federal definition of ADC.[5] Over half of these were Federally funded demonstrations. The average patient load was 40; the modal attendance was three to four days per week. Over half of the patients lived alone, 25 percent with a spouse, and 16 percent with a child. In most cases, admittance to the program was contingent on having a stable home environment (thus possibly indicating the key role of the "relevant other"), displaying no harmful behavior, not being bedridden, being able to pay for a portion of the care provided, and having a physician available in the community. Both the Kiernat study and the Massachusetts data discussed earlier indicate that large numbers of ADC clients

---

[4] The reports and censuses of Edith Robbins of HCFA provide us with virtually the only overall source of information on the characteristics of ADC programs and clients. These thorough and clearly presented internal sources of information might serve as the basis for further research on the costs and effectiveness of ADC programs.

[5] See the discussion of the Kiernat study in Doherty, Segal, and Hicks (1978).

live alone. Perhaps some ADC clients may not be as disabled as commonly believed. Research is definitely indicated in this area. Weissert's studies cover, first, some older, established programs and, second, a series of Section 222 experiments (under P.L. 92–603) mandated by Congress in 1972. These experiments and research first covered 10 sites and, later, six projects under 222 Medicare waivers. The latter were analyzed in great detail (Weissert, 1980; Weissert et al, February 1980, June 1980, Fall 1980). In both sets of experiments, the following questions were central to the analysis:

- Would the provided services reduce institutionalization?
- What would their impact be on the costs and use of other Medicare-supported services?
- Would the services be effective in maintaining or improving physical, psycho-social, and/or ADL functioning?
- Would the services postpone death?

In the earlier study of 10 sites and 300 clients, emphasis was placed on cost comparisons with nursing homes. In the latter, it was on a cost-effectiveness analysis of ADC. The former study did not explicitly sort clients for nursing home vulnerability, but Weissert (1976) claims that need for Medicaid eligibility, the thrust of some ADC programs as facilitators of inpatient release from rehabilitation facilities, and the mission of others as recipients of deinstitutionalized mental patients ensured comparability of the type desired. In general, he found that ADC daily costs exceeded those of nursing homes but that the costs per *episode* of care were lower for ADC than for nursing home patients, largely because the former used fewer days of care. ADC care cost, therefore, could be lower than nursing home costs by as much as 37 to 60 percent, at least to the third-party payers. Recognizing that nursing homes provide shelter, food, and warmth (cooling), as well as care, Weissert added an amount taken from the Bureau of Labor Statistics (BLS) budget estimates for a retired couple to derive a social cost of provision (though one excluding some of Doherty's secondary and tertiary costs; see Chapter VII), which showed annual cost savings ranging from about $860 to over $2,400 per year for ADC compared to nursing home care. The range of social saving from using ADC was thus 12 to 35 percent contrasted with nursing homes.

Although these numbers seem impressive and suggest that ADC should be explored further on cost grounds alone, this particular study of Weissert's raises a number of problems. First, the assumption that ADC clients in these experiments were comparable in medical, socio-psychological, or functional terms with those otherwise destined for nursing homes is dubious. Also, although Weissert

426

explicitly limits his comparison to clients who stay for a full year of care, Grimaldi (1979) makes the valid point that comparing costs for episodes of care may require the analyst to look at nursing home patients who stay for less than a year with ADC clients who stay for a longer period. Part of the cost comparison may thus be of time as well as money. Grimaldi also notes that the relevant comparison may really be that between ICFs (not SNFs) and ADC. In addition, the wide range of cost figures among facilities is not adequately explained by the use of medians in the cost comparisons. The size of the variance is statistically and analytically important. Indeed, sources of great cost variation must be examined in some detail before reliance can be placed on medians or other measures of central tendency for comparison purposes. Grimaldi also points out that the cost-of-living component in ADC may be underrated, since ADC clients may well run up costs beyond those incurred by a self-supporting, urban, reasonably healthy, and ADL-competent couple, the entity for which the BLS cost of living figures are developed.

Notwithstanding criticisms of this type, Weissert's analysis offers one of the first rigorous attempts to cost out the ADC/nursing home comparison in terms of the magnitudes which must be considered. The main policy and analytical point is that ADC and other alternative programs may be add-ons rather than substitutes for existing regimes of care, especially the nursing home. This conclusion is even more emphasized in Weissert's later work. Grimaldi puts the point well when he says that, if this is so, the key question may be whether society is interested in enhancing the lives of the elderly, not whether one form of care is more cost-effective than another. The applicability of this observation to the whole range of alternatives is obvious.

Section 222 ADC Experiments

Originally, for the second set of reports, almost 1,900 elderly Medicare eligibles were to have been included in a series of experiments at four ADC sites in 1978. Approximately half of the group was to be offered ADC and/or homemaker services, and half were not (Weissert et al, February 1980, June 1980, Fall 1980). Only 1,153 individuals were finally analyzed for all types of services, however, because of data problems. Both the experimental and the control (that is, those not receiving services) groups were determined by health professionals to be able to use such services. The intent of the experiment was to see whether the provision of ADC services emphasizing rehabilitation and medical care made any difference in terms of institutionalization and certain health and psycho-social outcomes (including death) and to explore differences in costs. Data were analyzed with both univariate and multivariate techniques.

Data from the four ADC sites indicate that there were seemingly few major differences in personal characteristics between the ADC experimental and control groups (384 people overall), although some subtle variations may underlie anomalies discussed below. The average age of the groups was 74–75; most were female (over 55 percent); three-quarters of them lived with others; most were moderately or severely dependent (requiring help from others with two or more ADL functions); most had not been recently hospitalized. The ADC experimental group had slightly more members under 75 and living with others, but they were less likely to have been hospitalized than the controls. Average attendance was 70 times per year (1.3 days per week) although the frequency range was very wide, from five times per week to once during the whole year. The most regular attenders were severely disabled, white females, most of whom had been hospitalized just prior to the program's onset. They attended an average of 100 sessions during the year and were probably custodial care patients rather than rehabilitation candidates. Among special therapies, physical therapy was used by 54 to 100 percent of patients (depending on site) and occupational therapy by 35 to 100 percent.

In terms of outcomes, the ADC group experienced a lower rate of use of SNFs: four versus nine days. Also, among those who actually went into institutions, the experimental group averaged 37 days in an SNF versus 42 for the control group. Weissert believes, however, that the low rates of use of SNFs by both the experimental (11 percent) and control groups (21 percent) indicate that most of the people in the demonstrations were not destined for institutionalization anyway. Therefore, his general conclusion for ADC is that it would be an additional benefit under Medicare rather than a substitute for the SNF, as is often claimed.

Physical functioning among ADC users was better maintained or improved than among the controls, even after allowing for those who died. The data seem equivocal, however, on two grounds: (1) when those who died are excluded, the difference in ADL is not quite statistically significant, and (2) data for the interval between the fourth and fifth quarters of the experiment show slight functional improvements among the control group but a continuation of decline in the group receiving ADC services. One clear finding did emerge: increased ADC utilization was associated with greater improvement in ADL. This was especially true when ADL results were lagged by one or two quarters after receipt of services. On the other hand, if clients who died are excluded from the analysis, the improvement in ADL functioning did not remain. Furthermore, both Weissert and Grimaldi-Sullivan noted that heavy ADC users may have self-selected

428

themselves, that is, they may have been better able to use ADC in the first place (Weissert et al, June 1980; Grimaldi and Sullivan, 1981).

A somewhat equivocal finding in the Weissert analysis was that ADC may reduce mortality among users, but just exactly how is not clear. It should be noted that Weissert's mortality findings may derive from methodological problems, since 25 percent of the original experimental group refused the ADC services and was excluded from the analysis. Because non-users were reported to be older, more likely to be in institutions, and had a higher death rate than users, the mortality rates among the original experimental group may have been understated. Overall, some 38 percent of all people originally scheduled to participate in the Section 222 experiments (including receipt of home care) were excluded from the final analysis (Stassen and Holahan, 1981). ADC users also seemed more contented than non-users and seemed to have higher levels of activity and mental functioning. These outcomes may be the most important from the perspective of enhanced quality of life, reinforcing the claims of some ADC supporters.

Weissert's cost analysis was couched solely in terms of Medicare-reimbursed costs, both for ADC services and all others. ADC costs per person came to $3,235 per year. Medicare costs for services other than ADC were $543 higher ($3,809 versus $3,266) among the control group than among the experimental group; however, when ADC costs are added in, the experimental group cost $2,692 or 71 percent more ($6,501 versus $3,809) then the controls. Note that no attribution was made for family costs or other secondary or tertiary costs. Medicaid costs were not included, although they were discussed in the analysis. Their inclusion might have altered the cost-effectiveness comparisons significantly (Stassen and Holahan, 1981). On the other hand, some of Weissert's earlier work comparing nursing home costs with ADC plus home support costs showed that ADC could be 12 to 35 percent cheaper if offered by more socially oriented ADC facilities. Average daily ADC and other Medicare costs (based on pooled data) in the earlier study were about $25 per day versus $52 per day in the later one. What is suggested is a study comparing social ADC support with that provided by an SNF regime, an ICF regime, or both. This would, of course, require some degree of Medicaid involvement and would have to recognize the possible add-on nature of ADC.

Steven Clauser has provided a strong internal agency critique of the Weissert report.[6] His criticisms relate mainly to the design

---

[6] Clauser's critique is also being published in Home Health Care Services Quarterly, forthcoming.

429

of the intervention being assessed and to shortcomings in method. Regarding the former, Clauser noted the relatively short time of the experiments (12 months), particularly in relation to the time frames of most long-term care problems. He also noted gaps in information provided about the availability of services to both experimental and control groups under Title XX (especially in California), as well as the fact that over 49 percent of the control group used no services at all and that the attrition rate in the project was over 25 percent. Methodologically, he criticized the asymmetry of assessments across sites, the number of clients omitted from the study for reasons of data weakness, and the lack of data on input costs and cost of living differences among ADC site areas. Perhaps most forceful was the observation that family and other ancillary costs were omitted from consideration. Given the presumed central role of the family in the success of ADC and other alternatives, this could be a significant omission. Clauser also believed that the conclusions of the report are not nationally applicable because of concentration on projects in the Northeast, California, and Kentucky, and because of little consideration of skill or quality differences among providers. (Weissert, in personal communication, claimed that there were no significant differences.) Potential client awareness of the short-term and experimental nature of the projects may have reduced utilization. (It should be noted that all demonstrations and experiments are subject to this shortcoming.)

Clauser also focused heavily on the shortcomings of the cost analysis and the alternatives questions raised by Weissert himself. On the former, Clauser claimed that average cost data were employed with no attempt to isolate sources of site-specific differences in marginal costs, a very important omission when variations among observations are as large as in this case. Also, the fact that experimental costs were so much higher than costs of similar programs reimbursed under Medicaid may be relevant. Certainly this type of difference is important, since it raises doubts about the necessity of the high costs found under the 222 experiments and about the impacts of different reimbursement systems on the findings of research and experiments of this type. As to the alternatives issue, Clauser noted that these experiments were aimed (at least implicitly) at the more medically dependent client; yet no attempt was made to use the assessment process to obtain this type of client. One may speculate, in light of this comment of Clauser's, whether the low levels of institutionalization found in the experimental and control groups did not reflect a lack of effective "targeting" for ADC services. Indeed, Weissert (1981) argues that targeting on small groups is needed if ADC or other alternatives are to make much difference.

430

Overall, Clauser doubts that Weissert's conclusions can be accepted without further analysis on the 222 data. He also argues for research and demonstration programs focusing on Medicaid-eligible populations and for true randomization of placements, longitudinal studies, implementation and data quality control, and the analysis of more broadly based systems of provision.

Grimaldi and Sullivan (1981) have a similar set of comments about these Weissert studies. In the first place, they note (as do Weissert et al) that the providers in the study were not randomly selected, so their service costs may differ widely from those of other providers. Second, the participants may not have represented those who would have been covered had ADC (and homemaker services) been more widely available. Third, the findings might well have differed under real life circumstances compared to the experimental conditions employed for the studies. Grimaldi and Sullivan additionally believe that the widely available social ADC programs might add to the net cost of long-term care. The argument rests on the belief that the social ADC model might serve more as an addition than as a substitute for nursing home care. Weissert shares this view. They conclude, however, that ADC programs, even though creating more costs, might still be desirable because of their demonstrated influence on feelings of contentment among the users. The analysis thus closely parallels those of Clauser and Weissert himself in certain particulars.

Because of the complex nature of long-term care dependency, Weissert and colleagues undertook a multivariate analysis of patient outcomes in different long-term care modes. Their data were essentially those of the earlier 222 studies, and their focus was the impact of ADC and home care on patient well-being. Their use of multivariate techniques is all the more important, since their other research was based essentially on bivariate analysis (Wan, Weissert, Livieratos, 1978; Weissert et al, June 1980).

Clients were assessed on ADL; their orientation to time, person, and place (using a Mental Status Quotient assessment instrument); their happiness; their social activities; and their individual activities. These assessments yielded 26 variables, organized in five categories. The first—socio-demographics—encompassed age 75 and older, sex, race, living status (alone, with others), and marital status. Social indicators were those on contentment, mental activity, and personal activity. Physical status was largely examined in terms of chronic conditions. Prognoses measures, based largely on physical condition, were also used. Last, researchers analyzed use of health services, that is, when and how intensely the patient had used hospitals, SNFs, home care, hospital outpatient services, and/or ambulatory care services.

431

The researchers then linked these variables to perceived patient outcomes for those clients involved in ADC and home care programs versus those who were not. Although it appeared that, on a single variate basis, a more intense use of both services led to an improvement in some outcomes (as shown by improved functional capacity, greater happiness and contentment, etc.) the multivariate analysis showed that factors other than use of experimental services were more effective in explaining outcomes. Very significant were primary diagnoses, impairment prognoses (based on ADL assessments), and the number of inpatient hospital days. In particular, positive outcomes appeared related to living status (living with others was beneficial), whether the patient had a high activity level and/or mental health function at the beginning of the experiment, whether the patient had a digestive or traumatic problem, whether the patient had a prognosis of decline in ADL functioning and of increases in bedfast disability and bed utilization, whether the patient had a prognosis of maintenance or improvement in ADL functioning, and whether the patient used a high volume of ADL and/or hospital based ambulatory care.

Because of data contamination and the necessity of excluding a number of potential candidates from the pools of both ADC users and controls, Weissert and his research group later analyzed their ADC data in three sections (Weissert, Wan, Livieratos, and Katz, 1980; Weissert *et al*, Fall 1980). The first analysis essentially replicated the one just described. The second analysis included those people who had been chosen for the experimental group but who had not used the ADC services. It also included members of the control groups (that is, those to whom ADC services were not to be given under the experiment) who had used the services. Essentially, the comparison was between all users and non-users, regardless of their assignment to the experimental or the control groups. On a single variate basis, that is, correlating only ADC with outcomes, it appears that use of ADC enhanced survival probabilities and functioning and reduced the probability of institutionalization. On the other hand, if other variables (such as demographic, psycho-social functioning, various prognostic measures, etc.) were included through use of a Multiple Classification Analysis (MCA), the impact of ADC dropped markedly, and the relationships were found not to be statistically significant.

A similar type of analysis comparing all members of the experimental and control groups, regardless of their actual use or non-use of the ADC services, was undertaken to control for the greater likelihood of death among assigned ADC users who did not use the services than among other groups in the study. The most interesting result in this analysis was that the probability of death was higher among older members of the experimental groups than

432

among the control group. For patients under 75, the reverse was true. However, the size of this influence was small and found to be non-significant when subjected to MCA types of analysis.

From this analysis, it is clear that the impact of ADC (and home care, for that matter) is not single-valued and that, again, one is confronted with both the complex interaction of determinants of dependency and with the intricacies of time-related influences—in short, both patient and system dynamics. Also, it must be recognized that some of the determinants of outcomes were also some of the outcomes sought, for example, change in ADL functioning.

On balance, it appears that this type of experiment shows several things. ADC by itself does not determine outcomes. Also, a pattern of continuing care must be provided on a patient-specific basis to achieve maximum results from regimes of ADC and home care. Furthermore, ADC and home care appear related to enhanced feelings of mental well-being and contentment and to a feeling of physical well-being. Their impact, alone, on physical activity appears limited.

In terms of further research on the cost-effectiveness of ADC and home care, socio-demographic, physical health, and health care utilization factors must all be controlled for. Moreover, much preliminary theorizing must be undertaken in relation to the mechanisms and circumstances relevant to dependency; this theory must be especially sensitive to dynamic considerations. At the risk of being unduly repetitious, these methodological and theoretical structures must be considered in connection with research on all modalities of care (including institutional care) and are especially relevant to long-term care.

Some Preliminary Conclusions

Brahna Trager's report (1979) on the 1977 and 1978 conferences on ADC provides a useful summary for this discussion. She observes that a number of characteristics and requirements are common to all ADC programs. All must be carefully planned, yet amenable to criticism and change. All should have clear goals and objectives for their services, most particularly those which see ADC as part of a spectrum of care rather than an answer in itself. The auspices of care, as well as the organization of financial and staff support, must be clearly understood and their limitations expressed in the program undertaken. Care setting requirements and availability must be previously determined, as must staff training and administrative and organizational procedures. Coordination with other care modes must be emphasized, as must the involvement of clients and families in the design and delivery of services. This last is important because patients' needs must be clearly understood, because family

433

support may be crucial to the success of an ADC program, and because family assumption of responsibility may be highly influential in determining outcomes for disabled family members. For many of the same reasons, community support is important in determining outcomes for the dependent. Hence, community support must also be solicited and incorporated into the ADC effort. Finally, in order that maximum benefit be derived from an ADC program, and in order that necessary changes may be made in a timely fashion, data collection must be designed in advance, data systems must be efficient, and standards and regulations must be clear and direct. These mandates of course apply to all long-term care modes.

In light of these strictures, a number of research areas are especially relevant. Clearly, we need to sharpen our knowledge about the population, either in the community or in other care settings, which might benefit from ADC. This demands more knowledge about the determinants of vulnerability and the interactions among various care modes in ministering to vulnerability, an issue raised earlier. So also we need to know the labor force and space requirements for individual ADC sites and for an ADC system, especially one which is a part of a larger long-term care system. Likewise, we need to know about the design of regulations which will help to produce the outcomes desired from ADC in a long-term care system. We also need to determine the minimum data needs and the means for integrating ADC records with larger sets of long-term care data, especially those related to assessment and patient characteristics. As indicated earlier in relation to the operation of ADC programs in Massachusetts, and as we have stated in previous parts of this chapter, analytically precise methods of reimbursement and costing should be identified as a matter of research. The effect of reimbursement and costing methods on outcomes and on the operation of ADC programs must be understood so that perverse effects, not related to patient needs, may be eliminated.

A Final Caveat

As a result of his own and his colleagues' research, and after a review of four sets of alternative demonstration results (Connecticut Triage, Wisconsin Community Care Project, Georgia Alternative Health Project, and Prof. Katz's use of home health aide teams), Weissert comes to a set of conclusions much at variance with conventional wisdom (1981, forthcoming). In the first place, he believes that all of these data indicate that the development of alternatives will add to health services utilization rather than serve as substitutes for more expensive modes of care. In many cases, the individuals served were already at very low risks of institutionalization (from a low of 1.6 percent to a high of 22 percent). If users of ADC and other alternatives were not likely to be nursing home candidates, a correct alternatives program should ensure that they would receive some benefit from the services received. The trouble, according to Weissert, is that neither his own research nor the research he reviewed seems to show that users' health conditions, functional status, or mortality rates showed much effect from the services received. Only feelings of contentment (quality of life, perhaps) were enhanced, although there may have been some effects on mortality as a result of receiving home care services. (This finding is considered in Chapter IX.) It should be noted that Stassen and Holahan (1981) come to the same conclusions regarding mortality or functional improvements from receipt of ADC services.

In Weissert's view, these findings suggest two imperatives: (1) to ensure that alternatives ". . . provide beneficial impacts on health status or that they reduce costs" by substituting cheaper for more expensive care, and (2) to target alternatives for those most likely to benefit while precluding use by those who would not. In one sense, we face the technical problem of serving existing clients in new ways. In another sense, the practical reality lies in the politics of adding new client groups while ensuring that those groups will really benefit. A complicating factor would be later findings that added services accomplish little, since removing them would be a formidable political task indeed. He argues that we should not give up trying to find new ways to serve present clients and to assist those who might benefit from new services. Our main obligation is to pursue lines of research which will develop better criteria so that we will serve those most likely to benefit. We should also develop indicators to identify benefits and to determine their existence before we embark on new care programs.

References

California Health and Welfare Agency, Department of Health Services, "Response to 'A Review of Adult Day Care Pilot Projects' by California Department of Finance, Report D 79–6," Sacramento, May, 1979. See also other reports on ADC by same agency.

Clauser, Steven B., "Comments on the Section 222 Adult Day Care and Homemaker Experiments," *Home Health Care Services Quarterly*, forthcoming.

Doherty, Neville, Joan Segal, and Barbara Hicks, "Alternatives to Institutionalization for the Aged: Viability and Cost Effectiveness," *Aged Care and Services Review*, January/February 1978, pp. 1–16.

Grimaldi, Paul L. and Toni Sullivan, *Broadening Federal Coverage of Noninstitutional Long Term Care* (Washington, D.C.: American Health Care Association, 1981).

Grimaldi, Paul L., "The Costs of Adult Day Care and Nursing Home Care: A Dissenting View," and Weissert's "Rebuttal," *Inquiry*, Summer, 1979, pp. 162–166.

Kilgore, Gloria and Gabriel Salmon, *Technical Notes: Summaries and Characteristics of States' Title XX Social Services Plans*, U.S. DHEW, Assistant Secretary for Planning and Evaluation, June 15, 1979.

Klapfish, Anne, "Adult Day Care in Massachusetts," in U.S. DHEW, Health Care Financing Administration (HCFA) 79–20021, February 1980, pp. 31–36.

Klapfish, Anne, "Adult Day Health Services, Massachusetts Medical Assistance Program Year End Report for Fiscal Year 1978 (July 1, 1977—June 30, 1978)," in Trager, 1979.

Stassen, Margaret and John Holahan, *Long-Term Care Demonstration Projects: A Review of Recent Evaluations* (Washington: The Urban Institute, Working Paper 1227–2, February, 1981).

Trager, Brahna, "Adult Day Health Care—A Conference Report," Arlington, Virginia, September, 1977, and Tucson, Arizona, September, 1978, under Grant No. 1 R13 HS 10580–01, National Center for Health Services Research, OASH, May, 1979.

Wan, Thomas T.H., William G. Weissert, and Barbara B. Livieratos, "Determinants of Outcomes of Care in Two Geriatric Service Modalities: An Experimental Study," paper delivered at the November 1978 meeting of the Gerontological Society.

Weissert, William G., Thomas T.H. Wan, Barbara B. Livieratos, and Julius Pellegrino, "Cost Effectiveness of Homemaker Services for the Chronically Ill," *Inquiry*, Fall 1980, pp. 230–243.

Weissert, William G., "Costs of Adult Day Care: A Comparison to Nursing Homes," *Inquiry*, March, 1978, pp. 10–19.

Weissert, William G., Thomas T.H. Wan, and Barbara Livieratos, *Effects and Costs of Day Care and Homemaker Services for the Chronically Ill: A Randomized Experiment*, DHEW (PHS) 79–3258 (Hyattsville, Maryland: National Center for Health Services Research, February 1980).

Weissert, William, Thomas Wan, Barbara Livieratos, and Sidney Katz, "Effects and Costs of Day-Care Services for the Chronically Ill," *Medical Care*, June 1980, pp. 567–584.

Weissert, William G., "Rationales for Public Health Insurance Coverage of Geriatric Day Care: Issues, Options, and Impacts," *Journal of Health Politics, Policy, and Law*, Winter 1979, pp. 555–567.

Weissert, William G., "Toward a Continuum of Care for the Elderly: A Note of Caution," *Public Policy*, Summer 1981, forthcoming.

Weissert, William G., "Two Models of Geriatric Day Care: Findings from a Comparative Study," *The Gerontologist*, October 1976, pp. 420–427.

436

Chapter XII

Domiciliary Care: A Semantic Tangle

by Hans C. Palmer

Many Settings: Many Services

The final "alternative" to be considered in long-term care is domiciliary care. Actually, this term refers to a number of different arrangements for providing shelter, food, and some modicum of supervision. Unfortunately, these combinations of settings and services are characterized by wide divergences in provision and by greatly differing terminologies. In some cases, room, board, shelter, recreation, and sheltered work supervision are all provided, while in other situations, only room and board and a minimum of supervision (designed to keep residents from harming themselves, their surroundings, or others) are offered. Some settings provide personal care, assistance with medication, etc; others give none. This range of provision renders client identification, regulation, and possible reimbursement (especially cost-related reimbursement) very difficult to design and implement. As a type of service, domiciliary care represents some elements of possible supervised living arrangements, which include congregate housing.

Complicating matters further is the wide variety of terms used in connection with the provision of food, shelter, and supervision. Not only do these terms vary among providers, users, policymakers, and analysts, but they also vary among the States, and in some cases, within States. Federal definitions are also imprecise. In some cases, the applicable term is domiciliary care; in others, it is board and care; in others, personal care facilities (where presumably there is no care—"three hots and a cot").[1] In some instances, there is even confusion as to whether it is the nature of the services provided, nature of the setting, number of clients per setting, or number of people per bedroom which is a (the) criterion of identification.

The multiplicity of categories in one State, New York, is shown in a February 1978 study by Community Research Applications (Steinbach, Holmes, and Holmes; 1978). In that State, at least five terms are used to describe domiciliary care facilities, depending on the size, ownership, and nature of the facility: foster home (for one

---

I wish to thank Leonard Gruenberg for his helpful suggestions for this chapter.

[1] These semantic issues are carefully discussed in Gebran (1979) and in Steinbach *et al* (1978).

client), private proprietary home for adults (PPHA; two or more adults receiving no medical or nursing care), home for the aged (non-profit PPHA), family care home (no more than six adults), and community residences (primarily for deinstitutionalized mental health patients).

Given this confusion, the following definition from a Temple University study of board and care homes in Philadelphia may be useful:

> . . . any facility, operated for profit or otherwise, which accommodates or is designed to accommodate two or more adults unrelated to the owner or operator and which provides room and board on a 24 hour basis to primarily non-transient aged or handicapped (physically or mentally) persons who require some personal care, supervision, or assistance in daily activities such as bathing, dressing, or the taking of medicine prescribed for self-administration. (Temple University, 1977, p. 3.)

This lengthy statement covers those services, offered in a quasi-institutional setting, which most analysts find in the modal type of domiciliary care. In this light, we will use it as a base of reference. We will also use the term "domiciliary care facility" (or DCF) as the umbrella for all these types of services/settings. Note that, among other things, the definition omits any mention of skilled nursing care or medical supervision. Although, as we will see, many DCF residents are mentally and/or physically disabled, the concept of the DCF does not encompass rehabilitation services for such people even though many DCFs may act as brokers with providers of such services. Note also that the DCF operator is not related to any of his/her clients. In fact, current public policy precludes any family relationship between clients and operators if support is to be forthcoming from public sources, a circumstance which often interferes with satisfactory provision of care for dependent people who need little else besides food, a home, some supervision, and some care and consideration.

Two factors must be considered in any discussion of DCFs: size and the complexity of State regulation. DCFs vary greatly in size, from very small (three or fewer clients) to very large. Different size homes are clearly suitable for different types of people. Also, the nature and amount of public oversight and regulation depend on the number and size of homes.

States differ greatly in their regulations and administrative structures applicable to DCFs. Some States merely license; others only license DCFs after they are certified. In some States, DCF clients must be screened and evaluated. In some cases, controlling agencies are integrated into one supervisory body, while in others, the various program elements (licensure, supervision, regulation) are found in many agencies. Some States separate aged, disabled,

438

mentally ill, and mentally retarded clients, while others combine the different groups for mutual support. The relative effectiveness of these differing administrative and regulatory structures has yet to be analyzed.

Concern with the DCF issue has recently arisen because of a number of fatal fires, notably those in Washington, D.C. and New Jersey. These incidents have increased Federal concern with facility regulation and certification and have sharpened interest in the circumstances of DCF residents, many of whom are supported by different Federal income maintenance programs, especially SSI. As we will see, one major focus of Federal attention has been the Keys Amendment (Section 1616e of the Social Security Act), which mandates State development of DCF regulatory programs for those facilities serving recipients of SSI payments.

More generally, however, the DCF issue relates to some fundamental questions about the spectrum of long-term care settings/ services and about services for weak, vulnerable people who may not need much medical care but who may require the basics of food, shelter, and supervision. The DCF question also meshes with broad issues of deinstitutionalization, especially of the mentally ill and mentally retarded.

In one sense, the DCF, to the extent that it caters to the dependent elderly, may actually be an extension of the poor homes, poor farms, county homes, or old people's homes of an earlier era.[2] Our society may have, in the DCF, found a surrogate for the "old folks home," one which is less subject to the negative judgments of a former time and which is significantly less "institutional." Public support for the residents of such homes through SSI and various mental health programs makes the analogy more complete, although, in current circumstances, payment is made by public authorities to the user, not the provider.

Secondly, the DCF is increasingly being considered as an alternative site for care/support for those elderly and mentally ill/retarded people who do not need institutionalization and/or medical care. To some analysts, the DCF is already filling this role; to others, the DCF may well be the wave of the future as a cost-effective alternative to the nursing home (New York State Moreland Act Commission, 1976). Certainly, DCFs already provide "homes" for many elderly people who do not need nursing care on a daily basis. If DCFs are to be meaningful alternatives, however, they must have linkages to key community resources. For example, deinstitutionalized mental patients may need community mental health services, while the

---

[2] See Manard et al (1977) and Vladeck (1980) on this aspect of DCFs and on the role which DCFs may play if policy moves away from support for institutionalization in SNFs and ICFs.

chronically impaired elderly may need visiting nurse and transportation services. Whether DCFs will also serve as cost-effective alternatives to the nursing home still remains to be analyzed.

On a third level, the DCF is entwined in the vagaries of Federal income maintenance, social services, and medical services programs. On the one hand, many DCFs are filled with SSI recipients; on the other, many Title XX programs could provide service to DCF dwellers. So also, there remains the distinct possibility that the Medicaid payment system might, directly or indirectly, come to be a source of support for DCF provision, especially to the extent that social services are to be provided (Noble and Conley, forthcoming), as in the current pilot foster care program at the Massachusetts General Hospital. At a more systematic level, support of DCF residents and the quality of DCF care are linked to the structure and consequences of Federal reimbursements and eligibility regulations and provisions. Specifically, the reduction of benefit payments for SSI recipients living with families and the inflexibility of State and Federal Title XX and Medicaid regulations dictate patterns of provision inappropriate for, or even harmful to, DCF residents.

Reasons for the Emergence (Resurgence?) of the DCF as a Setting for Care

Three major factors appear to be responsible for the recent growth of the DCF as a setting of support: rapid growth in the numbers of people in the age groups most likely to need care (the 75+); the emergence of Federally-supported programs of income maintenance for the elderly, blind, and disabled (SSI); and the waves of deinstitutionalization which have washed many elderly and other mental patients out of state mental health institutions (Noble and Conley, forthcoming).

Under SSI, many States pay supplements to individuals in DCFs. These payments can be administered by the Federal government through the Social Security program. This option may have reinforced the SSI stimulus.

Leonard Gruenberg of the University Health Policy Consortium (in a private communication) suggests that a fourth factor is the inability of many dependent elderly (or their families) to find nursing home beds. Again in Massachusetts, the State has initiated a foster care program, using Medicaid funding, to relieve hospitals (and public funds) of the "administrative days" problem which has kept many elderly people in hospitals because they cannot be placed in nursing homes. A similar situation has developed in New Jersey (Steinbach et al, 1978).

Most studies have emphasized deinstitutionalization as the reason for the growth of DCFs. The interaction between the emerging large

440

numbers of frail elderly and the SSI program has not, to our knowledge, been the focus of as much analytical attention. It should be added that the possibilities of substituting the DCF for the nursing home have not been rigorously analyzed.[3]

According to the GAO study of DCFs in November, 1979, the main reasons for deinstitutionalization were the following:

- concerns over deplorable conditions in many mental health and mental retardation institutions,
- new treatment methods and philosophies,
- development of tranquilizing drugs,
- development of the SSI and other income support programs,
- inducements to the States to save costs by placing persons in facilities in which costs are lower than they would be in mental hospitals, and
- court decisions mandating the return of institutionalized persons to the community (GAO, 1979).

These reasons largely echoed those advanced in the 1976 report of the U.S. Senate's Special Committee on Aging (U.S. Senate, 1976).

Limited Data

Despite the emerging concern with DCFs, and in spite of their evident importance in the spectrum of care, data about DCFs are very scanty. Although several studies are now underway (namely, the HRCA and CRA efforts cited earlier), few hard figures now exist.

Perhaps the most complete data available relate to deinstitutionalization. Numbers cited in the referenced 1976 Senate study show that between 1969 and 1974, the total number of inpatients in State mental hospitals declined from 428,000 to 238,000. Among the age group 65 and over, the decline was even more startling: from 135,000 to 60,000. A recent study conducted by Region III of the Department of Health and Human Services (DHHS) claimed that between one half and one million people had been released since 1955 (Mellody and White, 1979). Among the leaders in the deinstitutionalization of the elderly in the Senate study were Alabama, California, Illinois, Massachusetts, and Wisconsin, in which the percent of decline ranged from 76 percent to 98 percent. These people, together with an unknown number of elderly drawn from the community and from nursing homes, formed one of the major ingredients in the expansion of the board and care sector. Unfortunately, we have no idea of their magnitude.

Some related data which may also indicate the potential for expanding the DCF population has been drawn from the GAO

---

[3] Forthcoming studies by the Hebrew Rehabilitation Center for the Aged (HRCA) in Boston, and by Community Research Applications (CRA), both under grants/contracts from AoA, will shed some light on these questions.

"Cleveland Study," the source of much data on placement of the elderly and a document often cited in this chapter (GAO, 1977). These data appear to show that in Cleveland some 18 percent of the elderly not in institutions could use congregate housing, a type of housing similar to DCFs in that some form of help with at least one function of the activities of daily living (ADL) is required. This is the proportion of significantly impaired people whose conditions would make them candidates for congregate housing.[4] (In fact, many of them are already supported in their own homes and/or by their families, thereby reducing the need for congregate housing support to perhaps 2 to 4 percent of the elderly according to Leonard Gruenberg).

DCFs may provide more services, for example, shopping, cooking, and supervision, but the parallels may be quite close. Among the institutionalized elderly, that is, those in nursing homes, approximately 11 percent could have used congregate housing, a relatively small number, no doubt reflecting the greater medical and nursing dependency of this group. If these numbers were extrapolated to the nation, they imply a need for many more spaces than are currently available in congregate housing units, perhaps as many as four million. Of course, not all of this requirement would be met in DCFs, since many congregate housing units would not provide that much care. Also, many congregate units would feature independent living with some monitoring of health status while others would provide a much more comprehensive life care environment. Furthermore, many people would simply not choose to live in a DCF. Overall, the question of which type of supervised housing is suitable for which type of person requires more research and policy analysis. These numbers may give us some orders of magnitude, however.

The Region III Study

Since no surveys of the actual national number of DCF residents have been completed, it is necessary to resort to educated estimates such as those prepared by DHHS Region III in its 1979 survey of eight States (Mellody and White, 1979). This survey estimated that, nationwide, 600,000 to 800,000 people were housed in DCFs. Of these, 72 percent were white, 49 percent were over age 50, about half (47 percent) had a tenth grade education, and about half were women. The DCF population thus appeared to be younger and have more men than the population in nursing homes, no doubt reflecting the effect of mental hospital releases among the younger elements of the population. This survey also noted that younger people, many with alcohol and drug abuse problems, were increasingly frequent

---

[4] Letter from Comptroller General of U.S. to Senate Special Committee on Aging, dated October 15, 1979.

among the residents, often having come into the DCFs fairly recently. The impact of mental hospital releases on the DCF population can be inferred from the fact that an estimated 365,000 of those sent into the community from mental hospitals annually were in need of DCF support.

Disabilities reported among the DCF clients were largely mental. About 40 percent had been in mental hospitals for five years or more, but one-third had been hospitalized for less than a year. The one-time recidivism rate was about 40 percent, and the multiple rate was 30 percent, although some caseworkers felt that a return to the hospital was therapeutic and not so traumatic. These mental hospital stays reflect the fact that half of the DCF residents are mentally ill, and one in eight is retarded. Many also have multiple impairments. The great majority take medications, among them the potent psychotropic, Thorazine. Perhaps 70 percent of DCF residents are physically and/or mentally disabled. What is not shown in the Region III survey, however, is the frequency of mental and physical infirmity among those under 65 in contrast with those who are older. (Again, this should be a topic for research.) Unfortunately, rehabilitation programs were rare, despite the high levels of disability. Quite possibly, public policy creates few incentives and provides little means for such programs among DCF dwellers. Even where therapeutic and social services are available, dental, medical, nutritional, educational, and transportation services were rare. Recreation and mental health services were the most common in the DCF environment.

Caseworkers were responsible for about half of the placements of residents in DCFs, with families accounting for about one in seven. About 58 percent seemed to have no choice of a home. Despite the central role of caseworkers in placement, few residents were prepared for the transition from the mental or acute care hospital, and relatively few were visited frequently by their caseworkers.

Average facility size was 17 to 18 beds, although some had as many as 200. Most of the DCF operators were middle-aged (55 percent being 41 to 60 years of age) and female (by 2 to 1). About 41 percent were black. More than one-half had been in the "DCF business" for five years, more than 25 percent for more than 10 years. Most had had some training in the provision of health and social services, though often this was of a rudimentary type. (Less than half had been trained by health care or mental health institutions.) Many of the facilities were clean, but many were in poor physical condition, frequently sharing the same dilapidated conditions as their ramshackle neighbors in decaying, urban "psychiatric" ghettos. Residents of DCFs had little to do except watch television or take long walks, and few were asked or wanted to help with household chores, an act which might have had some therapeutic value. Only

443

14 percent participated in community mental health centers (CMHCs). Some were apathetic, others were lazy, and others were never surveyed because providers feared suits alleging the invasion of residents' rights.

Families might have supported some of these people, since approximately one-half were, or had been, married, and one-third had children. Among those with families (two-thirds of residents sampled), about 90 percent saw their families once a year, and about one-third, once a week. (This latter figure was probably optimistic.) In many cases, it appeared that families could not help much with care or financial support because of restrictions on SSI payments. In other cases, it was surmised that some families could have managed a DCF resident at home, had home care or respite care been available.

About 60 percent of DCF residents in the Region III survey were heavily dependent on SSI, which generated an average monthly income of about $215. About 58 percent turned their SSI checks directly over to the providers, receiving small amounts for spending money as their "change."

Whether this "market-type" use of income has any application to an analysis of vouchers or income supplements by users of long-term care and their families might be an interesting research topic. Although the constraints faced by potential users of DCFs may differ from those faced by long-term care users in general, the pattern of use of income as well as the supply-side response by providers should be better understood than they are currently.

The Temple Philadelphia Study

A smaller scale study of Philadelphia DCFs by Temple University revealed situations similar to those in the Region III survey. The Temple study estimated that Philadelphia held 1,500 DCFs, housing 15,000 residents. Of these, 52 to 59 percent were over 60 years old; about one half were women; 70 percent were white; half had never been married; 45 percent had only mental handicaps; only 5 percent had only physical disabilities, and 20 percent had multiple handicaps (Temple University, 1977). Although the characteristics varied from those found in the wider eight State study of Region III, the same general outlines of physical and mental dependency appeared, as did the limited roles which DCFs could play. A notable finding in the Philadelphia study was the very high proportion of black (94 percent) and female (88 percent) proprietors of the DCFs analyzed. Most of these proprietors had taken in boarders for an average of six years at the time of the survey; 25 percent had worked as practical nurses, and most desired more training (Temple University, 1978).

A notable common finding in most studies was that DCFs were not means to quick enrichment for most proprietors. In fact, the combination of increasingly stringent regulations and inflation was driving many facilities out of business. The advantages lay with DCFs which were members of chains and/or linked with nursing homes. This was particularly true in areas with an abundance of places and high vacancy rates. In Michigan, for example, when licensing was established, the number of homes dropped by 25 percent. Also, increasingly stringent regulations directly stimulated provider organizations. While adequate regulation and certification may be necessary to ensure at least a minimum quality of care, administrators and policymakers must recognize that there may be a tradeoff between quality control and the availability of spaces for the type of dependent residents usually served by DCFs (Mellody and White, 1979).

New York State Data and the Complexity of DCFs

Recent findings by New York State's Moreland Act Commission, the body responsible for oversight of nursing and residential facilities, shed some interesting light on the problems of building facilities without adequate analysis and planning and on the resultant problems of excess capacity in providing long-term care. The findings also illuminate the complicated relationships between DCFs and other long-term care providers (New York State Moreland Act Commission, 1976).

Because of rapid increases in long-term costs in the context of State fiscal stringency, the Commission surveyed New York facilities in the 1970s. Essentially, it found that long-term care costs were rapidly escalating, in part because of increases in the State's 65+ population, but more importantly as a result of a strong institutional bias in long-term care provision. Although nursing homes and DCFs were being built faster than the 65+ population was growing, occupancy rates in nursing homes continued to remain at 90 to 95 percent. Only in the DCFs were there substantial vacancies. By contrast with the nursing home situation, home care, day care, and foster care had been allowed to atrophy. The Commission alleged that the reasons for excessive institutionalization lay in the urge to fill beds that already existed and the inability of those with placement responsibility to use alternatives properly. In addition, new construction had been approved on rudimentary and arbitrary grounds. The Commission called for a moratorium on approving new long-term care construction and review of existing building permits. Additionally, it advocated much more careful and stronger planning for the provision of long-term care, as well as for construction.

Key data elements in the Commission's thinking were surveys from upstate New York, one in the Rochester region in 1969–71, the other in Monroe County in 1974–75. Both showed extensive misplacement of patients. For example, the Rochester figures showed that almost

445

27 percent of patients in skilled nursing facilities (SNFs) could have been in intermediate care facilities (ICFs) and almost 5 percent in DCFs; however, almost 4 percent of the DCF patients should have been in SNFs. The numbers in the Monroe County survey also showed misplacement, although the SNF misallocations were much lower. Most interesting in 1974–75 was the fact that perhaps 34 percent of the patients in a health related facility (HRF), New York's analog to the ICF, could have been in DCFs but that almost 44 percent of the DCF patients should have been in HRFs. One might conclude that DCF surplus beds offset HRF deficit beds, but the situation apparently was much more complicated.

In its census of facilities, the Commission found that there were 27,000 beds in 542 DCFs and about 25,000 in HRFs. (Steinbach *et al*, (1978) found roughly the same number of DCF beds.) Many of these had been built as communities attempted to adjust to the deinstitutionalization of mental patients. (In 1966, there were only 5,000 DCF beds and about 16,000 HRF beds. SNF beds rose by 65 percent in the same period.) Given the extent of estimated misplacement and the number of new DCF beds approved for construction, the Commission argued that the DCF vacancy rate by 1980 would be about 54 percent. It recommended suspension of permits to construct 11,700 DCF beds. In simple terms, it would appear that DCF addition should probably have been stopped. However, the Commission seemed to consider that, since New York standards for DCFs were so high, some DCF beds could be used for HRF patients. Perhaps the DCF should have been emphasized over the HRF on cost-effectiveness grounds. This consideration indicates that the boundary between these two sites of care is very imprecise and that choices about long-term care sites are not simple. In New York, such speculation was based on fiscal considerations, but the reality in care terms was much more complicated, revealing the effect of uncertain assessment procedures, past regulatory history, and the nature of the existing system.

The HRCA Pennsylvania Study

An ongoing study begun in 1976 by the Boston Hebrew Rehabilitation Center for the Aged is analyzing programs of domiciliary care placement and provision in the Commonwealth of Pennsylvania. The Center is also assessing DCFs on a multi-state basis. As of mid-1979, an extensive analysis of candidates for admission had been completed (Sherwood and Gruenberg, 1979). It considered applicant characteristics from the perspective of differences in referral agency sub-groups (that is, the aged, mental health patients, mentally retarded applicants, and an undefined group of others). Additionally, the researchers looked at specific problems of institutionalized applicants and at health, functional, mental, and social

446

differences among the institutionalized, those living in the community, and those living in foster homes about to be converted into State-supported DCFs. They also analyzed specific placement difficulties for certain sub-groups and for services.

The study was undertaken in connection with Pennsylvania's proposed domiciliary care program, focusing on providing noninstitutional alternatives for large numbers of chronically ill, physically and mentally handicapped, and marginally adjusted adults in the population. Two groups of homes were to be included in the program: foster homes, housing one to three clients, and group homes, housing four to 13 clients. Supplementary payments were offered to persons receiving SSI payments and judged incapable of living independently in the community though not in need of nursing home care. By providing adequate financial incentives, the State hoped to induce boarding house and foster care home operators to upgrade facilities and enter training programs. The purpose of the study was to provide a data base to monitor progress, devise guidelines for targeting services, identify the hard to place, develop criteria for training providers, and fashion DCF planning tools. The completed Pennsylvania study report was part of a large evaluation developed by DHHS Region III.

In mid-1978, six pilot areas, urban and rural, generated 494 subjects making up the total sample. These people were rated on seven scales: physical health, capacity to carry on ADL, intellectual functioning (to identify cognitive impairment), personal adjustment, social supports for all needs, social participation, and the quality of the physical environment. These data described the applicant group and were sorted by attributes of specific applicant sub-groups. They were linked to degree of success in placement. The aging (A) constituted the largest group, about 42 percent; mental health (MH) patients composed 34 percent; mentally retarded (MR), 17 percent, and other (O), 8 percent. (The aged and other groups shared many characteristics.) About 37 percent of the sample came from institutions, 34 percent from the community, and 30 percent from foster homes applying to convert to DCFs. The A and O groups were more community-based than the MH group, which was more institutionalized.

Overall, about 55 percent of the entire group was placed in DCFs, with small differences among the various characteristics of the groups (aging, etc.) but with major residence group differences. About 87 percent of the conversion-foster home residents were placed, versus only about 44 percent from the community and 40 percent from institutions. This skewing of placement introduced data problems and required a partial redirection of the analysis.

People over 60 accounted for 63 percent of the entire group. This was older than the Temple University sample discussed earlier (only

447

52 percent over 60), possibly reflecting the larger proportions of aging in the non-Philadelphia components of the HRCA sample. Among the aging sub-group, people 75 and older accounted for 59 percent. Clearly, the sample population resembled much of the LTC population generally. The high proportion of women corresponded to the group's advanced age (56 percent among the mental health sub-group and 67 percent among the aging). Again, this group was more female than the Temple group. Among the aging, over two-thirds were widowed, divorced, or separated; by contrast, 57 percent of the MH and 96 percent of the MR had never been married. Only 25 percent had one or more children close at hand. SSI payments went to 48 percent, with highest proportions (67 percent) among the conversion-foster home residents and community residents (54 percent). These last socio-economic findings indicate that the study groups were economically and socially vulnerable people. Their social weakness was also shown by the fact that, although 56 percent had made no more than one move in the five years prior to data gathering (thus suggesting a high degree of residential stability), the remaining 44 percent had moved more than twice. Moreover, for the entire group, the most common household arrangements were living alone, living with non-relatives, or living in a boarding home. Quite expectedly, large proportions among the MH (58 percent) and MR (36 percent) groups had been institutionalized over the past two years, but only about 25 percent of the aging and other groups had been in LTC institutions (including mental health facilities).

Many individuals had one or more major chronic physical conditions, with almost 80 percent of the aged and other groups showing an average of almost three conditions per person. The majority of the MHs and MRs also had multiple conditions. Nonetheless, over 50 percent of the total group was in good health or only mildly physically impaired, but 42 percent had painful diseases which required extensive medical treatment. On the other hand, only 14 percent of the sample group said that they had been too sick to function in any period of two or more weeks over the last three months. Clearly, the study sample was not in robust health, but significant numbers could probably be supported with a modest amount of medical help. This proposition is borne out by a subsequent analysis of medical need which indicated special major health requirements only for physical therapy and for the checking and maintenance of appliances.

Since medical/physical diagnosis is less important in LTC than capacity to function in ADL or IADL, the finding that only small percentages of the group were ADL-dependent was quite important, in that it indicated that this DCF-prone group does not need large amounts of intense personal care. Even among the aging sub-group,

448

only 37 percent were dependent in one or more functional ADL areas. Functioning in the community, however, also demands a certain amount of stamina, mobility, and capacity to carry out IADL tasks. Based on these indicators, the group was very dependent: 78 percent were not able to do heavy work around the house, 28 percent had some limitation in mobility (48 percent among the aging), and 64 percent (77 percent among the aging) required help with two or more functions of IADL (shopping, preparing meals, handling money, etc.). The composite need based on medical/physical condition, ADL, stamina, mobility, and IADL weaknesses was mainly for housekeeping support, not high technology or heavy nursing care. In almost all indexes of needed support, it was the aging who demonstrated a great deal of vulnerability. For example, 54 percent of them showed severely or completely impaired functional capacity, versus 36 percent for the MH (53 percent for MR).

The nature of the study group and of DCF candidates in general suggests that intellectual, mental health, and social adjustment problems may be crucial determinants of need. On the intellectual level, about 41 percent of the total group needed some personal supervision and help or 24-hour nursing supervision because of memory defects or disorientation. The MR group was highest in need, 80 percent falling in that category. In terms of personal adjustment, almost half, 49 percent, of the total group displayed only modest neurotic symptoms or none at all. The MH sub-group (with 29 percent having severely or grossly disturbing psychotic symptoms), showed the most impairment in this area, yet only 11 percent of the aged were in this category.

Social isolation was related to the group's relatively major intellectual and adjustment problems. Only one-fourth saw friends or neighbors as often as once per week, although the aged were less isolated. Overall, 53 percent of the sample was dissatisfied with social contacts or was extremely isolated. The entire picture is even more consistent, since 76 percent of the total group showed inadequate available social support. Again, the aged seemed better off than the rest of the group.

Quality of the physical environment was assessed for non-institutionalized applicants living in the community, including those in foster homes converting to DCFs. Many (53 percent) were living in quarters deemed physically adequate, a finding which very likely reflects the number of foster homes applying to convert. At the same time, many DCF residents (17 percent) were living in substandard homes, leading to a suspicion that many other people not reached by DCF programs may be in seriously substandard facilities.

Researchers in the HRCA study attempted to draw a combined physical/mental status profile to identify people with individual weaknesses or combinations of weaknesses making them likely candidates for DCF placement. The two major weakness areas identified in the sample were medical and physical functioning problems (24 percent of the group) and physical and intellectual functioning problems (17 percent of the group). A small proportion (10 percent) had no serious problems in any one area, but the cumulative effects of their separate problems were disabling. For the aging, the major problem areas were medical plus physical functioning (40 percent), whereas among both the MH and MR, the intellectual/social difficulties were relatively more important. Most telling, however, was the combination of mental and physical problems across all groups. Aging agencies thus must be prepared to summon mental health supports, while MH and MR groups must be sensitive to physical health and functioning dimensions as they support their clients in the DCF setting.

It should be noted that CRA found similar circumstances in a New York/New Jersey review (Steinbach *et al,* 1978). That review documented the "mingling" of mentally ill elderly with "normal" elderly. Many types of New York facilities included many elderly MH clients, some of whom were roommates of non-MH clients whose well-being often was adversely affected as a result. This may have fostered mental illness in the otherwise mentally healthy. Sufficient follow-up to MH placements was often lacking, a particular problem when many DCFs had sprung up near State mental hospitals during massive deinstitutionalization. In addition, in New Jersey especially, State and county agencies would vie for scarce beds, sometimes placing clients/patients without due regard for their MH or other care needs. In many instances, proprietors sought MH clients because they could be more easily ignored. In such instances, the probability of getting an MH roommate would be greatly heightened for a normal resident.

The HRCA group also analyzed differences between the placed and unplaced applicants. Overall, applicants from conversion foster homes were successfully placed, not surprising since these people were already on-site. In all, 87 percent of them were placed within a few months; they constituted 29 percent of the total sample but 46 percent of all placements. Because of data problems and the heavy representation of certain characteristics among given subgroups, HRCA did not attach much weight to the relationship between success in placement and certain socio-demographic variables: sex, children nearby, SSI status at application, and residential mobility within recent years (the variables linked to placement in cross-tabulations).

No major relationships were found between placement success and medical problems, except for number of medicines taken, regular taking of prescription medicines, and number of days of incapacitation. The last may have been an artifact of the number of residents

450

in conversion foster homes, however. Applicants better able to handle IADL tasks (shopping, cleaning, cooking, etc.) were less likely to be placed. Overall, it appeared that less needy patients were less likely to be placed when analyzed on physical/functional grounds.

Although the overall judgments about intellectual functioning were seemingly not related to placement success, people with personal adjustment or emotional problems seemed less likely to be placed than those without such problems. This finding characterized all residence sub-groups as well as the referral sub-groups. Available social supports (on an overall basis) similarly did not seem linked to placement, although applicant confidence in having someone close at hand was negatively linked, and illness of a person close to the applicant was positively linked. The former may have reflected the large conversion foster home element in the overall sample, since people in those homes showed low confidence in their available help. Again, social workers probably had already placed people whose social supports were shown to be weak. Participation in activities did not seem to have any significant links to placement. On the other hand, the need for analysis of services showed that persons with less need for meal services, transportation, and light housekeeping were less likely to be placed. Most importantly, persons were more likely to be placed if they had no need for personal adjustment services, including psychiatric counseling. Persons with poorer physical environments were less likely to be placed, possibly because such people may have had mental problems.

The data were also extensively analyzed without conversion foster home applicants. Among socio-demographic characteristics, only the presence of nearby children exerted any influence (positive) on placement. The linkage to the presence of children (whether as advocates or supports) suggested that a DCF program could benefit from enlisting informal family supports. When the reduced sample (without conversion foster home residents) was further analyzed for various sub-groups, only institutionalization within the past two years showed any significant links to placement success. Overall, while length of institutionalization was negatively related to DCF placement, it was not a deterrent to placing the MH population. The needs to coordinate mental health and physical health programs and to prepare the institutionalized elderly for DCF living were clearly demonstrated.

Assessment of the global physical/mental status links to placement success shows that the least successful were those with no serious mental/physical problems and those with personal adjustment difficulties. The clear implication is that, again, special attention must be paid to personal adjustment problems, perhaps through special incentive programs for DCF providers. The urgency of the

451

mental health/personal adjustment issues was underscored by the finding that, within the conversion foster home group of applicants, those with severe personal adjustment disturbances and those who had been receiving mental health or group clinic counseling were less likely to be placed. On the other hand, people from this same group who had ADL, IADL, or intellectual (not personal adjustment) problems were more likely to be placed.

The final portion of the HRCA study considered the non-institutional need for services and the extent of unmet needs (both as determined by professional opinion). The most consistent requirement was for housekeeping, other IADL supports, periodic casework, counseling and advocacy, recreational therapy, information and referral, friendly visiting, transportation/escort, and checking/emergency response. Specific physical and mental health related services were also widely needed. Not surprisingly, the aged required, on average, more IADL and physical health related supports.

The analysis showed that the percentage of unmet IADL need was not great. The absolute amount of unmet IADL need may, however, be considerable, given Pennsylvania's large population. Specific physical health related unmet needs were high: 26 percent of those needing home nursing had unmet needs, as did 90 percent of those needing physical therapy. If we accept professional judgments, this finding and others with respect to occupational therapy (75 percent unmet need) suggest a greater requirement for home health services in general. Unmet need for mental services was also great, showing a lack among 66 percent of those needing recreational therapy, 41 percent of those needing psychiatric counseling, and 21 percent of those needing counseling and advocacy. In general, there was significant unmet need for the aging and other sub-groups for psychiatric services and counseling.

Although conversion foster home residents seemed to have more of their needs met than did persons living in the community, even those facilities show an apparent lack of physical health related services and some social services (notably recreational therapy). That lack in all non-institutional settings will probably hinder the development of a successful DCF program unless service delivery can be coordinated.

Because of the special problems encountered in placing the elderly who had been long-term residents of institutions, the HRCA group devoted special attention to identifying problems associated with such institutionalization and to recommending ameliorative measures. Researchers found that poor motivation, fear of independence, and institutional attachment were the main sources of trouble. To remedy these conditions, the group suggested special programs aimed at the elderly in institutions to help prepare them

452

for an eventual life outside, most probably in a domiciliary care facility.

This discussion of the HRCA study has been quite extensive because of its importance as part of a larger analysis of DCFs. The study also is the source of some of the most comprehensive data ever gathered on applicants for DCFs. It represents one of the most extensive analyses of placement determinants and of service requirements. The data should be further analyzed for provider characteristics and by means of multivariate techniques to establish some models of client, provider, and social worker behavior and to sort out complex interactions among various indicators. The last type of analysis is particularly important because of the roles which the researchers identify for the social worker in making placement decisions.

Public Policy: Perverse or Inadequate?

As noted earlier, concern with safety and living conditions in DCFs led to the adoption of the Keys Amendment to the Social Security Act in 1976. This legislation was intended to protect DCF residents by forcing the individual States to develop standards of quality for those DCFs housing SSI recipients and to designate a single agency to monitor them. Unfortunately, the States' responses to this mandate were equivocal and inadequate in most cases. The April 1979 Gebran report, cited earlier, pointed to a lack of definition of facilities to be regulated, to multiplicities of State agencies, and to greatly varying standards among the States which had managed to come up with monitoring programs. In addition, somewhat paradoxically, the provisions of the Keys Amendment which called for a reduction in SSI payments to clients in "inadequate" DCFs may have been responsible for the failure to improve living conditions in DCFs. While Gebran recognized that many DCF residents and providers would resist further bureaucratic intrusions into their affairs, stronger Federal and State roles were recommended to ensure better quality control. This mandate was strongly laid on DHHS, since its regulations contained an enormous escape clause through which many facilities could evade any type of regulation under the Keys Amendment. Specifically, Department regulations stated that the Keys Amendment does not apply to facilities not offering care other than board and room. As a consequence, numerous facilities claimed exemption because they were providing only board and room, or "Eats and Sheets" to quote the Region III study (Mellody and White, 1979).

Regulating DCFs is difficult, largely because they are hard to find. For example, the referenced Temple University study was able to locate only about one-half of the DCFs they estimated to be in

453

Philadelphia. Many DCFs are invisible because they are small scale operations, run on a "Ma and Pa" basis without any claims on the Medicare/Medicaid apparatus or on Title XX or Title III funds. Similarly, many of these facilities make no demands on State or local governments' social services agencies. Essentially, this invisibility stems from the fact that DCF residents, in theory, are independent individuals who use their SSI (or other welfare) checks to support themselves in the community in a pattern consistent with the whole deinstitutionalization philosophy. While some States and counties require DCFs (or boarding houses, for that matter) to register and to be licensed, many States do not. Even in those States which do have such requirements, small homes may easily evade them.

Problems of DCF Administration at the State Level: The CRA and GAO Reports

Reimbursement problems abound in DCF provision. The CRA report notes three sets of reimbursement issues in New York alone: the difficulty of determining a fair DCF rate; the need to differentiate facility rate levels on the basis of the clientele being served, facility size, and services provided; and the need for flexibility in Federal administration of State supplementation of SSI payments (Steinbach, *et al,* 1978). Reimbursement determination (as of 1978) had been marked by acrimonious exchanges between DCF operators and State authorities over charges of bureaucratic interference, allegedly discriminatory admission practices, blocking of inquiries, and non-accountability for service provision. Although New York reimbursement rates far exceeded those in most other States, the State Comptroller found that many homes could not cover expenses on the $387 (1977) the State provided. On the other hand, some homes had much higher costs than homes very similar to them, allegedly because of excessive lease payments to companies with which the DCF operators were involved. Homes also varied in costs for perfectly legitimate reasons, such as the need to provide 24-hour services to the elderly in some homes, while other, similar DCFs had lower costs because their MH residents attended mental health clinics during the day. Overall, the CRA researchers concluded that the New York data base was inadequate to sustain judgments about the financing of the industry or the level of adequate DCF reimbursement.

CRA also found that more than one or two rate levels were needed. Specifically, rates should be related to level of resident impairment, facility service provision (especially special services), and general cost reimbursement. Of course, this assertion leads to many of the same reimbursement issues considered in connection with nursing homes, especially quality of care and patient condition.

454

Federal administration of SSI supplementation came in for some criticism because of alleged lack of flexibility on the part of DHHS and Congress. In addition, under the Federal rules, New York found itself unable to restrict payment of funds to DCFs on the grounds of inappropriate client placement or need for better standards of enforcement, except by decertifying facilities. To draw distinctions among facilities, the State might have had to withdraw from the system of combined Federal SSI and State supplementation.

CRA also found that certificate-of-need policy in New York required some revision. As with the Moreland Commission cited earlier, CRA found extensive evidence of excess capacity in certain areas of the State (6 percent in western New York versus 25 percent in New York City) and a state-wide average of 19 percent. Approval of all new beds being considered by the authorities could have resulted in a state-wide vacancy rate of 28 percent, ranging from 37 percent in New York City to 14 percent in the Finger Lakes District. The main problem with the certificate-of-need policy was that it was blind to special circumstances, for example, size of facility, impacts on neighboring communities, concentration of homes in specific areas of a county or city. Overall, there had been little coordination among the various responsible State agencies or between the State's mental health, welfare, health care, and health planning bodies.

In New Jersey, CRA found that certificate-of-need procedures, in general, resembled those for medically-oriented LTC facilities (SNFs and ICFs) and therefore did not consider characteristics unique to DCFs and their potential residents, including clients' social mobility and relative independence. Furthermore, DCF clients were counted as receiving care in their county of residence even though they may have been "away from home." Consequently, northern New Jersey, formal residence for many clients, had excess bed capacity, while Atlantic County in the south, where many residents had gone for the better weather, had excess bed demand. Nonetheless, the State formula could not take this location shift into account, and more beds were approved for the north. This problem aggravated yet another problem, that of shortage of LTC Medicaid beds. In many areas which were short of beds, LTC patients/clients were placed in unlicensed, unregulated boarding homes. In areas with excess DCF capacity, licensed DCFs often kept residents who could have moved into an SNF or ICF.

Other administrative and regulatory difficulties found in both States concerned case review and supervision, standards enforcement, placement criteria, and resident rights. Both States suffered from staff shortages, making case review difficult, and both found it hard to monitor unlicensed facilities (as was also true in the Temple

455

University study). Even the Keys Amendment did not help because DCF operators could claim that they were offering only hotel type services, precluding State intervention for "protective oversight." Although the Keys Amendment could have forced New Jersey authorities to identify DCFs, that State had a special problem: the widespread practice of many DCF operators of accepting SSI recipients and then transferring them to unlicensed facilities to clear yet another bed. This practice was made all the more possible by the general shortage of LTC beds in many parts of the State. Both States also suffered from the general lack of gatekeepers and supervisors. Paradoxically, the system of Federal administration of State supplementation aggravated these problems because it removed the need for SSI and supplementary payment recipients to be in contact with State authorities who would arrange rates and placements with county authorities. Under the Federal system, individuals could arrange DCF accommodation on their own without any oversight.

Enforcement of standards in both States again suffered from lack of staff and lack of sanctions applicable by the public authorities. Inspection schedules often could not be met, facilities could prepare for inspections in advance, and there were no effective mechanisms for resident complaints.

Neither State had clear-cut placement criteria. Although clients with medical problems supposedly were not to be placed in DCFs, many medically dependent people were placed in those facilities with doctors' certifications. Citing the Moreland Commission, CRA found that time pressures precluded effective assessment, making the entry to the LTC support system haphazard. Also, certificate-of-need procedures may have complicated placement by aggravating excess supply or demand for LTC beds. In the former case, operators would not wish to lose clients with medical needs to LTC facilities; in the latter case, clients may have been shunted into care which was at too low a level for their needs. Neither State had utilization review procedures for DCFs, means to assess needs of prospective clients, gatekeepers to DCF care, or widespread transfer policies among operators which would facilitate movement of clients among sites as their needs changed. Perhaps most telling was the fact that there had never been a determination of what type of DCF may be most beneficial to a particular type of resident. The question of resident rights was recognized as a pervasive problem but one which was difficult to resolve. Overall, it was found difficult to protect clients from operators who treated them as children and who abused them, often taking their money or possessions. The latter was a particular problem for clients completely reliant on SSI, whose monthly checks were often turned entirely over to the proprietors who resisted State attempts to provide residents with a modicum of private spending money.

456

This review of administrative and policy questions in these States sharply emphasizes the myriad administrative and implementation difficulties associated with such a multi-faceted type of LTC provision and demonstrates the awesome problems in framing all-embracing DCF policies.

In its recent report, GAO proposed a computer-assisted system for finding DCF residents and DCF facilities without violating either the Privacy or Freedom of Information Acts of 1974 (GAO, 1979). The very simple GAO system involves computer sorting of SSI recipients to identify clusters of such people living at the same address. After determining that these people are not independently living in the same hotel, apartment house, or congregate care facility, searchers would attempt to link the residents to the DCFs in which they may be living. If they can determine that the common address is a DCF, the local and State authorities can move in to inspect and license, if necessary.

Some Policy Questions: The Noble-Conley Analysis

John Noble and Ray Conley posed some provocative questions about deinstitutionalization and DCFs and proposed some policy shifts which could provide an excellent basis for a research program (Noble and Conley, forthcoming). In addition, their questions and suggestions have general applicability to the broadest issues in long-term care. Specifically, for DCFs, they seem to be asking if the DCF can be a humane alternative to the mental hospital. We might extend that question to ask if the DCF can be a humane alternative across the spectrum of long-term care, for the nursing home, for example. To answer either question, we need data on the numbers of people who have been (and could be) deinstitutionalized. We also need to know the extent of domiciliary care resources available. We also need information about present or potential DCF linkages to community services, such as community mental health centers, visiting nurse associations, or transportation services. At present, we have little information of this type.

On more particular grounds, Noble and Conley address the issues of the perverse effects of certain provisions in the SSI legislation. They point, first, to the average waiting time of 60 days before SSI eligibility can be determined for many DCF candidates. Not surprisingly, many of these people find themselves rejected by DCF operators who cannot wait for their money. In other instances, providers skimp on services until they are assured of payment. In either situation, the dependent person suffers. This suffering is especially acute if the patient is retained in an institution in which dependency may be increased even more by frustration and forced incarceration. Additionally, this type of delay is not cost effective.

457

One study cited by Noble and Conley shows that the average cost of an unnecessary day in a mental hospital was $56 versus $25 for SSI and health and social support services in less restrictive settings. One escape from this situation would be to amend the Social Security Act to allow for presumptive disability, and thus SSI payment, on the grounds of certification by a competent professional, at least until eligibility can be definitely established. Although rejected claims would not require return of the "temporary" SSI payments, the total cost would, allegedly, be modest.

In a similar vein, the Noble-Conley article mentions eliminating the one-third reduction of SSI payments now levied against SSI recipients who live within the household of another (usually a family member). It also mentions a proposal to eliminate any further deductions from SSI payments because of services received in kind. The additional cost of eliminating these provisions was estimated at $380 million. Both proposals, it is argued, could reduce the anti-family aspects of current SSI policy, although the authors acknowledge that more research is needed on effects of current SSI policy on the actions of family members and potential DCF candidates. At the other end of the deinstitutionalization process, Noble and Conley recommend that SSI payments be continued for three months in the event of reinstitutionalization. This would eliminate the anguish and bureaucratic problems connected with reducing payments to $25 per month as now required when a DCF resident has to return to the mental hospital or another facility.

Summary

Domiciliary care defies any attempt at definition. More complicated and diverse than home care, it lacks even the general focus on nursing care characterizing nursing homes. Furthermore, the purposes and intentions of domiciliary care are complex. To some analysts and policymakers, DCFs are halfway houses for deinstitutionalized elderly or young people; to others they are community-based, old people's homes of a non-institutional type; to still others, they may be sheltered homes for the frail. Perhaps it is safest to say that DCFs are all of these and more. In this circumstance, the role and purpose of any individual DCF is not always clear, nor is the function of the DCF sector in the spectrum or matrix of LTC support uncomplicated. At present, DCFs seem to constitute a set of flexible, reasonably safe, community-based facilities providing low-intensity, non-institutional care—supervision, meals, rooms—to groups of vulnerable people who literally may have no other place to go and would find living on their own in the community extremely difficult. Because of this general specification, however, DCFs confront the analyst with tough conceptual, methodological, and empirical questions.

458

As has been shown in the discussion of the highly disparate studies considered in this chapter, DCF clients come virtually in all sizes, shapes, and descriptions. Many are aged; many are discharged from mental health institutions; others are mentally retarded, and still others are just weak or handicapped. Almost all have some physical and/or mental functional disability. All studies indicate that most DCF residents suffer from more than one condition; a frequent finding is that mental health problems and physical disability combine to hinder ability to care for oneself or to function in the community. DCF clients may not all be physically weak, but interaction among their conditions—mental, personal adjustment, and physical—makes ADL and IADL functioning difficult for many of them. Disabilities and functional problems differ among client groups: the aged tend to be more physically debilitated than the MHs or MRs; the latter obviously suffer from relatively more mental and personality disorders. What is clear, however, is that all DCF groups share most types of infirmities to a greater or lesser degree, as do most LTC users. Interactions among infirmities must therefore be made a special focus of analysts', policymakers' and providers' concerns. This diversity among disabilities and DCF residents makes disability specification, nature of interventions, and desired outcomes all very difficult to identify. It also further complicates the already troublesome patient condition-quality-outcomes issue discussed in connection with the nursing home.

Diversity among clients is mirrored by variety among providers. Some facilities, usually private pay, resemble high quality hotels offering some supervision in a sheltered environment together with good quality food and accommodations. Others are dirty, dark, and overcrowded, providing little other than "three hots and a cot." Most probably lie in between, providing adequate food and lodging in a supervised, reasonably clean environment. Many proprietors claim to deal with their clients on an arm's length business basis, in which SSI checks or other financial support are exchanged for services. Actually, many clients come to the DCF under public auspices and through public placement, with provision often resulting from the intervention of public authority. DCFs differ not only in size and quality but also in purpose. Some cater to the elderly, others to mental health or mental retardation victims. For yet others, their clientele is defined by proximity to State mental hospitals and/or by the amount of excess demand or supply for beds in the vicinity. Many DCFs are not licensed or regulated, despite the Keys Amendment, and many DCF providers are not trained in providing adequate care and supervision. Many providers are, however, whether trained or not, very skilled at caring and at supervising.

Public policy, in many cases, has both complicated and worsened the DCF situation. It has also, through the SSI program, State supplementation, and State welfare, health, and mental health financial support, made possible both access to DCF provision and the growth of a DCF industry. Although SSI payments have ensured care for many people who would otherwise be unprovided for, the presumed personal and financial independence of SSI recipients has left many of them unsupervised in relations with DCF providers. Furthermore, Federal administration of State supplementation has further widened this supervisory gap. The Keys Amendment and the GAO recommendations may alleviate this situation and help lead to better licensure and supervision, but even this outcome is uncertain. Additionally, regulation and administration of the SSI program at the Federal level has delayed access to DCF provision for many would-be users.

State action in the DCF area parallels the jumbled nature of Federal policy and administrative action. Licensure standards vary widely from no control to highly exacting, perhaps excessive, regulation. Standards differ greatly among and within States, and placement criteria are rare. Even where criteria exist, time pressures, staff shortages, and bed shortages may make them ineffective.

An analyst attempting to place DCFs within useful categories will be frustrated from the outset by their complexity of type, purpose, and clientele. Definition of appropriate clients can be only very general, interventions too various to specify, desired outcomes too individually tailored, and relevant costs, benefits, and effectiveness too diverse to identify or quantify. At this stage of the analysis, therefore, attention must be focused on problems of definition and on public intentions. Clear description, accurate assembly of data, and policy clarity must all be provided before the techniques of scientific analysis can be applied to the DCF problem in an overall sense. In the meantime, individual analyses of specific types of DCF provision must identify outcomes, measure effectiveness of interventions, and appropriately assess cost-effectiveness.

References

Gebran, Gail, "Board and Care Homes: Analysis of the Issues," prepared for the Office of Policy Research and Analysis for Social Sciences and Human Development, DHEW, Office of the Secretary, April 1979 (mimeo).

Manard, Barbara B., Ralph E. Woehle, and James M. Heilman, *Better Homes for the Old*, Lexington, Mass.: Lexington Books, 1977.

Manard, Barbara B., Gary S. Kart, Dirk W. L. van Gils, *Old Age Institutions*, Lexington, Mass.: Lexington Books, 1975.

Mellody, James F. and Joseph G. White, *Service Delivery Assessment of Boarding Homes*, Philadelphia: U.S. DHEW, Office of the Principal Regional Official, DHEW Region III (May 1979).

New York, State Moreland Act Commission, *Nursing Homes and Domiciliary*

Facility Planning, Decisions on the Back of an Envelope, Report 4. (Albany: February, 1976).

Noble, John H. Jr. and Ronald W. Conley, "The Policy of Deinstitutionalization: Search for Fact Amidst Conjecture," Health Policy Quarterly (forthcoming).

Sherwood, Sylvia and Leonard Gruenberg, "A Descriptive Study of Functionally Eligible Applicants to the Domiciliary Care Program," with Executive Summary (Boston: Hebrew Rehabilitation Center for Aged, 1979, prepared in connection with HEW Contract No. 130-76-12.)

Steinbach, Leonard, Monica Holmes, and Douglas Holmes, "Domiciliary Care in New York and New Jersey" (New York: Community Research Applications, Inc., February 1978, developed for the Office of the Principal Regional Official, DHEW, Region II under Contract No. 120-76-0002).

Temple University, Center for Social Policy and Community Development, "Boarding Homes in Philadelphia: Findings, Policy Implications." Philadelphia: December, 1977.

Temple University, Center for Social Policy and Community Development, "Boarding Homes in Philadelphia: Summary of Findings and Implications for Policy," Philadelphia: January, 1978.

United States Comptroller General, General Accounting Office, Identifying Boarding Homes Housing the Needy Aged, Blind, and Disabled: A Major Step Toward Resolving a National Problem, HRD-80-17 (Washington, D.C.: November 19, 1979).

United States Comptroller General, General Accounting Office, The Well-Being of Older People in Cleveland, Ohio (Washington, D.C.: April 19, 1977).

United States Senate, Special Committee on Aging, Subcommittee on Long-Term Care, Nursing Home Care in the United States: Failure in Public Policy, Supporting Paper No. 7, "The Role of Nursing Homes in Caring for Discharged Mental Patients (and The Birth of a For-Profit Boarding Home Industry)" (Washington: U.S. Government Printing Office, March 1976).

CHAPTER XIII

Transportation and Dependency

by Steven G. Thomas

This chapter examines transportation as a necessary long-term care service. It begins with an overview of the characteristics and travel behavior of the "transportation handicapped" and continues with a summary of the major transportation problems affecting the chronically impaired. It then analyzes the Federal government's efforts to fulfill the special transportation needs of those elderly who require long-term care. It concludes with an analysis of the Federal perspective and presents recommendations for improving current programs and policies to enhance the vital relationship between transportation and long-term care.

Immobility and the Need for Adequate Transportation

A primary objective for long-term care services is to improve and maintain the mobility of a functionally disabled, older person. Arthritis, heart disease, frailness, and other debilitating conditions make it very difficult for an elderly person to climb stairs, walk a few blocks, kneel and stoop, and keep pace with a crowd. Also, these physical limitations can create hardships for the dependent elderly as they seek access to essential services and social activities (U.S. Senate, Special Committee on Aging, 1980). In general, long-term care providers must realize that mobility significantly influences an older person's physical and psychological well-being.

Adequate transportation is one of the most important mechanisms for improving the mobility status of the dependent elderly. Suitable transportation programs can help to fulfill essential long-term care functions, such as ensuring the provision of necessary personal and medical services and enhancing the independence and self-esteem of the individual. Furthermore, adequate transportation, by helping to maintain the health and social well-being of the individual, can forestall the need for institutionalization.

The Transportation Handicapped

To appreciate and understand the significance of transportation as a long-term care service, one must examine the characteristics and travel behavior of the chronically impaired population. This overview will introduce a more complete analysis of the relationship

463

between transportation and long-term care for the dependent elderly. The statistics for this review are from the U.S. Department of Transportation's *National Survey of Transportation Handicapped People*, released in 1978. DOT's survey provides useful and detailed information concerning the transportation behavior and requirements of the chronically impaired.[1] The survey's primary shortcoming is that its sample was limited to people living in urban areas, and no attempt was made to measure the transportation needs of the chronically impaired who are homebound. From the perspective of long-term care, it is unfortunate that these specific data do not exist because the care needs of the rural and homebound dependent elderly are usually more acute.

DOT defined the transportation handicapped as people who:

- lived in urban area households and were five years of age or older
- experienced general problems in the past 12 months such as a need for visual, hearing, or mechanical aids
- perceived they had more difficulty in using public transportation than persons without their general problem
- were not homebound (could go outside at least once a week with or without help).

Characteristics of the Transportation Handicapped Population

- 7.44 million or 5 percent of the urban population five years or older are transportation handicapped.
- Specifically, among the 7.44 million,
  1,938,600 (2.61 percent) use mechanical aids (braces, canes, crutches, etc.),
  1,572,800 (21.1 percent) have a hearing impairment,
  1,566,000 (21 percent) have a vision impairment,
  409,200 (5.5 percent) use a wheelchair, and
  3,502,300 (47.1 percent) have other problems, such as difficulty with stairs, stooping, walking more than one block, etc.
- 47 percent of the transportation handicapped are 65 and over; 67 percent are 55 and over.
- 21 percent of the total elderly population (65 or older) are transportation handicapped.
- 63 percent of the transportation handicapped are female.
- 4,940,000 live in mass transit areas (areas within one-half mile of a fixed route service), and 2,500,000 live in non-mass transit areas.

---

[1] This DOT survey is the most recent and thorough study of the travel behavior of the dependent elderly. Similar studies published before 1978 include Cantilli and Shmelzer, eds., 1970; Mark Battle Associates, 1973; and Miklojcik, 1976.

464

Travel Behavior of the Transportation Handicapped

- 98 percent, or 7,276,000, take an average of 29.5 trips per person per month.
- 96 percent of the elderly transportation handicapped take trips for a monthly average of 20.4 trips per person per month.
- 34 percent of all monthly trips are taken for shopping and personal business.
- 28 percent of all monthly trips are for leisure/recreation.
- 11 percent of all monthly trips are for medical/therapy services.
- 18 percent of all monthly trips are for work.
- 9 percent of all monthly trips are for school.

Travel Modes Used by the Transportation Handicapped

Eighty-three percent (6.175 million) of the transportation handicapped use a car as their principal means of transit. Of this group, 33 percent drive a car themselves, and 67 percent are driven. Sixty-eight percent of the transportation handicapped have a car available. However, 14 percent of this group use public transportation.

For the transportation handicapped who do not have access to a car (32 percent), 42 percent use public transit. Twenty-two percent (1,612,000) use public transit buses, and 223,000 of the transportation handicapped rely on the bus as their only means of transportation. Thirteen percent (927,000) use a taxi in an average month, and 2.2 percent (165,000) use the subway.

Throughout this review, these survey results will help to define the transportation problems and provide valuable information to analyze current programs and possible future policy reforms.

The Major Transportation Problems Confronting the Dependent Elderly[2]

Accessibility

Due to physical impairments caused by chronic conditions, many dependent elderly are unable to use most types of public transportation. DOT's survey found that because of their physical problems, 19 percent (1,405,000) of the transportation handicapped cannot use public transportation at all; 30 percent (2,175,000) can only use public transit with much more difficulty than a person without their physical problems; and 57 percent (3,860,000) have a little more difficulty than people without their physical problems. The primary bus barriers that prevented the chronically impaired from using a

---

[2] The reader may want to consult the following sources for a fuller and more detailed review of the major transportation problems of the dependent elderly: Institute for Public Administration, 1975; Mark Battle Associates, 1973; U.S. Department of Transportation, 1973; and Abt Associates, 1969.

bus were the need for a seat and difficulty in getting on and off. Taxi barriers included difficulty getting in and out of the taxi and difficulty in opening and closing doors.

The accessibility problem is not only associated with vehicular barriers. Within the entire transportation system, there are a variety of barriers, any combination of which can hinder or prevent maximum mobility. ". . . it is necessary to take an entire system approach rather than a vehicle and service approach in solving transportation handicapped people's problems. Removing vehicle barriers only helps a limited number of transportation handicapped who are currently prevented from using existing transportation systems" (U.S. Department of Transportation, 1978). For example, 49 percent of the transportation handicapped living in mass transit areas had difficulty getting to the bus stop. Moreover, the chronically impaired require some form of assistance from another person while they travel. DOT's survey data revealed that while 61 percent of the transportation handicapped do not require assistance when traveling, 39 percent (42 percent of the elderly) do require assistance throughout the entire trip. Overall, the dependent elderly require an accessible system which caters to all of their mobility needs.

Availability

For most dependent elderly, there is no such thing as an accessible and suitable transportation system. Even if a chronically impaired older person has access to a barrier-free public transit network, it is likely that, because of infrequent schedules and limited routing, the individual will still find it difficult to travel. Many functionally disabled elderly would be better served by a demand-responsive, door-to-door, transportation service. Yet, because of various program inefficiencies and usage restrictions, these special transportation systems fail to use their full service potential. (The program deficiencies associated with these services will be discussed later.)

The problem of availability is especially severe for those who do not own or have access to an automobile. Thirty-three percent of all transportation handicapped in urban areas do not own a car, and 32 percent do not have access to a car. As the DOT survey revealed, the transportation handicapped rely overwhelmingly upon the car to meet their transit requirements. Furthermore, American society is dependent upon the automobile as its primary means of transportation. Given this situation, the transportation handicapped who do not have cars are vulnerable to rapid isolation from essential services and social interaction.

466

Affordability

According to DOT's survey, ". . . transportation handicapped people come from lower income households." Thirty-four percent of the transportation handicapped live in households with incomes under $4,000, while only 15 percent of the total urban population has incomes below this level. Also, while 54 percent of all urban households earn over $10,000 per year, only 29 percent of the transportation handicapped are from households that earn more than $10,000. Lower incomes can directly affect the ability of a dependent elderly person to acquire adequate transportation and thus maintain a limited degree of mobility.[3]

In addition, many elderly who are transportation handicapped require special, more expensive modes of transit because they are physically incapable of using mass transit. For instance, DOT's survey data indicate that taxis are one of the most accessible and practical forms of public transportation for the chronically impaired. The obstacle which prevents most transportation handicapped from using taxis, however, is their cost. Forty-five percent of all people surveyed claimed they could not afford the service.[4]

In short, many dependent elderly confront a cruel paradox as they budget a limited income. Use of expensive transportation depletes precious resources needed for essentials such as food and medical care. And yet, if a dependent older person does not use an accessible but costly transit service, he or she will experience difficulties in obtaining food and medical care.

Rural Living and Few Transportation Alternatives

"For the rural elderly in particular, mobility difficulties . . . (are) compounded by the simple fact of distance and, consequently, high travel costs. A lack of adequate transportation in rural communities translates into greater isolation, which in turn produces poorer physical and mental health for the rural elderly" (U.S. Senate, Special Committee on Aging, 1980). The problem of obtaining necessary services and maintaining a socially active lifestyle in rural areas is even more serious for the dependent older person who does not own or drive a car because there are few public programs which provide special, demand-responsive transportation.

Statistics from the White House Rural Development Initiatives

---

[3] Gillan and Wachs (1975) found that, unless economic barriers are eliminated, improving a transit system will not increase the mobility of many elderly. For another discussion of the importance of affordable transportation, see Transportation Research Board, 1974.

[4] The inability to purchase taxi service and suggested remedies are reviewed in Urban Institute, 1975; Lovdahl, 1974; and Karash, 1975.

467

(1979) can help to convey the dimensions of the transportation difficulties of many chronically impaired, rural elderly.[5]

- 31 percent of Americans in 20,000 towns with a population of 50,000 or less are served by a public transit system.
- About 50 percent of America's towns of 50,000 or less are served by intercity bus lines.
- An estimated 60 percent of the nation's towns with less than 2,500 people have no taxi service.
- 45 percent of the rural elderly do not own an automobile.
- 30 percent of all rural residents (compared with 10 percent of all urban residents) must travel more than half an hour to obtain medical care.

Finally, the problem of inadequate transportation for the rural, dependent elderly is compounded by their lower than average incomes. For example, the incidence of poverty is higher for the rural elderly than for those older people living in urban areas. In 1977, the U.S. Census Bureau reported that 18.7 percent of all persons 65 or older living in non-metropolitan areas had incomes below the poverty level. This rate was greater than the 11.4 percent of all elderly living below the poverty level in metropolitan areas.

An Uncoordinated and Fragmented Transportation Planning and Delivery System

"Transportation services have traditionally been provided to the elderly and handicapped by health and social service agencies and organizations on an *ad hoc*, piecemeal, and uncoordinated basis. This had resulted in duplicated, underused, and expensive services" (U.S. Department of Transportation, 1979). As practical as it seems, agencies offering transportation to the dependent elderly do not share resources, services, or equipment. As a result, many dependent elderly are denied adequate door-to-door or fixed-route transportation.

The House Select Committee on Aging presents a good example of "the scope and magnitude of the duplication and fragmentation" that exist among community transportation projects created to serve the dependent elderly (U.S. House of Representatives, Select Committee on Aging, 1976). In 1975, Pinellas County, Florida had 26 different projects serving the elderly and handicapped. Among all the projects there were over 40 vehicles (not including taxis and private

---

[5] A more extensive review of the transit problems of the rural elderly can be found in U.S. Department of Transportation, 1976, and McKelvey and Dueker, 1974. Recommended strategies for addressing this problem are reviewed in McKelvey, 1975; Notess, Eakes, Popper *et al,* 1975; and Transportation Research Board, 1976.

468

cars driven by volunteers) and "26 separate budgets, maintenance bills, drivers, and administrations."

Although the potential benefits from a centralized and coordinated transit system may appear obvious, there are many barriers to consolidation. One analysis prepared for DOT found that social service agencies felt coordination was a "good idea" but the agencies were afraid that actual implementation of the concept would threaten "their control of program funds, client allegiance, and visibility in the community" (U.S. Department of Transportation, 1979). The study also found that labor problems, planning delays, and competition with private transit operators were some of the coordination problems confronting transit operators. Furthermore, the study revealed that barriers to coordination also exist in Federal statutes and program regulations (U.S. Department of Transportation, 1979).

Along with consolidated program efforts, cooperation between transportation and social service planners is required. As mentioned earlier, transportation is an important long-term care service for improving the mobility status of the chronically impaired. An adequate transportation service requires a systems approach to planning which recognizes the physical, social, and psychological requirements of the dependent older person. Such an effort will not be realized, however, unless all the transportation planners, providers, and operators in a given location cooperate by sharing their expertise.

The Federal Perspective

Federal regulations, program funding, and demonstration projects have a tremendous influence over the development and provision of adequate transportation for the dependent elderly. Given the significance of the Federal role, a review of the major government transportation programs and policy objectives is necessary to understand the transportation issue. Specifically, it is important to analyze these Federal programs to see if they exhibit an appreciation for the long-term care requirements of the dependent elderly.

Department of Transportation Programs
Section 3, Urban Mass Transportation Act of 1964 as Amended

Under Section 3, there was an estimated $1.38 billion available in fiscal year 1980 to help State and local public transit agencies finance transportation projects in urban areas. Through grants or loans administered by the Urban Mass Transit Administration (UMTA), Section 3 will fund up to 80 percent of the capital costs for the acquisition, construction, or improvement of mass transit facilities and equipment. Of the estimated $1.38 billion, $255 million was to be used to finance bus-related capital expenditures in fiscal year 1980. Section 3 does not fund operating costs. Although this program exists to meet the transit needs of the entire urban population, it is an UMTA policy to give priority to projects assisting the elderly.

Section 5, Urban Mass Transportation Act as Amended in 1975

Section 5 funds can be used by a State or local public transportation agency for capital purchases or to offset up to half of a transit system's operating costs. Most of the funds have been used by transit authorities to finance operating expenses. An estimated $1.37 billion for fiscal year 1980 was distributed by UMTA to various States, based on urban population and population density. Section 5 also requires Section 5 recipients to charge half fares to elderly and handicapped riders during non-peak hours.

Section 6, Urban Mass Transportation Act of 1964 as Amended

Section 6, with an estimated $14.5 million in fiscal year 1980, allows UMTA to finance a variety of research and demonstration projects. Although the funding is relatively insignificant, Section 6 grants are important for funding innovative techniques to transport the chronically impaired.

Section 16(b)(2), Urban Mass Transportation Act of 1964 as Amended in 1978

This provision distributes grants or loans to buy vehicles and equipment for transporting the elderly and handicapped.[6] Recipients must be private, nonprofit organizations and pay a cash share of 20 percent of the capital costs. Operating expenses must be covered by funds from other sources. This program was supplemented by an estimated $20 million of Section 3 money in fiscal year 1980 which was dispersed to the States in proportion to their numbers of elderly and handicapped residents.

Section 18, Urban Mass Transportation Act of 1964 as Amended

Initiated in 1979, this program provides operating and capital funds to improve rural and small urban area transportation. In fiscal year 1980, an estimated $85 million was available, up from $75 million in 1979. Projects must provide maximum coordination to rural transportation services. Both public and private non-profit transportation agencies are eligible for funding, and the program operators have enough flexibility to define the type of transit service to be provided (for example, demand-responsive or fixed-route service). While the

---

[6] For a case study of how New York State activated programs under Section (16)(b)(2), see Brunso, 1975.

transportation must serve the general public, the dependent elderly are likely to benefit most from any rural transportation initiatives.

Section 16(a), Urban Mass Transportation Act as Amended

Two of the most influential and controversial transportation initiatives for the dependent elderly have been promulgated through DOT regulations. The first provision to be examined, 16(a), was enacted in 1970 and it states:

It is hereby declared to be the national policy that elderly and handicapped persons have the same right as others to utilize mass transportation facilities and services; that special efforts shall be made in the planning and design of mass transportation facilities and services so that the availability to elderly and handicapped persons of mass transportation which they can effectively utilize will be assured; and that all Federal programs offering assistance in the field of mass transportation (including the provisions under this Act) should contain provisions implementing this policy. (Public Law 91–453, 49 U.S.C. 1601 *et seq.*).

In April 1976, the Urban Mass Transit Administration and the Federal Highway Administration jointly issued regulations to meet the Congressional requirements enacted under 16(a). The 1976 regulations provided planning guidance and established design criteria for vehicles and facilities funded under Federally-assisted mass transit projects. Local transportation agencies were also required to make regular transit services more accessible to the elderly and handicapped; efforts to achieve this purpose would serve as the basis for allocation of Federal transportation funds.

Upon entering office, DOT Secretary Brock Adams deferred implementation of these regulations because of the controversy surrounding UMTA's bus design standards. In short, critics felt that UMTA's criteria would not make vehicles and facilities fully accessible to the elderly and handicapped. As a result, the DOT Secretary announced in May 1977 that full-size transit buses purchased with Federal funds after September 30, 1979 were required to have a maximum floor height of 22 inches, be capable of "kneeling" to 18 inches at bus stops, and be equipped with wheelchair lifts or ramps and tie-downs. "The effect of this decision was to mandate Transbus, a fully-accessible bus that had been designed through UMTA's research and development program" (U.S. Department of Transportation, 1979).

When bids were solicited to build a vehicle to meet the Transbus specifications, however, no manufacturers submitted bids. They contended that the technological and commercial aspects surrounding the specifications "made the risk of bidding too great" (U.S. Department of Transportation, 1979).

471

Section 504, Rehabilitation Act of 1973

Greater implications for the design and cost of public transportation vehicles and facilities arose following DOT's issuance of regulations implementing Section 504, which declares:

No otherwise qualified handicapped individual in the United States . . . shall, solely by reason of his handicap, be excluded from the participation in, be denied the benefits of, or be subjected to discrimination under any program or activity receiving Federal financial assistance (U.S. Senate Special Committee on Aging, 1979, p. 145 and Public Law 93–112, 29 U.S.C. 790 *et seq.*).

Issued on May 31, 1979, these regulations required that all public transit buses purchased with DOT funds after July 2, 1979, had to be wheelchair accessible and that within 10 years, 50 percent of the rush-hour buses had to be wheelchair accessible. Similar accessibility requirements and time limits were set with respect to rapid transit, light rail, and commuter rail facilities. Also, any Federally-assisted transit system not made accessible by July 1982 must provide interim accessible service until the entire transportation network is barrier-free.

These final regulations have generated a great deal of controversy, primarily due to the projected costs. Opponents argue that "the regulations are unlawful because the broad congressional policy of non-discrimination in Section 504 neither authorizes nor requires sweeping affirmative actions, costing billions of dollars . . ." (U.S. Department of Transportation, 1979). Opponents also contend that special, door-to-door services would be the most effective and efficient transit system. They also argue that even when public transit vehicles and facilities are made accessible, many of the chronically impaired will be unable to travel from their homes to the transit stops.

Advocates for DOT's regulations claim that Section 504 is civil rights legislation which demands equal, not separate, transportation for all. They argue that special services stigmatize the user and are inherently unequal because of their high user costs and restrictions in service. In short, the handicapped have a civil right to be incorporated into the mainstream of society, and a fully accessible transit system would make this possible.

Department of Health and Human Services Programs

Title XX—Social Service Amendments of 1974 as Amended,
Social Security Act

Title XX assists States in providing social services to the poor. Individual States receive $2.5 billion through formula grants, which

can be used to pay up to 75 percent of the cost of providing necessary services to those persons receiving Federal income assistance.
"Of the $2.5 billion, about $42 million, or 1.7 percent is expended for
transportation, but no data exist to show how much of that amount
is going to older persons" (U.S. House of Representatives, Select
Committee on Aging, 1976).

Title III—Older Americans Act of 1965 as Amended 1978

Under Title III, funds are allocated on a formula basis to State and
local aging offices to develop systems of comprehensive and coordinated social services for the elderly. "In fiscal year 1975, approximately 20 percent of all Federal funds for area planning and social
services, or about $16 million, was spent on transportation" (U.S.
House of Representatives, Select Committee on Aging, 1976).

Title XIX—Social Security Act as Amended

Medicaid regulations require that States must ensure necessary
transportation of Medicaid recipients to and from the providers of
health services. There are, however, no accurate estimates concerning the amount of Medicaid funds spent on transportation.

Federal Transportation Objectives and the Government's Interpretation of the Problem

A review of the Federal transportation programs for the dependent
elderly reveals that the government's primary objective is to develop
a more accessible and affordable urban public transit system. Furthermore, DOT has established regulations to ensure all chronically
impaired persons equal access to every public transit vehicle and
facility. A secondary but important transportation objective has been
to encourage the research and development of innovative vehicles
and systems for transporting the functionally disabled.

Apparently these objectives address what Federal officials believe
are the major transportation problems of all dependent persons. For
instance, the government presumes that a major problem for most
functionally disabled persons, is the inability to use public transportation because of vehicular and facility barriers. Another problem, from
the Federal perspective, is that inaccessible public transit systems
violate the civil rights of a chronically impaired individual. Finally,
the government feels that many dependent elderly and handicapped
people desire special, demand-responsive transportation, but such
services are rarely adequate.

Federal Transportation Objectives and Long-Term Care for the Dependent Elderly

None of the major Federal transportation programs focuses on
long-term care. Nevertheless, most of the government's efforts to

473

assist the transportation handicapped population fulfill, to some degree, the mobility requirements of the dependent elderly. The dependent older people who are not homebound and who are living in urban areas would obviously benefit from a more accessible and affordable transit system. Also, special, door-to-door transportation services could enhance the mobility of the chronically impaired elderly who are only able to travel with great difficulty. These general assumptions, however, cannot be substantiated, primarily because DOT never evaluates the transportation programs from the perspective of long-term care.

UMTA's efforts to improve all public transportation vehicles and facilities may in fact assist a significant number of elderly people who require some level of long-term care transit service. But a sensitive, adequate system can only evolve if the transportation planners and policymakers recognize and appreciate the specific long-term mobility requirements of the dependent elderly. Present transportation policies for the elderly and handicapped would be more effective if it were understood that these initiatives could also provide an important long-term care service.

There are several indications that a long-term care perspective would enhance the effect of transportation policy objectives and programs. First, transportation policymakers have failed to study the mobility requirements of the elderly who are homebound or living in institutions. Moreover, planners have not examined the transit network associated with delivering long-term care services (such as home health care) to homebound individuals. The transportation needs of this segment of the dependent, elderly population have been overlooked, principally because policymakers do not recognize the value of transportation as an essential long-term care service.

A second example of how a proper understanding of long-term care would improve transportation programs for the functionally disabled is a product of DOT's transportation handicapped survey. The results indicate that current transportation programs may not constitute the most effective or efficient approach for serving the chronically impaired. Those interviewed were more interested in a subsidized, demand-responsive transit system than an accessible, fixed-route system.[7] The subsidized, door-to-door alternative would remove many more travel barriers than a fully accessible public transit system could eliminate. One result which is particularly in-

---

[7] DOT's survey indicates that the combination of a separate, door-to-door service and individual subsidies has the widest appeal among potential users who are transportation handicapped; 75 percent expressed an interest. In contrast, 59 percent indicated an interest in using a fully accessible, fixed-route system.

474

teresting from a long-term care perspective is that 42 percent of the elderly who are transportation handicapped require assistance while traveling.

These results suggest that the dependent elderly require much more than simply an accessible public transit system. Not only do they desire a more personal system, but their health conditions require an alternative to public transit. Enlightened transportation policy objectives and programs are required to address the real transit needs of the dependent elderly. Policymakers, however, must understand the long-term mobility problems of the functionally disabled before they can develop more effective objectives and programs.

Analysis and Recommendations

DOT's Regulations Implementing Section 504 Must be Revised

Currently, it is not economically feasible for public transportation agencies to abide by DOT's regulations. The American Public Transit Association contends that an expenditure of $3 to $5 billion would be required to make existing transit systems fully accessible. The Congressional Budget Office reported that if the DOT regulations were enacted, they would cost an estimated $6.8 billion over the next 30 years. Moreover, such an accessible system would serve no more than 7 percent of all severely disabled persons living in urban areas (Congressional Budget Office, 1979). As previously mentioned, DOT's own survey revealed that the greatest number of transportation handicapped people desire and would be able to use a subsidized, demand-responsive transit system.

As an UMTA report states, ". . . the issue today is not whether or not to accommodate the special transportation needs of elderly and handicapped persons but how to accommodate them and at what cost" (U.S. Department of Transportation, 1979). The current regulations issued by DOT are not the type of sensitive and enlightened rules which will encourage and support the creation of an efficient, effective transit system for the functionally disabled.

More Research is Needed Concerning the Transportation and Mobility Requirements of the Dependent Elderly

As a whole, UMTA's research and demonstration efforts are respectable and useful. These efforts, however, must be expanded to include the transportation handicapped people living in all parts of the country and in all types of facilities. For example, a detailed survey of the urban transportation handicapped exists, but there is virtually no information on the transportation needs of the rural dependent person. Overall, policymakers must study more thor-

475

oughly the transit requirements of those impaired persons who do not have access to public transportation.[8]

Second, the mobility and transportation requirements of the homebound and institutional care residents must be studied. In fairness to DOT, its 1977 survey did include a quota sample of dependent persons living in group living facilities (boarding homes, congregate living quarters, etc.). Yet a complete analysis cannot be based on these results, since the sample was not chosen randomly, and residents in only certain types of facility were interviewed.

Third, the transportation problems experienced by the providers of long-term care in the home should be examined. Is transportation a significant problem for these providers? Do transportation problems hinder the efficient and effective delivery of services to the homebound? More information is needed to determine whether these questions are pertinent. Finally, transportation for the chronically impaired must be analyzed with a long-term care perspective. Policymakers and analysts must evaluate transportation as a long-term care service to determine the function and importance of transportation in improving the mobility status of the functionally disabled.

The Implications of a Transportation Handicapped Person Owning or Having Access to an Automobile Must be Recognized

It appears that transportation planners have taken for granted the predominant role of the car in servicing the transportation needs of the chronically impaired. Practically all transportation planning and policy for the functionally disabled is focused on mass transit or special transportation services. Yet the overwhelming majority of the transportation handicapped will continue, in the immediate future, to rely on the automobile as their primary mode of transit.[9] This reliance could generate some very difficult problems, however, especially for the dependent elderly.

As older people live longer, the aging process and chronic conditions increase the likelihood that an older driver will no longer be capable of operating the vehicle safely. Also, rising gasoline prices will certainly hinder the travel behavior of those dependent, elderly drivers with limited or fixed incomes. The automobile is important, but because of this dependency on the car, future trends may decrease the mobility of many functionally disabled drivers. Transportation planners must realize and contend with the implications of these potential problems.

---

[8] The following studies review methods for determining transit needs and measuring the latent demand for transportation by the dependent elderly: Miller, 1976; Yukubousky and Politano, 1974; and Hoel et al, 1968.

[9] For a profile and analysis of elderly drivers, see Planek and Overend, 1973.

The Transportation Handicapped Must Become Active Participants in the Planning of Transportation Policies and Programs

Transportation policymakers cannot rely on their own perceptions of the problems confronting the elderly and handicapped. Both the dependent elderly and the handicapped must be consulted and given the opportunity to contribute toward the development of adequate transit systems. By expressing their transportation and mobiliy requirements, the transportation handicapped can help to create an effective and efficient system of barrier-free vehicles and facilities.[10]

Transportation Programs Must Be Coordinated and Consolidated

At the delivery level, agencies serving the transportation handicapped should pool and share their transportation resources (equipment, personnel, maintenance, administration). Such a recommendation, however, will be very difficult to implement until some human and institutional barriers are removed. One problem is that agencies are constantly seeking to protect their realm of the social service arena. Scarce funds and agency pride can create a highly competitive environment which makes it difficult to cooperate and share resources. Moreover, franchise problems and friction between agency providers, public transit authorities, and taxi companies are major roadblocks to a more efficient transportation system.

A primary cause for the friction and fragmentation at the local level is Federal transportation policies and regulations. There are at least "30 major sources of Federal funds financing transportation services to the elderly . . ." (U.S. House of Representatives, Select Committee on Aging, 1976). Every one of these funding sources is governed by program restrictions which stipulate user characteristics, income restrictions, health requirements, and service area. This hodgepodge of Federal programs and regulations inevitably creates a variety of agencies at the local level providing transportation services to essentially the same target group.

Ultimately, the best approach for improving coordination is to thoroughly revise government transportation regulations and programs. The 30-odd programs which are scattered across different Federal agencies must be consolidated. Program regulations must be reformed so that the rules complement the intent and purpose of creating a complete and adequate transportation system for the functionally disabled.

---

[10] Providers may find these two handbooks useful for planning and operating a transit program for the dependent elderly: Institute of Public Administration, 1975, and Brail, Hughes, and Arthur, 1976. It is essential, however, that the planning process include the elderly (recipients) as active participants.

The Potential of Volunteer Services as a Transportation Resource Must Be Recognized and Used

Volunteers play a significant role in delivering transportation services to the dependent elderly.[11] Most social service agencies depend, to some degree, on volunteer labor to operate transportation programs for the functionally disabled. One can also assume that many neighbors and friends volunteer their time on an unorganized basis to transport the dependent elderly. During these times of fiscal restraint and less "big" government, volunteers constitute one of the most valuable transportation resources of the dependent elderly population. Every effort must be made to offer incentives and to publicize the need for volunteers. One of the most important incentives to volunteer could be to offer attractive income tax deductions to those persons who offer their cars and time to transport the functionally disabled.

Transportation for the Chronically Impaired Should be Provided, Not According to Age, but According to Need

Age-based transportation programs are probably not the most effective mechanisms for improving the mobility status of the dependent elderly. The transportation handicapped, as a whole, encounter mobility barriers regardless of their age. Chronic conditions, although most prevalent among the elderly, hinder persons of all ages; there are rarely any transportation problems which are unique to the dependent elderly. Therefore, special transit policy should serve all persons who encounter transportation barriers. When such legislation is formulated toward a specific age group, it prevents the creation of a well-financed, coordinated system of accessible transportation because limited funds are used inefficiently, resulting in a fragmented delivery network.

Transportation Must Be Perceived As a Social Service Which Is Required to Improve the Mobility Status of the Functionally Disabled

A total systems approach is needed to develop an adequate transit network that would truly serve the chronically impaired. Engineers, legislators, program administrators, and user-group advocates must all expand their understanding of the transportation problems confronting the handicapped. The issue is not simply accessible transportation because limited funds are used inefficiently, mand-responsive services. Ultimately, the transportation provided must enhance the well-being of the user.

---

[11] The value and importance of volunteers has been highlighted in various studies. See Millar and Kline, 1975; Teixeira and Karash, 1975; and Crain and Associates, 1974.

478

Conclusion

The most immediate solution for improving the mobility status of the transportation handicapped is to provide subsidized, demand-responsive transportation. Both DOT's survey and the CBO report indicate that providing door-to-door transit services, along with subsidized fares, would be the most efficient and effective form of service,[12] but several factors must be considered. Many elderly and handicapped expressed the need and/or desire for assistance while they travel. A major problem with taxi service is that the assistance one receives (if any) is not adequate. Furthermore, transporting dependent individuals is just one component of servicing mobility needs. Transportation handicapped people must also be able to move around effectively once they have reached their destinations.

The present demand-responsive system of transit services must be thoroughly restructured and replaced by a more centralized service network. This consolidated social service transportation must then be supplemented by subsidized taxis (where they exist). In addition, incentives are required to encourage the participation of many more volunteers.

Finally, policymakers must weigh the costs and benefits of making public transportation more accessible. All mass transit users would no doubt benefit from improved vehicle and facility design. But some very difficult decisions must be made to determine how extensive these alterations should be. Nonetheless, the transportation handicapped do have a right to an accessible and dignified mode of transportation. A well-conceived, extensive system of demand-responsive transit services, operated by conscientious individuals, would substantially improve the mobility of all transportation handicapped persons.

References

Abt Associates Inc., "Transportation Needs of the Handicapped," August 1969, for U.S. Department of Transportation, Office of Economics and Systems Analysis, PB 187327.

Brail, Richard K., James W. Hughes, and Carol M. Arthur, "Transportation Services for the Disabled and Elderly," Rutgers University, Center for Urban Policy Research, New Brunswick, New Jersey, 1976.

---

[12] Many researchers have reviewed the planning and operation of demand-responsive transit programs in various areas of the country. This wealth of information is a valuable resource for expanding and improving demand-responsive transit services. For example, see Notess and Paaswell, 1972; Dewey and Mikkelsen, 1973; McLaughlin, 1975; Cantor and Rosenthal, 1975; Florida State Department of Transportation, 1974; Duffy and Shanley, Inc., 1975; and Lincoln-Lancaster Commission on Aging, 1975.

Brunso, Joanna M., "Transportation for the Elderly and Handicapped. A Prototype Case Study of New York State Experience in Activating an Element of a Federal Grant Program," Washington University, August 1975, for U.S. Department of Transportation, Urban Mass Transportation Administration, PB 249105.

Cantilli, Edmund Jr., June L. Shmelzer, and Staff Administration on Aging, eds., *Proceedings of the Interdisciplinary Workshop on Transportation and Aging, Washington, D.C.—Transportation and Aging Selected Issues,* Polytechnic Institute of Brooklyn, Department of Transportation Planning, 1970, DHEW Pub. No. (SRS) 7220232.

Cantor, Marjorie H. and Karen Rosenthal, "Dial-A-Ride: The New York City Experience—An Alternate Transportation System for the Elderly," New York City Department for the Aging, Bureau of Research Planning and Evaluation, May 1975, for U.S. Department of Health, Education, and Welfare, Administration on Aging, PB 251135.

Congressional Budget Office, *Urban Transportation for Handicapped Persons: Alternative Federal Approaches* (Washington: U.S. Government Printing Office, November 1979).

Crain and Associates, "Para-Transit Survey, Component of MTC Special Transit Needs Study," April 1974, for Metropolitan Transportation Commission, San Francisco Bay Area and U.S. Department of Transportation, Urban Mass Transportation Administration.

Dewey, Michael and Betty Mikkelsen, "Grand Rapids Model Cities Dial-A-Ride Summary Report on Design and Implementation," Ford Motor Company Transportation Research and Planning Office, October 1973.

Duffy and Shanley, Inc., "Cranston Transvan," February 1975, for U.S. Department of Transportation, Urban Mass Transportation Administration, PB 244639.

Florida State Department of Transportation, "Transportation of the Elderly (TOTE)—A Pilot Project to Develop Mobility for the Elderly and the Handicapped," April 1974, for U.S. Department of Transportation, Urban Mass Transportation Administration, PB 233593.

Gillan, Jacqueline and Martin Wachs, "Life Styles and Transportation Needs Among the Elderly of Los Angeles County," University of California at Los Angeles, School of Architecture and Urban Planning, February 1975, for U.S. Department of Transportation, Urban Mass Transportation Administration, PB 243631.

Hoel, Lester A., Eugene D. Perle, Karel J. Kansky, Alfred A. Kuehn, Ervin S. Roszner, and Hugh P. Nesbitt, "Latent Demand for Urban Transportation," Carnegie-Mellon University, Pittsburgh, Pennsylvania, May 1968, PB 178979.

Institute for Public Administration, "Transportation for Older Americans—The State of the Art," March 1975, for U.S. Department of Health, Education, and Welfare, Administration on Aging, PB 243441/3G1.

Institute for Public Administration, *Planning Handbook—Transportation Services for the Elderly,* November 1975, for U.S. Department of Health, Education, and Welfare, Administration on Aging, PB 247958.

Karash, Karla H., "Analysis of a Taxi Operated Transportation Service for the Handicapped," Executive Office of Transportation and Construction, Massachusetts, December 1975, 8600-24-225-1-76-CR.

480

Lincoln-Lancaster Commission on Aging, "Lincoln Experimental Transportation Demonstration Project," Lincoln, Nebraska, October 1975, for U.S. Department of Transportation, Urban Mass Transportation Administration, PB 248735.

Lovdahl, J. Leonard, "Transportation for the Elderly and the Handicapped, Special Report 154," Transportation Research Board, 1974.

Mark Battle Associates Inc., "Transportation for the Elderly and Handicapped," July 1973, for the National Urban League, New York, New York, PB 225283.

McKelvey, Douglas J. and Kenneth J. Dueker, "Transportation Planning: The Urban and Rural Interface and Transit Needs of the Rural Elderly," University of Iowa, Institute of Urban and Regional Research, Center for Urban Transportation Studies, August 1974, Technical Report 26.

McKelvey, Douglas J., "Considerations in Planning and Operating Transportation Systems for Older Americans and Public Systems in Rural Areas," University of Iowa, Institute of Urban and Regional Research, Center for Urban Transportation Studies, May 1975, Working Paper Series 15.

McLaughlin, Bruce, "City of Cleveland Neighborhood Transportation Project, Dial-A-Bus," City of Cleveland, May 1975, for U.S. Department of Transportation, Urban Mass Transportation Administration, PB 248903.

Miklojcik, Jacob L., "Mobility and Older Americans: An Analysis," *Transit Journal,* May 1976.

Millar, William W. and William R. Kline, "Operating Costs and Characteristics of Selected Specialized Transportation Services for Elderly and Handicapped Persons," Pennsylvania Department of Transportation, August 1975.

Miller, Joel A., "A Hierarchical Model of Latent Demand of the Handicapped and the Elderly," *AMV Tech Notes,* Vol. III No. 5, March 1, 1976, Alan M. Voorhees & Associates, McLean, Virginia.

Notess, C., E. Eakes, R. Popper, R. Zapata, E. Pittelkau, D. Rajala, S. R. Vermuri, L. Chavis, and P. Davis, "Transportation of Elderly to Rural Social Services."

Notess, Charles B. and Robert E. Paaswell, "Demand Activated Transportation for the Elderly," *Transportation Engineering Journal,* November 1972.

Planek, Thomas W. and Robert B. Overend, "Profile of the Aging Driver—Who He Is, . . . When, Where, How He Drives," *Traffic Safety,* Vol. 73, No. 1, January 1973.

Public Law 91-453, 49 U.S.C. 1601 *et seq.*

Public Law 93-112, 29 U.S.C. 1601 *et seq.*

Teixeira, Diego B. and Karla H. Karash, "An Evaluation of Councils on Aging Dial-A-Ride Systems in Massachusetts," *Transportation 4,* 1975.

Transportation Research Board, "Transportation for the Elderly, the Disadvantaged, and Handicapped People in Rural Areas," *Transportation Research Record 578,* 1976.

Transportation Research Board, "Transportation for the Poor, the Elderly, and the Disadvantaged," *Transportation Research Record 516,* 1974, PB 239281.

The Urban Institute, "Implementing Shared Taxicab Services—A Case Study in Arlington, Virginia," for U.S. Department of Transportation, Urban Mass Transportation Administration, PB 245645.

481

U.S. Department of Transportation, "Summary Report of Data from National Survey of Transportation of Handicapped People" (Washington: U.S. Government Printing Office, June 1978).

U.S. Department of Transportation, "Coordinating Transportation Services for the Elderly and Handicapped" (Washington: U.S. Government Printing Office, May 1979).

U.S. Department of Transportation, "Elderly and Handicapped Transportation" (Washington: U.S. Government Printing Office, September 1979).

U.S. Department of Transportation, "Transportation Systems Center, The Handicapped and Elderly Market for Urban Mass Transit," October 1973, Urban Mass Transportation Administration, PB 222828/6.

U.S. Department of Transportation, Technology Sharing Program Office, Transportation Systems Center, "Rural Passenger Transportation—State of the Art Overview," October 1976.

U.S. House of Representatives, Select Committee on Aging, "Senior Transportation: Ticket to Dignity" (Washington: U.S. Government Printing Office, May 1976).

U.S. Senate, Special Committee on Aging, "Developments in Aging: 1979" (Washington: U.S. Government Printing Office, 1980).

White House Rural Development Initiatives, "Improving Transportation in America" (Washington: U.S. Government Printing Office, June 1979).

Yukubousky, Richard and Arthur Politano, "Latent Travel Demand of the Elderly, Youth, and Low Income Population," New York State Department of Transportation Planning and Research, August 1974.

Chapter XIV

Mental Illness and the Elderly

by Marni J. Hall

This chapter discusses (1) the extent and causes of mental disorders in the elderly, (2) utilization of services by the mentally ill elderly, (3) barriers to the receipt of appropriate mental health services, (4) the major mental disorders of the elderly and their prognoses, (5) possible policy changes in Medicare and Medicaid psychiatric coverage, and (6) ideas for future research.

Need for Mental Health Services for the Elderly

Glasscote (1977) and others state that old age puts one at a high risk of psychiatric disability. From 15 to 25 percent of the elderly living in the community have moderate or severe mental health problems (Epstein, 1975). "Psychopathology, in general, and depression, in particular, rise with age. The World Health Organization reports that the highest incidence of new cases of psychopathology of all ages is found in persons 65 and older, with the rate of new cases approximately 2½ times that found in the next highest age group" (Pardes, 1979). One quarter of all reported suicides in the United States are committed by the elderly (Cohen, 1977).

Some of the factors believed to be related to the greater need for mental health services by the elderly include (1) the presence of chronic physical ailments limiting activity and frequently resulting in pain and isolation, (2) loss of age peers (including spouse) through death or institutionalization, (3) diminished and often inadequate financial resources, (4) changes in identity brought on by retirement, and (5) the fear of serious debilitating illness and death. Some suspected causes are drug interactions, inappropriate drug dosages, and nutritional deficiencies. However, there is limited empirical evidence on factors which increase the risk of mental illness for the elderly. Blazer (1980) points out that mental illness in the elderly is undoubtedly caused by a number of interacting factors. Most older people experience multiple stresses and yet do not become mentally impaired. His research suggests that stressful life events "are not important risk factors for the development of mental health impairment in the elderly when physical health and social support are controlled." Additional research is needed to identify contributing factors and the characteristics of those elderly persons who seem to be most vulnerable to mental illness.

Utilization of Services by the Elderly Mentally Ill

Mental Health Settings

Use of mental health services by the elderly differs from that of the general population. Although the elderly compose 11 percent of the population and have a greater need for these services, they are under-represented in admissions to mental health settings. Table XIV–1 indicates that elderly admissions accounted for only 4.8 percent of total admissions to the mental health services listed for 1971 and 1975. The highest admission rates were for the institutional settings, that is, the private and public mental hospitals and general hospital psychiatric units; the lowest rates were for the outpatient settings (the community mental health centers and outpatient services). Data on services provided by private psychiatrists indicate that only 2 percent of their time is spent serving the elderly (Ronch and Maizler, 1977), in what is frequently believed to be primarily an assessment rather than a treatment capacity.

Non-Mental Health Settings

The utilization statistics for the settings in Table XIV–1 would present a fairly complete description of mental health care received by the under 65 age group, but the elderly have been described as being "on the periphery of mental health care" (Cohen, 1976). A large proportion of the elderly mentally ill never come in contact with mental health professionals. Many are cared for by physicians who are not psychiatrists; others receive care in nursing homes.

Cummings (1977) estimated that as many as 60 percent of Medicare beneficiaries' visits to their physicians were for emotional distress, rather than for physical illness. Mental health professionals acknowledge the role of the general medical practitioner in treating the mentally ill of all ages (Health United States, 1978). In the over 65 group, this role is even more important because of this age group's tendency to define problems as physical rather than mental. Often physical and mental illness are very closely related; for example, a chronic disabling condition can lead to serious depression. The precise number of mentally ill elderly seeking care from their physicians for mental health problems is unknown, but it is believed to be considerable.

In 1977, approximately 22 percent of the nursing home population (288,000 persons) was listed as mentally ill or senile. This is compared to 170,000 in mental hospitals (Division of Biometry and Epidemiology, 1980). Since only those persons with a primary diagnosis of mental illness are included in this figure, it is a very conservative estimate. Including all of the elderly with mental or behavioral problems would increase the figure to at least one-half

484

TABLE XIV-1
Admissions 65 Years of Age and Over as a Percent
of Total Admissions to Selected Mental Health Services,
U.S., 1971 and 1975[1]

	1971	1975
All Services	4.8	4.8
State and County Mental Hospitals	8.5	5.3
Private Psychiatric Hospitals	11.5	9.9
General Hospital Inpatient Units	7.0	7.4
Community Mental Health Centers	3.6	4.0
Outpatient Psychiatric Services	2.1	3.8

[1] Data provided by the Division of Biometry and Epidemiology, National Institute of Mental Health, Alcohol, Drug Abuse and Mental Health Administration, U.S. Department of Health and Human Services.

to two-thirds of the total number of nursing home residents (Redick, 1974). It is only within the past 10 years that nursing homes have become common settings for the elderly mentally ill. The reasons for this, and nursing homes' appropriateness for treating this group, are discussed in the following sections of this chapter.

The Effect of Deinstitutionalization on the Utilization of Mental Health Services by the Elderly

The deinstitutionalization movement had far-reaching effects on the treatment of the mentally ill. Four major reasons (Comptroller General, 1977) for this massive shifting of patients out of mental hospitals were: (1) humanitarian concerns about the poor conditions prevalent in these facilities and the lack of adequate treatment; (2) changes in the current psychiatric philosophy which favored community treatment; (3) the discovery and increasing popularity of psychotropic drugs; and (4) court decisions against involuntary commitment and in favor of treating patients in the least restrictive environment. The goal of the deinstitutionalization movement was to reduce the population of State mental hospitals by at least half. This goal was to be achieved both by relocating the current population and by restricting new admissions.

In 1963, P.L. 88-164, Title II, authorized the establishment of community mental health centers (CMHCs). These centers were to provide a comprehensive array of mental health services in the community, regardless of the patient's ability to pay for care. It was anticipated that the centers would serve many of the individuals who were deinstitutionalized, but resources were insufficient to care for this most difficult group. Frequently, there was little coordination between the centers and State and county mental hospitals. The elderly have generally made up only about 4 percent of the centers' caseload (Department of Health and Human Services, 1978). In 1975, P.L. 94–63 added specialized services for the mental health of the elderly to the comprehensive services centers were to provide, but no additional funds were made available. Serious financial problems, as well as the mandate to become self-sufficient after initial Federal support, impeded special efforts by the centers to serve hard-to-reach groups including the elderly.

The deinstitutionalization movement changed the mental health service system from one composed primarily of long-term inpatient care in public facilities to one increasingly oriented toward short-term, acute, outpatient care in the private sector (Health United States, 1978). From 1963 to 1971 the utilization rates of outpatient services for the population as a whole more than doubled (Birren and Renner, 1975). Deinstitutionalization had a very different effect upon the elderly. Their rate of utilization of outpatient services increased only slightly. While the younger age groups were being moved out of institutions and into the community, the elderly were being moved to nursing homes. Between 1969 and 1973, the number of elderly persons in public and private mental hospitals decreased by about 40 percent, while the mentally ill in nursing homes increased more than 100 percent from 96,000 to 194,000. In recent years, more mentally ill individuals resided in nursing homes than in public mental hospitals (Division of Biometry and Epidemiology, 1980).

Factors Encouraging Placement of the Mentally Ill Elderly in Nursing Homes

A number of factors explain the massive shifting of the elderly mentally ill from mental hospitals to nursing homes. One of the most important was the availability of Federal matching funds, primarily through the Medicaid program, to support patients in nursing homes. Glasscote (1976) and others contend that "without the advent of federal financing for nursing home care the elderly population of state hospitals would have increased substantially rather than declined." The costs of caring for the elderly mentally ill, which had been borne entirely by the States, could now be shared with the Federal government. In addition, nursing homes were generally less expensive than mental hospitals. The availability of this new reimbursement alternative was especially important because financing for other community alternatives was often lacking.

In a variety of ways, it simplified matters to place patients in nursing homes. These settings, like mental hospitals, provided a number of services designed to meet the patients' basic needs, that is, housing, food, medical or nursing care, and supervision. The

486

difficult task of locating, coordinating, and arranging financing for each of these services separately in an ill-prepared community setting was thereby avoided.

Placement in nursing homes not only eliminated the State hospitals' initial coordination of essential services but also often eliminated, in the hospitals' view, the need for follow-up. All responsibility for the patients was transferred to the new institutional setting. In many cases, the records of the newly discharged patients were not even forwarded to the nursing homes.

Appropriateness of Nursing Homes for the Treatment of the Mentally Ill

For some elderly patients, nursing home placement could be justified. Largely due to advanced age, a number of patients were suffering from severe chronic physical impairments in addition to mental problems. Others had spent decades in the protected setting of the hospital and could not have been placed in a less sheltered setting in the community. Because of their extended institutionalizations, many had no homes or families to return to. A number had conditions considered irremediable, so the absence of psychiatric treatment in the nursing homes was not considered a problem. Also, there frequently were no other types of facilities in the community where these people could receive care. This lack of appropriate community facilities and services is still a major problem.

There is considerable controversy over the advisability of placing mentally ill patients in nursing homes rather than mental hospitals. In some ways, nursing homes are seen as beneficial for patients, for example, they are less isolated, smaller, and less stigmatized (Stotsky, 1970). On the other hand, the mental patient is essentially moved out of the mental health system and into a setting designed almost exclusively to meet patients' physical needs. It has been contended that mental patients in nursing homes "suffer in the sense of increased and unnecessary dependency, identification with terminal patients, social isolation, unnecessary depression, and lack of activity with a rehabilitative focus" (Glasscote et al, 1976). There is also evidence to suggest that individuals with mental conditions are placed in lower quality homes. Other homes discriminate against them, since they can disrupt the normal routine of the home (Manard, 1975).

An estimated 50 to 66 percent of nursing home residents have some type of mental or behavorial problem, yet nursing homes rarely offer mental health services. Patients are admitted by general practitioners or other physicians who rarely call in a psychiatrist or other mental health professional for consultation. The U.S. Senate Special Committee on Aging (1975) estimated that "80–90 percent of the care afforded the elderly in nursing home settings is provided by aides and orderlies." These people have little or no training dealing with mentally ill individuals. The only "treatment" which many nursing homes provide is drug therapy. Even this may be less for therapeutic purposes than for maintaining order and serenity in the homes (Butler and Lewis, 1977). A large proportion of Medicaid drug expenditures for nursing home patients are for psychotropic drugs (Glasscote et al, 1976). Mental health services are not specifically required under existing nursing home regulations, and funds are generally not available to pay for them.

Barriers to the Receipt of Appropriate Mental Health Care by the Elderly

Problems in Diagnosing and Treating the Major Mental Disorders of the Elderly

The lack of appropriate mental health treatment for the aged in nursing homes and in the community can be partially explained by the widespread confusion among physicians (including some psychiatrists) about the major mental disorders of the elderly. Most harmful is the belief that the elderly mentally ill cannot benefit from treatment. In this section the major mental disorders afflicting the elderly are discussed. The discussion will specify whether these disorders are generally considered to be reversible or irreversible.

Butler and Lewis (1977) divide the major mental disorders of old age into two categories: 1) the organic disorders which have a physical cause, for example, abnormal and identifiable changes in brain tissue, and 2) the functional disorders which have no known physical cause and which appear to be related to the individual's personality and life experience. The organic disorders can be either acute and reversible or chronic and, at present, irreversible.[1] The symptoms of both reversible and irreversible conditions are very similar, consisting of confusion, forgetfulness, impaired intellectual functioning and judgment, labile or shallow affect, disorientation, and, in very severe cases, loss of the ability to walk, or to control bowels or bladder (Glasscote et al, 1977).

Too frequently, both physicians and laymen readily classify the mental disturbances of the elderly as "senility." This term generally covers two chronic disorders: the first is senile dementia, formerly known as chronic brain disease associated with senile brain disease. This condition, also known as Alzheimer's disease, is characterized by the dying off of brain cells and shrinkage of the brain. Its cause is unknown. Although onset may be gradual, the disease can progress rapidly, and death may occur within only a year or two.

---

[1] The International Classification of Diseases no longer retains the distinction between acute and chronic conditions.

The second condition often simply labeled "senility" is chronic brain syndrome resulting from hardening of the arteries of the brain, either a non-psychotic organic brain syndrome with circulatory disturbance or psychosis with cerebral arteriosclerosis (Glasscote *et al*, 1977). At present, both of these conditions, believed to cause as much as 50 percent of the mental disorders in old age, are incurable. However, since these conditions frequently co-exist with depression, anxiety, and psychosomatic disorders, treatment can have a significant, positive effect on the patient (Butler and Lewis, 1977).

Senility in its severe form affects more than one million older persons and reduces longevity by two-thirds after onset. An estimated additional two million older persons may have mild to moderate forms of this devastating disease. The prevalence of the disorder increases with advancing age (Group for the Advancement of Psychiatry, 1979). "Senile dementia alone afflicts more than 50 percent of nursing home residents and probably accounts for a sizable number of nursing home admissions, although physical health problems are commonly listed as the primary diagnosis" (Division of Biometry and Epidemiology, 1974).

Senility is a serious and significant mental disorder of the elderly, but mental health professionals feel it is "one of the most overdiagnosed and misdiagnosed disorders of the mind" (Cohen, 1979). Robert Butler, Director of the National Institute on Aging, states that "there are over 100 reversible syndromes that may mimic senile dementia" (1977).

Many physicians are not familiar with the mental problems common among the elderly and may diagnose confusion and forgetfulness as symptoms of organic brain disease. As was indicated previously, acute organic brain syndromes often have symptoms very similar to chronic conditions, such as senile dementia, but acute syndromes are reversible. These acute conditions can be caused by trauma or injuries to the head, infections, side effects of drugs, metabolic malfunctions brought on by thyroid trouble, inadequate nutrition, anemia, tumors, circulatory problems, or neurological states (Cohen, 1979). If acute brain syndromes are not properly diagnosed and treated, they may develop into irreversible conditions (Secretary's Committee on Mental Health and Illness of the Elderly, 1979). Another major mental problem for the elderly, depression, can also have symptoms similar to chronic brain syndrome. Depression, however, is "among the most treatable of all mental disorders" (Glasscote *et al*, 1977).

Although the elderly may have a number of disorders which affect younger persons (for example, schizophrenia, neurosis, alcoholism, etc.), the two most frequent diagnoses for all admissions to specialty mental health inpatient and outpatient settings in 1975 were depression (35 percent) and organic brain syndrome (31 percent; Health United States, 1978).

The failure of many physicians, including psychiatrists, to differentiate among the reversible and irreversible mental disorders of the elderly often results in inappropriate treatment or no treatment at all. According to Dr. Herbert Pardes, Director of the National Institute of Mental Health, the results of a recent study indicated that "more than 60 percent of elderly patients who are admitted to State mental hospitals have received no previous psychiatric care . . . Rather than being the most conservatively applied link in the chain of treatment provision, and an alternative of last resort, institutionalization often is used as a first-choice intervention for elderly persons" (1979). Institutionalization in nursing homes can be particularly harmful since few homes offer mental health care. Even the acute reversible conditions under these circumstances can become steadily worse, and may develop into irreversible syndromes. Premature death may also occur.

Attitudes of Mental Health Professionals Toward Treating the Elderly

Many of the above-mentioned problems have occurred because of the lack of interest among mental health professionals in treating the elderly. Most mental health professionals have little training or experience in caring for the elderly. The Group for the Advancement of Psychiatry cites the following reasons for the disinterest in serving the elderly: (1) the unjustified belief that elderly people cannot change and that their problems are always due to untreatable organic brain disease; (2) the fact that they're nearing death anyway and may even die during treatment; (3) the perceived stigma attached to treating the elderly; (4) negative myths about the elderly; (5) fear that the large number of problems that the elderly have will be overwhelming; (6) cultural insensitivity to this age group; and (7) therapists' fear of facing the inevitability of their own death and possible disability (1971).

Cohen (1976) feels that psychiatrists should be made aware of the rewarding and challenging aspects of serving the elderly due to the "interplay of the psychological, social, and biomedical factors" influencing their mental health. Special knowledge and expertise is required to differentiate among several common conditions that manifest themselves in similar ways and to determine an older person's sensitivity to psychotropic drugs (Glasscote et al, 1977). It is also important for psychiatrists and other mental health professionals to lay to rest the notion that the elderly will not or cannot respond to treatment.

Additional training for psychiatrists and other mental health professionals in the diagnosis, care, and treatment of the elderly mentally ill is needed.

490

Negative Stereotypes about the Responsiveness of the Elderly to Mental Health Treatment

Contrary to beliefs held by mental health professionals and the general public, research findings suggest that the elderly are just as responsive, or even more responsive, to psychiatric treatment than other groups. Clinical depression in the elderly has been found to "respond to treatment, whether in the form of talking about problems, pharmacotherapy, improved family and social supports, or, when indicated, electroconvulsive therapy" (Cohen, 1977).

Bryson (1977) reports that in a Texas county with an outreach information and referral program in effect from September 1973 to August 1977, the mean length of hospital stay of elderly patients was reduced from 111 days to 53 days. This substantial decrease resulted in a cost reduction of $1.1 million. In a control county (also in Texas) without an outreach program, the mean length of stay during the same period was 114 days.

A report entitled *Mental Health and the Elderly: Recommendations for Action* states that numerous innovative and experimental programs have evidence that early detection and appropriate treatment of the elderly's psychiatric problems can "minimize their debilitating effects and prevent or delay more serious illnesses from developing" (Secretary's Committee on Mental Health and Illness of the Elderly, 1979).

When qualified individuals thoroughly assess the elderly, the provision of mental health treatment required for the maximal level of functioning possible in view of the diagnoses is more assured.

Attitudes of the Elderly Toward Mental Health Services

The elderly often accept the widespread notions that their conditions (mental deterioration or emotional instability) are inevitable and irreversible consequences of aging. Many also share the belief that they are "too old to change" or to be treated.

Perhaps because of these negative views, the elderly are less likely to define their problems as mental problems. Their psychological problems are often manifested through physical symptoms. Many of their psychological problems may be directly related to, or caused by, physical conditions. They seek care in the more familiar and socially acceptable doctor's office or from family, friends, or clergy.

This age group tends even more than their younger counterparts to define mental illness as a stigma and as a personal failure. Memories are still vivid of insane asylums where "crazy" people were "put away." Because of the common negative image, one community mental health center's staff serving this age group carefully avoided mentioning their affiliation with the center until their clients clearly accepted them. This center also found a much greater willingness among the elderly to accept the center's mental health counseling from a nurse because of her clear identification with the medical system (Paterson, 1976).

These attitudes present a significant barrier to the receipt of mental health care by the elderly and undoubtedly partly explain their low utilization of mental health services. Vigorous outreach programs are often needed to overcome the hesitancy of the elderly to recognize the value of, and need for, mental health treatment. Goldensohn (1977), in an article discussing the utilization of mental health services in the Health Insurance Plan of New York, felt that adequate numbers of mental health staff delivering care in the centers where the aged receive their other medical care were necessary to reach this normally under-served population.

Limited Financing for Psychiatric Care

Another barrier to the receipt of care by the elderly could be the prohibitive cost of this treatment and the limited Medicare psychiatric coverage. Some experts feel that the lack of sufficient financing for ambulatory mental health services provides incentives for unnecessary hospitalization and for receipt of general medical services not designed for the treatment of mental disorders (Cummings, 1977).

Medicare reimbursement for physician services is limited to a maximum of $250 per year for outpatient psychiatric treatment. A 50 percent copayment by the beneficiary is also required. Only those services provided by a physician, or those under the direct supervision of a physician, are covered. Coverage for psychiatric hospitals is subject to a lifetime limitation of 190 days.

More liberal coverage for psychiatric care is provided for patients in psychiatric units of general hospitals, and for physicians' services delivered to these inpatients. Inpatients in general hospitals are subject only to general Medicare provisions (e.g., spell of illness) and have no special psychiatric limitations.

Lack of Needed Support Services for the Elderly Mentally Ill

This chapter has already discussed the need for greater interest on the part of mental health professionals in serving the elderly. Even if mental health services to this age group are made available, some problems would remain. Outreach services are needed to identify the elderly in the community who need care. Some of these individuals, particularly those with mobility restrictions, will need transportation to bring them to care and treatment. The availability of other support services in the community (for example, home health care, homemaker services, meals on wheels) could enable the mentally ill who are receiving outpatient treatment to remain in their homes or with their families longer or even indefinitely. One of the important reasons cited for the increase in readmissions to mental hospitals has been "the failure of existing systems of community care to address the problems of the population in need" (Department of Health and Human Services, 1980). The placement and then abandonment of the elderly in substandard boarding and rooming houses and other unsuitable settings is common due to lack of alternatives. Residences similar to the intermediate care centers for mental health (mentioned later in this chapter) are needed, either supported by Medicaid or other funding sources. These centers, or some other designated agency, need to act as case managers for the elderly mentally ill. Community mental health centers may be the most appropriate coordinators of services needed in some cases. However, the centers would need adequate resources and other incentives to assign this task a high priority.

Possible Changes in Medicare and Medicaid Psychiatric Coverage Which Might Encourage Appropriate Provision of Services to the Elderly Mentally Ill

The following sections will discuss proposed changes in Medicare and Medicaid which might encourage more appropriate provision of psychiatric care. It should be noted, however, that changes in financing alone could not be expected to end the low or inappropriate utilization of mental health services by the elderly. A demonstration project in Colorado tested the effects of reimbursing for clinical psychologists' care and of allowing more generous outpatient psychiatric coverage and a lower copayment. The results showed very low utilization of these services in spite of the coverage expansion. The Mental Health Service of the Health Insurance Plan of Greater New York (HIP) offered psychiatric coverage to subscribers without a coinsurance or deductible. Even under these circumstances the utilization by the elderly of these services was low. The consultation rate for the Medicare population was 5.8 per 1,000 in 1975. The rate for those below age 65 was 14.3. The rate of services received by Medicare beneficiaries (83 per 1,000) was also low compared to the rate for the under-65 age group (221 per 1,000; Goldensohn, 1977). Just as important as changes in financing are additional training programs for psychiatrists and other mental health professionals in the diagnosis, care, and treatment of the elderly mentally ill, along with outreach and education programs to encourage the elderly to use mental health services.

Medicare

Outpatient Psychiatric Care

Outpatient psychiatric coverage under Medicare is currently very limited for physicians' services. The beneficiary is responsible for

493

a 50 percent copayment for treatment of mental conditions, and the program will not reimburse more than $250 a year for this care. Outpatient care for other conditions has no similar limitation and only requires a 20 percent copayment.

There are a number of problems with the psychiatric limitation. First of all, particularly due to inflation, fewer services can be bought now than in 1965 when Medicare was enacted. Second, combined with the liberal coverage of inpatient psychiatric hospitalization in general hospitals and inpatient physicians' services, this limitation encourages the use of more costly and not necessarily more appropriate inpatient care. Third, the high copayment may significantly deter the receipt of needed psychiatric care in the early stages of illness. This neglect could lead to steadily worsening conditions which can only be treated in an institution by the time the person enters the health care system for treatment. In the interim, a reversible condition could become irreversible. Fourth, even if we assume that the high copayment is no problem for the elderly, the ceiling on program payment strictly limits the number of visits which are covered. This reimbursement limitation, in addition to being a disincentive for the patient, could also act as a disincentive for psychiatrists to treat the elderly.

In view of these considerations, President Carter's Commission on Mental Health recommended that the maximum allowable program payment for psychiatric services be increased to $750 and that the copayment be lowered from 50 percent to 20 percent. The National Plan for the Chronically Mentally Ill (Department of Health and Human Services, 1980) also endorsed these modifications.

Inpatient Psychiatric Coverage

Medicare was designed to cover only active treatment for psychiatric conditions, rather than custodial care. Because psychiatric hospitals were primarily custodial in nature when this legislation was enacted, a 190-day lifetime limit on care received in these facilities was written into the law. Psychiatric care received in general hospitals was not subject to this special limitation, since those facilities offered short-term psychiatric treatment. Since the passage of Medicare, the essential character of mental hospitals has changed. They are no longer custodial institutions with high average lengths of stay. Rather, they provide treatment for acute episodes of mental illness. Lengths of stay are short and readmissions common. "In 1950, only 25 percent of admissions to State hospitals were readmissions. By 1972 this figure had increased to 64 percent" (Department of Health and Human Services, 1980).

In view of changes in the functions of the mental hospitals, the 190-day limitation may no longer be appropriate and may be encouraging more costly treatment in psychiatric units in general

494

hospitals. It is probable that mental hospitals would be better able to deliver needed specialized care to many elderly mental patients. Critics of the 190–day lifetime limitation argue that equal coverage of psychiatric inpatient care in mental and general hospitals would lead to placement decisions based on the needs of the patients rather than on financial concerns.

For these reasons, President Carter's Commission on Mental Health recommended that the 190-day limitation be eliminated. Instead, psychiatric hospitals would remain subject only to the spell of illness provisions which also govern care received in general hospitals.

Community Mental Health Center (CMHC) Reimbursement

Present Medicare policy makes it difficult for community mental health centers to receive reimbursement for all of the services they offer. Currently CMHCs are reimbursed for both Parts A and B of Medicare if they are operated by a hospital which qualifies for provider status. Only 15 percent fit into this category. A number of other CMHCs have agreements with provider hospitals to provide inpatient care to CMHC patients. But for CMHC outpatient services in facilities not operated by a hospital, there are serious impediments to reimbursement. Fee-for-service reimbursement is available for services provided by or under the direct supervision of a physician. However, a number of services offered by centers are provided by non-physicians without direct physician supervision, and hence are not covered by Medicare. One proposal to extend Medicare mental health coverage would offer provider status, or some other form of cost-based reimbursement, to CMHCs so that more of the services they offer can be covered.

A recent report to Congress (Department of Health and Human Services, 1978) discussed the advantages and disadvantages of this proposed extension of Medicare. Included in the advantages was the fact that expanded CMHC coverage could result in greater accessibility of mental health services to the elderly, probably at reduced cost. Appropriate assessment, treatment, follow-up, and ancillary social services could be made available to the elderly. The outreach program staff would also have more of an incentive to serve the elderly. The increased exposure of the elderly to CMHC services could lead to earlier outpatient treatment of their conditions, which might prevent unnecessary inpatient care and institutionalization. To be most effective in the above-mentioned ways, the extension of Medicare coverage to CMHCs would have to be coupled with an increase in the $250 limit on outpatient psychiatric benefits and a decrease in the 50 percent coinsurance for these services.

Among the disadvantages of extending Medicare coverage are (1) the difficulty of monitoring care provided in CMHCs by non-

495

physicians, (2) possible increases in overall costs if CMHCs are inappropriately substituted for informal caregivers who have previously offered sufficient support for the elderly, and (3) lack of CMHC personnel who are adequately trained and experienced in care of the elderly.

A demonstration project is now underway to study the utilization, costs, and quality of care provided in community mental health centers. This Department of Health and Human Services project is being directed by the Health Care Financing Administration, along with the Office of the Assistant Secretary for Planning and Evaluation and the National Institute of Mental Health. Guidelines for standards for eligible providers offering care in the absence of on-site physician supervision are being developed, as is a methodology for determining appropriate cost-related reimbursement policies for centers.

Partial Hospitalization

Partial hospitalization (also called psychiatric day care) involves treatment for mental disorders within an organized setting for from four to eight hours a day up to seven days a week. It is widely believed that partial hospitalization programs prevent or delay institutionalization, or facilitate release to the community following institutionalization. Medicare reimbursement for this care is frequently through hospital outpatient departments. This system may not yield equitable reimbursement, since items which would be covered in an inpatient setting are often excluded. Also, higher quality and lower cost programs may be ineligible for reimbursement just because they are independently operated and not associated with a hospital, or because the services are not provided in "physician-directed clinics."

To gain needed information about partial hospitalization programs, an ongoing demonstration project will assess the utilization, costs, and quality of care provided to Medicare beneficiaries in a variety of partial hospitalization settings. This project will yield a uniform definition and standards which could apply to eligible partial hospitalization programs, along with more equitable reimbursement techniques.

Home Health Care Benefits

Medicare benefits for home health services were designed primarily for the treatment of acute illness. Part A benefits were contingent upon prior hospitalization, and Parts A and B required that a beneficiary need "skilled care" and remain "homebound." To qualify for Part A or B home health care, a beneficiary had to be confined to the home under care of a physician and require intermittent skilled nursing care or physical or speech therapy. If a beneficiary fit into these categories, he or she was also eligible for

496

other home health services, including occupational therapy, medical social services, and the part-time or intermittent services of home health aides. But if a patient did *not* require intermittent skilled nursing or physical or speech therapy, he or she would not qualify for these other home health services (Department of Health and Human Services, 1980). These policies strictly limit the number of beneficiaries eligible for these services and the utilization of this care. It is particularly difficult for the mentally ill to qualify. These policies also ignore the less intensive needs of patients which, if met, could keep them in their own homes longer. Many States model their Medicaid program after Medicare provisions; consequently, frequently neither of these programs offer the types of services required to prevent institutionalization of the mentally ill and other elderly patients.

Some modifications of the home health care provisions under Medicare were recently made by the Omnibus Reconciliation Act of 1980 (P.L. 96–499). This law provides for Medicare coverage of unlimited home health visits, eliminates the three-day prior hospitalization requirement for home health services under Part A, eliminates the $60 deductible for home health services under Part B, and permits participation of proprietary home health agencies in States not having licensure laws.

These expansions of home health care benefits are expected to discourage unnecessary hospital admissions and result in more of the needs of the elderly, including the mentally ill, being met in the home. Appropriate use of home health benefits could also significantly reduce unnecessary admissions to nursing homes and could lead to earlier discharge for those requiring some inpatient care.

Other changes in home health care policies which unnecessarily restrict coverage of the mentally ill are required. After the effects of the above modifications on the mentally ill are determined, additional recommendations for changes in home health care policy should be drafted. Estimates of the cost of expansions of services to the mentally ill should be included in the recommendations.

Medicaid

General Provisions in Medicaid

The Medicaid program was designed to give the States significant leverage, within broad Federal guidelines, to decide about the eligibility and scope of coverage. Federal cost-sharing is available for most types of care required to treat mental illness, including inpatient hospitalization in a general hospital, outpatient services (including partial hospitalization), clinic services, skilled and intermediate nursing services, physicians' services, and drugs. The program prohibits discrimination in the State Medicaid plans on the basis of

497

diagnosis for required services. However, many States have chosen to follow very strict eligibility criteria, set very low rates of payment for some services, and severely limit the number and types of services covered. States also differ in the extent to which they cover non-physician providers. Some basic changes in Medicaid were recommended by the President's Commission on Mental Health under President Carter. The Commission recommended broader eligibility for the needy under Medicaid, mandatory mental health benefits in every State plan, equitable reimbursement rates, and removal of provisions limiting mental health benefits on the basis of age. The next section will discuss the restriction of coverage for individuals from 21 to 64 years old in institutions for mental diseases. The treatment of individuals in this age group has implications for their condition and service needs after age 65.

Exclusion of Federal Matching Funds for Individuals Age 21 to 64 in Institutions for Mental Diseases

The Medicaid statute authorizes the States to provide, as optional services, inpatient hospital services, skilled nursing facility services, and intermediate care facility services for individuals 65 years of age or over in an institution for mental diseases (IMD) and inpatient psychiatric hospital services for patients under age 21. There is no provision for Medicaid coverage of services for patients in IMDs who are 21 to 64 years of age.

There is no statutory definition of an IMD in legislative history. The definition in Medicaid regulations states that an IMD is "an institution that is primarily engaged in providing diagnosis, treatment or care of persons with mental diseases, including medical attention, nursing care, and related services. The classification of a facility as an institution for mental diseases is determined by its overall character as that of a facility established and maintained primarily for the care and treatment of individuals with mental diseases, whether or not it is licensed as such" (42 Code of Federal Regulations 435.1009(e)).

Eight criteria have been included in the guidelines for identifying IMDs, including whether a facility:

(1) is licensed as a mental institution,
(2) advertises or holds itself out as a mental institution,
(3) has more than 50 percent of its patients with a disability in mental functioning,
(4) is used by mental hospitals for alternative care,
(5) accepts patients directly from the community who may have otherwise entered a mental hospital,
(6) is in proximity to a State mental institution (within a 25-mile radius),

498

(7) has an age distribution uncharacteristic of nursing home patients,

(8) has as the basis of Medicaid eligibility for patients under 65 the presence of a mental disability, exclusive of services in an institution for mental disease.

These guidelines are not contained in the regulations, but rather in the Field Staff Information and Instruction Series. Some experts consider them to be of questionable value. For this reason a new, more specific definition of an IMD may be needed. This definition could be used by the States in deciding upon the appropriateness of coverage of care to individuals in nursing homes. It is frequently argued that only accredited or licensed psychiatric hospitals were intended by lawmakers to be classified as IMDs, and nursing homes were inappropriately included in the definition and guidelines adopted by Medicaid administrators.

Originally, the 21 to 64 exclusion was adopted because the treatment of the mentally ill was seen solely as a State responsibility. But the exclusion, as defined by Medicaid, has been criticized because many individuals are left without appropriate care, and because institutions are believed to manipulate diagnoses to have the patients qualify for Medicaid reimbursement. Permitting payment for these individuals could be a first step toward ensuring that they receive appropriate care and, if possible, are rehabilitated at an early age. An increase in costs would probably occur if this restriction were eliminated, but it is difficult to estimate these costs since we do not know how many of the individuals are already being supported by Medicaid under other diagnoses. The National Plan for the Chronically Mentally Ill recommended that the age restrictions that currently apply to patients in institutions for mental diseases, except public mental hospitals, be removed (Department of Health and Human Services, 1980).

Emphasis on Institutional Care

Medicaid, like Medicare, is strongly biased in favor of coverage in institutional settings. Almost 70 percent of the mental health care reimbursed through Medicaid in fiscal year 1977 was for institutional services. This number would have been even higher if Federal matching funds had been available for persons age 21 to 64 in institutions for mental disorders.

Fundamental changes in Medicaid outpatient coverage might eliminate inappropriate utilization of institutional care. Broader coverage of community mental health centers under clinic services is one possible expansion of service. Existing incentives which favor institutional care (for example, nursing homes) should be eliminated. Home health and other community support services

499

might be further expanded. Either through Medicaid or other financing, appropriate housing must also be financed.

Conditions of Participation for Nursing Homes

Present nursing home standards relate to care provided to physically ill patients. Nursing home patients with chronic mental impairments are therefore not assured appropriate care. The National Plan for the Chronically Mentally Ill (Department of Health and Human Services, 1980) mentions the following four problems with nursing home care for the mentally ill: (1) absence of the necessary psychosocial environment, (2) failure to develop plans for rehabilitating patients, (3) insufficient numbers of trained staff, and (4) heavy reliance on physical and chemical restraints.

The National Plan recommended that standards be developed for nursing homes serving the mentally ill. Because of the large number of mentally ill individuals in nursing homes and the large number at risk of developing mental illness, services should be available to meet their needs. Psychiatric services provided by the nursing home staff or under contract should be reimbursed under Medicaid.

Recent Federal Legislation Affecting Care for the Elderly Mentally Ill

The Mental Health Systems Act

The Mental Health Systems Act, P.L. 96–398, which was enacted in October, 1980, can be expected to affect the care and treatment of the elderly mentally ill. Federally-funded community mental health centers are to provide, after a three-year period, a program of specialized services for the elderly, including a full range of diagnostic, treatment, liaison, and follow-up services. CMHC provision of care must be coordinated with services provided by other health and social service agencies (including public mental health facilities).

This legislation makes grants available to State mental health authorities, community mental health centers, and other public or non-profit organizations, to provide mental health and related support services for the chronically mentally ill, which could include the elderly. Coordination among the various involved agencies is stressed, as well as coordination of the many funding sources for services to the chronically mentally ill.

Grants for projects serving the elderly are specifically encouraged. Grantees would have appropriate personnel who would be responsible for (1) providing or arranging services for the elderly, or coordinating the provision of such services with area agencies on aging and other community agencies providing mental health and support services, and (2) providing services available under Titles XVI, XVIII, XIX, and XX of the Social Security Act, the Older

500

Americans Act, the U.S. Housing Act, and other relevant Federal and State statutes.

These or similar grant programs can be used to expand services to needy groups if fundamental changes in Medicare or Medicaid, both open-ended insurance programs, are not made.

Research—Current Projects and Future Needs

Some of the research needed in the mental health area is already underway. Basic research in the area of senile dementia and other mental disorders of the elderly is being sponsored by the National Institute on Aging and the Center for the Studies of Mental Health and the Aging in the National Institute of Mental Health. This research will provide information on fundamental issues such as the causes, prevention, and appropriate treatment of these conditions. It is also important to support more research on depression and on the interrelationships of mental disorders. Some research on the effects of psychotropic drugs on the elderly is currently underway, but further work in this area is needed.

On-going demonstration projects previously mentioned in this chapter are the community mental health center and the partial hospitalization projects. Another project, conducted by the Departments of Health and Human Services and Housing and Urban Development, will provide living arrangements and appropriate services for the chronically mentally ill. The evaluation of the project will indicate the success of these efforts to maintain the chronically mentally ill in residential settings in the community. Information will also be gathered on the costs of providing needed services and the effectiveness of various types of services as these relate to quality of life. Although the channeling agency demonstration projects are not specifically addressed to the mentally ill, many of the findings from this research should also be relevant to this subgroup of functionally impaired elderly. Additional information about demonstration projects is included in Chapter VI.

One idea for a future research project would be to assess the effects of establishing a number of CMHCs as channeling agencies for the mentally ill. Most of the 700 CMHCs already have established linkages with health and social service agencies which would prove valuable to them in this new role. These demonstrations could test a series of incentives to promote care of the chronically mentally ill. The costs of CMHC case management could be assessed in such projects, along with the ability to prevent, delay, or shorten institutionalization. These projects could provide model programs for CMHCs attempting to set up specialized services for the elderly mandated in their 1975 and 1980 enabling legislation.

Another possible demonstration project could feature a CMHC serving nursing home patients. This project, if successful, could remedy the shortcomings of CMHCs in serving chronically ill elderly patients, and of nursing homes in providing psychiatric services to their residents. The CMHC staff could assess and treat clients and could also train nursing home staff. Financing for psychiatric services would be expanded for the duration of the project. This project would provide information on the costs of operation and the effectiveness of treatment provided under this program. The Center for Studies of the Mental Health of the Aging is sponsoring an on-going training program which is developing cooperative programs between CMHCs and nursing homes for the provision of case consultation services, in-service training of nursing home staff, and program development. Other CMHCs have developed innovative programs for treating the elderly, and these efforts should also be evaluated.

The Administration on Aging also supports research on mental illness of the elderly. One project is examining the interrelationships between the aging network and the mental health system. Further research in this area is needed.

According to the National Plan for the Chronically Mentally Ill (Department of Health and Human Services, 1980), "the lack of an alternative to the conventional nursing home for patients without somatic problems [is] the single biggest gap in community based service systems." To fill this gap, the plan first proposed a demonstration project, and then the inclusion of intermediate care centers for mental health (ICC-MH) under Medicaid as an optional service. These centers would be adapted to the needs of the individual community. They would serve as residences for individuals who do not need acute care or a highly protective environment. Services could be provided either within the residence or in the outside community. In certain cases, the ICC-MH would be closely linked to the area's community mental health center. The ICC-MH would provide, or arrange for others to provide, housing, food, transportation, and treatment by qualified mental health professionals and support personnel. These residences could serve patients discharged from State hospitals, nursing homes, or boarding homes who need psychosocial services. These patients could compose a crisis population, a transitional rehabilitative population, or a long-term population. These centers would be part of a planned, integrated, community service system. They would be linked to the State's discharge planning and patient assessment system (Department of Health and Human Services, 1980).

In some respects, demonstration projects to test the ICC-MH would yield data similar to the demonstration project being conducted by the Departments of Health and Human Services and Housing and Urban Development mentioned earlier. However, the ICC-MH demonstration would test the impact of a single funding source on the provision of care to the chronically mentally ill. Also, there would be more intensive monitoring of services in the ICC-MH and greater attention to measuring the quality of services delivered. In addition, the demonstration would examine the feasibility of using Medicaid funds to support housing.

References

Birren, James E. and V. Jayne Renner, "A Brief History of Mental Health and Aging," *Issues in Mental Health and Aging* 1, Research, Proceedings of the Conference on Research in Mental Health and Aging, sponsored by U.S. Department of Health, Education, and Welfare, Public Health Service, Alcohol, Drug Abuse, and Mental Health Administration, National Institute of Mental Health, Center for Studies of the Mental Health of the Aging, November 10–11, 1975.

Blank, Marie L., "Meeting the Needs of the Aged: The Social Worker in the Community Health Center," *Public Health Reports* 92, 1 (January-February 1977).

Blank, Marie L., "A Perspective on De-institutionalization of Older Patients and a Proposal for Community-Based Services," *Journal of Gerontological Social Work* 1, 2 (Winter 1978): 135–45.

Blank, Marie L., "Raising the Age Barrier to Psychotherapy," *Geriatrics* 29 (November 1974): 141–48.

Blazer, Dan, "Life Events, Mental Health Functioning and the Use of Health Care Services by the Elderly," *American Journal of Public Health,* 70, 11 (November 1980): 1174–1179.

Bryson, Brent J., "Cost Effectiveness Analysis of TRIMS Geriatric Services," Data compiled especially for the Task Panel on the Elderly, President's Commission on Mental Health by the Texas Research Institute of Mental Health, Houston, Texas, December 2, 1977.

Butler, Robert N., "Psychiatry and the Elderly: An Overview," *American Journal of Psychiatry,* 132, 9 (September 1975): 893–900.

Butler, Robert N., "The Need for Geriatric Medicine," Background paper prepared especially for the Task Panel on the Elderly, President's Commission on Mental Health, Washington, D.C., 1977.

Butler, Robert N. and Myrna I. Lewis, *Aging and Mental Health,* St. Louis, Missouri: The C. V. Mosby Co., 1977.

Code of Federal Regulations, 42, 435.1009(e).

Cohen, Gene D., M.D., "Mental Health Services and the Elderly: Needs and Options," *American Journal of Psychiatry* 133, 1 (January 1976): 65–68.

Cohen, Gene D., M.D., "Approach to the Geriatric Patient," *Medical Clinics of North America* 61, 4 (July 1977): 855–66.

Cohen, Gene D., M.D., *Senile Dementia (Alzheimer's Disease),* Rockville, Maryland: U.S. Department of Health, Education, and Welfare, National Institute of Mental Health Fact Sheet, Center for Studies of the Mental Health of the Aging, 1979.

503

Cohen, Gene D., M.D. *et al,* "Geriatric Psychiatry Training: A Brief Clinical Rotation," *American Journal of Psychiatry* 137, 3 (March 1980): 297–300.

Comptroller General of the United States, General Accounting Office, *Returning the Mentally Disabled to the Community: Government Needs to Do More,* Washington, D.C.: U.S. Government Printing Office, No. HRD-76-152, January 1977.

Cummings, Nicholas, "The Anatomy of Psychotherapy under National Health Insurance," *American Psychologist* 32, 9 (September 1977).

Eisdorfer, Carl, "Evaluation of the Quality of Psychiatric Care for the Aged," *American Journal of Psychiatry,* 134, 3 (March 1977): 315–17.

Eisdorfer, Carl and Donna Cohen, "The Cognitively Impaired Elderly: Differential Diagnosis," *The Clinical Psychology of Aging,* Edited by Martha Storandt *et al,* New York: Plenum Publishing Corporation, 1978.

Epstein, Leon J., "Open Forum: The Elderly Mentally Ill: Finding the Right Treatment," *Hospital and Community Psychiatry,* 25, 5 (May 1975): 303–306.

Glasscote, Raymond M. *et al, Old Folks at Homes: A Field Study of Nursing and Board and Care Homes,* Washington, D.C.: American Psychiatric Association and Mental Health Association-Joint Information Service, 1976.

Glasscote, Raymond M. *et al, Creative Mental Health Services for the Elderly,* Washington, D.C.: American Psychiatric Association and Mental Health Association-Joint Information Service, 1977.

Goldensohn, Sidney S., "Cost, Utilization, and Utilization Review of Mental Health Services in a Prepaid Group Practice Plan," *American Journal of Psychiatry,* 134, 11 (November 1977): 1222–1226.

Grad de Alarcon, Jacqueline, "Social Causes and Social Consequences of Mental Illness in Old Age," Chapter VII in *Recent Developments in Psychogeriatrics—A Symposium,* Edited by D. W. K. Kay and Alexander Walk, British Journal of Psychiatry Special Publication No. 6, 1971, 75–86.

Group for the Advancement of Psychiatry, *The Aged and Community Mental Health: A Guide to Program Development* 8, Series 81 (1971).

Group for the Advancement of Psychiatry, *Toward a Public Policy on Mental Health Care of the Elderly* 7, 79 (1979): 657–700.

Manard, Barbara B. *et al, Old-Age Institutions,* Lexington, Mass.: Lexington Books, D. C. Heath and Co., 1975.

National Institute of Mental Health, *De-institutionalization: An Analytical Perspective,* Washington, D.C.: U.S. Government Printing Office, DHEW Publication No. (ADM) 76-351, 1976.

Pardes, Herbert, M.D., Statement to National Conference on Mental Health and the Elderly, A Conference sponsored by the Select Committee on Aging, U.S. House of Representatives, Ninety-Sixth Congress, First Session, April 23 and 24, 1979, Washington, D.C.: U.S. Government Printing Office, Committee Publication No. 96-186, 1979.

Paterson, Robert D., M.D., "Services for the Aged in Community Mental Health Centers," *American Journal of Psychiatry* 133, 3 (March 1976): 271–73.

504

Raskind, Murray A. et al, "Helping the Elderly Psychiatric Patient in Crisis," Geriatrics 31, 6 (June 1976): 51–56.

Redick, Robert, Patterns in Use of Nursing Homes by the Aged Mentally Ill, Washington, D.C.: National Institute of Mental Health, Division of Biometry and Epidemiology, Statistical Note #107, 1974.

Ronch, Judah and J. S. Maizler, "Individual Psychotherapy with Institutionalized Aged," American Journal of Orthopsychiatry 47, 2 (April 1977): 275–83.

Roth, Martin, M.D., "The Psychiatric Disorders of Later Life," Psychiatric Annals 6, 9 (September 1976): 57–76.

Secretary's Committee on Mental Health and Illness of the Elderly, Mental Health and the Elderly: Recommendations for Action, Washington, D.C.: Department of Health, Education and Welfare, Federal Council on the Aging, DHEW Publication No. (OHDS) 80-20960, 1979.

Stotsky, Bernard A., The Nursing Home and the Aged Psychiatric Patient, New York: Appleton-Century-Crofts-Meredith Corporation, 1970.

U.S. Department of Health and Human Services, Alcohol, Drug Abuse and Mental Health Administration, National Institute of Mental Health, Division of Biometry and Epidemiology, 1980.

U.S. Department of Health, Education, and Welfare, Report Required by P.L. 95–210 on the Advantages and Disadvantages of Extending Medicare Coverage to Mental Health, Alcohol, and Drug Abuse Centers, Unpublished report. October 1978.

U.S. Department of Health, Education, and Welfare, Public Health Service, National Centers for Health Services Research and Health Statistics, Health United States, Washington, D.C.: DHEW Publication No. (PHS) 78-1232, December 1978.

U.S. Department of Health and Human Services, Report to the Secretary, National Plan for the Chronically Mentally Ill, Washington, D.C., August 1980.

U.S. Senate Special Committee on Aging, Mental Health and the Elderly. Washington, D.C.: U.S. Government Printing Office, 1975.

CHAPTER XV

A Legislative History of Nursing Home Care

by Saul Waldman

Legislation supporting nursing home services can be classified into three major types: (1) legislation providing direct payment for the cost of nursing home services on behalf of residents, (2) legislation providing income maintenance to aged and disabled persons, enabling them to purchase nursing home care from available facilities, and (3) legislation providing loans and grants to providers of nursing home services to build and improve facilities.

The Origin of Nursing Homes

To understand the effect of these types of legislation on nursing homes, it is useful to study the historical origins of the present nursing home industry. These origins can be traced to developments, mostly in the late 19th and early 20th centuries, in five types of facilities—the county poorhouses, the State mental hospitals, the voluntary homes for the aged, the early proprietary boarding houses, and the hospital-affiliated nursing homes.

Before the Depression, a major form of government support for institutional care of the elderly was the county poorhouse, alternately known as the county "almshouse," "home," or "farm." Operated and financed by local governments, these institutions originally supported children and adults of various ages and in various health and financial circumstances, including the poor, the old, the disabled, the retarded, and the mentally disturbed. Over time, however, specialized institutions were established to care for many of the groups previously confined to the poorhouses, so that these institutions primarily became residences for the aged and disabled. The poorhouses were widely known for their dilapidated appearances and poor living conditions, and this reputation was generally well deserved.

The disappearance of poorhouses in the 1930s and 1940s was partially due to the efforts of reformers to close these institutions. But even more significant in the long run were the effects of the 1935 social security legislation, which provided income maintenance for the aged and disabled and made it possible for residents of the poorhouses to pay for alternative living arrangements. A few of the former poorhouses have been converted and have survived as publicly-operated nursing homes.

The growth of the present nursing home industry was also influenced by developments affecting mental hospitals over the past half century. The mental hospitals, most of which were State institutions, had long been important facilities for the institutionalization of the aged. In the 1940s, for example, about one-quarter of the institutionalized aged were confined to mental hospitals. To some extent, aged persons who did not suffer mental illness were placed in mental hospitals because such hospitals were the only facilities available for persons needing institutional care. With the advent of psychotropic drugs and other developments in the care of the mentally ill, it became possible to discharge many patients from mental hospitals. In the 1960s and 1970s, a large proportion, probably about one-half of the population of mental hospitals, was discharged. In fact, some observers believe that many of these discharges were inappropriate, and there have been accusations of wholesale "dumping" of patients from mental hospitals. While many of the discharged patients have been able to live independently or with relatives, many others have been sent to other institutions, including nursing homes (U.S. Department of Health and Human Services, 1980). Placement of these patients in nursing homes was facilitated by the availability of financing for nursing home care under the vendor payment provisions of old age assistance and later under the Medicaid program.

Another predecessor of the present nursing home industry comprised the homes for the aged established by immigrant groups and voluntary and religious organizations, notably Lutheran, Methodist, and Jewish organizations in the late 19th and early 20th centuries. These voluntary homes for the aged were generally established to provide shelter and maintenance to elderly persons of limited financial means who were without family (Dunlop, 1979). Over the years, additional personal and nursing services have been added in many of these institutions, and these homes have evolved into the voluntary, non-profit sector of the nursing home industry.

The largest segment of the nursing home industry today, however, is the proprietary sector (National Center for Health Statistics, 1979). Much of this segment began in the late 19th and early 20th centuries as boarding home accommodations for persons needing room, board, and limited personal care. Many of the boarding homes started with the conversion of existing one-family homes, and these homes often began to provide additional personal and nursing services as the residents continued to age. A report of the Senate Committee on Labor and Public Welfare (1960) describes the origins of the proprietary nursing home industry:

Some actually started as nursing homes. Some started as boarding homes for elderly people. But in historical back-

508

ground, even as in contemporary operations, the line between homes which offered nursing care and those which provided domiciliary services was not sharply drawn. With the passage of time, homes which had begun as room-and-board enterprises gradually, and sometimes imperceptibly, assumed responsibility for meeting the personal and nursing needs as these areas arose among their aging residents. Thus, many of today's nursing homes are yesterday's small private boarding homes for older people.

Another component of the nursing home industry is the hospital-affiliated nursing home established by hospitals, mostly in the 20th century, as an adjunct to regular hospital services (Dunlop, 1979). The establishment of these nursing homes reflects in part the increasing specialization of hospitals as centers for the treatment of acute illness. The construction of separate nursing home facilities by hospitals received considerable encouragement under the provisions of the Hill-Burton Act, described later in this chapter. Most of these hospital-affiliated nursing homes are governmental or voluntary institutions reflecting the ownership status of the hospitals themselves.

Income Maintenance Legislation

The Social Security Act of 1935 played an important role in aiding the growth of nursing homes by providing an additional source of income for purchasing nursing home care. The Act provided a program of old age assistance (OAA) under which monthly payments were made to persons age 65 and over who qualified under a means test, with eligibility and benefit amounts largely determined by the States. The Federal government shares the cost of the program with the States. The legislation specifically forbade payments to "inmates of a public institution" to prevent the program from supporting residents of the county poorhouses (Vladeck, 1980).

By providing funds to pay for care, the OAA program was especially important in the further development of the proprietary nursing home industry in the 1930s. The OAA payments also helped support residents of religious and other voluntary homes for the aged and thus helped to maintain these homes during the Depression years, when charitable contributions declined and financing became more difficult (Vladeck, 1980).

Legislation enacted in 1950 provided for aid to the disabled (AD) on a means-tested basis similar to the OAA program. The 1950 amendments also removed the prohibition on assistance payments for residents of public institutions, apparently with the hope that what remained of the county poorhouse systems would be improved and brought up to acceptable standards (Vladeck, 1980).

Under the 1972 amendments to the social security law, the OAA and AD assistance programs were abolished and replaced by the Supplementary Security Income (SSI) program. Like the assistance programs, SSI provides monthly payments to aged and disabled persons, but SSI is a Federal program and is financed and administered by the Federal government (Social Security Act and Related Laws, 1978). Some States provide supplementary payments to resident SSI recipients. Some of these States pay an additional amount to persons receiving domiciliary care. When a person enters a nursing home under the Medicaid program, the Federal SSI payment is reduced to $25.

While the OAA program represented the most important income maintenance program for the aged in the 1930s, the social security law also provided for payment of retirement insurance benefits to aged persons beginning in 1940. Over the succeeding years, as additional persons have become insured under the program, it has become, by far, the most significant income maintenance program for the aged. Also, in 1956 the social security law was amended to provide disability insurance benefits to disabled persons insured under the program (Social Security Act and Related Laws, 1978).

Expanding the Supply of Nursing Homes

As use of nursing home care increased in the 1940s and 1950s a shortage of nursing home beds was developing (Vladeck, 1980). Several Federal laws were enacted during the 1950s to encourage the construction and modernization of nursing homes in all three sectors of the nursing home industry—the non-profit, the public, and the proprietary.

The original Hill-Burton Act of 1946 provided for grants, loans, and loan guarantees to non-profit and government hospitals for construction and modernization, if a survey of available facilities indicated that additional facilities were needed in the community (Dunlop, 1979). Legislation enacted in 1954 extended Federal financial support to non-profit and government nursing homes, also based on a survey of facilities to establish need. Financial assistance under this legislation was limited to nursing homes capable of providing a high level of skilled nursing care. In this connection, the legislation established standards for physical construction, facility design, medical supervision, staffing patterns, and other matters relating to the quality of nursing home care (Vladeck, 1980).

The financial assistance available under the Hill-Burton Act significantly affected the development of the voluntary, non-profit segment of the nursing home industry. The appendix of this chapter analyzes the role of voluntary nursing homes in the industry.

510

In testimony before Congress in the 1950s, representatives of the proprietary nursing home industry indicated that the nature of the industry was such that private capital from banks and other financial institutions was not readily available. Consequently, the industry had difficulty in obtaining funds necessary for expansion (Reiss, 1980). In 1956, under its general loan authority pertaining to small business, the Small Business Administration (SBA) inaugurated a loan program for qualified nursing homes (Reiss, 1980). To be eligible, a nursing home had to meet the overall criteria of the SBA as a small business. For eligible homes, loans were available for new construction, expansion, equipment, supplies, and working capital. Besides making direct loans, the SBA also guaranteed commercial loans to qualified nursing homes.

For a variety of reasons, the SBA program apparently did not fully satisfy the need of proprietary nursing homes for capital and loans. The representatives of the proprietary industry stated the following in testimony on the proposed Housing Act of 1959:

The Hill-Burton benefits are restricted to non-profit and tax-supported institutions which are for only 29 percent of the people in nursing homes. The (existing) FHA program does not contain adequate provision for nursing care on a continuing basis and was not designed to support nursing homes per se. The Small Business Administration loan policy, in keeping with its general policy, is far too short a loan period and far too low a Federal participation. This prevents the great majority of the proprietary nursing-home owners from obtaining such loans and makes it difficult for them to compete with the nonprofit home supported by finance programs existing within the Government (U.S. Senate Committee on Banking and Currency, 1960).

To further help meet the needs of proprietary homes, Congress enacted Section 232 of the Housing Act of 1959, which provides a program of mortgage insurance for proprietary nursing homes. Under this program, the Federal Housing Administration (FHA) insures lenders against loss for loans for construction or rehabilitation of nursing homes. The FHA insurance covers 75 percent of the estimated value of the improvements for loans which could extend over a period of 20 years (Dunlop, 1979). (Under later amendments, the insurance was increased to 90 percent and the loan period to 40 years.) Interest rates charged on these insured loans are comparable to prevailing interest rates. A condition of the loan insurance is that the proposed project receive a certificate of need from the appropriate State agency indicating that a need exists for the proposed beds. Over the years, the FHA mortgage insurance program has become the most important Federal program assisting in the construction and development of proprietary nursing homes.

An additional source of financing for nursing homes in rural areas is the Farmers Home Administration of the Department of Agriculture. The Farmers Home Administration makes loans under the Consolidated Farm and Rural Development Act to build or improve community facilities providing essential services (including health benefits) to rural residents (Reiss, 1980).

The Appalachian Regional Commission has broad authority under the Appalachian Regional Development Act of 1965 to make project grants to State and local governments and non-profit organizations for demonstrations for health related activities, including nursing homes (Reiss, 1980).

Medical Vendor Payment Programs

From the beginnings of the OAA and AD assistance programs, States were permitted to use funds from the assistance programs to pay for medical care, including nursing home care, for recipients. Initially, the method used to pay for medical care under the programs was to include the cost of the medical care in the cash allowance of the recipient and have the recipient pay the provider of the medical services (Dunlop, 1979).

The 1950 amendments to the Social Security Act permitted welfare agencies to make direct payments, termed medical vendor payments, to providers of medical service to recipients (Social Security Act and Related Laws, 1978). The funds available for medical vendor payments were limited under the sharing formula used to determine Federal sharing in the cost of the assistance program.

Under the 1950 legislation, vendor payments were available only to persons whose income was at or below the eligibility level for the assistance program. At their option, States used two major methods for determining the income level at which eligibility began. Some States used the "in or out" method, under which only persons whose income fell below the specified level were eligible for either money payments or medical care. Other States used the "spend-down" method, under which persons whose income was above the specified level were ineligible for money payments but could become eligible for medical vendor payments if the amount they spent for medical care from their own funds brought their net income down to the eligibility level. Because of the relatively high cost of nursing home care, many persons in the "spend-down" States who were not eligible for money payments qualified for nursing home care.

The methods of reimbursing nursing homes under the medical vendor program were left to the States. Most States reimbursed on a flat rate basis, paying a single rate state-wide, several flat rates for different levels of care, or flat rates negotiated at the county level. In some States, the nursing home was required to accept the

512

State reimbursement as full payment, while other States permitted the home to charge a supplemental amount to the resident or his or her family.

The 1950 social security amendments mandated that States making vendor payments to nursing homes must establish licensing requirements for those homes (Vladeck, 1980). These Federal licensing requirements were very general and did not specify licensing standards or indicate how they were to be enforced. Most States did not have any licensing requirements for nursing homes at that time, and the 1950 legislation promoted the enactment of such requirements. These State laws, however, generally contained minimal requirements and made little provision for enforcement.

Medical Assistance for the Aged

The Medical Assistance for the Aged (MAA) program, enacted in 1960, was initially proposed as a possible substitute for the Medicare program then under consideration (Vladeck, 1980). The MAA program was essentially an expansion of the vendor payment program under OAA, but with several major improvements. Most importantly, the program permitted the States to provide eligibility for the medically indigent, that is, persons whose income was above the OAA standard but who were considered as having insufficient income to pay for medical care. As in the OAA vendor payment program, some States tested eligibility on an "in or out" basis, while others used the concept of the "spend-down." The MAA legislation did not forbid relative responsibility requirements, that is, requirements that specified that relatives contribute toward care for the applicant if they were determined to be financially capable of doing so.

The Federal government contributed 50 percent to 80 percent of the cost of the MAA program, with the higher contributions going to States with the lower *per capita* income. Unlike the OAA vendor payment program, the Federal contributions for medical care under MAA were open-ended, with no limit based on individual payments or total State expenditures.

There was considerable variation among the States in the extent to which the MAA program was implemented. Most States with a program included nursing home care among the services covered. Overall, the program had a significant effect in increasing expenditures for nursing care, and by 1965 some 300,000 persons were receiving nursing home care under that program (Vladeck, 1980).

The Medicaid Program

The 1965 amendments to the Social Security Act created the Medicare and Medicaid programs, both of which have had far reaching effects on public financing of nursing home care. The Medicaid program replaced the medical vendor and MAA programs and substituted for them a uniform medical assistance program for persons of all ages (Social Security Act and Related Laws, 1978).

The Medicaid program covered persons eligible for cash assistance payments (and later SSI) and, at the option of the State, persons above the income standard who were determined to be medically indigent. States considering the medically indigent as eligible generally determined eligibility using the "spend-down" method. In the case of married couples, where one spouse was in a nursing home, eligibility was based on the cost of the nursing home care plus a specified amount which is protected for the maintenance of the spouse remaining in the community.

The Federal law governing the Medicaid program prohibits the States from applying financial responsibility requirements to relatives when determining the financial resources of applicants. Only spouses and parents of children under age 21 could be held financially responsible. (For example, an elderly applicant could not be rejected on the basis of his or her children's income.)

The 1965 Medicaid law required the States to provide five specified types of medical care, one of which was skilled nursing home care. In addition to the five services, other types of services could be provided at the option of the State.

The Federal government contributes 50 percent to 83 percent of the cost of the Medicaid program, according to State *per capita* income (Social Security Act and Related Laws 1978). As for the MAA program, Federal payments for Medicaid are open ended, with no limit on spending based on individual payment or total State expenditures (Social Security Act and Related Laws 1978).

Under a special provision included in the 1972 amendments to the social security law, the Federal government pays 100 percent of the administrative cost of certain State enforcement activities. This provision was designed to encourage State activity in investigating and prosecuting cases of fraud and abuse (Vladeck, 1980).

Under Medicaid, providers of services are required to accept the Medicaid payment as payment in full (Dunlop, 1979). Thus, the provider cannot charge the patient or his/her family an additional amount for covered services.

The original Medicaid law did not specify methods of reimbursement to be used by the States to pay nursing homes (Dunlop, 1979). States were advised by the Department of Health, Education, and Welfare (DHEW) that methods of reimbursement based on reasonable cost were preferable, although not required. Many States used a reasonable cost method of reimbursement but placed a relatively low maximum on the amount of the payment, in effect converting their reimbursement systems into a flat rate system. Other States

514

paid uniform flat rates to all nursing homes or used other methods of reimbursement (Dunlop, 1979).

The 1972 amendments to the social security law required the States to reimburse nursing homes on a reasonable, cost-related basis using cost-finding techniques and methods approved by DHEW (Social Security Act and Related Laws, 1978). However, these reimbursement provisions were never fully implemented, and 1980 legislation repealed them. This latter legislation permitted States to develop their own reimbursement methods with the provision that the rates be reasonable and adequate to cover the costs of an efficiently operated facility. Each State must file its method with the Department of Health and Human Services (DHHS), which is given authority to approve or disapprove the States' proposals (HCFA Administrator's Report, 1981).

The 1965 Medicaid legislation did not authorize the Federal government to establish standards for participation of nursing homes in the program (Dunlop, 1979). Legislation enacted in 1967, known as the Moss Amendments, first provided such authority (Social Security Act and Related Laws, 1978). Among the more important Federal standards for nursing homes established by later regulations were staffing requirements which called for 24-hour nursing service, services of an RN, and services of a charge nurse (the nurse in charge of nursing services on each shift) who met certain qualifications as a licensed practical nurse. These staffing requirements became relatively controversial and were revised several times over the years (Dunlop, 1979). Other significant regulations dealt with fire safety standards, medical supervision, drug dispensing, dietary matters, and sanitation (Vladeck, 1980).

Intermediate Care Facilities

Intermediate care facilities (ICFs) are facilities which regularly provide health-related care to individuals who do not require the degree of care and treatment of a hospital or skilled nursing home but who, because of their mental or physical conditions, require care and services above the level of room and board which can be made available to them only through institutional services (Social Security Act and Related Laws 1978). The 1967 amendments to the Social Security Act included provisions, known as the Miller Amendment, which provided vendor payments for care in ICFs under the cash assistance titles of the Social Security Act (Dunlop, 1979).

This ICF provision supported residents of many nursing homes which did not meet the standards of skilled nursing homes, residents of homes for the aged, and the institutionalized mentally retarded. In some cases, residents who were classified as needing skilled nursing care under Medicaid were reclassified as needing only intermediate care, and facilities previously classified as Medicaid skilled nursing homes were reclassified as ICFs.

Legislation enacted in 1971 transferred the ICF benefit provisions to the Medicaid program. With this transfer, States could now permit eligibility for ICF care on the basis of medical indigency. Reimbursement to ICFs under Medicaid could not exceed, on the average, 90 percent of the state-wide rate for skilled nursing facilities. Federal standards for ICFs were established for staffing, safety, and other matters as described for SNFs, but they were related to a lower level of care than the SNF standards (Dunlop, 1979).

The Medicaid program is, by far, the most significant government program for financing nursing home care. According to the 1977 National Health Survey, Medicaid was the primary source of payment for almost 48 percent of all residents of nursing homes. Other government programs were the primary support for about 8 percent of the residents. (Most of the remaining residents were supported by their own or family resources.)

The Medicare Program

The Medicare program, enacted in 1965, provides hospital, physician, nursing home, and other health services to persons age 65 and over who have acquired sufficient credits under social security to qualify for insurance benefits under the social security law. In 1972, Medicare eligibility was extended to disability insurance beneficiaries under social security who had been on the rolls for at least two years.

The nursing home provision of the Medicare law is carefully designed to provide a limited period of highly skilled nursing home care to persons recently discharged from a hospital. Under this provision, persons who require continued care, but at a less intensive level then that provided in the hospital, can be moved to a skilled nursing home. It was believed that providing arrangements for such care, which was termed "extended care," would result in a net savings for the Medicare program (Vladeck, 1980).

The original Medicare law made care in skilled nursing facilities available to persons who had spent at least three days in a hospital and were transferred to a nursing home within 14 days of discharge from the hospital. The 14-day requirement was changed to 30 days by legislation enacted in 1980. The maximum stay covered by Medicare is limited to 100 days. Medicare covers the first 20 days in full, with any additional days being subject to a deductible equal to one-eighth of the hospital deductible.[1]

In the first few years of the Medicare extended care program, use of extended care increased substantially beyond original expecta-

---

[1] The hospital deductible is an amount calculated to be equal to the average cost of one day of hospital care for beneficiaries of the program.

516

tions (Vladeck, 1980). By 1968, expenditures for extended care exceeded $500 million a year. It was thought that considerable care was being provided to beneficiaries not in need of the kind of high-level extended care intended by the Medicare legislation (Vladeck, 1980). As a result, revised instructions were issued in April 1969, clarifying and redefining the circumstances under which benefici-aries would be eligible for extended care. These instructions pro-vided a revised and narrowed definition of skilled nursing and spelled out with great specificity those services that must be pro-vided if the qualifications for extended care were to be met. These revised instructions significantly reduced the number of beneficiaries eligible for extended care benefits. For example, the number of extended care bills approved for payment fell from over one million in 1968 to fewer than 400,000 in 1972 (Vladeck, 1980).

One problem in administering the nursing home provision was the retroactive denial of eligibility of patients already admitted to nursing homes. Legislation enacted in 1972 established a "presumptive period of coverage" so that, in many cases, persons with certain diagnoses would be "presumed" eligible for nursing home care for a specified period of time after discharge from the hospital. How-ever, 1980 legislation eliminated this provision.

Under the 1965 Medicare law, skilled nursing homes, like hospitals, were paid on the basis of their costs, with no upper limit on the amount of reimbursement. In 1969, additional cost control regula-tions were introduced, including the "prudent buyer" concept which limited reimbursement for nursing home services to levels no higher than a prudent buyer would pay for similar services in a given geo-graphic region (Vladeck, 1980). The formula for determining reim-bursement made provision for a return on investment for proprietary facilities, with the amount of the return tied to the rate of return on long-term Federal securities.

To participate in the Medicare program, a nursing home must meet certain standards as an extended care facility, including the requirement that it be formally affiliated with a hospital or maintain a written "transfer agreement" for transfer of patients and their records from the hospital. The standards for extended care facili-ties also established staffing requirements, including 24-hour nurs-ing service, a full-time RN, and a charge nurse meeting requirements as a licensed practical nurse. Other standards related to medical supervision, fire safety standards, sanitation, dietary matters, and drug dispensing.

When the Medicare program went into effect, it was believed that the number of hospitals and extended care facilities meeting the exacting standards of the program would be insufficient to deliver the benefits promised to Medicare beneficiaries (Vladeck, 1980). Therefore, by regulation, hospitals and extended care facilities were

517

permitted to participate in the program by meeting a standard of "substantial compliance," although they might not meet all the standards required for full compliance. The majority of nursing homes participating in the program, in fact, qualified as extended care facilities on the basis of substantial rather than full compliance (Vladeck, 1980).

Additional Legislation

Some of the nursing home legislation applies to both the Medicaid and Medicare programs. For example, under a provision of the 1972 amendments to the Social Security law, the classification of nursing homes was consolidated by combining extended care facilities under Medicare and skilled nursing homes under Medicaid into a new classification known as skilled nursing facilities (SNFs). DHEW then developed a single set of standards for this new classification. Legislation passed in 1980 requires the Department (now DHHS) to study the availability of SNFs under Medicare and Medicaid and the effect of requiring joint participation.

The 1972 law also established the Professional Standards Review Organizations (PSROs), a system of local organizations to monitor the quality and necessity of services under the Medicare and Medicaid programs. This review activity includes nursing home services.

The Medicare and Medicaid Antifraud and Abuse Amendments of 1977 incorporated numerous provisions to prevent and punish fraud and abuse under the Medicare and Medicaid programs. Most of the provisions of these amendments apply to nursing home as well as to other services.

Characteristics of Federal Legislation on Nursing Homes

This study of the Federal legislative history of nursing home care reveals three major characteristics of the Federal legislation. First, the legislative process has been an evolutionary one, with Federal involvement growing and expanding over a half century. Second, the provisions for nursing home care have been largely tied to the nation's welfare systems with eligibility based on demonstration of need. Third, the nursing home systems established by the Federal legislation have followed the medical model and have been part of a broader medical care program.

The first step in the evolutionary process of this Federal legislation was the indirect support of nursing homes in the 1930s, resulting from the OAA and social security programs which provided funds to purchase nursing home care. Direct support of nursing home care was first provided in 1950 under the vendor payment program of OAA. A further step in the evolutionary process was the enactment in 1960 of the MAA program which introduced the concept of

518

medical indigency and, for the first time, permitted open-ended Federal financial participation in the cost of service. These principles of the MAA program were later incorporated in the Medicaid low of 1965 which extended coverage on this basis to the entire population.

With the exception of the Medicare program, which provides only a limited nursing home benefit, nursing home care has been provided as part of the nation's welfare program under the public assistance titles of the Social Security Act. Eligibility is thus based on meeting a test of need, although in the States using the concept of the "spend-down," eligibility has been extended to those somewhat above the lowest income level.

Finally, the provision of nursing home care has followed the medical model, with nursing home care included along with hospital care, physician services, and other medical services in a broad medical care program. Both SNFs and ICFs are required to meet standards based on medical considerations.

Appendix
The Role of Voluntary Nursing Homes in the Nursing Home Industry

The forerunners of the present voluntary, non-profit nursing home were the homes for the aged, founded in the later years of the 19th century and the early years of the 20th century by immigrant self-help organizations. These early homes were built largely by ethnic and religious groups; for example, Scandinavians and Germans built Lutheran homes, and Jews and Methodists built their own facilities. Over the years, these homes evolved into the present church- or synagogue-affiliated nursing homes.

In more recent years, voluntary nursing homes began with the establishment of nursing homes by voluntary hospitals as an adjunct to their hospital facilities. These hospital-affiliated nursing homes were often built with Hill-Burton funds which were made available for nursing home construction beginning in 1954.

Size of the Voluntary Nursing Home Industry

Considerable information on the characteristics of voluntary nursing homes, as compared to proprietary and government homes, is available from the 1977 National Nursing Home Survey published by the National Center for Health Statistics (NCHS) in 1979. Table XV–A–1, taken from that survey, compares voluntary facilities with proprietary and government facilities.

The NCHS data show that voluntary nursing homes supplied about one-fifth of the total number of nursing home beds in 1977. As

TABLE XV-A-1
Number of Nursing Homes and Beds, by Type of Ownership, 1977

Ownership	Nursing Homes		Beds	
	Number	Percent Distribution	Number	Percent Distribution
Total	18,900	100.0	1,402,000	100.0
Proprietary	14,500	76.8	971,000	69.3
Voluntary	3,400	17.1	296,000	21.1
Government	1,000	5.5	136,000	9.7

Source: National Center for Health Statistics, *The National Nursing Home Survey: 1977 Summary for the United States* (Washington: U.S. Government Printing Office, 1979).

indicated, proprietary homes composed the largest segment of the nursing home industry, with the voluntary homes second and the government facilities last.

Table XV–A–2 gives the certification status of nursing homes under Medicare by type of ownership. Many nursing home beds, referred to as swing beds, are certified by more than one program or for more than one level of care, so that the figures in Table XV–A–2 overlap and do not add to the total. These data show that, overall,

TABLE XV-A-2
Certification Status of Nursing Homes, by Type of Ownership, 1977

Ownership	Total Beds	Certification Status [1] (percent)		
		Medicare Skilled	Medicaid Skilled	Medicaid Intermediate Care
Total	1,402,000	25.3%	45.4%	52.1%
Proprietary	971,200	24.7	45.0	53.1
Voluntary	295,600	26.9	47.1	49.6
Government	135,700	27.0	44.5	50.4

[1] Percentages do not add to 100 percent because beds are certified by more than one program or for more than one level of care.
Source: National Center for Health Statistics, *The National Nursing Home Survey: 1977 Summary for the United States* (Washington: U.S. Government Printing Office, 1979).

voluntary home beds are certified at a slightly higher skill level than proprietary homes.

Data on occupancy rates from the NCHS survey showed that the occupancy rate for all nursing homes in the survey averaged 89.0 percent, with the rates at 89.8 percent, 87.4 percent, and 87.4 percent for proprietary, voluntary, and government facilities, respectively.

Employees and Wage Rates

Voluntary nursing homes used more employees per 100 beds than did proprietary or government nursing homes, including greater numbers of nursing personnel. More personnel, especially nursing staff, is often considered one indication of a higher quality of care. The number of full-time equivalent employees of nursing homes and the rate per 100 beds, by occupational category, is shown in Table XV–A–3. As these figures indicate, the overall rate of employees per 100 beds for voluntary nursing homes was nearly 25 percent greater than for proprietary homes and about 15 percent greater than for government homes. The voluntary home rate was greater than that of both proprietary and government homes for nearly all the occupational categories shown here. The rate was especially high for registered nurses, for whom the rate averaged 50 percent greater than for proprietary homes and 10 percent greater than for government homes.

The wages paid to employees by voluntary nursing homes were generally somewhat higher than those paid by proprietary homes and slightly lower than those in government facilities. The hourly wages for full-time employees by occupational category are shown in Table XV–A–4. By occupational category, the wages for voluntary homes were slightly greater than for proprietary homes for the various categories of nurses and substantially greater for administrative, medical, and therapeutic staff. Wages for nurses in government homes were the highest of the three classes of ownership.

Revenues and Costs

The revenues of voluntary nursing homes are derived largely from patient revenues, with a relatively small part received from charitable contributions and other non-patient sources. Table XV–A–5 shows the revenues per patient day in 1976 of nursing homes by type of ownership. In this table, patient revenues include direct payments from the patient (often derived from social security or other sources) and payments from Medicare, Medicaid, and other public assistance or welfare programs. Non-patient revenues include financial contributions, grants, and subsidies received from churches, foundations, voluntary agencies, government agencies, and similar sources for general operating purposes. Non-patient revenues also include

521

TABLE XV-A-3
Number of Employees of Nursing Homes and Rate per 100 Beds, by Occupational Category and Type of Ownership, 1977

Ownership	All Employees	Occupational Category			
		Administrative, Medical, and Therapeutic	Registered Nurse	Licensed Practical Nurse	Nurse's Aide
		Number of Employees			
Total	647,700	66,900	66,900	85,100	424,900
Proprietary	421,500	44,500	40,300	55,300	281,300
Voluntary	158,700	19,200	18,800	19,500	101,300
Government	67,500	6,900	7,800	10,300	42,400
		Rate per 100 Beds			
Total	46.2	5.0	4.8	6.1	30.3
Proprietary	43.4	4.6	4.2	5.7	29.0
Voluntary	53.7	6.5	6.4	6.6	34.3
Government	49.7	5.1	5.8	7.6	31.2

Source: National Center for Health Statistics, *The National Nursing Home Survey: 1977 Summary for the United States* (Washington, U.S. Government Printing Office, 1979).

522

TABLE XV-A-4
Hourly Wages of Employees of Nursing Homes,
by Occupational Category and Type of Ownership, 1977

		Occupational Category			
Ownership	All Employees	Administrative, Medical, and Therapeutic	Registered Nurse	Licensed Practical Nurse	Nurse's Aide
Total	$3.64	$7.48	$5.59	4.04	2.76
Proprietary	3.47	7.20	5.49	4.01	2.64
Voluntary	3.95	8.25	5.54	4.07	2.91
Government	3.97	7.03	6.07	4.13	3.15

Source: National Center for Health Statistics, *The National Nursing Home Survey: 1977 Summary for the United States* (Washington, U.S. Government Printing Office, 1979).

TABLE XV-A-5
Revenues per Patient Day Received by Nursing Homes,
by Source of Revenues and Type of Ownership, 1976

Ownership	Total Revenues	Source of Revenues	
		Patient Care	Non-Patient Sources
		Amount per Patient Day	
Total	$23.89	$22.78	$1.11
Proprietary	22.63	22.33	.30
Voluntary	26.91	24.37	2.53
Government	26.66	22.68	3.97
		Percent Distribution	
Total	100.0	95.4	4.6
Proprietary	100.0	98.7	1.3
Voluntary	100.0	90.6	9.4
Government	100.0	85.1	14.9

Source: National Center for Health Statistics, *The National Nursing Home Survey: 1977 Summary for the United States* (Washington: U.S. Government Printing Office, 1979).

sources of revenue not directly related to providing nursing care to patients, such as revenue from beauty and barber services and vending machines.

These data indicate that non-patient revenues accounted for about 9 percent of the total revenues of voluntary nursing homes. Of course, the data do not consider construction costs which, for voluntary homes, are sometimes financed from charitable contributions.

Table XV-A-6 shows the amount and distribution of nursing home costs per patient day, by type of cost, for 1976. These data clearly indicate that labor costs are the largest item of cost for nursing homes in all three ownership categories.

Table XV-A-7 provides data on the revenues, costs, and net income in the nursing home industry, in total and per resident day. The data indicate that voluntary nursing homes accounted for almost one-quarter of total revenues and of total costs of the nursing home industry. The net income data in this table indicate that voluntary homes had a loss of $61 million in 1976 or about $0.66 per resident day.

524

TABLE XV-A-6

Cost per Patient Day of Nursing Homes, by Type of Cost and Type of Ownership, 1976

Ownership	Total Cost	Type of Cost			
		Labor	Operating	Fixed	Other
		Amount			
Total	$23.84	$14.23	$5.14	$3.40	1.08
Proprietary	21.97	12.46	4.65	3.76	1.09
Voluntary	27.56	16.93	6.49	3.03	1.11
Government	29.54	21.33	5.80	1.49	.92
		Percent Distribution			
Total	100.0	59.7	21.6	14.2	4.5
Proprietary	100.0	56.7	21.2	17.1	4.9
Voluntary	100.0	61.4	23.5	11.0	4.0
Government	100.0	72.2	19.6	5.0	3.1

Source: National Center for Health Statistics, *The National Nursing Home Survey: 1977 Summary for the United States* (Washington, U.S. Government Printing Office, 1979).

525

TABLE XV-A-7
Revenue, Cost, and Net Income of Nursing Homes
by Type of Ownership, 1976

Ownership	Revenue	Cost	Net Income
		Amount (in millions)	
Total	$10,821	$10,796	$25
Proprietary	7,164	6,954	211
Voluntary	2,513	2,574	−61
Government	1,144	1,268	−124
		Per Resident Day	
Total	$23.89	$23.84	$.06
Proprietary	22.63	21.97	.67
Voluntary	26.91	27.56	−.66
Government	26.66	29.54	−2.89

Source: National Center for Health Statistics, *The National Nursing Home Survey: 1977 Summary for the United States* (Washington: U.S. Government Printing Office, 1979).

Sources and Amount of Payment

Table XV–A–8 shows the distribution of residents of nursing homes by the primary source of payment. The category "All Other Sources" refers to patients primarily dependent on religious organizations, foundations, volunteer agencies, Veterans Administration contracts, and initial-payment life care funds, as well as patients for whom no charge was made.

These data indicate that almost one-half of the residents of voluntary homes were primarily dependent on their own income (often from social security payments or other sources of income) or on family support for payment of their nursing home care. The proportion paying from their own or family resources was greater for voluntary homes than for proprietary or government homes. About 40 percent of the patients of voluntary homes were financed through the Medicaid program, and this proportion was lower than for proprietary or government homes, each of which had about 50 percent of their patients under Medicaid.

Table XV–A–9 shows the total monthly charge paid by, or on behalf of, residents of nursing homes, according to the primary source of payment. These data indicate that the monthly charges were higher for patients of voluntary homes paying from their own resources than for patients of proprietary or government homes.

526

TABLE XV-A-8

Source of Payment of Nursing Homes, by Type of Ownership, 1977

Ownership	Total	Source of Payment					
		Own Income or Family Support	Medicare	Medicaid		Other Government Assistance or Welfare	All Other Sources
				Skilled	Intermediate		
Number of Residents							
Total	1,303,100	500,900	26,200	260,700	362,600	83,400	69,200
Proprietary	888,800	133,400	14,900	178,400	263,300	65,200	33,600
Voluntary	281,800	130,200	7,300	52,100	60,300	10,400	21,600
Government	132,500	37,300	[1]	30,200	39,100	7,900	14,100
Percent Distribution							
Total	100.0	38.4	2.0	20.0	27.8	6.4	5.3
Proprietary	100.0	37.5	1.7	20.1	29.6	7.3	3.8
Voluntary	100.0	46.2	2.6	18.5	21.4	3.7	1.7
Government	100.0	28.1	[1]	22.8	29.5	6.0	10.6

[1] Information is not available.
Source: National Center for Health Statistics, *The National Nursing Home Survey: 1977 Summary for the United States* (Washington, U.S. Government Printing Office, 1979).

527

TABLE XV-A-9
Monthly Charges for Nursing Home Care, by Type of Ownership, 1977

Ownership	All Sources	Own Income or Family Support	Monthly Charges				
			Medicare	Medicaid Skilled	Medicaid Intermediate	Other Government Assistance or Welfare	All Other Sources
Total	$689	$690	$1,167	$873	$610	$508	$440
Proprietary	670	686	1,048	798	596	501	562
Voluntary	747	721	[1]	1,023	645	[1]	373
Government	700	619	[1]	1,061	655	[1]	[1]

[1] Information is not available.
Source: National Center for Health Statistics, *The National Nursing Home Survey: 1977 Summary for the United States* (Washington, U.S. Government Printing Office, 1979).

TABLE XV-A-10
Number of Voluntary Homes Established,
by Ten Year Intervals

Period of Establishment	Number of Homes
Before 1900	171
1900 – 1909	64
1910 – 1919	71
1920 – 1929	99
1930 – 1939	45
1940 – 1949	67
1950 – 1959	149
1960 – 1969	288
1970 – 1979	198

Source: Tables XV-A-10 through XV-A-16 are reprinted, with permission, from *The American Association of Homes for the Aging: A Profile*, copyright 1980.

Please note that the Profile data were based on a 1978 survey and therefore, cannot be presumed to present an accurate picture of the association and its members in 1984.

AAHA Survey of Voluntary Homes

Additional information about the characteristics of the voluntary nursing home industry is available from a survey of its membership conducted in 1978 by the American Association of Homes for the Aging (AAHA; 1980). Founded in 1961, the AAHA represents the voluntary sector of the nursing home industry in the United States. The organization has a membership of nearly 1,700 homes.

Among the AAHA data is the year in which its member homes were established. The first voluntary homes go back to the beginnings of the nation when the very first home, the Christ Church Hospital-Kearsley Home, was established in 1772. By the start of the Civil War, 21 homes had been established and, at the turn of the 20th century, some 171 homes were providing services. The number of homes continued to increase in the early part of the 20th century but declined during the Depression and war years. After the war and into the 1960s and 1970s, the number of homes continued to increase significantly. The increase was due in part to the additional funding available from the Hill-Burton program and Federal mortgage insurance programs (American Association of Homes for the Aging, 1980) and the growth of reimbursement under the Medicaid and Medicare programs. Table XV–A–10 shows the number of homes established in 10-year intervals.

The member homes of the AAHA are sponsored by a variety of religious and other organizations. Table XV–A–11 gives a breakdown of sponsoring organization by type.

TABLE XV-A-11
AAHA Sponsoring Organizations

Type of Organization	Percent of Homes
Religious Organizations	76%
Community Organizations	6
Private Foundations	6
Fraternal Organizations	3
Government Agencies	3
Private, Non-Profit Groups	2
Unions	0.4
Other Organizations	5

Source: American Association of Homes for the Aging (1980).

Levels of Care

The AAHA classifies its homes into three categories for statistical purposes. Nursing care homes are those which provide some level of nursing care, either skilled, intermediate, or other (such as acute care). Personal care homes are those facilities which provide personal assistance for residents, including help with bathing, walking, eating, and other activities, but provide no nursing care service. Independent living facilities provide activities, meals, housekeeping, and other services but do not provide any personal or nursing care services. Single level homes are defined as homes which offer only one level of services (nursing care, personal care, or independent living). Multi-level facilities offer more than one level of services. About three-fifths of the voluntary homes are multi-level.

About eight out of 10 of the homes in the AAHA survey, with over one-half the total beds, offered nursing care to their residents. About 58 percent of the nursing care beds were classified as skilled, 38 percent as intermediate, and 4 percent as other.

Most nursing care homes had fewer than 200 nursing care residents. Table XV-A-12 indicates the size of homes providing nursing care services.

In general, the voluntary AAHA nursing care facilities served a relatively old population, with the average age being 81.8 years. The breakdown by age of residents is contained in Table XV-A-13.

The occupancy rate for nursing care beds in the AAHA survey was 96.7 percent, with over one-third reporting 100 percent occupancy and another one-third reporting over 95 percent occupancy. In computing these figures, beds not occupied but reserved and unavailable were considered as occupied beds. These occupancy figures

530

TABLE XV-A-12
Distribution of Nursing Care Residents in AAHA Homes

Number of Nursing Care Residents	Number of Homes	Percent
1 – 49	297	28.6%
50 – 99	365	25.2
100 – 199	276	26.6
200 +	100	9.6

Source: American Association of Homes for the Aging (1980).

therefore differ from those obtained from other sources, such as the National Center for Health Statistics, which compute occupancy rates on different bases.

By comparing the number of nursing care beds under construction to those already in existence, we can compute an expansion rate for the nursing care facilities. Almost 9,600 nursing care beds were being built at the time of the 1978 survey, representing an expansion rate of 8.5 percent for nursing care beds in non-profit facilities.

Personal Care Facilities

About three out of 10 AAHA homes provided personal care beds (as defined earlier). The 22,000 personal care beds reported represented about 11 percent of the total beds of facilities in the survey.

The average number of personal care beds in homes with these services tended to be smaller than for nursing care facilities. Table XV–A–14 shows the distribution of personal care patients in AAHA homes.

The average age of personal care residents was 81.5 years, slightly lower than for nursing care residents (81.8) and higher than for independent living residents (79.0).

TABLE XV-A-13
Age Distribution in AAHA Nursing Care Homes

Age	Percent of Residents
Under 65	3.1%
65 – 74	11.0
75 – 84	41.3
85 and older	44.6

Source: American Association of Homes for the Aging (1980).

TABLE XV-A-14
Distribution of Personal Care Residents in AAHA Homes

Number of Personal Care Residents	Number of Homes	Percent
1 – 49	271	65.5%
50 – 99	103	22.8
100 – 199	31	7.5
200 – 299	9	2.2

Source: American Association of Homes for the Aging (1980).

The occupancy rate for personal care beds shown in the survey was 93.7 percent computed according to the criteria described earlier. About one-third of the homes reported 100 percent occupancy for these beds, and other 20 percent reported over 95 percent occupancy.

About 2,500 personal care beds were reported under construction at the time of the survey, representing an expansion rate of 11.2 percent. This rate is somewhat higher than the rate for nursing care beds.

Independent Living Facilities

In the 1978 survey, four out of 10 AAHA facilities reported offering some sort of independent living arrangement. Such arrangements include three types of facilities: congregate housing units where at least one meal per day is provided, housekeeping units where residents do their own housekeeping but central dining is available, and housekeeping units without central dining. Of the 70,200 independent living units reported, 57 percent were congregate housing apartments, 28 percent were housekeeping units with central dining, and 15 percent were housekeeping units without central dining.

Of the total number of independent living facilities, 13 percent offered only independent living with the rest being multi-level facilities also offering personal and/or nursing care.

About one-half of the independent living arrangements served fewer than 100 residents, and about one-third between 100 and 199 residents. Table XV-A–15 gives the distribution of these homes by number of residents.

The occupancy rate for independent living arrangements in 1978 was 96.8 percent. Over 45 percent of the facilities reported 100 percent occupancy, and almost 30 percent had 95 percent occupancy.

Independent living units were being built at a greater rate than either personal care or nursing care facilities. More than 14,500 independent living units were under construction at the time of the

TABLE XV-A-15
Distribution of Independent Living Residents in AAHA Homes

Number of Residents	Number of Homes	Percent
1 – 49	146	27.0%
50 – 99	113	20.9
100 – 199	170	31.5
200 +	111	20.5

Source: American Association of Homes for the Aging (1980).

survey, representing an expansion rate of 20.6 percent. Over 11 percent of the homes in the survey reported that they were in the process of building or adding independent units.

Outreach Services

The AAHA survey also collected information on the extent to which the member homes offered services to persons not living in the home itself. By providing such services, termed outreach services, to members of the community, these facilities support and enable aged persons to live more independently in their own homes.

Four out of 10 AAHA facilities offered at least one outreach service to elderly persons in the community. Of those facilities providing outreach services, 60 percent offered two or more services, 20 percent offered five or more services, and 12 percent offered between six and 10 services.

Among the types of outreach services offered, Meals on Wheels for the homebound elderly was the most frequent type provided. The recipient usually pays for these meals, but many homes reported using public and private funds to finance the cost. Other types of outreach services are funded by the home itself, and these most frequently include religious activities, information and referral, recreational activities, transportation/escort services, and counseling. A listing of the more common outreach services and the number of homes offering them is given in Table XV–A–16.

Boards of Directors

One of the special characteristics of voluntary homes is that they are commonly governed by a volunteer board of trustees or directors. The AAHA survey indicated that a total of 22,000 persons were serving as volunteer board members at the time of the survey. A typical AAHA home has 18 persons on the governing board, with a range of as few as three and as many as 100. The smallest homes

TABLE XV-A-16
Outreach Services and Number of AAHA Homes Offering Them

Outreach Service	Number of Homes	Percent of Total
Meals on Wheels	202	15%
Religious Services	172	13
Information and Referral	151	11
Recreational Activities	132	10
Physical Therapy	129	10
Transportation/Escort	95	7
Adult Day Care	92	7
Congregate Meals	90	7
Counseling	83	6
Occupational Therapy	61	5

Source: American Association of Homes for the Aging (1980).

averaged 16 members on the board, and the largest averaged 22 board members. The majority of boards (86 percent) met at least four times a year, with almost one-third of the boards holding monthly board meetings.

Many voluntary homes have established resident councils, that is, councils composed of residents of the home. These groups allow residents to participate in the decisions that affect their lives and to influence the homes' administrations and philosophies. The AAHA survey showed that 69 percent of the voluntary homes had resident councils, with large homes more likely to have such councils than small ones.

Minority Residents

The survey also collected some information on minority residents living in the homes. In total, 3 percent of the residents of the voluntary homes in the survey were members of an ethnic minority. Of these, black residents composed 2 percent. The balance of the minority residents were Hispanic, American Indian, or Oriental American. There were a few homes in the survey where at least 50 percent of the residents were black (10) or Hispanic (4).

References

American Association of Homes for the Aging, *A Profile Report Based on 1354 Responses to a 1978 Survey of AAHA Member Homes* (Washington: AAHA, 1980).

Dunlop, Burton D., *The Growth of Nursing Home Care* (Lexington, Toronto and London: D.C. Heath and Company, 1979).

534

National Center for Health Statistics, *The National Nursing Home Survey: 1977, Summary for the United States* (Washington: U.S. Government Printing Office, 1979).

Reiss, Kay, *Nursing Homes: An Overview, Including A Summary of Legislative Proposals in the Ninety-Sixth Congress* (Washington: Congressional Research Service, Library of Congress, 1980).

U.S. Department of Health and Human Services, Undersecretary's Task Force on Long Term Care, *Report of the Work Group of Nursing Home Bed Supply*, processed, 1980.

U.S. Department of Health and Human Services, Health Care Financing Administration, *Administrator's Report*, Number 30, January 9, 1981, processed.

U.S. Senate, Committee on Banking and Currency, *Hearings*, 86th Congress, 1st Session, January 22–28, 1959 (Washington: U.S. Government Printing Office, 1960).

U.S. Senate, Committee on Finance, *The Social Security Act and Related Laws*, December 1978 edition (Washington: U.S. Government Printing Office, 1978).

U.S. Senate, Committee on Labor and Public Welfare, *The Aged and Aging in the United States: A National Problem, Summary and Recommendations* (Washington: U.S. Government Printing Office, 1960).

Vladeck, Bruce C., *Unloving Care: The Nursing Home Tragedy* (New York: Basic Books, 1980).

CHAPTER XVI

Models of the Nursing Home

by Hans C. Palmer and Ronald J. Vogel

An economic model[1] of the behavior of providers of nursing home care is an important tool in understanding such behavior. Here we formulate a simple, heuristic model of the nursing home. Using that model as a base, we will analyze the behavior of other types of providers of long-term care. Although differences exist among nursing homes for purposes of regulation and reimbursement, this exposition will treat them all as a single type of facility. The more complex analytics of sets of presumably differing facilities will be presented subsequently.

Our analysis begins with the assumption that the nursing home is a profit-seeking, imperfectly competitive firm, offering a specific set of services to clients with similar levels of dependency.[2] The production of varying amounts of these services in a given facility is subject to diminishing relative returns in the short run and is characterized by rising average costs as production expands in the long run. In other words, both the short-run and long-run average cost curves are U-shaped. The case of proprietary facilities selling care to so-called private pay patients (those who pay for care out of their own or their families' pockets) is first considered. We extend the analysis to private pay care in non-profit facilities and then consider the impacts of the Medicaid system of financing care on the behavior of providers. The influence of private and Medicare insurance will follow, and the exposition will end with the problems of so-called

The authors would like to thank Philip G. Cotterill, William J. Lynk, and Robert L. Seidman for their critical comments on a previous draft of this chapter that was presented at the Annual Meeting of the Southern Economic Association, November 5–7, 1980.

[1] Economic models do not purport to be exact descriptions of reality. Rather, they represent a manner of thinking about a real-world phenomenon in a precise fashion. Their degree of abstraction makes them more or less applicable to the real-world, but more often than not they yield important insights into aspects of reality and provide important policy direction. (See Friedman, 1953, pp. 3–47.)

[2] The term "imperfect competition" does not connote a value judgment which implies that something is "wrong" with a market. It is simply economic terminology for a market which is neither perfectly competitive nor perfectly monopolistic. Firms in imperfectly competitive markets are often termed "price makers" (that is, they can determine or influence price through output decisions). Firms in perfectly competitive markets are "price takers;" they take the price as given by the market.

537

"subsidies" by private pay patients to recipients of publicly financed care and with the issue of "substandard" care.

For-Profit Nursing Homes

Seventy percent of the nursing homes in the United States are profit-oriented, proprietary enterprises. It seems safe to assume that these enterprises seek to maximize their profits and thus the income and wealth of their owners. (We will ignore the complications introduced by other forms of maximizing behavior on the part of administrators, managers, etc. We will also ignore the effects of low occupancy penalties and other similar regulations.)

Figure XVI–1 shows the demand and cost situation of a profit maximizing home in the short run. We will assume that all patients in a given home and in a given type of home are of the same level of disability and receive the same type of care and volume of services (that is, the product is homogeneous). The output of the firm (nursing home) is bed days per year, shown as Q on the horizontal axis; price (P) and average total costs and marginal costs (ATC and MC) are measured on the vertical axis, as is marginal revenue (MR). Under conventional assumptions, the profit maximizing firm would in the short run produce at point E, that is, where marginal revenue (MR) equals marginal cost (MC). The corresponding quantity would be Q_1 and the price would be P_1. If the home produced more bed days than Q_1, the cost of an additional bed day (marginal cost) would be greater than the additional revenue from that additional day (marginal revenue), thus reducing profit (revenues minus costs). Since marginal cost does not equal price (marginal value to the consumers), the home is not economically efficient at the margin. This is, of course, true of all imperfectly competitive firms. On the other hand, if the home produced fewer than Q_1 days of care, some profit would be forgone, since up to output Q_1, MR exceeds MC. To be sure, levels of output other than Q_1 would not necessarily produce losses, but profits would not be *maximized*. A firm may actually end up generating losses if its total costs exceed total revenues, but a loss-minimizing strategy would dictate the same $MR = MC$ type of behavior to the proprietor(s) of the nursing home[3] (unless

---

[3] It should be noted that, in the long run and without legal impediments, profit rates greater than those in other lines of activity in the economy will attract new firms and resources to the industry (possibly through the expansion of existing firms), while losses will drive resources and (probably) firms from the industry. Note also that Q_1 is not necessarily a least cost level of output for a nursing home of a fixed bed capacity, given the absence of perfect competition. Even if the equilibrium level of output is also a least-cost level of output, price will exceed average and marginal cost, and the firm will be economically inefficient. In the short run, firms making losses will produce as long as price covers average variable cost (AVC, not shown). In the long run, losses would imply closing the firm.

538

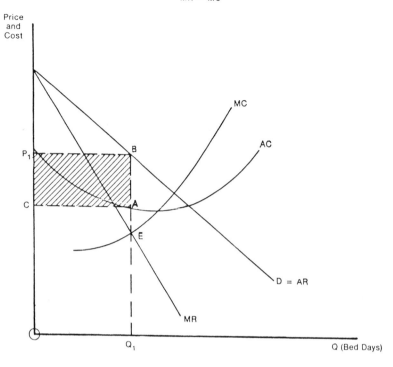

FIGURE XVI-1
Profit Maximizing Nursing Home
No Price Discrimination
MR = MC

revenues do not cover variable costs, in which case the firm closes). In this situation, if we assume a single set of demanders (no possibility of splitting the market based on differences in customers' incomes, tastes, locations, etc.), at output Q_1 the firm would earn profits denoted by the area P^1BAC.

If underlying conditions were to change, for example, because of increased labor costs, the firm's cost curves would move upward, while the profit-maximizing price and quantity would increase and decrease, respectively. (This assumes no changes in demand conditions.) Conversely, price could drop and quantity increase if the firm became more efficient or if inputs became cheaper, and unit costs dropped. Shifts in the demand and in the marginal revenue curves would cause similar price and output effects, assuming no changes in costs. Upward shifts in demand, for example, because of increases in household incomes or the numbers of dependent aged in the home's "marketing area" could cause P and Q to increase; the reverse could be true of decreases in demand.

Since profit maximizing behavior requires the equalizing of marginal cost and marginal revenue by the firm, the ultimate price and quantity effects of changes in demand or cost will depend on the shifts in demand and cost curves in relation to each other. They also hinge on changes in the corresponding marginal revenue and cost curves and upon resulting shifts in their equilibrium intersections.

Non-Profit Nursing Homes

Various organs of government, as well as a number of private organizations, operate nursing homes oriented not to profit but rather to the maximization of some other magnitude, for example, quantity of service, usually at some previously determined "high" standard of quality. Alternatively, non-profit firms may attempt to provide some given quantity of care (for example to the members of a given ethnic, income, or religious group) at as high a level of quality as possible, within budget limits. In general, it is assumed that such organizations will try to cover all operating, if not capital, costs or that they will try to operate within limits set either by external subsidies or by their internal capacity to generate contributions. In the case of nursing homes, the conventional wisdom suggests that the main objectives are maximum quantity of care of a given quality, provided under break-even conditions.[4]

Figure XVI–2 presents a picture of the price and output decisions of a non-profit facility in an imperfectly competitive market. (The

---

[4] See Joseph E. Newhouse, (1970) for a discussion of the quantity-quality trade-offs in hospital care. Karen Davis (1972) offers a somewhat more skeptical view of the behavior, if not the assumptions, of non-profit care providers.

540

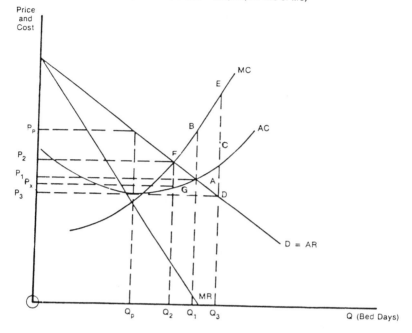

FIGURE XVI-2
Non-Profit Nursing Home
No Price Discrimination
Possible Subsidy

(AR = AC) or (AR = MC) or (AR < AC or MC)

541

notation of Figure XVI–2 corresponds to that of Figure XVI–1, with which it is to be compared.) If we assume a quantity-maximizing model with a given quality of care, and costs of providing care presumably the same as those of the proprietary home of Figure XVI–1 (an assumption common to all that follows), the marginal cost-equals-marginal revenue imperative no longer applies. Instead, the facility will choose among three different rules for the determination of price and output.

Rule 1: An entity desiring to break even in its operations would produce at point A where demand or average revenue equals average cost, and total revenue equals total cost.[5] The non-profit firm would produce Q_1 bed days and charge price P_1, whereas the profit maximizer will produce Q_p at a price of P_p, that is, $MC = MR$. Assuming the same technology and type and quality of care as in the proprietary case, the non-profit firm will offer more care at a lower price than will proprietary ones. Such a price-quantity combination, while possibly catering to the non-profit home's goals, would not be socially efficient, since bed-day consumers value the marginal unit of care by the amount Q_1A, the price they pay, while production of the marginal unit of care adds Q_1B to total costs (marginal cost).

Rule 2: If the non-profit facility's trustees or managers wish to offer more care than a proprietary firm, yet wish to be economically and socially efficient, they would find equilibrium at point F, corresponding to P_2 and Q_2. Although, since MC (marginal cost) = AR (average revenue or price), this point may be economically efficient in equating society's marginal valuation with marginal costs, it may yield either a "profit" (net return) or a loss to the supposedly non-profit institution.[6] In Figure XVI–2, the facility is making a profit of FG per unit and a total profit of P_2FGP_x, a situation incon-

---

[5] If the facility treats capital as costless, for example, because of charitable provision and/or because capital is provided through fund-raising campaigns conducted by volunteer groups at no cost to the facility, average and total revenues may have to only cover average and total variable costs. If capital has a positive cost, the non-profit firm may continue to operate in the short run, provided that variable costs are covered by revenues. This is true also for the proprietary firm following a loss-minimizing strategy. In both cases, if variable costs are not covered, both types of firms may shut down unless subsidized. In the long run, if both types of firm must operate under break-even conditions, then losses will force exit of resources from the industry.

[6] Price ($P = AR$) equals consumers' marginal evaluation of the product. Marginal cost (MC) equals the additional cost to society of generating one more unit of the product. Therefore, when $P = (AR) = MC$, society is efficiently balancing marginal resource use against the gain in value from having the additional product produced by those marginal resources.

sistent with the institution's own goals, unless profit is to be used for altruistic purposes in the future.

Rule 3: If the firm wishes to practice "altruistic" pricing, possibly to encourage consumption of its care by especially needy groups, it might choose a P_3 price and Q_3 quantity. Such a price-quantity combination, would, however, produce losses and require a subsidy equal to CD per day just to break even. Also, Q_3 would represent an inefficient short-run position, since the marginal valuation placed on care (its price) is less than its marginal cost.

Medicaid Demand

At this point we expand the analysis to consider the effects of governmental assistance in gaining access to care, presumably of requisite quality. In the United States, this assistance is largely provided via financial support rather than through government delivery of services. Medicaid, a system of Federally matched, State payments, is the most important vehicle for such financial support. To the facility providing care for Medicaid-eligible beneficiaries, the Medicaid-financed demand appears as a horizontal demand function at a price equal to the so-called reimbursement rate, the price which the government says it is willing to pay for care.

Figure XVI–3 shows the short-run, profit maximizing situation for a proprietary nursing home "selling" care to the government as the payer for users of care. This facility has no private pay patients. Again, the profit-maximizing equilibrium occurs where marginal revenue (MR) equals marginal cost (MC). Note, however, that in this case the demand curve is horizontal, not negatively sloped, and that marginal revenue equals price over the relevant range of outputs.[7] (That range would be determined either by the capacity of the facility or by the willingness of the government to buy care from that facility, arguably an amount of care greater than bed capacity.) Under these circumstances, the facility in the short run would provide Q_M bed days of care at the Medicaid rate, R. If the rate covers average total costs, the facility is in long-run, as well as short-run, equilibrium; if the rate exceeds AC, there are profits, perhaps inducing entry to this facility's market area, possibly forcing up costs because of competition for inputs. If the rate falls below costs, the home may close in the short run if average variable costs (AVC, not shown) are not covered and in the long run if average total costs are not covered.

The analysis is much the same for the non-profit firm selling care only to the government for Medicaid beneficiaries. In this instance,

---

[7] The demand curve is not that of the user of care but rather is that of the payer who is ready to pay for a limited or unlimited amount of care at the rate (price) R.

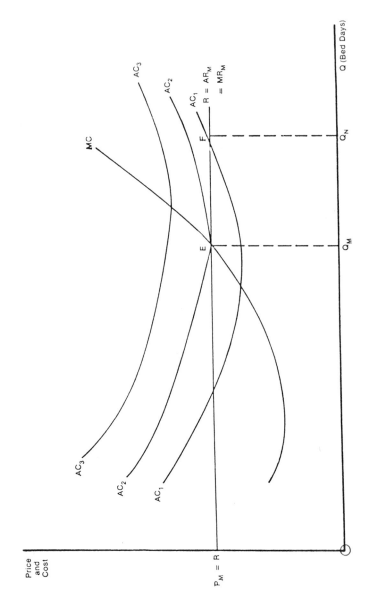

FIGURE XVI-3
Proprietary or Non-Profit Homes
Selling Care to the Government
at a Fixed Reimbursement Rate

if the non-profit facility seeks to cover costs (Rule 1), and if the MC equals R, the intersection is at the same point as the minimum of the ATC (or the AVC) with AC_2, and the proprietary and the non-profit firms will produce the same quantity of care. Otherwise, the non-profit facility will produce care up to the point where the rate equals cost, that is, at Q_N, as with cost curve AC_1. (This will be the AVC in the short-run, ATC in the long.)

Under these conditions, if both types of firms have cost curve AC_2, the non-profit will produce more bed days of care than will the proprietary one at a given reimbursement rate, Q_N versus Q_M. With AC_3, the position of the equilibrium for the non-profit firm is essentially indeterminate unless some subsidy rule is specified, unless the facility strives for lowest average costs, or unless some other external rule is given.

Private Demand Plus Medicaid Demand

Most actual nursing homes cater to private pay clients and to public pay clients. Indeed, much evidence shows that many private pay patients become Medicaid eligible as they "spend-down" their assets to the requisite indigency levels. Under these circumstances, where the private pay market will adjust quantity demanded to price charged and where the public price is fixed, the provider faces two demand curves, each with a different elasticity. In such cases, we would expect the provider to adjust prices and quantities produced to maximize profits for the proprietary firm and presumably, quantity of service (or some other magnitude) for the non-profit facility.

Figure XVI–4 shows the situation of a proprietary facility facing a combined private pay and Medicaid market.[8] Actually, the facility is facing two markets simultaneously and will simultaneously seek to determine gross output, the allocation of that output between markets, and the price to be charged to the private pay patients. It should be stressed that this set of decisions develops together and not in sequence and that the decisions emerge jointly as a result of the firm's desire to maximize profit. In Figure XVI–4, the curves labeled D_p and MR_p, respectively, refer to the private pay market. The horizontal line, $D_{MD} = AR_{MD} = MR_{MD}$, is the demand and marginal revenue curve for Medicaid bed days. The line is at the level of reimbursement rate, R, set by the Medicaid authorities in the State in which the facility operates. This, in effect, is the price per bed day which those authorities will pay. The quantity $Q_Z Q_M$ represents the

---

[8] This exposition follows that of Sloan, Cromwell, and Mitchell (1978); Scanlon (1978); Bishop (1979); Yett et al (1980); and Scanlon (1980), although our geometric exposition more explicitly combines demand and marginal revenue consideratoins. We are indebted to Philip Cotterill for significant clarifications of this model and of the subsidization argument following.

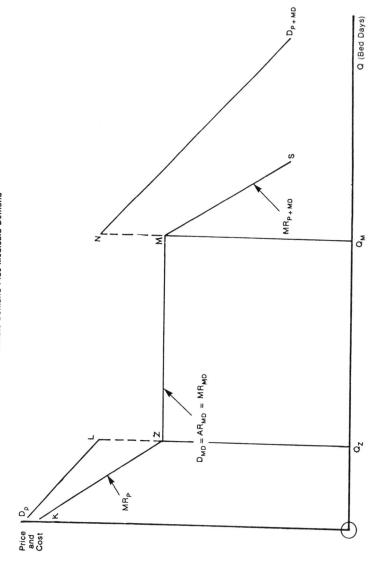

FIGURE XVI-4
Private Demand Plus Medicaid Demand

total number of Medicaid eligibles in this nursing home's "marketing area."[9] If the spend-down phenomenon occurs, the number of eligibles may increase regardless of State policy in the short run. In that case, the State may have to increase its Medicaid budget allocations, and/or reduce the reimbursement rate, and/or tighten the eligibility rules.

In Figure XVI–4, the demand and marginal revenue curves for private pay and Medicaid bed days are summed horizontally. With the horizontal summation, the revenue curves assume shapes different from those in either the pure private pay or pure Medicaid cases, in effect showing the combination of the two markets. As perceived by the supplier, the demand curve in this combined market is traced out by the line $D_P LZMND_{P+MD}$. It thus appears to be discontinuous for the vertical distances LZ and MN.[10]

In effect, the ND_{P+MD} portion of the private demand curve is shifted by the insertion of the Medicaid demand curve which expands the total market for the nursing home. The marginal revenue curve becomes the line $KZMS$ because the ZS portion of the original marginal revenue curve is displaced. The horizontal portion of the new marginal revenue curve reflects the coincidence of the demand and marginal revenue functions over the range $Q_Z Q_M$ because of a fixed level of reimbursement by Medicaid.

In this situation, the average revenue curve is no longer the demand curve but lies above and to the right of the latter, reflecting the combined effects of private pay prices and the fixed level reimbursement rate. The new AR curve would approach the fixed reimbursement rate as Medicaid patients became a larger portion of the total patient load for the given facility. If, however, the total amount of Medicaid bed days is fixed by public policy, the AR curve would begin to fall below the reimbursement rate as total output exceeds Q_M. This last situation is considered in the following discussion of marginal cost curves intersecting marginal revenue to the right of Q_M.

Again, the profit-maximizing rule of marginal cost equals marginal revenue determines the equilibrium level of output. In this combined case, however, the complex marginal revenue curve embodies the separate marginal revenue curves from the two sub-markets. In determining the equilibrium, therefore, we must consider the position

---

[9] Eligibility is a function of income and asset position. It varies by State. Eligibility rules usually do not allow patients to divest themselves of assets by gift to become eligible.

[10] Note that in the absence of the Medicaid reimbursement system, the demand curve would appear as that in Figure XVI–1. It is only because of the peculiar conditions of the joint market that the demand function appears discontinuous. The reasons for the discontinuity are found in the equal marginal revenue conditions discussed subsequently.

547

of the relevant marginal cost curve in relation to the relevant portions of the complex marginal revenue curve.

If the cost situation of the proprietary firm can be described by MC_1 in Figure XVI-5, the profit-maximizing home will not participate in the Medicaid market at all (assuming no legal mandates to do so.) In this case, private patients will absorb all the bed days of output, Q_1, for each unit of which they will pay price P_1.

If the home's cost curve is MC_2, both Medicaid and private pay patients will be served.[11] In this situation the firm (home) faces two different markets with differing price elasticities and can engage in price discrimination in pursuit of profit maximization.[12] Because the State sets R, the Medicaid reimbursement rate, the home becomes a price taker for Medicaid patients; yet it remains a price maker for private pay patients. Following the conventionally assumed behavior for price discriminators, the home will want to equalize the level of marginal revenue (and of marginal cost) in the two markets. Otherwise it could increase total revenue, hence profits, by shifting sales from the low to the high marginal revenue market. This behavior follows line R, which coincides with the rate (public price) line and thus with the demand curve and the marginal revenue curve over the range $Q_Z Q_M$. In this range the firm will seek to produce Q_2 units of care, allocating OQ_Z to the private pay market and $Q_Z Q_2$ to the Medicaid market. The price received in the Medicaid market will be R per bed day; in the private pay market it will be P_Z.

The case of marginal costs intersecting marginal revenues to the right of Q_M in Figure XVI-5 can be divided into two other cases: one in which the intersection yields a private price higher than the Medicaid rate and one lower. Both share the characteristic that the equal marginal revenue principle cannot be applied across the two markets (private pay and Medicaid), mainly since the proprietor cannot reallocate output to the Medicaid market (the one with the higher marginal revenue) because of the State-imposed limits on Medicaid expenditure. If the marginal cost curve intersects the marginal revenue curve over the Q_M to Q_W range of outputs, the private pay price will still exceed the Medicaid reimbursement rate. In this circumstance, the total output will be, for example, OQ_3, of which $OQ_Z + Q_M Q_3$ will go to private pay and $Q_Z Q_M$ will go to

---

[11] The marginal cost curves are those for operators with different productive capacities.

[12] The term price discrimination refers to charging two (or more) different prices for the same good in two different markets. It is practiced because profit can be increased by charging buyers in the less elastic market a higher price than that paid by buyers in a market with higher demand elasticity. It can persist only when the buyers in the two markets cannot trade the commodity with each other but must buy from the seller. For a formal discussion, see Ferguson and Maurice (1978), pp. 358–366.

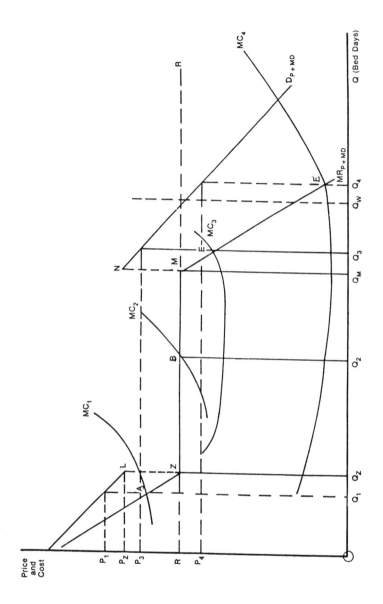

FIGURE XVI-5
Alternative Equilibria, Private Pay and Medicaid Reimbursement, Proprietary Home

549

Medicaid. The private pay price will be P_3, greater than the Medicaid rate, R. If the $MC = MR$ intersection lies to the right of Q_W, for example, at Q_4 (corresponding to MC_4), $OQ_Z + Q_M Q_4$ will go to private pay and, again, $Q_Z Q_M$ to Medicaid.

Note that with an MC_3 type of curve, one could argue that, in the short run, private pay patients are subsidizing Medicaid patients. With an MC_4 type of curve, that is, one that intersects MR to the right of Q_W, the private patients are arguably being subsidized by Medicaid in the short run.[13] To restate an earlier position, in neither the MC_3 nor the MC_4 case is the firm operating at maximum profit or social efficiency, inasmuch as marginal revenues cannot be equated in all markets.

The region to the right of output Q_M is also interesting because of its policy implications in a financially constrained environment. Conventionally, one assumes that the private pay price will always exceed the Medicaid rate, usually because of the historically rapid growth of the demand for nursing home beds, itself associated with the emergence of the Medicare-Medicaid system. It is, however, conceivable that a combination of increasing scale of enterprise and related falling cost curves could dictate an output level to the right of Q_W. If the public authorities constrain total Medicaid budgets (because of taxpayer pressure), and yet must keep reimbursement rates around R (because of proprietor, professional, and political pressure), the potential for a Medicaid-subsidized system becomes very real indeed. The implications for the inconsistency between the intended and actual results of a public program of financial provision for nursing homes are complex and troublesome.

Non-Profit Providers and the Medicaid Market

Not surprisingly, public payment systems complicate the theoretical models of behavior for the non-profit providers just as for the profit-oriented firms. The picture is even more complex because of the multiplicity of non-profit pricing and output "rules" as noted above.

Figure XVI–6 shows a set of possible alternative equilibria for a non-profit home seeking to maximize output (Rule 1). Because Rule 1 aims at equalizing average costs and revenues, it is necessary to construct an average revenue curve (AR) which differs from the

---

[13] The concept of a subsidy will be developed later in this chapter. In particular, one should note that in the long run the subsidy may run to the higher priced market from the lower priced market, since the larger market may be needed to allow economies of scale, possibly associated with lower costs of production.

FIGURE XVI-6
Alternative Equilibria for Non-Profit Facilities, Combined Private Pay and Medicaid

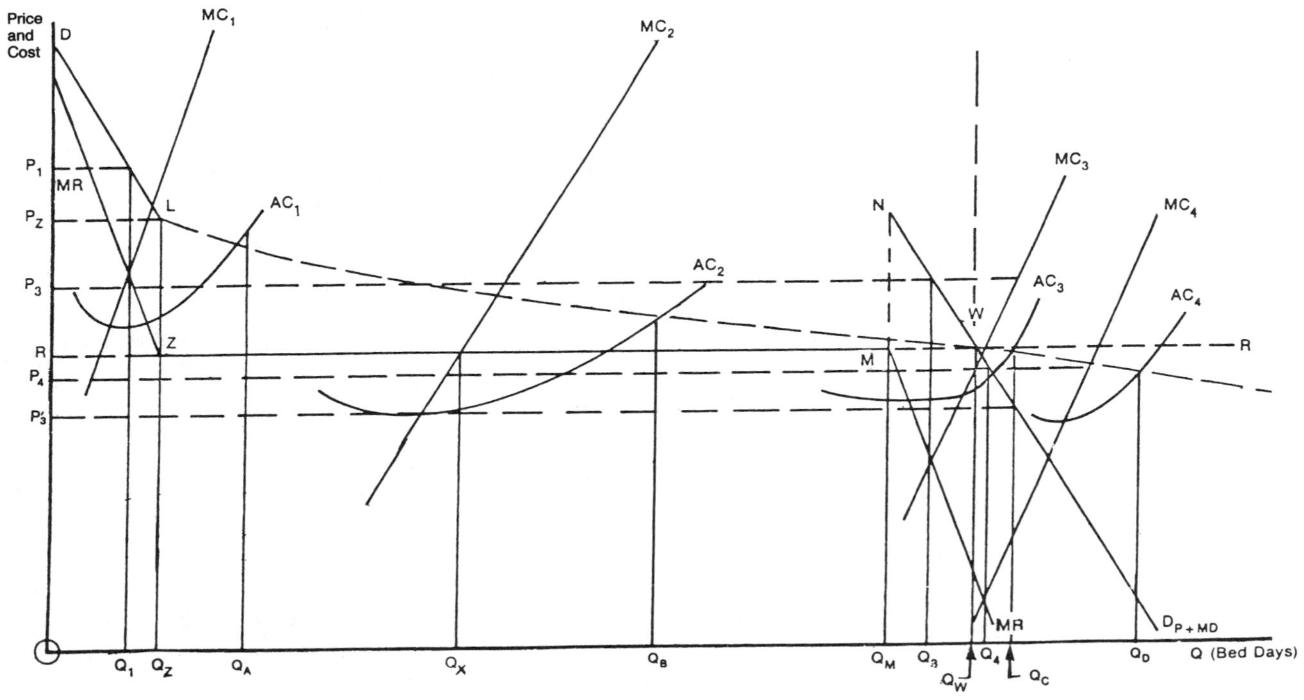

demand curve, reflecting the combination of the fixed Medicaid rate and the private pay price for output above Q_Z.[14]

Note that the average revenue curve, as distinct from the demand curve, begins at the point of the first discontinuity of the demand curve, intersecting the R line at the point where the displaced portion of the demand curve also cuts the R line (point W), that is, where $P = R$.[15] Also note that the level of the Medicaid rate, R, determines that position of the average revenue curve, just as it determines the level of private output and price because of the equal marginal principle.[16]

Consideration of the various marginal and average cost curves in Figure XVI–6 produces some provocative speculations with important policy implications. For example, if the relevant marginal revenue curve is MC_1, corresponding to AC_1, it appears that a proprietary firm would not accept Medicaid patients (MC intersects MR to the left of LQ_Z), but that an output maximizing, non-profit home might do so if its average cost curve intersected its average revenue curve in the appropriate region, namely, to the right of line LQ_Z. For the proprietary firm, total output equals OQ_1, all sold at P_1, in the private market. For the non-profit firm (with the same cost curves), total output is OQ_A; OQ_Z goes to private pay at price P_Z, and Q_ZQ_A goes to Medicaid users at rate R. Of course, again, a non-profit firm would not be economically efficient, in the sense of $MC =$ price. The private pay price, P_Z, charged by the non-profit firm, would be lower than that of the proprietary firm (assuming the same private market for both types of facilities), and the "average" price would be lower because of a greater number of Medicaid patients.

---

[14] As noted earlier, the average revenue curve can be derived for the proprietary facility as well as the non-profit ones; however, since the proprietaries make their decisions on the basis of $MR = MC$, the average revenue curve is irrelevant in the short run. In the long run, average revenue must cover cost if the proprietary home is to avoid losses and not go out of business. See Scanlon (1978) p. 157ff, for a discussion of average revenue defined in this way.

[15] Algebraically, AR is the arithmetic average of the Medicaid rate and the private pay rate, calculated by summing the total days of care at the private rate and the total days of care at the Medicaid rate and dividing the grand total by the number of days provided to both categories of patients. Since, with a given Medicaid rate, there would be no Medicaid days of care provided before point Z (corresponding to Q_z), the average revenue curve would coincide with the demand curve between the origin, O, and Q_z. At point W, the Medicaid rate and the private pay price (shown by the $D_{P + MD}$ private pay demand curve) would coincide; beyond W, the Medicaid rate lies above the private pay price, and the AR curve lies below R.

[16] For a non-profit, output-maximizing home, the maximization of output requires that average cost equal average revenue and that the marginal revenue from the private pay patients be at the same level as that for Medicaid patients.

In effect, the non-profit firm is using profit (excess of revenue over cost) from the private pay to subsidize the expansion of Medicaid care.

If the relevant curves are MC_2 and AC_2, the non-profit home will provide OQ_B of care versus OQ_X for the proprietary one. In this instance, the private pay price would be the same, P_Z, for the two types of providers, but average revenue again would be lower, reflecting the larger share and absolute amount of Medicaid care, than would be true with profit-oriented provision.

The region to the right of the line NQ_M presents something of a conundrum for the non-profit facility. If the profit-maximizing rule is followed, with MC_3 and AC_3, the $MC = MR$ rule implies an equilibrium output of OQ_3, with a private pay price of P_3. In that case, private pay patients could "subsidize" Medicaid patients (again, the meaning of "subsidy" will be subsequently developed). With the non-profit output-maximizer, the equilibrium level of output is OQ_C, with Q_ZQ_M allocated to Medicaid and $(OQ_Z + Q_MQ_C)$ to private pay. In this circumstance, the private pay price is P'_3, below the Medicaid rate. This implies a subsidy from Medicaid patients to private pay, an uncommon outcome for presumably altruistic facilities whose Medicaid population is their most dependent.

If the MC_4 and AC_4 curves apply, the degree of Medicaid subsidy to the private payers is even greater. Again, the policy implications vary somewhat from the expected.

Medicare Demand and Private Demand

At this point, we further expand the analysis to consider the effects of the Medicare program. We do so only briefly, however, because the analysis of the model for the Medicare case is not unlike that for Medicaid. The following analysis uses comparative statics.

The Medicare program provides nursing home care for up to 100 days, after at least a three day stay in a short-stay hospital. Figure XVI-7 depicts the aggregate demand curve ($D_{ME}D_{ME}$) for Medicare bed days by consumers and the conditions under which the Medicare entitlement might be exercised.[17] During time T_0 (0–20 days), no copayment is required on the part of the consumer, and, if enough beds were available, Q_ZQ_0 bed days would be consumed. For the next time period, T_1 (21–100) days, the consumer

---

17 We have chosen this form of exposition for the sake of simplicity. The number of stays of x length demanded is a function of the number of persons willing to pay copayment for x days and the persons eligible for x days. It could be that patient demand is inelastic, given the severity of condition. Scanlon believes that coverage decisions probably play the major role in affecting the number of days demanded. Also, for the sake of simplicity in this exposition, we assume that all Medicare patients are homogeneous and have similar consumption histories.

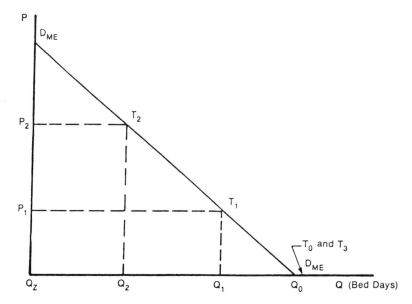

FIGURE XVI-7
The Medicare Demand Function for Bed Days, Consumers

T_0 (0-20 days): Q_ZQ_0—no payment on the part of the consumer

T_1 (21-100 days): Q_ZQ_1—$22.50 per day copayment by consumer

T_2 (101 + days): Q_ZQ_2—full payment by consumer

T_3 (21 + n days): Q_ZQ_0—arrival at Medicaid "spenddown"

must presently pay a fixed daily copayment ($22.50 per day in 1980).[18] Given the aggregate demand curve, patients would consume $Q_Z Q_1$ bed days. In the following time period, T_2 (101 +) days, Medicare coverage ceases, and the individual consumer must pay the full cost of a bed day if he/she remains in a nursing home. On the aggregate demand curve, quantity $Q_Z Q_2$ of bed days would be consumed. Finally, T_3 (21 + n) days denotes the arrival at the so-called "Medicaid spend-down," that point at which the patient becomes medically indigent and qualifies for Medicaid coverage. Given the shape, slope, and height of the aggregate demand curve, $Q_Z Q_0$ bed days would be consumed, if available. Note that T_0 and T_3 are analytically similar in that in these two situations, the consumer faces a zero price.

Figure XVI–8 shows the comparative statics of T_0 through T_3, *as perceived by the nursing home firm*.[19] At T_0 and T_1, just as was the case for Medicaid, the Medicare-financed demand (D_{ME}) appears as a horizontal demand function at a price equal to the Medicare reimbursement rate, R, which is the price that the Federal government is willing to pay for Medicare patients.[20]

As with the private demand-Medicaid demand analysis, we can use similar reasoning for the private demand-Medicare demand analysis. From Figure XVI–7, $Q_Z Q_0$ in Figure XVI–8 represents the amount of Medicare bed days demanded at a zero price to the consumer, and $O Q_Z O_0 Q$ represents private demand. The analysis for price and output determination parallels that of the Medicaid cases presented previously. T_1 only differs in that the pool of Medicare eligibles $(Q_Z Q_1)$ to the nursing home is now smaller, because of the co-payment provision.[21]

---

[18] The nursing home copayment has now been pegged to one-eighth the average daily charge in a short-stay hospital.

[19] Again, for the sake of simplicity of exposition, we assume that all Medicare patients are *uniform* and *move uniformly* through consumption periods T_0, T_1, T_2 or T_3. A more realistic portrayal would have the firm considering the admission of patients with differing propensities to stay or leave, to go on Medicaid, or remain private-pay after Medicare benefits have been exhausted. The firm's own policies about admission selection, discharge, and acceptance of Medicaid, as well as private price, affect the progression of patients through the different consumption states. The firm's expected marginal revenue is also affected by the progression. This whole set of issues is presently being modeled by Christine Bishop and Thomas Willemain, using expected revenues under different provider strategies.

[20] R is the same in both T_0 and T_1 because the nursing home receives R in T_0 and $(R - CP) + CP$ in T_1, where CP is the co-payment, paid by the consumer and not by the government.

[21] Some of the previous Medicare demanders have dropped out of the market.

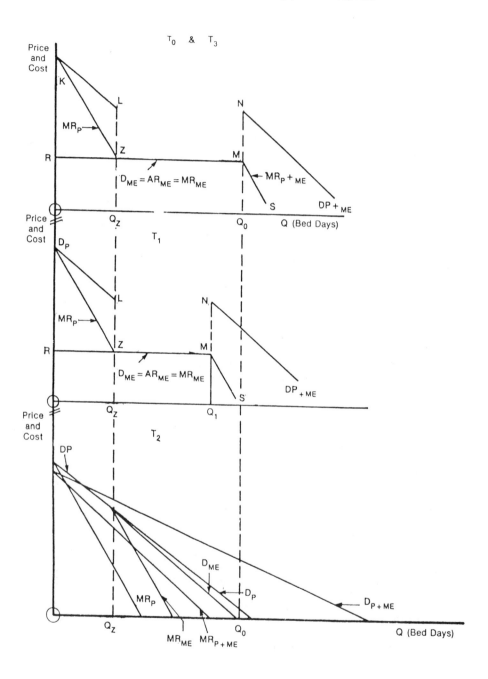

FIGURE XVI-8
The Demand Function for Medicare Bed Days, Perceived by Firm

556

TABLE XVI-1
The For-Profit Firm Price and Output
Pricing Rule
Marginal Revenue = Marginal Cost

	MC_1	MC_2	MC_3	MC_4
(1) Price to Private Patients	P_1	P_Z	P_3	P_4
(2) Quantity to Private Patients	Q_1	QQ_Z	$OQ_Z + Q_M Q_3$	$OQ_Z + Q_M Q_4$
(3) Price from Medicaid Patients	None	R	R	R
(4) Quantity to Medicaid Patients	None	$Q_Z Q_2$	$Q_Z Q_M$	$Q_Z Q_M$
(5) Price from Medicare Patients (0–100 days)	None	R	R	R
(6) Quantity to Medicare Patients (0–100 days)	None	$Q_Z Q_2$	$Q_Z Q_M$	$Q_Z Q_M$

Again, the previous analysis for Medicaid price and output determination is applicable here. By T_2, the government has stepped out of the picture completely and the demand function faced by the firm is the familiar down-sloping one. In panel T_2 of Figure XVI–8, we have summed the private and previous Medicare patients' demand curves horizontally to arrive at demand curve D_{P+ME}, with its attendant marginal revenue curve MR_{P+ME}. In this case, the price and output decision would be similar to those for Figures XVI–1 and XVI–2. Finally, T_3 becomes the Medicaid case because of the spend-down, and price and output are determined exactly as in Figures XVI–5 and XVI–6.

In the previous pages we have arrived at a multiplicity of possible pricing and output determinations. Basically, these determinations depend upon whether the provider of long-term care is a for-profit or non-profit firm. But they also depend upon the payment source, whether that be private, Medicaid, or Medicare, and the shape and position of the relevant cost curves. Tables XVI–1 and XVI–2 give a systematic presentation of all of the cases considered thus far in this chapter.

TABLE XVI-2
The Non-Profit Firm Price and Output
Pricing Rule
Average Revenue = Average Cost

	MC_1	MC_2	MC_3		MC_4	
			(a)	(b)	(a)	(b)
(1) Price to Private Patients	P_Z	P_Z	P_3	P'_3	P_4	P lower than P'_3
(2) Quantity to Private Patients	QQ_Z	QQ_Z	$QQ_Z + Q_M Q_3$	$QQ_Z + Q_M Q_C$	$QQ_Z + Q_M Q_4$	$QQ_Z + Q_M Q_D$
(3) Price from Medicaid Patients	R	R	R	R	R	R
(4) Quantity to Medicaid Patients	$Q_Z Q_A$	$Q_Z Q_B$	$Q_Z Q_M$	$Q_Z Q_M$	$Q_Z Q_M$	$Q_Z Q_M$
(5) Price from Medicare Patients (0–100 days)	R	R	R	R	R	R
(6) Quantity to Medicare Patients (0–100 days)	$Q_Z Q_A$	$Q_Z Q_B$	$Q_Z Q_M$	$Q_Z Q_M$	$Q_Z Q_M$	$Q_Z Q_M$

Subsidies

Much of the professional and policy literature on nursing homes refers to processes of subsidization. Much of this literature, however, fails to define subsidy in a technical sense. In addition, many of the definitions differ from each other; yet the differences are often inadequately understood by the users. In some cases, a subsidy presumably arises when two groups of consumers pay different prices for the same commodity, as in the nursing home serving both private pay and Medicaid beneficiaries. Arguably, there is some type of income or wealth transfer from the high price payers to the low price payers, probably because it is believed that the service would not be provided to the low price users without the resource transfers from the high price users.

In yet other approaches, subsidies are said to arise from economies of scale realizable through access to the large, low price, presumably publicly financed segment of the market. Furthermore, if the assumption of a uniform quality of care for all patients is relaxed, some analysts argue that low cost patients are subsidizing high cost patients, even though both may be paying the same price for care. The concept of subsidization also is extended to the possibility that the existence of a large publicly financed sector allows proprietors to offer private pay patients a wider and richer set of amenities than would otherwise be possible, thus enhancing their attractiveness to private pay clients.[22]

Of course, all of these subsidy definitions relate to what, using Grimaldi's term, can be called internal subsidies, that is, the transfer of resources or entitlements from one group of users to another. They do not refer to the basic external subsidization process, namely, public payments of charges or private charitable provision, nor do they refer to altruistic transfers from the operators of facilities to their patients/clients, for example, the forgoing of certain amounts of profit or the acceptance of low wages by volunteers.

Consider first the arguments about alleged internal subsidization of one group of patients by another arising from a two-price discriminatory pricing policy on the part of the facility. Most arguments focus on private pay and Medicaid patients, the latter presumably being subsidized by the former. Figure XVI–9 illustrates this type of subsidy situation. Take the case of a proprietary home for which the $MC = MR$ equilibrium level of output is Q_E and which has cost curves MC_2, AVC_2 (not shown), and ATC_2, VC and TC referring to variable and total costs, respectively. The Medicaid rate is R_1, which at Q_E

---

[22] These and other approaches to the concept of subsidy can be found in Scanlon (1978), Bishop (1979), Fraundorf (1977), and Grimaldi (1978).

FIGURE XVI-9
Proprietary Facility Experiencing Losses on Medicaid Provision
and Profits on Private Pay

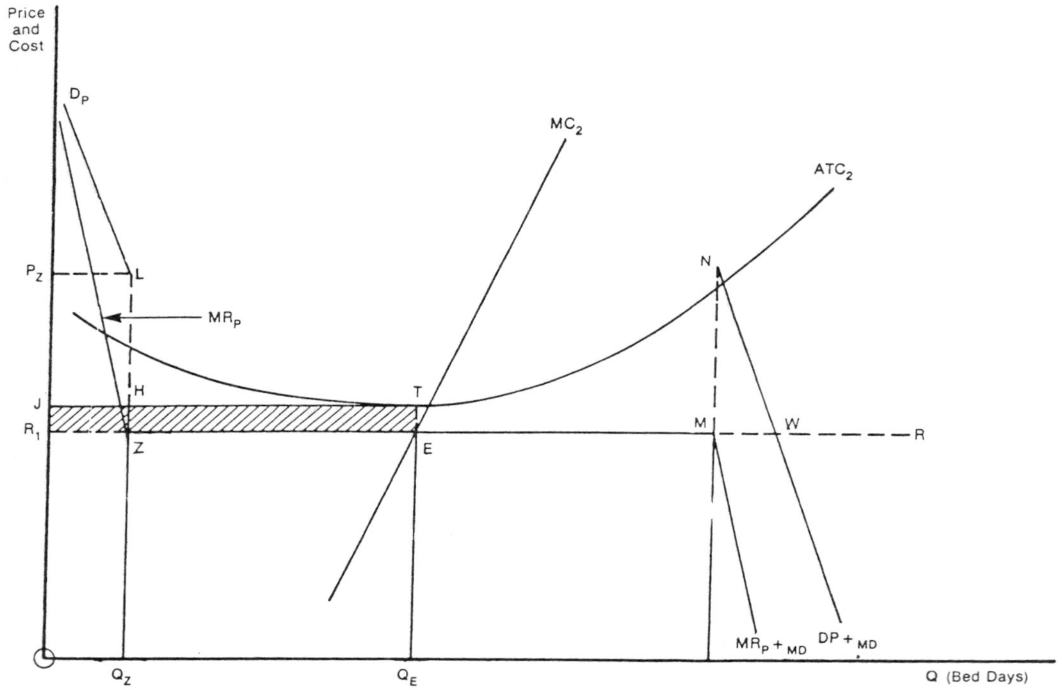

falls below the level of average total cost. On the Medicaid patients, the home "loses" an amount TE per patient, totaling to $HTEZ$ on all Medicaid patients served. For the private pay patients, however, the price P_Z exceeds average cost by the amount LH, yielding a "profit" equal to P_ZLHJ. According to the usual analysis, this profit offsets the Medicaid losses, thus, in effect, permitting the home to continue in the Medicaid program. Without the private profit, the Medicaid patients supposedly would not be served at all, at least not by this facility. Recall that both types of patients receive care of equal quality.

Some analysts have argued that, in the short run at least, the existence of a surplus on private pay and the subsidization of Medicaid patients is unneeded as long as the Medicaid rate covers average variable costs at the equilibrium level of output. All variable costs would thus be covered, and some part of fixed costs would be offset. In the long run (which may be the life span of the physical plant), however, failure to cover total costs might compromize the firm's viability, unless fixed costs as well could be recouped. While this argument is analytically valid for a conventional firm, the nature of the nursing home clientele requiring care for long periods of time may, on the one hand, force the firm to think in total rather than variable cost terms. Of course, it may take long enough for providers to "run facilities into the ground" that patients could still be provided with a relatively stable environment for a long time. This argument assumes, of course, that providers are concerned about stability for patients, possibly for competitive reasons. In fact, Medicaid patients may have to take what they can get. In any event, the relatively large share of variable costs in total costs may make variable costs a more important consideration for long periods of time for most nursing home operators. Their sensitivity to the home's fixed costs may be somewhat further diluted because of the opportunity for gains from real estate and other transactions ancillary to the operation of the home itself. McCaffrey *et al* (1975) and Baldwin (1980), among others, have pointed to the opportunities for gain afforded by tax shelters, capital gains, real estate transactions, construction company operations, and other ancillary operations. In some cases, they argue, these ancillary activities account for more gain and profit than does the operation of the home.[23]

Fraundorf takes another line of argument, claiming that there is no subsidy as long as the reimbursement rate covers marginal costs. Unless he is referring to the linkage between marginal costs

---

[23] McCaffrey *et al* (1975) extensively discussed the phenomenon of "trafficking" in homes, made possible by the various public pay reimbursement practices. See also Baldwin (1980), Vladeck (1980), and Fraundorf (1977) for discussions of these ancillary gains.

and average variable costs in the short run, it is hard to understand his position, since output equilibrium for the firm is determined by the $MC = MR$ intersection and thus the equivalence of marginal costs and the reimbursement rate. It would only be possible for R not to equal MC if the firm were constrained (or constrained itself) to produce at an output level other than that of profit-maximizing (or loss-minimizing) equilibrium.

Obviously, if the reimbursement rate just covers average total costs at the equilibrium level of output, the question of two-price subsidization becomes moot, although as shown below, the role of the Medicaid market in sustaining operations of a given scale may be crucial. The Medicaid rate, however, may be set for a class of homes to which a particular firm belongs, yet because of internal efficiencies or highly localized, low-price factor markets, that particular home may reap profits on Medicaid as well as on private pay. With a non-profit market, these profits may well persist. In this circumstance, the firm enjoys the profit-maximizing position of, perhaps, a regional monopolist, the converse of its loss-minimizing position where R does not cover costs.

The policy aspects may be non-symmetrical, however. If we accept the proposition that the private payers are essential in providing care to the Medicaid patients in the loss situation, what is their function from the standpoint of public policy in the case of positive profit in both markets? One could conceivably argue that such homes should accept only Medicaid patients if they are to take any at all. Such an extreme position may be tempting for a policymaker concerned about asserted bed shortages for Medicaid patients. If he or she believes that proprietors are making money on Medicaid anyway, why let them have the added profit of the private pay as well? Although this view may be tempting for the short run (or the relevant policy horizon), in the long run it would be harmful to the interests of indigent patients. If proprietors are not allowed to make money on their private pay patients, they may well not partici-pate in the industry, or at least in the public pay portions of it; thus the supply of beds might be further reduced. This danger would be even greater if the proprietors were especially fearful of government intervention of the type considered here.

This discussion of the private pay subsidy to public pay patients necessarily applies to the reverse case. (See Figure XVI–10.) Should the equilibrium level of output, given the fixed reimbursement rate, R, yield a private pay price below average cost, the Medicaid patients would, in effect, be "subsidizing" the private payers. Should the high Medicaid rate be sustained because of political pressure, for example, the implications of this situation for public policy would be interesting, indeed. If private payers tend to come from higher

FIGURE XVI-10
Differing Scales of Operation,
With and Without Medicaid Market, Proprietary Facility

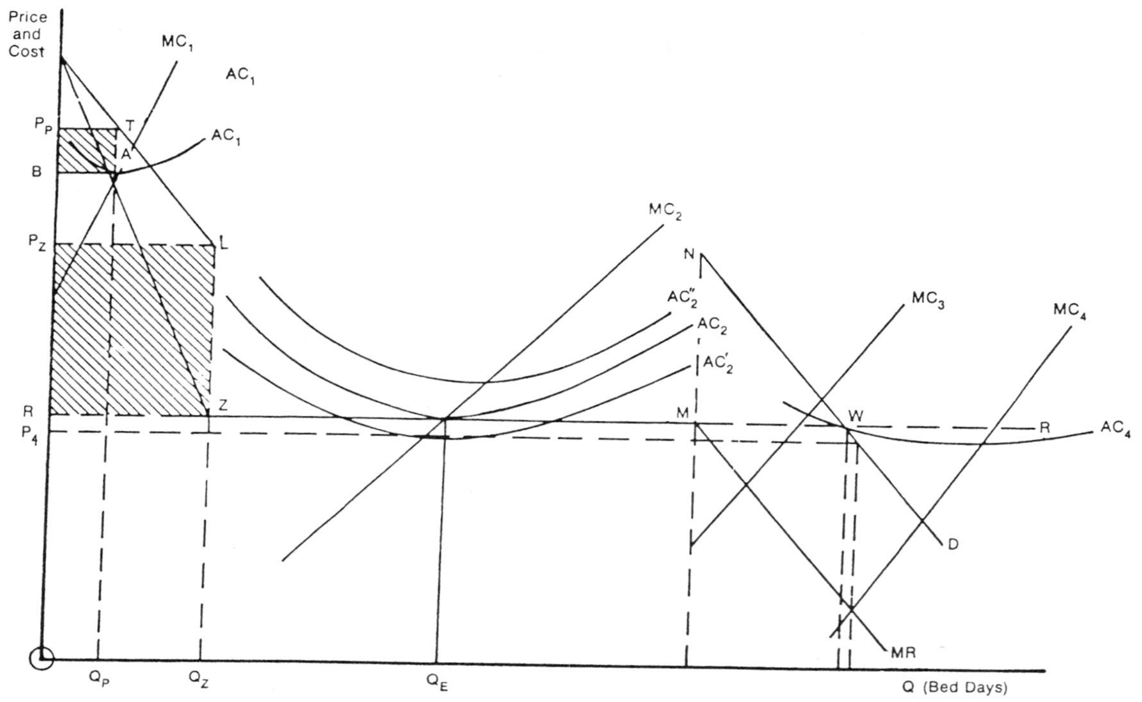

income strata than do Medicaid patients, or if they are more affluent than the average taxpayer, then such an outcome might be seen as regressive in its effects. Of course, if the private pay group is poorer than Medicaid clients and/or the taxpaying public, the reverse may be true. This latter case may be particularly relevant for the facility which caters to an identified poor part of the population.

Another form of subsidy often alleged to exist is that provided by a large Medicaid market. This argument holds that if private payers constituted the only market for nursing home services, the scale of operation would be so small that only high cost-high price services could be supplied. In Figure XVI–10, an exclusively private pay market is characterized by marginal and average cost curves MC_1 and AC_1. If the Medicaid market did not exist, the scale of operations would be small, and the price correspondingly very high (P_p). When the government undertakes a system of financial support, the Medicaid market appears, offering an additional range of potential sales and outputs. Assuming that the introduction of Medicaid involves a large enough increase in demand, the firm now enjoys a scale of operations corresponding to the cost curves MC_2 and AC_2. (Abt [1979] and others doubt this.) Had the firm been constrained to sell only in the private market, not only would few people have been served at a very high price, but the possibility of losses even at a small output might have raised doubts about much provision at all.[24] With Medicaid, however, production can occur at a larger scale, the total volume of care can increase, and both the indigent and the more affluent, private payers can be supplied, the latter at a lower price than before $(P_z$ versus $P_p)$. Not surprisingly, in a large market the firm's total profits may increase (especially if the new cost curves are such as AC_2). Even if there are losses on Medicaid patients, the enlarged profit potential from the much larger numbers of private patients may enable the firm to cover Medicaid losses and still make a profit.[25]

---

[24] Under normal market theory assumptions, there would be nothing inherently wrong about high prices or even a non-existent provision, unless we assume that the provision of nursing home services is *ipso facto* a "good thing" and/or unless there exists widespread community distress because of the absence of a commodity (bed days of care). Federal policy appears to subscribe to both of these beliefs.

[25] Of course, this situation is similar to many others in which an expanded market makes larger outputs and lower costs/prices possible. As in similar cases in which government purchases have created the new, larger market, the private market might not, of its own accord, have permitted such expansion. Two factors must, however, be considered: the private market *may* have, on its own, undertaken the search for larger scale, lower cost production, and government action is not socially costless in alternate uses of revenues and in the resources going into the nursing services.

Even if all the results of this shift in scale are positive and even if it appears that firms and users are "better off" in some sense, one cannot really speak of a subsidy from the public pay patients to the private pay, except in the sense that meeting the needs of the former provides the occasion for advantaging the latter. Actually, what has occurred here is the creation of a new market situation as a result of a political decision, that is, to provide bed days of care to public beneficiaries. We thus have a circumstance in which the taxpayers, in pursuit of a public purpose, have provided benefits to a nominally non-targeted group whose welfare may or may not be a matter of public concern. Also, these larger amounts of provision are not costless, even if more efficiently produced than at a smaller scale.

Two other so-called subsidy issues should be considered. First, the large Medicaid market with its associated profit potential allows some homes to "sweeten" their private pay care offerings to attract a larger number of private pay patients, that is, to shift their private pay demand curve to the right.[26] If the home is successful in this endeavor, and if the equilibrium level of output is still the same (there are no shifts in the marginal or average cost curves as a result of the changed demand situation), the Medicaid patients who made possible a larger, more profitable scale of operations may be displaced to some extent by the private pay patients. (The Medicaid share shrinks by the distance $Q_\chi Q'_\chi$.) Figure XVI–11 shows how this might happen. Should this be true, the seeming objective of public policy, to expand access to care via Medicaid, would be self-defeating. As with the economies of scale, this situation is not one so much of subsidy as of possibilities created by the existence of a market-expanding governmental program. It may be even more at cross-purposes with public policy, however, in that the indigent population ironically may be less able to find care, as the Medicaid program expands.

Subsidies Among Patients in the Non-Profit Facilities

Definitionally, non-profit facilities are offering some amount of subsidized consumption to all or part of their clienteles. As with government financing of care, this type of supported provision can be denoted an external subsidy. One may, however, reasonably ask if there are not internal subsidies or at least inter-group transfers in the non-profit case as well.

Figure XVI–12 shows various alternative equilibria for a non-profit facility. Consider an output maximizing facility operating with a break-even rule. Under those circumstances, equilibrium output would be Q_3, of which OQ_χ would be provided to private pay patients

---

[26] See Bishop (1979) on this point.

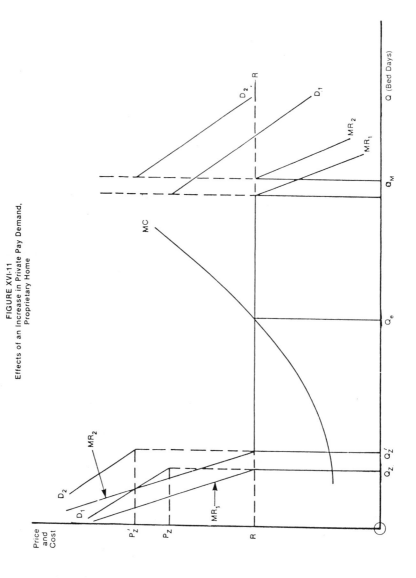

FIGURE XVI-11
Effects of an Increase in Private Pay Demand,
Proprietary Home

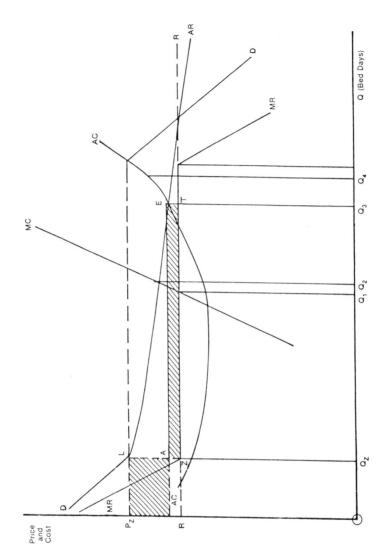

FIGURE XVI-12
Inter-Group "Subsidies,"
Non-Profit Facilities

567

at a price of P_Z. Medicaid would absorb $Q_1 Q_3$ more than would be available were the facility operating on a for-profit basis. Per unit Medicaid losses (price less than average cost) of ET would have to be offset by per unit private pay profits of LA. Indeed, if $AR = AC$ (and $TR = TC$), profits on private pay would have to offset losses on Medicaid.

As with the proprietaries, the non-profit homes can only offer care to the Medicaid patients if they can transfer revenues to cover the costs of Medicaid provision. In the non-profit situation, however, a given amount of private pay surpluses have to be spread over a greater number of Medicaid patients than in the proprietary case.

If the facility follows Rule 2 (marginal cost pricing), the equilibrium output could be either Q_1 or Q_2, depending on the interpretation of "price." If it is construed as the Medicaid rate, R, the home will offer Q_1; if the home strives for some sort of average between public and private marginal valuations (as reflected in the Medicaid rate and private pay price, respectively), equilibrium will be at Q_2. With the average cost curve AC, either level of output will yield a profit on both types of pay, a questionable outcome for a putatively non-profit entity. It is, of course, conceivable that the average cost curve shows costs greater than the Medicaid rate, thus yielding losses presumably offset by gains on private pay.

An "altruistic" output level such as Q_4 almost definitionally involves losses, possibly on the private pay as well as the Medicaid pay. These could only be overcome by the surplus (if any) on the private pay or, if such surplus is unavailable, from an outside source.

Overall one might expect that non-profit facilities would be subject to the same advantages from expanded markets as would proprietaries. It is likely, however, that a non-profit facility seeking to maximize output would take even more advantage of the opportunities offered by the increase in the size of the market due to the government payment system. Also recall that the non-profits may well require a smaller expansion of the market to induce participation in the Medicaid segment than would a proprietary facility faced with the same cost curves. For example, consider AC_1 in Figure XVI-13. Facing such a curve and with a marginal cost curve such as MC_1, a proprietary facility would not enter the Medicaid market. An output maximizing facility, however, would enter the market because of the difference in its decision rule, that is, it maximizes output rather than profit. As a result, the non-profit would produce OQ_T (versus OQ_1 for the proprietary), of which $Q_Z Q_T$ would go to the Medicaid market. Under the same cost structure the proprietary would have offered nothing to the Medicaid market.

FIGURE XVI-13
Alternative Scales of Operation,
Private Pay and Medicaid Markets, Non-Profit Facility

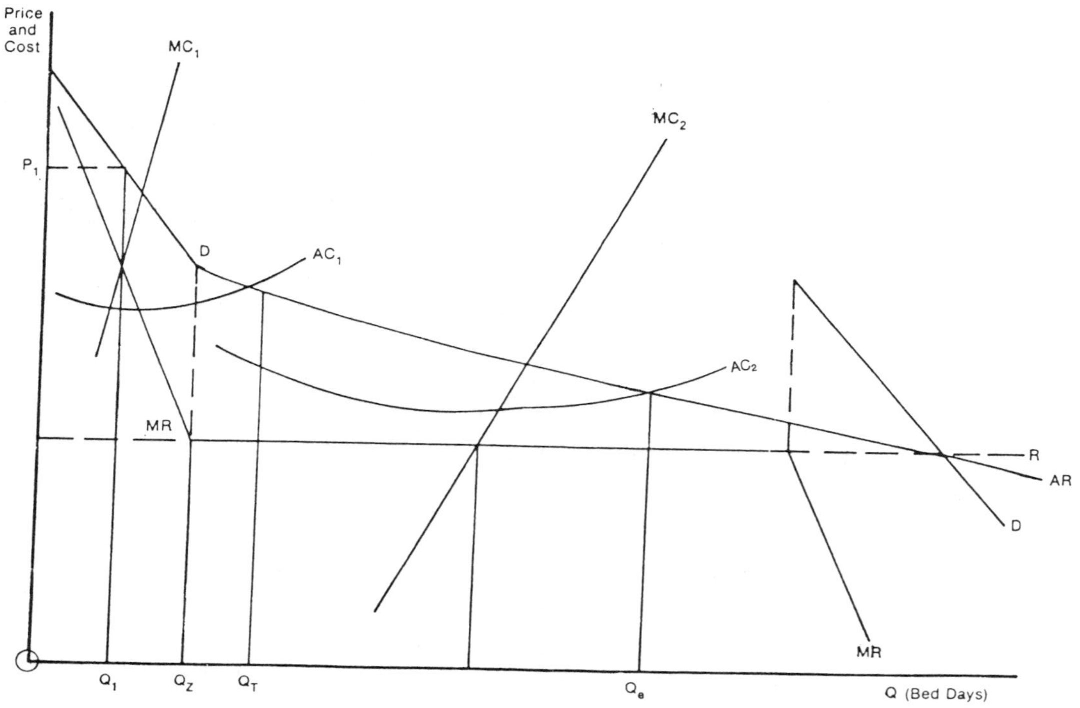

569

Access for the Medicaid Patient

Up to this point we have shown that a provider, proprietary or non-profit, would under certain circumstances offer services to Medicaid as well as private pay patients and that different groups of payers may internally transfer revenue. Grimaldi (1978) raises the important dynamic question of whether a provider, especially a profit maximizer, would have admitted a Medicaid patient in the first place, setting the question in the context of a provider whose private pay clientele did not "exhaust all patient days." In a static sense, of course, the equilibrium level of output will determine the availability of bed days to Medicaid patients. The facility, in seeking to maximize either profit or output, will allocate that output jointly among various categories of patients in accordance with the equal marginal revenue rule analyzed earlier. Search costs associated with private patients (with which Grimaldi is specifically concerned) could be subtracted from average and marginal revenues for private pay, thus reducing their share of total output.

Grimaldi's analysis does, however, raise an important question, namely, would a provider offer care to Medicaid patients if, by waiting, the facility could fill beds with more private pay patients? Presumably the temptation to wait would arise because private pay patients generate higher net profits than Medicaid patients or because the Medicaid rate is set below average cost (total or variable) at the equilibrium output level. Essentially, Grimaldi is asking the question: Can a provider shift the private pay demand curve to the right and under what circumstances would the facility be willing to do so, restricting Medicaid provision in the process? The answer suggested by Grimaldi, quite appropriately, is framed in terms of the losses and gains from the two alternatives. Basically, he argues that a provider would be indifferent between a Medicaid and private admission if the net income generated over time by the two types of patients were the same. Normally, this net income would be the arithmetic difference between average revenue and average cost for the two types of patients; however, the potential search-time cost for additional private patients would reduce their production of net income. On the other hand, the provider may also perceive that Medicaid patients, in addition to paying a lower rate (or having the rate paid on their behalf), may reside at the home longer than do private pay patients. In the Grimaldi formulation, then, all of these aspects of revenues, costs, search time (and costs), and residency period combine into a decision rule. Of course, as Bishop and Willemain suggest in an ongoing project, the optimal strategy for a private operator should be framed in terms of optimal number of beds allocated to private patients, given rates at which they arrive, their lengths of stay, etc. All of these, in turn, depend on the nature of the private demand curve and the level of the public rate, R. These factors cannot be precisely determined, however. Rather, they must be considered in stochastic terms because of unpredictable patient arrival and turnover.

To illustrate, let us denote the Medicaid rate as AR_M, the private pay rate as AR_P, the lengths of stay as X_M and X_P, respectively, the average costs as AS_M and AC_P, respectively, and the lost "search-time revenue" as ALR_P. The provider would then be at equilibrium, that is, be indifferent between admitting a Medicaid patient and leaving a bed vacant until a private pay patient can be found, if the net income from the private pay $[(AR_P - AC_P - ALR_P) \cdot X_P]$ equals the net income from a Medicaid patient $[(AR_M - AC_M) \cdot X_M]$. If the net income from private pay patients is greater than for Medicaid patients, the latter will not be admitted. The reverse, of course, is also true.

Substandard Care

Much of the critical literature on nursing homes asserts that size-able amounts of the care provided is substandard, in that it falls below some agreed upon threshold level of quality. This level is usually defined by a set of standards emanating from one or another professional group, or it is set with reference to vaguely specified canons of "humane treatment." Assertions about sub-standard care are generally made regarding Medicaid and other forms of public provision (though not about Medicare, for reasons to be discussed later). For example, Fraundorf (1977) claims that one result of the States' penuriousness in providing financing for Medicaid has been steady erosion in the quality of care provided to public pay patients. Vladek (1980) seems inclined to much the same position. Actually, some of the evidence indicates that funding shortfalls have been reflected more in reduced access to care than in reduced quality (Scanlon, 1978 and 1980), at least with respect to the quantity that would be demanded at a low price to the user. Clearly, the substandard question has a quantitative as well as a qualitative aspect: access versus adequacy. Actually, the data are somewhat unclear. While numbers of hours of service provided may have increased, we know little about the quality of those hours or about the quality of other services.

While conceding that the quality of care may fall below some ideal level proposed by health professionals, Grimaldi and others have shown that the amount and quality of care provided through govern-ment funding may well accord with the preferences of voters and, implicitly, of the public at large (Grimaldi, 1978). Starting from the familiar proposition that voters, like everyone else, balance costs and benefits, Grimaldi develops a model which includes the long-term

571

care provided to public pay patients, together with income, in the taxpayer's set of preferences (utility function). His formulation depends on two crucial assumptions: one, public pay patients and taxpayers are mutually exclusive groups; and, two, majority vote decides the extent of taxes levied to support long-term care. Subject to these assumptions, Grimaldi argues that the median (the ith) taxpayer receives utility or satisfaction (denoted by U_i) from his/her own after-tax income (denoted by Y_i) and from the long-term care (denoted by C_j) provided to the jth patient who is not the taxpayer. Utility to the taxpayer is thus a function of the utility derived from take-home income and from the care provided to others through the taxes which he/she pays. Thus, $U_i = F(Y_i, C_j)$. Clearly, taxpayer utility depends upon taxpayer preferences which, in the case of perceptions about long-term care, relate to a matrix of supports to treat, rehabilitate, and maintain long-term care patients. These supports have qualitative as well as quantitative dimensions.

Taxpayer willingness to support long-term care through additional taxes depends on the marginal balance between benefits and costs (that is, additions to total benefits and total costs). To the taxpayer, the benefits are those derived from responses to increased quantity and quality of care. The costs are those associated with reduced satisfaction through the loss of income. Marginal benefit can be expressed as

$$MB_i = \sum_{j=1}^{P} \frac{\partial U_i}{\partial C_j}$$

Usually one assumes that the value of marginal benefits decreases with qualitative or quantitative increases in the item from which the benefit is derived; that is, a graph of the marginal benefit curve would show it as downward sloping. Therefore, at some point the additional benefit (marginal benefit) associated with increases in the quality (or quantity) of care would become zero. Up to that point, however, increases in the number of patients (or number of bed days of care provided) would increase total utility to the taxpayer arising from his/her seeing taxes go to support such services. Likewise, utility would increase from improvements in the quality of service being provided.

The taxpayer will, however, not be able to gratify wishes to get utility from C_j in a costless manner. Taxes must be paid to provide support, and the payment of taxes involves loss of utility, since the taxed money cannot be used to satisfy private wants. If we can assume that all public pay patients receive identical care bundles, and that taxpayers share equally in paying taxes to cover care, then the marginal cost to the taxpayer will be

$$MC_i = \frac{\partial U_i}{\partial Y_i} \times \frac{P}{N}$$

where $\partial U_i/\partial Y_i$ represents the loss of utility from the loss of taxed income P = number of public pay patients, and N = number of taxpayers. Note that MC_i will increase with C_j if the marginal utility of income after taxes rises with every tax increase to support more C_j. Also, the marginal cost will increase with every rise in the number of public pay patients relative to the number of taxpayers.

Equilibrium for the individual taxpayer is reached when the marginal benefit equals marginal cost. For the individual taxpayer this can be shown as

$$\sum_{j=1}^{P} \frac{\partial U_i}{\partial C_j} = \frac{\partial U_i}{\partial Y_i} \times \frac{P}{N}$$

that is, the addition to total utility from the sum of all utilities gained from serving j long-term care patients equals the loss to total utility from the loss of income because of having to pay for the individual taxpayer's share of support for P patients.

These individual (ith taxpayer's) benefits and costs can be aggregated over the tax-paying and care-receiving publics, again recalling that the two groups are assumed to be mutually exclusive. Algebraically, the marginal benefit/marginal cost equality can be expressed as

$$\sum_{i=1}^{N} \sum_{j=1}^{P} \frac{\partial U_i}{\partial C_j} = \sum_{i=1}^{N} \frac{\partial U_i}{\partial Y_i} \times \frac{P}{N}$$

From this type of formulation, Grimaldi and others argue that the expenditure for long-term care (or for any other type of service provided by the government) can be considered "Pareto optimal." Since the benefit/cost conditions have been satisfied, society as a whole (and the taxpayers in particular) can be made no better by increasing expenditure either on the quantity or quality of care, since to do so would upset the equilibrium.

While acknowledging that a Pareto optimal formulation can be derived, Fraundorf (1978), as well as other critics of this approach to public expenditure analysis, argue that Grimaldi's assumptions are unrealistic and too restrictive. The main complaint turns on the failure to include the preferences (utility) of those receiving the care. By this failure, it is argued, an important element in the decision process and in the benefits (outcomes) is forgotten. This argument can be extended and further complicated by incorporating the preference functions of the families of potential and/or actual recipients of long-term care. Quite correctly, Fraundorf also notes that the lack of information for users, users' families, and taxpayers renders a marginal calculus highly artificial. It is also doubtful

573

whether a public goods formulation of the type used by Grimaldi is appropriate under these circumstances.[27]

Notwithstanding the criticism of Fraundorf *et al,* the public goods approach as used by Grimaldi provides a useful point to begin discussion of the issue of sub-standard care. In the first place, it forces consideration of the relative nature of the standards in question: who sets them, to what outcomes and services do they relate, and so on. Secondly, it forces recognition of the reality that the quantity and types of care provided are matters of choice on the part of those who make spending decisions—the taxpayers. By itself, however, the Grimaldi approach should be expanded to loosen the restrictive assumptions about uniformity of care across all receivers and about the equality of the tax burden across all payers. These are in addition to the need to include the preferences of the clients of the care system.

An amended version of the Grimaldi approach might include provision for the preferences of the clients in the social utility function. This might be added to the preferences of the taxpayers as a separate group.[28] In addition, the analysis should consider the income levels and distributions among the clients and the taxpayers. Furthermore, it might well address the different types and quality of care received by the patients.

At bottom, however, it must be recognized that there may be a quality of care below which vulnerable, dependent people cannot fall without some danger to their lives. It may also be true that the taxpayers' preference function may be such that they are unwilling to provide the level of financial support required to keep enough public pay patients at a standard of care adequate to fend off life-threatening conditions. If that is true, and it may well have been true before the advent of Medicare and Medicaid, we are faced with a policy dilemma. That dilemma may be resolvable only by changing the preference functions of the taxpayers through political action and/or mobilizing charitable efforts on the part of the public most concerned with these issues. Indeed, there is some evidence that

---

[27] A public good is one which is indivisible and excludes no one. Conventionally, public goods are provided or produced by governments because private markets fail to do so; that is, an equilibrium based on the equivalence of private benefit and cost would not incorporate all of the benefits and costs (private plus public) associated with the provision of the public good. Also, users cannot be forced to pay a price, so there is a free rider problem. In this instance, the free riders in a totally private pay care system would be the taxpayers who derived benefit from the knowledge that good care was being provided without their having to pay.

[28] Of course, the clients and the taxpayers may be partially overlapping groups. This would necessarily complicate the analysis.

574

the increased numbers and political effectiveness of older people in the United States may have helped secure Medicare and other medical welfare legislation.

Concluding Thoughts

Total public expenditures on nursing homes may be expressed as the product of two basic variables:

$$TE = B \cdot R, B = \min{(f(e), g(r))}$$

where
TE is total public expenditures
B is the number of nursing home beds for which public payment is made
R is the rate at which the government reimburses
e is the number of persons eligible for public payment.

In this formulation, B, R, and e become public policy variables. For example, total public expenditures may be kept low by restricting the supply of beds (B) through such legislation as Certificate of Need, by varying the public payments rate (R) downward, or by tightening eligibility criteria (e). Our analysis in this chapter has concentrated upon provider private price and output response to changes in an exogenous public R.[29]

Although our various analytic models are abstract, they clarify important central tendencies on the part of providers, given the types of demand that they face: both for-profit and non-profit providers should act in certain predictable ways in their pricing and output decisions, depending upon the level of and way in which public rates are set through the Medicare and Medicaid programs.

The models assume that the objective function of for-profit firms is to maximize profits, and that of the non-profit firms is to maximize output and/or quality of care provided, subject to a break-even constraint or some amount of external subsidy. The final output and quality results, given provider objective functions, may or may not coincide with the fulfillment of the public's objective function for the provision of nursing home care. What is clear, however, is that once a public objective function has been delineated, and once provider response to economic incentives is understood, the public objective function can be achieved through the proper use of incentive mechanisms in reimbursement policy.

As we have shown here, the government has an important policy instrument in its ability to adjust the rate which it will pay for public

---

[29] For more detailed analyses of the other policy variables, see Chapters XVII and XVIII.

patients.[30] At first blush, this conclusion appears trite. But, if government were able to ascertain the cost conditions under which each provider firm (or group of firms) operates, and if government were an effective agent of public patients for the assurance of given quality levels, rate levels for provider-firms could be theoretically manipulated to attain some kind of optimal outcomes.

In practice, however, ascertaining cost functions for each provider firm or debility levels for each patient poses formidable measurement and administrative difficulties, and there is no conclusive evidence that government has been an effective or efficient agent for the nursing home patient (Fraundorf, 1977). At best, some would argue, government's role in this area is more appropriately defined as providing information[31] and subsidizing those who are too poor to pay for their own nursing home care. But this does not imply that government has to pursue its present course of paying for nursing home care directly. If sufficient information about levels of provider quality were made available to the elderly and their families, some form of voucher might more closely approximate the social objective function for the elderly in need of nursing home care than what is presently being accomplished. Such a voucher system would not be difficult to design. The key to its desirability would be the levels of information, mobility, and lucid choice which one would be willing to assume or assign to the elderly, their families, and/or their agents.

---

[30] Similar theoretical analyses could be performed on cost-related or debility-related forms of reimbursement. Another possible form of reimbursement that has not been considered, to our knowledge, would be to auction the care of groups of patients to provider-bidders in a fashion analogous to the way in which Treasury bills are presently auctioned. The major difficulty with such a proposal is that Treasury bills are homogeneous, whereas patients are not homogeneous in their degree of debility. Although many public offerings and projects are done through auction or bid, they are generally homogeneous or of some easily measured standard of quality. Groups of patients with a known set of debility characteristics could be "offered" to bidders who would be required to provide a specific level of care for the distribution of debility of the group. However, such a scheme would create a host of administrative problems and would probably be repugnant to the citizenry in general, because it appears to treat human beings as commodities and effectively rob them of individual choice of location and environment.

[31] See Becker (1976, Parts 1 and 7) for a discussion of information costs.

References

Abt Associates, Inc., *Reimbursement Strategies for Nursing Home Care: Developmental Cost Studies*, Cambridge: Abt, 1979, HCFA Contract No. 600–77–0068.

Alchian, Armen, "Some Economics of Property," P2316, Santa Monica: RAND Corporation, 1961.

Alchian, Armen and Harold Demsetz, "Production, Information Costs and Economic Organization," *American Economic Review*, Vol. 62, December 1972, pp. 777–795.

Alchian, Armen and Reuben Kessel, "Competition, Monopoly, and the Pursuit of Money," in National Bureau of Economic Research, *Aspects of Labor Economics*, Princeton University Press, 1962.

Baldwin, Carliss Y., "Nursing Home Finance: Capital Incentives Under Medicaid," Background Paper, University Health Policy Cosortium, July 1980.

Becker, Gary S., *The Economic Approach to Human Behavior* (Chicago: University of Chicago Press, 1976).

Bishop, Christine E., "Nursing Home Behavior Under Cost-Related Reimbursement," University Health Policy Consortium Paper DP–13, Brandeis University, August 1979.

Borcherding, Thomas E. and Robert T. Deacon, "The Demand for the Services of Non-Federal Governments," *American Economic Review*, Vol. LXII, December 1972, pp. 891–901.

Davis, Karen, "Economic Theories of Behavior in Non-Profit, Private Hospitals," *Economic and Business Bulletin*, Winter 1972.

Ferguson, C. E. and S. Charles Maurice, *Economic Analysis: Theory and Applications* (Homewood: Richard D. Irwin, Inc. 1978).

Fraundorf, Kenneth C., "Competition and Public Policy in the Nursing Home Industry," *Journal of Economic Issues*, Vol. XI, September 1977.

Fraundorf, Kenneth C., "The Nursing Home Industry: A Reply," *Journal of Economic Issues*, Vol. XII, December 1978.

Frech, H. E., III, "The Property Rights Theory of the Firm: Empirical Results from a Natural Experiment," *Journal of Political Economy*, Vol. 84, February 1976, pp. 143–152.

Friedman, Milton, *Essays in Positive Economics*, Chicago, University of Chicago Press, 1953.

Furubotn, E. and S. Pejovich, "Property Rights and Economic Theory: A Survey of Recent Literature," *Journal of Economic Literature*, Vol. 10, December 1972, pp. 137–162.

Grimaldi, Paul J., "A Note on the Nursing Home Industry," *Journal of Economic Issues*, Vol. XXI, December 1978, pp. 911–921.

Grimaldi, Paul, *Cost, Utilization, and Reimbursement of Nursing Home Care*, Washington: American Enterprise Institute, 1982.

Kahn, Alfred E., *The Economics of Regulation: Principles and Institutions*, New York: John Wiley and Sons, Inc. 1970.

LaPorte, Valerie and Jeffrey Rubin, editors, *Reform and Regulation in Long-Term Care*, New York: Praeger, 1979.

Lee, Robert and Jack Hadley, "Supplying Physicians' Services to Public Medical Care Programs," Working Paper 1145–17 (Washington: The Urban Institute, October 1979).

Mansfield, Edwin, *Microeconomics: Theory and Applications*, Third Edition, New York and London: W.W. Norton and Company, 1979.

McCaffree, Kenneth M., Lawrence Muller, and R. P. Johnson, "An Economic Analysis of the Production Process in Washington State Nursing Homes," Seattle: Battelle Human Affairs Research Centers, 1975, NCHSR Contract No: HS01582.

Newhouse, Joseph P., "Toward a Theory of Non-Profit Institutions: An Economic Model of a Hospital," *American Economic Review*, Vol. LX, March 1970, pp. 64–74.

Scanlon, William J., "Aspects of the Nursing Home Market: Private Demand, Total Utilization, and Investment," Working Paper 5907–1. Washington: The Urban Institute, February 1978.

Scanlon, William J., "A Theory of the Nursing Home Market," *Inquiry*, Vol. 17, Spring 1980, pp. 25–41.

Sloan, Frank A., Jerry Cromwell, and Janet B. Mitchell, *Private Physicians and Public Programs*, Lexington and Toronto: D.C. Heath and Company, 1978.

Vladeck, Bruce C., *Unloving Care: The Nursing Home Tragedy* (New York: Basic Books, 1980).

Weisbrod, Burton A., *The Voluntary Non-Profit Sector*, New York, Toronto, and London: D.C. Heath and Company, 1979.

Williamson, Oliver E., "Corporate Control and the Theory of the Firm," in H. Manne, ed., *Economic Policy and the Regulation of Corporate Securities*, Washington: American Enterprise Institute, 1969.

Williamson, Oliver E., *Corporate Control and Business Behavior: An Inquiry into the Effects of Organizational Form on Enterprise Behavior*, Englewood Cliffs: Prentice Hall, 1970.

Yett, Donald E., William Der, Richard L. Ernst, and Joel W. Hay, "Blue Shield Plan Physician Participation," Human Resources Research Center, University of Southern California, Summer 1980, mimeo.

CHAPTER XVII

The Industrial Organization of the Nursing Home Industry

by Ronald J. Vogel

Introduction

An analysis of the market structure, conduct, and performance of the nursing home industry can provide insight into nursing home behavior and suggest policies to allow and/or encourage this sector to serve the public more effectively. Economists in the field of industrial organization make use of such analysis of particular industries to ascertain the extent to which they adhere to or deviate from the competitive norm,[1] and to offer policy prescriptions to rectify any deviations which detract from efficient exchange and consumer satisfaction. Table XVII–1 presents an outline of the industrial organization paradigm. In this chapter, this paradigm will be applied to the nursing home industry.

Market Structure

Sellers of Nursing Home Services

Because the degree of seller concentration does so much to shape industry conduct, it is necessary to first determine the number of producers and to investigate possible reasons for seller concentration and monopoly power, if it exists. The number and concentration of buyers in a market also affects industry behavior and must be considered. The nursing home industry may be characterized as one with many sellers and many consumers and with government as the predominant buyer for those consumers.

Table XVII–2 provides information on nursing homes, nursing home beds, and number of patients between 1967 and 1976; the data in Table XVII–2 also show growth rates for 1967 to 1971 and 1971 to 1976. Between 1967 and 1971, the number of nursing homes grew by

---

The author gratefully acknowledges the thoughtful and extensive comments of Christine E. Bishop, A. Mead Over, Jr., and Robert L. Seidman on previous drafts of this chapter.

[1] Under certain, well-defined assumptions, perfect competition is viewed as the ideal because it offers the achievement of "Pareto Optimality," that is, a long-run trading equilibrium where no one can be made better off without making someone else worse off (Samuelson, 1947; Henderson and Quandt, 1971).

TABLE XVII-1
The Industrial Organization Paradigm Adapted
to the Nursing Home Industry

Market Structure
  The Number and Degree of Concentration of Sellers
  The Number of Consumers and Buyers
  Government as Buyer
  Product Differentiation and the Geographical Structure of the
    Market
  The Condition of Entry

Market Conduct
  The Determination of Price and Output: Dual Pricing Mechanisms
  Subsidies
  Shortages and Lack of Equilibrium
  The Effects of Certificate of Need and Other Regulations
  Research, Innovation, and Legal Tactics

Market Performance
  The Problem of Quality
  Profitability and Growth
  Productive Efficiency

Conclusion and Policy Implications

---

15 percent, but it declined by 7 percent between 1971 and 1976. During the same time periods, the number of nursing home beds grew by 43.6 percent and 17.7 percent, respectively. As a consequence of these two divergent national trends, the average bed size of the nursing home grew from 43.7 beds in 1967 to 69.1 beds in 1976, a 58 percent increase. The national nursing home bed occupancy rate remained high relative to that of hospitals, although Table XVII–3 shows that there was some variation by State. Taking into account data from the 1977 National Nursing Home Survey (National Center for Health Statistics, 1979) on the number of nursing home residents, their number grew by 53 percent between 1967 and 1977. Yet Table XVII–3 indicates a wide interstate variability in the number of nursing home and related home residents per 1,000 civilian population age 65 and over in 1976, ranging from a high of 106.8 in Nebraska to a low of 21.3 in Florida. This wide disparity is difficult to explain, using conventional explanatory variables (Scanlon, 1980). But, because the nursing home industry comprises many

580

TABLE XVII-2
The Nursing Home Industry: Homes, Beds, Patients, 1967-1976

	1967	1969	1971	1973	1976	Percentage Change 1967–1971	1971–1976
All Nursing Homes	19,141	18,910	22,004	21,834	20,468	15.0	−7.0
Nursing Care	10,636	11,484	12,871	21,345	NA		
Personal Care	8,249	7,306	8,937	NA	NA		
Domiciliary Care	256	120	196	489	NA		
All Nursing Home Beds	836,554	943,876	1,201,598	1,327,704	1,414,865	43.6	17.7
Nursing Care Beds	584,052	704,217	917,707	1,107,358	NA		
Personal Care Beds	247,883	238,406	280,664	220,346	NA		
Domiciliary Care Beds	4,619	1,253	3,227	NA	NA		
All Nursing Home Residents	NA	849,775	1,075,724	1,197,517	1,293,285		20.2
Nursing Care Residents	NA	634,747	824,038	1,011,092	NA		
Personal Care Residents	NA	213,952	248,827	186,425	NA		
Domiciliary Care Residents		1,076	2,859	NA	NA		
Occupancy Rate—All Nursing Homes		90.0	89.5	90.2	91.4	24.9	2.1
Average Bed Size—All Nursing Homes	43.7	49.9	54.6	60.8	69.1		26.6

Source: National Center for Health Statistics, *Master Facility Inventory File*, unpublished data
NA = Not Available

	Number per 1,000 Aged Persons			Occupancy Rate[1]		
	Total Residents	Nursing Homes	Personal Care and Other Homes[2]	Total Residents	Nursing Homes	Personal Care and Other Homes
United States	56.1[3]	47.3	8.8	91.5%	92.4%	86.3%
Alabama	46.6	42.3	4.3	93.8	94.0	91.5
Alaska	78.3	68.1	10.2	90.1	88.8	100.0
Arkansas	63.3	59.9	3.8	93.6	93.4	97.4
Arizona[4]	23.9	22.1	1.8	94.8	95.3	90.0
California	59.1	46.0	13.1	90.1	91.1	87.3
Colorado[4]	87.4	81.2	6.2	83.9	86.3	61.4
Connecticut	71.2	58.1	13.0	96.4	96.8	93.5
Delaware	40.1	34.0	6.1	91.8	91.4	93.9
District of Columbia	34.6	26.9	7.7	86.7	85.7	90.6
Florida	21.3	18.8	2.5	89.5	89.5	92.6
Georgia	63.9	62.9	1.0	95.5	95.5	100.0
Hawaii	48.4	38.3	10.1	91.5	91.0	93.5
Idaho[4]	56.6	46.4	10.1	95.1	94.5	97.1
Illinois	68.5	57.8	10.7	91.3	91.8	89.2
Indiana	59.6	52.7	6.9	86.6	90.6	83.1
Iowa	83.6	67.6	16.1	93.4	94.2	91.0

TABLE XVII-3 (Continued)

	Number per 1,000 Aged Persons			Occupancy Rate[1]		
	Total Residents	Nursing Homes	Personal Care and Other Homes[2]	Total Residents	Nursing Homes	Personal Care and Other Homes
Kansas	73.6	65.3	8.3	94.5	95.5	87.4
Kentucky	50.0	33.4	16.6	90.7	90.8	90.7
Louisiana	51.2	48.7	2.5	95.3	95.3	96.2
Maine	64.4	48.9	15.5	95.4	96.8	91.2
Maryland	51.1	45.1	6.0	94.8	95.4	89.6
Massachusetts[4]	70.7	54.3	16.4	94.7	95.3	92.7
Michigan[4]	70.2	57.4	12.8	88.2	94.3	68.5
Minnesota[4]	92.4	78.3	14.1	95.6	95.6	95.3
Mississippi	32.5	31.0	1.5	94.2	94.5	83.3
Missouri[4]	50.3	43.0	7.3	91.0	92.1	83.9
Montana	65.7	58.0	7.7	95.5	95.1	98.7
Nebraska[4]	106.8	99.8	7.0	90.9	91.7	80.5
Nevada	28.9	25.0	4.0	86.3	85.9	90.9
New Hampshire	64.0	58.0	5.9	93.2	93.1	90.8
New Jersey	41.5	35.0	6.6	94.8	95.4	93.0
New Mexico	28.8	23.4	5.4	88.9	90.4	84.4
New York	46.2	34.8	11.3	93.2	94.1	89.7
North Carolina[4]	43.9	23.3	20.6	92.2	90.7	94.1
North Dakota	86.7	67.4	19.4	96.3	96.2	97.5

	Number per 1,000 Aged Persons			Occupancy Rate[1]		
	Total Residents	Nursing Homes	Personal Care and Other Homes[2]	Total Residents	Nursing Homes	Personal Care and Other Homes
Ohio	55.1	50.1	5.0	93.6	94.5	86.2
Oklahoma	70.2	67.0	3.2	91.2	91.2	91.4
Oregon	55.1	44.4	10.7	92.1	92.1	92.2
Pennsylvania[4]	41.6	37.6	4.0	91.2	91.0	90.9
Rhode Island	56.9	45.4	11.4	90.0	89.2	92.7
South Carolina	32.9	31.0	1.9	91.4	91.5	90.5
South Dakota	87.4	70.6	16.7	95.8	97.4	89.8
Tennessee[4]	42.5	39.1	3.5	95.9	96.3	94.6
Texas[4]	70.1	63.2	6.8	82.5	84.8	64.8
Utah	45.9	39.9	5.9	94.4	93.9	96.7
Vermont[4]	85.7	52.3	33.3	88.5	93.6	81.4
Virginia[4]	59.8	42.4	17.5	92.6	94.4	88.8

	Number per 1,000 Aged Persons			Occupancy Rate[1]		
	Total Residents	Nursing Homes	Personal Care and Other Homes[2]	Total Residents	Nursing Homes	Personal Care and Other Homes
Washington	74.1	65.7	8.4	92.2	92.9	86.6
West Virginia	23.5	19.0	4.6	90.0	92.7	83.6
Wisconsin[4]	91.7	83.2	8.5	91.2	92.1	82.5
Wyoming	48.7	42.6	6.1	92.4	93.6	84.7

[1] Calculated by dividing the number of residents per 1,000 aged persons by the number of beds per 1,000 aged persons.

[2] Includes personal care homes with nursing, personal care homes without nursing, and domiciliary care homes.

[3] Preliminary data.

[4] State reporting 1976 data in the Cooperative Health Statistics System; data may not always agree wih individual State reports, usually because of variations in imputation procedures or in time period over which the data were collected.

Source: Grimaldi, Paul L., Medicaid Reimbursement of Nursing Home Care, (Washington: American Enterprise Institute, 1981 forthcoming), and calculated from, U.S. Department of Health, Education, and Welfare, Office of Health Research, Statistics, and Technology, Health Resources Statistics, 1976–77 Edition, 1979, Tables 232 and 236.*

*Reprinted with permission of American Enterprise Institute.

relatively small providers,[2] one could reasonably infer that a potential for competition among sellers exists.[3]

Consumers and Buyers of Nursing Home Services

However, even though there are many individuals using nursing home services, there are certain characteristics of these users that may reduce their ability to elicit a competitive market response from providers. The picture that emerges from this combination of characteristics is that of a population that is, by and large, physically, mentally, and financially debilitated and dependent, a population whose stock of human capital is in a highly depreciated state (Grossman, 1972). These are hardly the characteristics of the well-informed, rational, and mobile consumer that economic theory would have making choices about how to spend his or her income and wealth constraints. On the other hand, one or two of the characteristics in this segment of the aged population do indicate that some do have ties to the community and can look for some form of help, advice, or financial aid from children, other relatives, or friends.

For an ideal competitive outcome, consumers must, at least at the margin, be able to make informed choices among suppliers. In the nursing home market, there appears to be only limited consumer information about service quality and alternatives. In the words of the U.S. Senate Subcommittee on Long-Term Care (1976):

Reliable guidance is scarce, thus forcing many to make a "blind" selection. To the prospective customer, the choice of a nursing home can be truly agonizing. Looks can be deceiving. . . . There

---

[2] Even though conglomerates continue to grow in the industry, as has the average bed size of the typical nursing home, the nursing home industry is by no means dominated by large conglomerates (Di Paolo, 1979), nor is the behavior of the few conglomerates in the business dissimilar to that of the smaller firms.

[3] But the great number of public utilities in the country does not prevent each from having considerable market power. The problem is that the different utilities are not very effective substitutes for one another. The high psychic costs imposed on consumers of nursing home care far from home may mean that nursing homes often have a quite perfect local monopoly, that is, the industry demand is the firm's demand. Thus, it would seem that the important question is the size of a typical home's "catchment area." More research must be done on this issue, but very little data presently exist for such research.

Another important consideration is the existence of care in the home as a substitute for nursing home care. The effective price ratio between the two should affect decisions on nursing home placement at the margin. It may be that the availability of such care in persons' homes is much more effective competition for many nursing homes than is the care of other nursing homes. The effectiveness of the competition would, of course, be enhanced if government reimbursement were available for caring for an individual in his/her home.

is virtually no way to tell what type of care is provided. Accordingly, patients and family must rely upon the judgments of physicians, social workers, and ministers who themselves are guided almost entirely by limited experiences and rumor (*Supporting Paper No. 1*).

Nursing homes very rarely advertise, except in the Yellow Pages, and, as Fraundorf (1977) observes, ". . . the absence of advertising competition (where products are heterogeneous) is consistent with the existence of market power" on the part of providers *vis-a-vis* consumers.

Moreover, consumers are not always in a position to use information to alter consumption choices. Table XVII–4 shows the age distribution of aged nursing home residents in 1977 compared to the aged in the general population. While only about 5 percent of the aged population was in nursing homes in 1977, almost 22 percent of those 85 years and over were living there.

These patients had the following characteristics:

- They were old or very old: their median age was 81; 87 percent were over 65, and 35 percent were over 85 years old (NCHS, 1979).
- Many were mentally deficient: 20 percent had "mental disorders and senility without psychosis" as a primary diagnosis at their last examination, but 32 percent were described as having senility as a chronic condition or impairment (NCHS, 1979).
- In general, nursing home patients had about four chronic or crippling disabilities (New York State Department of Health, 1971). Less than half of the patients could walk unassisted (34 percent); about 86 percent required assistance in bathing;

TABLE XVII-4
Comparison of U.S. Nursing Home Resident Population and General Population by Age, 1977

Age	Number in General Population	Nursing Home Residents	
		Number	% of General Population
65 Years and Over	23,494,000	1,126,000	4.8
75 Years and Over	8,910,000	914,600	10.3
85 Years and Over	2,079,000	449,900	21.6

Source: U.S. Department of Health, Education, and Welfare, National Center for Health Statistics, *The National Nursing Home Survey: 1977 Summary for the United States*, (Washington: U.S. Government Printing Office, 1979), p. 28

70 percent needed help in dressing, and 33 percent in eating; 45 percent were incontinent, and 23 percent were dependent in all six activities of daily living (bathing, dressing, using toilet room, mobility, continence, eating; NCHS, 1979).

- They consumed large quantities of drugs: the average nursing home patient took 4.4 different drugs per day, and some were ·taken two or three times; 70 percent took five or more drugs per day. (U.S. Senate, Subcommittee on Long-Term Care, 1976).
- Only a minority were married: 12 percent were married; 62 percent were widowed; 19 percent never married, and about 7 percent were divorced (NCHS, 1979).
- Some patients were alone, but many were not: 13 percent of nursing home patients did not have visitors, while 62 percent had visitors daily or weekly; about half of all visitors were children or other relatives (NCHS, 1979). Moreover, there is little evidence that families "dump" their aged into nursing homes (Brody, 1969; Pincus 1967, Kent 1965; see Chapter VIII). A member of the family, however, usually places the resident. Children placed other relatives 20 percent of the time, 12 percent were placed by a spouse or institutionalized themselves, and about 25 percent were placed by social workers or staff of previous institutions (NCHS, 1979).
- Many patients were Medicaid patients (Liu and Mossey, 1980) subject to the direction of overworked social worker "agents" whose time for any case may be severely limited.

The decision to enter a nursing home may be traumatic, made at a time of poor health. The search for a suitable home is probably often limited by being in a hospital and having an immediate need for a discharge plan.

- More than half of nursing home residents in 1977 were housed in another health facility prior to admission to a nursing home: 32 percent came from a general or short-stay hospital, 6 percent from State mental hospitals, 13 percent from other nursing homes, homes for the aged, boarding homes, or other housing; about 40 percent came to the nursing home from their own or relatives' homes (NCHS, 1979).

While individuals contemplating nursing home admission might appear to have many choices, in reality many providers may be effectively ruled out by strong consumer preferences for remaining close to the community of residence and by personal financial constraints.

- In 1972, most nursing home patients were placed in facilities close to their homes: five out of six nursing home patients were housed in facilities less than 25 miles from their community home (Day, 1972).

- Individual financial resources to pay for nursing home care were limited: the average monthly charge for a nursing home in 1977 was $689, and the average nursing home resident age 65 and over had a mean monthly income of $306 in 1976. However, 43 percent of outlays for nursing home care came from private sources in 1977 (NCHS, 1979; Department of Commerce, 1978; Liu and Mossey, 1980).

For many, entering a nursing home involves a decision about living situations. These patients give up community residences and thus reduce their options.

- The majority of them could expect to be in nursing homes for almost two years: the median number of days spent in a nursing home for those residing there in 1977 was 597 days. Of the 1,117,500 discharges in 1977, 73.9 percent were alive and 25.9 percent were dead, and the median duration of stay for those discharged was 75 days (NCHS, 1979).[4]

The salient aspect of this combination of statistics is that individual consumers in this market seem *qualitatively* different from consumers in many other economic markets, not only because of their physical and mental debility but also because of the seeming irreversibility of the decision to enter a nursing home for many elderly patients. Most of the services of a nursing home are not unlike those of a hotel. But for the traveler, who is healthy and mobile almost by definition, the choice of hotels is a continuous one, based on price and service. Even though many purchases in the health care sector are not done on a regular "shopping" basis, most of them lack the finality of choosing a nursing home because the average consumer of health services is more mobile and, therefore, probably better informed than the average aged consumer of nursing home services. Thus, even to the extent that children or relatives act as effective agents for the elderly, decisions to move can only be made after careful consideration.

Government as Buyer of Nursing Home Services

The two features of the structure of the nursing home industry which make it unique are the limited capacities of its consumers and the dominance of government as both payer for nursing home services and regulator of the activities of the industry. Tables XVII–5 and XVII–6 present a time series of nursing home expenditures. By the

---

[4] Grimaldi and Sullivan (1981) believe that the "length of stay difference strongly suggests that nursing homes contain at least two distinct populations: one with chronic conditions and little chance of discharge and the other in need of services for a comparatively short period of time."

TABLE XVII-5

Calendar Year Estimates of Nursing Home Care Expenditures by Source of Payment, 1948–64

(Millions of Dollars)

Year	1948[1]	1949	1950	1951	1952	1953	1954	1955	1956	1957	1958	1959	1960	1961	1962	1963	1964
Total	150	168	187	207	228	248	270	312	358	368	303	434	526	606	695	891	1,214
Private	150	162	170	182	197	211	227	260	297	330	314	343	419	432	420	554	834
Consumer[2]	148	160	168	180	195	208	224	257	293	295	308	336	441	422	409	540	814
Other	2	2	2	2	2	3	3	3	4	5	6	7	8	10	11	14	20
Public[3]	—	6	17	25	31	37	43	52	61	68	69	91	108	174	275	337	380

[1] Data prior to 1948 are not available.
[2] Includes direct payments and insurance benefits.
[3] Public assistance money; Federal and State/local funds are not separable in this source prior to 1965.

Source: *Compendium of National Health Expenditures Data*, HEW (ORS/SSA); January 1976.

TABLE XVII-6
Calendar Year Estimates of Nursing Home Care Expenditures by Source of Payment, 1965–79
(Millions of Dollars)

	1965	1966	1967	1968	1969	1970	1971	1972	1973	1974	1975	1976	1977	1978	1979
Total	2,072	2,356	2,776	3,380	3,805	4,697	5,635	6,457	7,217	8,567	10,105	11,390	12,810	15,102	17,807
Private Funds	1,360	1,400	1,404	1,640	1,640	2,421	2,798	3,418	3,581	3,960	4,424	5,054	5,478	6,463	7,705
Consumer Payments	1,339	1,378	1,382	1,616	1,616	2,387	2,759	3,370	3,529	3,906	4,362	4,984	5,402	6,373	7,598
Out-of-Pocket Payments	1,337	1,375	1,375	1,607	1,607	2,375	2,746	3,359	3,512	3,841	4,284	4,894	5,312	6,268	7,481
Private Insurance	2	3	7	9	9	12	13	11	17	64	78	91	90	105	117
Philanthropic Funds	21	22	22	24	24	34	39	48	52	54	61	70	70	90	107
Public Funds	712	956	1,372	1,740	1,740	2,276	2,837	3,039	3,636	4,607	5,681	6,336	6,336	8,639	10,102
Federal Funds	460	538	794	1,037	1,037	1,339	1,692	1,670	2,051	2,603	3,186	3,606	3,606	4,792	5,461
Medicare		34	233	356	356	259	195	175	192	244	291	334	334	353	313
Medicaid (Federal Share)		236	444	566	566	779	1,042	1,396	1,740	2,218	2,720	3,064	3,548	4,157	4,775
Veterans' Administration	6	21	30	37	37	58	82	99	120	141	174	208	248	282	313
State and Local															
Government Funds	251	418	579	703	703	938	1,144	1,369	1,585	2,003	2,496	2,730	3,171	3,848	4,642
Medicaid (State Share)		252	463	570	570	644	884	1,184	1,356	1,710	2,150	2,359	2,740	3,328	4,021
Other Public Aid	251	166	115	132	132	294	260	184	229	293	346	371	431	520	621
Total Medicaid		488	908	1,137	1,137	1,422	1,926	2,580	3,096	3,928	4,870	5,423	6,288	7,485	8,796
Public Expenditures as a Percentage of Total	34.4	40.6	49.4	51.5	51.5	48.5	50.4	47.1	50.4	53.8	56.2	55.6	57.2	57.2	56.7
Medicaid Expenditures as a Percentage of Total	0	20.7	32.7	33.6	33.6	30.3	34.2	40.0	42.9	45.9	48.2	47.6	49.1	49.6	49.4
Medicare Expenditures as a Percentage of Total	0	1.5	8.0	10.5	10.5	5.5	3.5	2.7	2.7	2.8	2.9	2.9	2.8	2.3	2.1

Note: Totals may not add because of rounding.
Source: Division of National Cost Estimates, Health Care Financing Administration.

late 1960s, government had become the predominant buyer of nursing home services through the Medicare and especially the Medicaid programs. Except in the much smaller end-stage renal disease program, government payments constitute a larger percentage of the total in the nursing home industry than in any other area within the health care sector. Given its financial dominance, government should be able to exercise a good deal of monopsonistic power[5] in this market and thereby compensate for the limited physical and mental capacities of the consumer of nursing home care.[6] We would expect this to be true especially in the latter part of the 1970s, as government's share of the market grew even larger. There is a paradox in this monopsonistic situation, however, because government pays and regulates, but under the "freedom of choice" provisions of Medicare and Medicaid, the patient can "buy" from whomever he/she chooses. This provision limits government's monopsonistic power. Also "government" is not merely one entity but consists of the Federal government, which has a single Medicare policy and rules, and 54 State and territorial Medicaid jurisdictions, that have widely varying policies and rules. Furthermore, to the extent that nursing homes tend to specialize in private or public patients, government monopsony power may be diluted or enhanced.

Product Differentiation and Geographical Structure of the Market

Many of the persons in nursing homes prefer to be in a home near their relatives and/or friends. Indeed, marketing research suggests that the effective radius of the nursing home's market is about 25 miles (Scott and Whitaker, 1975), and that homes differentiate their products by location (U.S. Subcommittee on Long-Term Care, 1976). Therefore, at least in metropolitan areas, one would suppose that nursing homes vigorously compete against one another. Yet the existence of continuously high occupancy rates (refer to Tables XVII–2 and XVII–3) supports Scanlon's empirical evidence (1980) that there exists excess demand for nursing home care. Dissatisfied customers may have no place else to go, although immobility may be a greater problem for public patients than for private-pay patients who can afford to spend more, and therefore may have a greater measure of mobility.

Nursing homes also differentiate their product by service type. Some choose to produce high levels of care for public patients and

---

[5] Monopsony is the other side of the coin of monopoly. With monopoly, one seller has the whole market or is powerful enough to control it. Where monopsony exists, one buyer holds a similar position *vis-a-vis* the market.

[6] Government as regulator will be reviewed in the market conduct section of this chapter.

thus become designated as "skilled nursing facilities" for purposes of the Medicare or Medicaid programs; others provide "intermediate care facility" levels of care, with less emphasis upon medical and nursing care. Some homes provide equivalent services, but remain uncertified by either the Medicare or Medicaid programs. Finally, other nursing homes remain at "personal care" and "domiciliary care" levels. In this regard, it has been said that, over time, ". . . institutional development follows the federal money" (Under Secretary's Task Force on Long-Term Care, 1980).

Quality differences may also stem from rural and urban locations and locations within these geographical units (Scott and Whitaker, 1975). Homes that market their product to more affluent private patients tend to emphasize in their advertising the ready availability of physician services and reliable and constant nursing care, as well as the quality of their housing, food, and recreational and transportation amenities.[7]

The Condition of Entry

Chapter XIX thoroughly analyzes the cost structure of the industry; suffice it here to say that there is nothing about its cost structure which would appear to impede the orderly working of a market, as is the case with public utilities. Because variable costs are so large a proportion of total costs, there appear to be no economies or diseconomies of scale.[8] There is no major vertical or horizontal integration in this industry, which is also true for the majority of the service industry.[9]

Moreover, equity requirements for investment in a nursing home have been minimal in the past (McCaffree et al, 1978; Baldwin, 1980). Little special skill is required to become a nursing home operator (U.S. Senate Subcommittee on Long-Term Care, 1976). Unlike hospitals, nursing homes have not sought accreditation from the Joint Commission on Accreditation of Hospitals which also covers

---

[7] The reader may consult the Yellow Pages of the telephone directory in most large cities or such magazines as the *Washingtonian* or *New York Magazine*.

[8] One possibility to note is that increasing regulation may be bringing about economies of scale for dealing with the regulation. Merrill Lynch (1979) argues that one explanation for the increasing size of the average nursing home and the growth of nursing home chains is that the so-called "Mom and Pop" operations can no longer cope with the complexity and extent of government regulations. Legal departments within chains, or a lawyer on retainer to a large home, are more easily able to specialize in such matters. The Life Safety Code is one example of the type of regulation that might also work to the detriment of small firms. Another example is Certificate of Need, which we will explore more fully later in this chapter.

[9] McCaffree et al (1978) found that profitability did not appear to be linked with either vertical or horizontal integration in the nursing home industry.

nursing homes; 95 percent of hospitals are accredited, whereas only about 4 percent of nursing homes are. Apparently nursing homes see no economic or professional advantage in being accredited (Fraundorf, 1977).

Prior to the enactment of certificate of need (CON) legislation in 1972, the only barrier to entry into the nursing home industry was licensure. In the majority of States, it was not difficult or expensive to obtain a license to open and operate a nursing home (Under Secretary's Task Force on Long-Term Care, 1980). Certificate of need represented the first major barrier to entry into this industry and seems to have had an impact upon the conduct and performance of nursing homes. We analyze the effects of CON in the sections that follow.

Market Conduct

The Determinants of Price and Output

Basically, the prices offered to private patients are set in a manner identical to the prices offered to the consumers of household appliances, for example, or to the consumers of the product or service of any monopolistically competitive industry. Price is set where marginal revenue equals marginal cost in the case of for-profit providers, and probably where average revenue equals average cost in the case of non-profit providers, depending upon non-profit objectives. The providers of nursing home care are "price takers" for public patients;[10] with cost or cost-plus forms of government reimbursement, the price taken becomes endogenous to some nursing home firms. Flat rate forms of reimbursement are exogenous to the firm. The level of public reimbursement determines how many patients will be admitted to the nursing home, and if rates are set too low, few, if any, public patients will be admitted.

In the absence of controls, it is assumed that markets will clear via the equilibrating mechanism of the price system: no shortage or surplus could exist in the long run. The dual pricing mechanism in the nursing home market allocates beds between private and public patients, and, in the short run, all of the public patients demanding care conceivably might not receive it. Therefore, we can speak of a "shortage" of beds for the residual public patients.

---

[10] There is the possibility that nursing homes might collude, tacitly or otherwise, to raise their reimbursement rates or to influence the legislative process in their favor. To the author's knowledge, no work has been done on this potential problem. Nursing home associations do lobby, but legal cases or data on such practices as price coordination, price leadership, or price following are difficult to find.

594

Shortages and Lack of Equilibrium

In the analysis of Chapter XVI, we made the public patient residual a function of the reimbursement rate that the government was willing to pay. Here we wish to develop further the mechanics of the reimbursement system as it exists under the Medicaid program. For each of the 54 State and territorial Medicaid jurisdictions, we can write:

$$TE_{MB} = (B_M \cdot R)(1-t)$$
$$B_M = f(R,e,Q_p(P_p))$$

where TE_{MB} is total State expenditures on Medicaid beds,

B_M is Medicaid beds supplied,

R is the public rate paid per bed,

t is the share paid by the Federal government,

e is the patient eligibility criterion, and

Q_p is the quantity of private beds demanded, which is a function of the private price, P_p. [11]

For the moment, we assume that planning agencies and certificate of need legislation do not exist. The State decides how much of its budget it will allocate to Medicaid nursing home beds (TE_{MB}) and then could set a perfect combination of the rate (R) and the eligibility criterion (e) such that the market would clear and there would be no shortage of Medicaid beds or private beds, according to the economic definition of shortage. In practice, it would be difficult for 54 separate entities to make such a perfect estimation of R and e; even if they could, there could still be a shortage for both private and Medicaid patients, according to the planning definition, based on need. If the eligibility criterion (e) were set too broadly, there could be a shortage according to both the economic definition and the planning definition.[12] Whatever the case, it remains true that R and e may be essentially established in a normative context.

---

[11] We would assume that, in most cases, $\partial B_M / \partial Q_p < 0$, and $\partial B_M / \partial_e > 0$.

[12] This could happen in the short run because all of the public eligibles face a subsidized price, but some of them would be denied entry into nursing homes due to the fact that operators of nursing homes set output decisions according to the criteria developed in Chapter XVI. If R were set high enough, the economic shortage would disappear in the long run, as operators expanded capacity. In fact, there are losses to the State from errors on either side of the "correct" R. This is important, because if losses from overestimating R were negligible, the shortage problem would be easily soluble. However, it is not at all clear that the States' loss function is at a minimum at the value of R at which excess demand is exactly zero. Given the opportunity cost to the State of expenditures on nursing home care, the optimal amount of excess demand from the States' perspective may be positive.

Figure XVII–1 illustrates the shortage problem. The *length* of the lines $ZMEMR$ or $Z'M'EMR'$ is a function of the public eligibility criterion; ZM could represent one set of public eligibles. Likewise, the *height* of the lines $ZMEMR$ or $Z'M'EMR'$ is a function of the public rate paid per bed; ZM would represent a higher public reimbursement rate than $Z'M'$. With ZM public bed days demanded (or "needed" in a planning sense) and at a public rate of R_1, Q_1 bed days would be produced, of which OQ_Z would go to private patients and $Q_Z Q_1$ to public patients; there would be an economic and planning shortage of $Q_1 Q_M$ bed days.[13] The shortage would be even greater if eligibility criteria were broadened and the line ZM became longer. If the public rate were lowered to R^2 and eligibility remained constant by the length ZM, the new equilibrium output would be OQ_2 bed days, of which private patients would receive OQ'_Z, and public patients $Q'_Z Q_2$. Private patients would replace public patients and the queue of public patients not receiving bed days would become even longer, by the amount $Q_2 Q_1 + Q_M Q'_M$. The only way in which this situation could be ameliorated, from the point of view of public patients, is if the supply curve of bed days were to shift outward, the private demand curve for bed days were to shift inward, or the public rate were to rise until ZM bed days were provided.

At equilibrium (R_1, Q_1), State expenditures on bed days would be $Q_Z Q_1 \cdot R^1 (1 - t)$ and at equilibrium (R^2, Q^2) they would be $Q'_Z Q_2 \cdot R_2 (1 - t)$. If the State budget constraint for nursing home public bed days is set exogenously as, for example, some percentage of total tax revenues received, then e and R may be manipulated as policy variables to meet that constraint. On the other hand, if the State budget constraint for nursing home public bed days is subject to debate and competes with other public expenditures such as education and highways, e and R may be set in a normative context.[14]

In this respect, one aspect of the political and normative atmosphere which is often ignored is the possibility that a State Medicaid jurisdiction may only allow the Federal minimum eligibility criteria, or even exceed the Federal minimum, but have low *effective* eligibility due to a failure to advertise eligibility and/or due to beneficiary

---

[13] Another definition of "planning shortage" could be that quantity demanded at zero price. Thus, while the economic shortage (excess demand) would be $Q_1 Q_M$ at $R = R_1$, the planning shortage would be Q_1 to that point where ND_{P+MD} touched the horizontal axis.

[14] Also, Federal restrictions affect how these policies are set, and there are multiple goals regarding access and quality, as well as cost, so that manipulations of e and R may not be able to achieve expenditure control without a shortage.

596

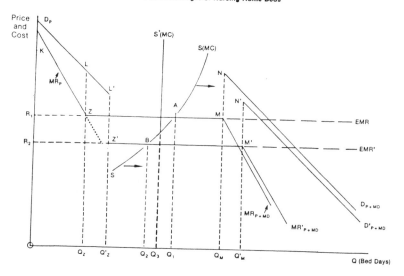

FIGURE XVII-1
Public Shortages of Nursing Home Beds

597

ignorance.[15] Not much work has been done on this potential problem, but Table XVII–7 illustrates its possible magnitude. In a sample study of 3,400 of Washington State's 546,000 elderly, 60 and above, researchers found that a large proportion were unaware of services available to them under the various State programs. What is equally interesting is the high percentage of those previously unaware who said that they would now use the services; this was particularly true for those persons with three or more chronic illnesses. For instance, 41.4 percent said that they would use homemaker and home health services, 39.4 percent, visiting nurse services, and 32.2 percent, at-home physical therapy. These could be three relatively expensive additional services to provide. If all the "unaware" who would use the service actually did, it could significantly enlarge Washington State's Medicaid budget. One can only speculate on the extent to which the national aggregate Medicaid budget could be enlarged if similar dormant demand exists and were activated in other States.

Finally, S (the supply function) may become a policy variable if e and R are politically sensitive, and no suitable substitutes for nursing home bed days exist or can be funded by the public sector. Returning to Figure XVII–1, consider the vertical supply curve $S'(MC)$. Certificate of need regulations (the full outcome of which we will shortly discuss) could result in the production of OQ_3 bed days by individual nursing home firms.[16]

If the nursing home firm depicted in Figure XVI–1 is representative of firms in the State, then certificate of need would create a state-wide shortage of $\sum_{i=1}^{n} (Q_3 Q_M)_i$ bed days, according to the planning definition of shortage (that is, the aggregation of the differences between the quantities demanded and the quantities supplied for all of the nursing homes in the State, at the rate and eligibility criteria established by the State).

Scanlon (1980) has found empirically that there is excess demand for nursing home beds, but this is due to the subsidy inherent in Medicaid and the fact that a smaller subsidy is extended to other forms of long-term care. Vladeck (1980) implicitly argues that there is a shortage of nursing home beds, largely because other forms of

---

[15] Although the following example pertains to the Medicare program, it is instructive, nonetheless. In a personal communication, the author was informed by a member of the Marketing Department at the Kellogg School of Northwestern University that, after careful study, it was his considered opinion that an elderly individual would have to be able to read at approximately the 12th grade level to understand the "Medicare Handbook" currently distributed to the elderly (a level at which only 25 percent of elderly individuals are likely to read).

[16] This assumes that some services or even some beds can be considered to be included under variable costs.

TABLE XVII-7
Percent of Washington State Citizens Age 60 and Over Unaware of Available Services

	(1) Percent of Total Sample Unaware of the Service	(2) Percent of Respondents With Three or More Chronic Illnesses Unaware of the Service	(3) Percent of Total Unaware Who Said They Would Use the Service	(4) Percent of Unaware with Three or More Chronic Illnesses Who Said They Would Use the Service
Home Repair or Chore Services	60.8%	65.8%	40.4%	56.1%
Homemaker or Home Health Services	55.3	59.3	28.2	41.4
Home Delivered Meals	32.5	34.4	22.6	31.2
Group Meals	31.2	32.7	18.4	16.7
Senior Centers or Recreation Programs	18.8	20.0	3.2	3.4
Day Care Programs	51.7	55.6	13.2	19.6
Telephone Visiting and Checking Services	54.5	62.9	22.5	31.8
Employment Services	48.1	50.9	11.3	7.1
Information and Referral Services	58.3	66.9	41.5	53.0
Legal Services	53.9	58.2	43.3	52.5
Telephone Bill Assistance	73.0	75.3	37.6	46.4
Laundry Service	77.3	81.6	18.3	22.5
Communication Service for Those with Impaired Hearing	70.7	81.6	18.3	22.5
Visiting Nurse Service	42.5	45.6	31.8	39.4
At-Home Physical Therapy	58.7	64.9	26.8	32.2
Counseling for Emotional Problems	60.0	67.6	14.2	14.8

Source: Washington State Department of Social and Health Services, *The Needs of the Elderly 1978.*

long-term care are not as heavily subsidized and because of problems of geographical and financial access. But to the extent that public-pay consumers receive some amount of subsidy for nursing home care or its alternatives, and producers receive a public rate that only covers average costs, the long-term care market will be out of equilibrium and there will be shortages, according to the economic definition.[17] This implies some measure of market power on the part of the sellers of nursing home services, even though there are many of them.

The Effects of Certificate of Need Regulations

By 1979, every State had passed certificate of need legislation. Alarmed by the rapid and seemingly uncontrollable escalation in health care costs, the States and the Federal government sought to control the building of new health care facilities and the purchase of new equipment by refusing to reimburse health care provided in facilities which had not first obtained a certificate of need before building or purchasing additional equipment.

Certificate of need (CON) is essentially a barrier to entry into a market. This kind of regulation is founded upon a basic premise that markets do not work "properly," and that institutionally-certified need, rather than the price mechnism, should perform the allocatory function. CON is seen to be necessary in the health care market because consumer demand, underwritten by health insurance, gives different market signals than if the consumer paid much of the cost out of his or her own pocket. As a consequence, much larger amounts of health care are consumed than would be the case in the absence of insurance. It could be argued that such a rationale is more convincing in the hospital sector where health insurance covers 85 percent of the bill (See Newhouse, 1978 and 1981) than it might be for the nursing home sector, where there is little private health insurance coverage. However, there is a significant amount of social insurance for nursing home care built into the Medicaid program.

Economic theories of regulation hypothesize certain outcomes that are usually inimical to the public interest (Stigler, 1971). One, the "capture theory," asserts that regulators are ultimately captured by the industry which they regulate.[18] While this process of capture need not necessarily be overt, it seems natural that regulators who come into daily contact with an industry would better understand its

---

[17] In the short run, the economic shortage would disappear if S (MC) crossed the EMR curve at point M in Figure XVII–1. There could *always* be shortages, according to the planning definition.

[18] According to this theory, the regulators *do* regulate after they have been captured. However, they no longer regulate in the public interest, but rather in the interest of existing firms.

problems and become sympathetic toward them. Frequent contact with industry executives in the course of the regulatory process, and a narrowing of the mental focus on the regulation of the industry to the exclusion of other concerns, creates an atmosphere where it becomes easier for the regulators to identify with the industry and to end up being concerned primarily with its welfare.[19]

One of the pieces of circumstantial evidence often used in support of the capture theory is that the regulated themselves often vociferously lobby for and support regulation. For example, when the Civil Aeronautics Board began the initial steps to deregulate the airline industry, it was the airlines themselves that posed the most objections.

Another more general theory of regulation is the "political-economic theory" (Noll, 1975). Its basis is the fundamental asymmetry between the information that the regulated industry possesses and that which is available to the regulatory agency. Moreover, the interests of the regulated industry are sharply focused on its own narrow concerns, whereas the consumers of its product or service have diverse interests in that they also consume many other products and services. Because of its narrowed focus, the regulated industry can devote more time and energy to pursuing its intrests by influencing legislators, regulators, and even its consuming public.

Finally, Grabowski (1976) has pointed out another asymmetry that exists in the regulatory process; his insight might be labelled the "risk" theory. The bureaucrat who inadvertently allows Thalidomide to slip through the regulatory screen will be remembered; however, he will incur little criticism, except from the industry, for demanding extremely thorough testing of a new drug. Likewise, nursing home fires attain widespread publicity and recrimination for supposedly lax regulators.

Given these generally-accepted theories and the empirical evidence which gives credence to them, the literature in economics tends to take a dim view of the ultimate efficacy of most forms of regulation. Certificate of need regulation for hospitals and nursing homes has been studied, and the outcome of this regulation has likewise been questioned.

In a much-cited study that attempted to assess the impact of CON regulations on hospital investment, costs, and use from 1968 to 1972, Salkever and Bice (1979) found that CON ". . . did not significantly affect total investment by hospitals but did alter its composi-

---

[19] In this respect, it is interesting to note that it is the practice of the United Nations and its sister agencies not to leave their personnel in any one country for too long a period of time, on the grounds that U.N. personnel tend to begin representing the host country's views and objectives rather than those of the U.N.

601

tion." In effect, the supply of hospital beds grew at a slower rate than would have been expected in the absence of CON regulations, but hospital plant assets grew at a faster rate. They also found that ". . . no significant savings in hospital costs were achieved through certificate-of-need programs." Any savings that were achieved through lower admission rates and total hospital days due to the slower growth of the bed supply were dissipated in the upgrading of the style of care through the use of sophisticated new technologies.

In another study, Sloan and Steinwald (1980) examined the effects of regulation on hospital costs and input from 1969 to 1975. Their evidence suggested ". . . that, as a group, regulatory programs did not meaningfully contain hospital costs during the first half of the 1970's." They conceded that this effect may be due to the fact that CON is a "piecemeal" form of regulation. Present evidence also suggests that even more comprehensive forms of regulation would not have achieved regulatory goals in the long run.

To determine the effects of certificate of need in the nursing home sector, Scanlon and Feder (1980) conducted an exhaustive set of interviews with Medicaid officials in eight States: California, Colorado, Georgia, Massachusetts, New Jersey, New York, Tennessee, and Washington. Approximately 40 percent of all Medicaid nursing home expenditures in 1977 occurred in these States. Research centered upon the following issues: (1) the State's methods and objectives in applying CON regulations to nursing homes, (2) problems faced in achieving their objectives, and (3) the consequences of the policies adopted for the availability and use of nursing home beds.

Scanlon and Feder emphasize that they are cautious about making global statements on these questions due to the varying intensity of their interviews in only eight States, and they prefer to analyze the experience in each State. But, the reader may draw certain general conclusions from their interviews and their analysis.

Their findings indicate that CON has been successful in limiting the supply of nursing home beds and that the States use CON primarily as a tool to limit their total expenditures on nursing home care. However, there are a number of ways in which a State may limit its expenditures on long-term care or nursing home care. As shown earlier in this chapter, a State may define strict eligibility requirements and thereby limit the number of eligibles or set its payment rate per patient at a low level.[20] Finally, it might use certificate of need legislation to strictly limit the supply of beds available.

---

[20] It should be noted that Section 249 of Title XIX of the Social Security Act creates problems of uncertainty for the States about what it does or does not allow.

Scanlon and Feder ask the logical question of why States seem to prefer CON to the other possible methods of limiting expenditures. Based upon their interviews, one may infer that the "political-economic" and "risk" theories of regulation explain this phenomenon in large part. Certificate of need regulation is a more subtle and a less visible form of expenditure limitation; as such, it offers a greater chance of avoiding public controversy. Ultimately the market mechanism might replace homes that had gone out of business because of rates set at too low a level for some, but the transitional risk is seen by State governments to be too great politically. Limiting eligibility could also invite public controversy. With CON, it is possible to pay higher rates per patient and still have lower total State expenditures on nursing homes than without it.

In the Scanlon-Feder analysis, CON produces winners and losers. If CON's only objective is to hold down total expenditures on nursing homes, the State wins. If, however, one considers expenditures in relation to services provided, the State may not win because CON does not ensure the provision of quality services, even at high rates per patient. Scanlon and Feder found that nursing home operators, and associations representing them, clearly recognized the value of the barriers to entry which CON imposes. They observe that ". . . whatever losses in efficiency CON restrictions impose on the State are gains in revenue and security to nursing home operators. The monopoly power CON restrictions create is apparently far more valuable to these operators than [the expected value of] any new investment they might forego."

Finally, it would appear that nursing home patients are net losers compared to nursing home operators and the States. Because CON reduces competition, private patients probably pay more than they would if there were competition, and they also have fewer choices. Public patients have less access to care, and CON reinforces the incentive for nursing home operators to choose relatively less difficult cases over the more difficult.

Research, Innovation, and Legal Tactics

We will only briefly touch upon the other aspects of this industry which affect market conduct. Research and innovation do not presently seem to be important; however, no data exist on this point. One could reasonably suspect that, with the proper financial incentives, more effort would be given to finding ways to rehabilitate patients in nursing homes and/or make their lives more fulfilling. Again, this pertains to the provision of quality care and all its attendant problems. Finally, legal tactics are largely employed against threats of lower reimbursement rates or pieces of legislation that the industry fears will be detrimental to its financial interests (Scanlon and Feder, 1980).

603

Market Performance

The Problem of Quality

For the most part, the economic models in Chapter XVI also assumed product or service homogeneity. One hotel room bought from a major chain will not be much different in quality from a comparably priced room bought from another; the competition for buyers assures this outcome. Yet, an examination of the market structure of the nursing home industry has revealed that the consumers of nursing home services have little information and limited capacities for choice and mobility. If government is an inefficient or indifferent surrogate buyer of nursing home services for its consumers, then nursing home quality becomes a dimension of nursing home output which the operator may be able to manipulate.

In our diagrammatic exposition of Chapter XVI, the manipulability of product quality would result in a lowering of the cost curves if the public rate were exogenous to the firm's cost structure, or, with cost-based forms of reimbursement, a falsification and/or a manipulation of the costs entering into the reimbursement formula. Again, the price and output decisions of providers would be determined by the marginal revenue equals marginal cost or average revenue equals average cost rules for the for-profit and non-profit providers, respectively. However, "bad" bed days, rather than "good" bed days, could now be produced.[21]

Indeed, flat rate forms of government reimbursement give the for-profit entrepreneur an even greater incentive to minimize cost or severely reduce quality than he or she would have under normal market conditions because in a competitive market, the product or output for all firms is homogeneous. In a service industry that is not confronted with the usual market demand constraints, it is easier to adjust the quality dimension of the service provided. Even a cost-related system of reimbursement does not assure the quality dimension of output; costs can be manipulated to maximize profits rather than to pay for the inputs technically necessary to provide some level of "adequate" care.

Hence, the reimbursement system can offer incentives to operators to provide a certain level of care to nursing home residents or, in the absence of sufficient or attainable incentives, government can draft regulations and enforce them vigorously. Such regulations by themselves will not ensure the desired quality and level of output, even when enforced vigorously, if the level of reimbursement is not sufficient to attain a fair rate of return on investment.

---

[21] Here "bad" or "good" days would be defined relative to some publicly determined norm.

Ruchlin (1977) believes that the regulatory process in long-term care has failed to achieve its major objectives. He groups the causes of this failure under two broad headings, the characteristics of the regulatory process itself and structural barriers. Inadequate financing of the enforcement process and a lack of objective criteria of quality to be enforced make the outcome of regulation in long-term care problematic. Moreover, bureaucratic apathy, the circuitous nature of the legal process, and the political influence of the regulated hinder the regulatory process. Ruchlin sees the fragmentation of agency responsibility and the shortage of beds as structural barriers. He cites the fact that in most States a facility is licensed and inspected by one agency, paid by another, and sent residents by still another. The shortage of beds impedes efforts to close facilities that grossly neglect quality to the physical and mental detriment of their inhabitants.

Table XVII–8 contains a compilation made by the Senate's Subcommittee on Long-Term Care on the incidence of the most common complaints against nursing homes as reported in general newspaper investigations. While it is true that newspapers have made similar anecdotal allegations about insurance companies, auto repair firms, home repair companies, and a variety of other suppliers of goods and services to the general population, these allegations must be weighed more carefully in the nursing home industry due to the debility and consequent immobility of the consumer of its services. In its report, the Subcommittee lists a "Litany of Nursing Homes Abuses:"

I. Abuse and Poor Treatment of Patients
II. Deliberate Physical Injury
III. Unsanitary Conditions
IV. Poor Food or Poor Preparation
V. Misappropriation and Theft
VI. Inadequate Control of Drugs
VII. Other Hazards to Life and Limb
VIII. Unauthorized or Improper Use of Restraints
IX. Reprisals Against Those Who Complain
X. Lack of Eye Care, Dental Care and Podiatry
XI. Assaults on Human Dignity
XII. Profiteering and Cheating the System [22]

Even though much of this information is anecdotal, the constant publicity about nursing home abuse and inadequate patient care over the last few years implies that nursing home providers do have

---

[22] Interestingly, Section XII of the report begins with the sentence: "The Subcommittee received far fewer examples, comparatively, of profiteering and abuse of the system than it received of patient abuse."

TABLE XVII-8
Incidence of Most Common Complaints Against Nursing Homes as Reported in the General Newspaper Investigations

	Negligence Leading to Death or Injury	Bribery	Intentional Physical Injury	Untrained Administrators	Poor Care	Non-Profit Homes are Better	Poor Food	Profiteering	Unsanitary Conditions	Refusing to Take Heavy Care Patients	Excessive Charges in Addition to Basic Rates	Fire or Other Hazards	Lack of Dental Care	Lack of Psychiatric Care	Lax Control of Drugs	Untrained and Inadequate Personnel	False Advertising	Absentee Ownership	Lack of Human Dignity	Lack of Activities	Theft	Lack of Podiatry	Doctor's Absent	Unnecessary or Unauthorized Use of Restraints	Ineffective Inspections—Lax Enforcement	Advance Notice of Inspections	Discrimination Against Minority Groups	Reprisals Against Patients Who Complain	Use of Unlicensed Homes to House Patients (the bootleg nursing home)
San Diego Union, 1971	X		X		X	X	X	X	X	X	X	X			X	X		X	X	X	X		X	X	X		X		X
Chicago Tribune, 1971	X		X	X	X		X	X	X	X	X	X			X	X			X	X	X		X	X	X			X	X
Philadelphia Bulletin, 1968							X	X	X	X		X		X	X	X			X	X			X	X	X		X	X	X
New York Daily News, 1962	X				X	X	X		X	X	X			X	X	X			X	X	X		X		X				
Milwaukee Sentinel, 1970		X			X	X	X	X	X	X	X		X	X	X				X	X			X	X	X		X		
Newsday, L.I., N.Y., 1970			X	X	X		X	X		X						X			X	X				X					
Boston Globe, 1968					X		X	X			X	X						X					X		X				
St. Petersburg (Fla.) Times, 1969	X		X	X	X		X	X	X		X			X	X	X	X		X	X	X	X	X	X	X		X	X	
Associated Press series, 1969	X		X		X		X	X	X			X		X	X	X			X		X		X	X	X				
Nashville Tennessean, 1965	X						X		X							X			X	X	X		X	X	X				X
Reader's Digest, 1972	X		X		X	X	X	X		X		X			X	X			X	X			X		X			X	
New York Times, 1970				X	X			X	X	X						X			X	X			X	X	X		X	X	
Boston Herald Traveler, 1971					X		X	X	X						X	X			X	X			X	X	X				
Baltimore Sun, 1971				X			X	X	X	X	X					X		X	X	X			X		X				

Source: U.S. Senate, Subcommittee on Long-Term Care (December 1974), *Supporting Paper No. 1*, p. 168.

some measure of market power that insulates them from the kind of competition that occurs in other markets where there are many buyers and sellers.[23]

Most empirical studies of nursing home quality have used input measures, such as the number of registered nurses or the number of patient contact hours. While these input measures give some indication of quality, they are nonetheless inferior to true output measures. No one, as yet, has been able to measure government's contribution to the quality of output, but Fraundorf (1977) contends that some indication is given in examining the process by which this monopsonistic buyer has attempted to affect the quality of care for both public and private patients. He analyzes the "confusing array of regulations" and how they have multiplied and changed over time, and also how they have become diluted by HEW (now HHS) policies. His conclusion is that: ". . . Medicare and Medicaid regulations . . . would do little to increase the quality of patient care." The Senate study described enforcement efforts as "haphazard, fragmented, and generally inadequate" (U.S. Senate Subcommittee on Long-Term Care, 1976). However, one government source believes that "impressionistic evidence suggests that regulatory initiatives by Federal and State governments have improved the quality of care in nursing homes in recent years" (HCFA, Office of Legislation and Policy, 1981).

Profitability and Growth

There have been many allegations of excessive profits in the nursing home industry (Mendleson, 1974; Townsend, 1971; Moreland Commission, 1976) and questions about the bed supply. As part of this section, we make a theoretical and an empirical effort to examine the question more carefully.[24]

Any investment decision can be characterized as one in which an individual gives up a certain amount of wealth in one time period to secure a greater amount of wealth in a future time period. A rational risk-neutral investor makes that decision on the basis of the expected, internal, real rate of return on the investment. Basically, the internal, real rate of return calculation yields information not

---

[23] In this same vein, there have been many complaints about the so-called "Medigap" problem. In the health insurance market, there are also many buyers and sellers, but it has been alleged that sellers take advantage of elderly consumers' ignorance of their Medicare coverage and sell them health insurance supplementary to Medicare that is in excess of what they would buy if they were well-informed, and that in many cases this insurance is actuarially unfair. Recently, Congress has passed legislation that may ameliorate this alleged abuse.

[24] Chapter XVI has already dealt with the short run theoretical considerations and Chapter XVIII will expand more fully on reimbursement issues.

607

only on whether an investment will be profitable, but also on by how much more or less than the prevalent interest rate.[25]

The internal real rate of return calculation can be expressed as follows:

$$Y_o = \sum_{t=1}^{n} \frac{R_t - C_t}{(1 + i)^t} + \frac{S}{(1 + i)^n} \tag{1}$$

where Y_o = the initial investment sum,

i = the internal real rate of return,

t = the number of years that the investment would be in existence,

R_t = receipts received in period t,

C_t = outlays incurred in period t,

n = productive life of an investment, and

S = the salvage value of the investment after n time periods.

It is assumed that R, C, n, and S are known, or can be empirically estimated, and the equation is solved for i.[26] Depreciation may be viewed as a non-recurrent cost which would be deducted from an earnings statement but is not included in an internal rate of return calculation.[27]

---

[25] The two standard references on this topic are Fisher (1930) and Lutz and Lutz (1951). Consideration of the prevalent interest rate is important for this reason: if the prevalent interest rate on a loan to a reputable bank is 10 percent, but the internal real rate of return on an alternative investment of similar risk is expected to be only 5 percent, then at the margin, the alternative investment would be profitable, but not as profitable as making the loan to the bank.

[26] This formulation is somewhat different, but basically follows that of McCaffree et al (1978) and standard textbook treatment.

[27] The internal rate of return calculation ignores depreciation for the following reasons. Assume for the moment a simple rate of interest of 10 percent per annum and no inflation. A bank deposit of $10,000 for five years at 10 percent per annum would yield the following financial profile:

Investment: $10,000

Year	1	2	3	4	5	
Net Income:	$1,000	$1,000	$1,000	$1,000	$1,000	= $5,000

Wealth at the end of year 5: $15,000

A competing investment might be in a machine which produces hats. This machine has an economic life of five years, so that at the end of the five years, it is used up and has no scrap value. For the investor to be indifferent between the bank deposit and the machine, the following financial profile would be necessary:

Investment in the machine: $10,000

Year	1	2	3	4	5	
Net Income:	$1,000	$1,000	$1,000	$1,000	$1,000	= $5,000

However, at the end of five years, the machine which originally cost $10,000

608

Whether a person is investing in a financial instrument or a real asset, he or she is giving up the use of Y_0 in period 1 and for the full period of the investment. What he/she is basically concerned with is the change in personal wealth at the end of the investment period.

Hence, equation (1) expresses the essential relationship whether one is considering a *financial* investment or a *real* investment. Assuming an initial Y_0 of \$10,000, in the case of a bank deposit, $S = \$10,000$, while in the case of a *machine, S* = 0.

The investor is also interested in his or her rate of return after taxes. Some investments have more favored tax aspects than others and, under a progressive tax system, the real rate of return on an investment might be low if the investor is in a high marginal tax bracket because the tax system is steeply progressive and/or because income from other sources is high. In general, we can express the after-tax real rate of return as:

$$Y_0 = \sum_{t=1}^{n} \frac{(R_t - C_t)(1 - \tau)}{(1 + i)^t} + \frac{S}{(1 + i)^n} \tag{2}$$

where τ is the investor's marginal tax rate. Moreover, the tax system does take depreciation into consideration as a cost of an investment in real assets as opposed to financial assets. Therefore, equation (2) must be modified:

$$Y_0 = \sum_{t=1}^{n} \frac{[R^t - (C_t + D_t)](1 - \tau)}{(1 + i)^t} + \frac{S}{(1 + i)^n} \tag{3}$$

where D is depreciation for tax purposes.

The investor's objective is to continue to make investments until he or she has driven i to zero, and in a competitive economy where resources are freely mobile, we would expect investor capital to flow into those industries which offer a high rate of return and flow out of those industries where the rate of return is low. In equilibrium, industries of similar risk would offer similar rates of return.

---

would have zero value. Assuming straight-line depreciation, it would deteriorate at the rate \$2,000 per year:

Year	1	2	3	4	5		
Depreciation:	\$2,000	\$2,000	\$2,000	\$2,000	\$2,000	=	\$10,000
			Net Income and Depreciation			=	\$15,000

Therefore, if the two investments are to be equivalent, gross revenue on the hat machine would have to be:

Year	1	2	3	4	5		
Gross Income:	\$3,000	\$3,000	\$3,000	\$3,000	\$3,000	=	\$15,000

In the above example, the net change in investor wealth at the end of five years would be \$5,000, whether the initial \$10,000 had been invested in a bank deposit or in a hat-making machine.

609

The comparative statics of this process are illustrated in Figure XVII–2, which shows a monopolistically competitive setting for one group (Group A) of three firms (Firms 1, 2, and 3; Firm 4 will enter the analysis shortly) and also depicts one firm in a competitive setting. Initially, the competitive firm in industry B and firms like it are only earning normal profits.[28] One of the firms in the monopolistically competitive group (Firm 2) is also earning normal profits, while Firms 1 and 3 are earning better than normal profits. Suppose now any firm in industry B decided that it would leave industry B and penetrate Firm 1 or Firm 3's market, as Firm 4. For a marginal firm in industry B, P might move to P′ (because of a slight backward shift in the industry supply curve) and D, for Firm 1, (in industry A) might drop to D′ because a new firm, Firm 4, has lured away part of Firm 1's market by producing a slightly different product. Firm 4 is now earning slightly better than a normal profit. We might also expect other investors to enter industry B now because greater than normal profits are being earned there, and more investors might well also enter industry A. In a dynamic economy, prices and costs shift continuously, so this process would go on continually.

The nursing home industry is one among many industries, and capital is generally mobile in the United States. Therefore, investors simply will not enter an industry such as the nursing home industry if they can find a greater real rate of return on their capital elsewhere. Medicare and, especially, Medicaid represented a large increase in the public demand for long-term care as a merit good, and investors responded to this increase in public demand, particularly in the early years of the two programs. Evidently, many investors believed that they could achieve a higher real rate of return on their capital in this sector than in other sectors of the economy.

State and Federal government funds now provide some 57 percent of all nursing home receipts (see Table XVII–6) so that changes in government reimbursement rate levels can have a profound effect upon the revenues and thus the profitability of the industry. Changes in government regulations can also affect the cost side and consequently bring about lower or higher rates of return. Indeed, any policy-induced change in any of the terms in equation (3) can affect the real rate of return on an investment in nursing home care relative to investments in other sectors of the economy.[29]

---

[28] In the language of the economist, "normal profits" are those just sufficient to keep a firm in business in the long run. Otherwise, it could place its assets in an interest-bearing bank account and earn the same rate of return or a little better. In a competitive setting, the marginal firm earns zero excess profits while inframarginal firms may earn excess profits greater than zero.

[29] The investment theory outlined in the previous pages is a pure theory which, in practice, is modified by accounting conventions and the availability of data for use in the computation of the real rate of return. For a more detailed discussion, see the Appendix to this chapter.

610

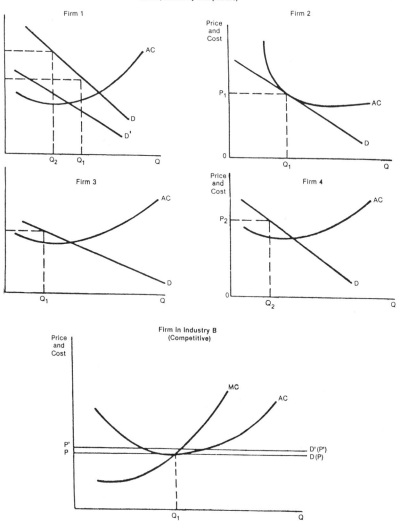

FIGURE XVII-2
Competition Among Firms
and Industries

Firms in Industry (or Group) A
(Monopolistically Competitive)

Firm In Industry B
(Competitive)

611

In reality, an investment in nursing home care is different from most investments in other forms of long-term care and from an investment in steel, precisely because government is a major reimbursor for nursing home care and the government reimbursement rate is determined not by market forces but by regulatory formulae. Following Baldwin (1980), one definition of revenue on a nursing home facility that houses only public patients and that receives cost-based retrospective reimbursement would be:

$$R = C_A + D + I + E \tag{4}$$

where R = revenue,

C_A = those operating costs which are allowable for reimbursement,

D = depreciation,

I = interest payments on debt, and

E = the return which the reimbursement authorities allow on owner equity.

In this formulation, components of cash revenue and cash expense which offset each other (such as nurses' salaries) are netted out. Adding a time subscript, substituting equation (4) into the first term of equation (3), adding a term for land value (L), and collecting terms yields:

$$Y_o = \sum_{t=1}^{n} \frac{(I_t + E_t + C_{A_t} - C_t)(1 - \tau)}{(1 + i)^t} + \frac{S(1 - \tau)}{(1 + i)^n} + \frac{L(1 - \tau)}{(1 + i)^n} \tag{5}$$

Equation (5) represents the fundamental formula for computing an internal real rate of return on an investment in nursing home care when only public patients are present.[30]

---

[30] In equation (5) the depreciation term D has been netted out: if the depreciation formula for tax purposes were different than that for the reimbursement formula, then a net D (either positive or negative) would remain. For example, if the tax laws allowed accelerated depreciation but the reimbursement formula paid straight line depreciation, then net D would be negative initially and become positive in later years. Equation (5) would then appear as:

$$Y_o = \sum_{t=1}^{n} \frac{[(I_t + E_t + C_{A_t} + D_{A_t}) - (C_t + D_{IR_t})](1 - \tau)}{(1 + i)^t}$$
$$+ \frac{S(1 - \tau)}{(1 + i)^n} + \frac{L(1 - \tau)}{(1 + i)^n}$$

where D_A was depreciation granted for reimbursement purposes and D_{IR}, depreciation allowed for tax purposes.

The Health Care Financing Administration (HCFA) has funded two studies which examine investment incentives for nursing homes. In a heuristic exploration of the finances of a single representative new nursing home in Massachusetts, Baldwin (1980) attempts to answer the following question: "given current reimbursement practices, what returns does a nursing home offer to private investors . . . and how do these returns compare to other investment opportunities . . . ?" Using a cash-flow analysis, which is the equivalent of a real rate of return analysis, she finds that this nursing home would not be competitive with other types of investments for investors in the 50 percent marginal tax bracket, if its occupants consisted solely of Medicaid patients. If Massachusetts were to allow a change in reimbursement upon sale of the facility, which it does not, then the facility might become profitable because the higher sales price would create a larger annual depreciation that enters into the reimbursement formula. However, allowance of this so-called "step-up-in-basis" may encourage the "trafficking" in nursing homes that many popular writers have deplored. (For example, see Mendleson, 1974). Baldwin then performed the same calculations, assuming that 30 percent of the home's patients were private-pay.[31] She found that the home would become an attractive investment if a premium of about $13.00 per day could be charged to private patients. This finding is interesting because it falls within the range of private-pay premiums now charged state-wide in Massachusetts.

McCaffree et al (1978) were primarily interested in finding evidence on four basic issues: (1) the relationships between profits, growth, and reimbursement systems; (2) rates of return to capital under various reimbursement systems; (3) the level of risk in investments in nursing homes; and (4) the impact of financial integration on nursing home profitability. They found that, with the exception of minimum occupancy rate regulation and a total payment limit on the per diem rate, cost-related reimbursement systems did not affect profitability and growth in the industry. However, most reimbursement methods contribute to an inefficient and costly use of capital resources. Furthermore, the level of risk in the nursing home industry appears lower than the risk of a portfolio of common stocks. Finally, neither vertical nor horizontal integration appears to affect profitability one way or the other.

As a result of their analyses, both Baldwin and McCaffree et al conclude with recommendations for reforming current public reimbursement systems. Their common argument is that reimbursement systems which more closely resemble the workings of the market have a better chance of achieving public policy goals than reimbursement systems which, so to speak, "buck" the market. Cost-based reimbursement systems that rely upon historical cost, all other

---

[31] Conventional wisdom within the industry itself maintains that a home must have at least 30 percent private-pay patients to be profitable.

terms in equation (5) held constant, do not recognize the current market value of capital, and thus reduce the potential returns to it. Under such circumstances, one would expect capital to flee elsewhere, or, as has happened in the past, one would expect owners of capital to subvert the intent of cost-based reimbursement by "trafficking" in nursing homes. Both studies recommend some form of market-rent reimbursement for capital in the nursing home industry.

However, the question of the profitability of the nursing home industry is far from settled. During the late 1960s and early 1970s, the industry seems to have expanded at a relatively greater rate than many other industries. Such expansion is usually a sign that there are above-normal profits to be made; indeed, entry into a high-profit industry is a desirable equilibrating process which eventually drives profits down to a "normal" level.

Other empirical research that has been done on nursing home profits has yielded mixed results. Fraundorf (1977) cites the results of two studies and an article in the March 1973 Barron's.[32] The AMS study found that the after-tax rate of return on sales for 228 nursing homes in a random sample averaged 6 percent, but there was wide variability around the mean. Six percent on sales seems high when compared to supermarkets, where the rule of thumb is one-half of 1 percent on sales, but "sales" *per se* is not always the most meaningful base, and most analysts would argue that equity is more suitable as a profits base.

On the other hand, the Morton study of a non-random sample of incorporated nursing home chains found lower returns on sales than did the AMS study and also found fairly low rates of return on equity. The Barron's article states that the 7.3 percent after tax rate of return on sales earned by one particular nursing home chain was "exceptionally high" (presumably relative to the risk involved). Another piece of evidence on nursing home profits is contained in the Batelle study done for HCFA (McCaffree *et al*, 1978). On average, Batelle did not find high rates of return in the four States studied but did find a large amount of variability around the mean: the average rate of return on equity was 14 percent for the 278 facilities studied, but 30 percent of these facilities suffered losses. Given the empirical evidence, it is difficult to draw firm conclusions about profitability in nursing homes. Controversy continues to exist about the computation of the base for profit comparison; McCaffree *et al*

---

[32] The two studies were Applied Management Systems, *A Business and Financial Analysis of the Long-Term Care Industry* (Silver Spring: A.M.S. 1974) and Morton Research Corporation, *The Nursing Home Industry: An Economic and Financial Study Analysis* (Merrick, N.Y.L. The Corporation, 1974).

(1978) argue that equity is the best base but that historical cost of equity can be deceptive for comparative purposes.

Finally, Merrill Lynch (1979) is enthusiastic about nursing home stocks, not only because of the large growth in nursing home demand that it anticipates due to demographic changes, but also because the outlook for chains seems to be favorable, given the growing amount of government regulation, the major thrust of which restricts supply.[33]

The large variability in profit rates may indicate that an inevitable "shaking out" of marginal firms in the industry is now taking place, after a period of extremely rapid growth; it may also indicate the absence of competition in the market. Or, it may indicate that government is becoming an increasingly effective monopsonistic buyer of nursing home services. Clearly, this is one area that needs further research.

Although we have analyzed profitability and growth as a national phenomenon, each State clearly has its own rules and regulations, enforcement mechanisms, and climate of profitability. Despite great effort, Scanlon (1980) was not satisfactorily able to explain variations in bed supply by State, but they do exist. Tables XVII–9 and XVII–10 show trend changes in the nursing home bed supply and changes in the bed population ratio between 1973 and 1976. Hopefully, future empirical research combining more recent data will give more insight into the reasons for these changes.

Productive Efficiency

As a concluding observation on the market performance of this industry, it is difficult to make statements about its productive efficiency. Very little empirical work has been done on the subject in the service sector. The currently accepted thought on productivity in the service sector is that it is difficult to achieve gains in productivity because the sector is so labor intensive; it is usually only in those sectors of the economy where large amounts of capital can be combined with labor that productivity gains may be achieved. A priori, one would suspect that cost-based forms of reimbursement would be likely to negatively affect efficiency. Nevertheless, Frech and Ginsburg (1980) have shown empirically that non-profit nursing home firms have higher costs than for-profit nursing home firms ". . . with a substantial part of the difference probably related to efficiency." They indicate that the robustness of their results ". . . implies that they are unlikely to be due simply to omitted patient mix and quality of care variables."

---

[33] Grimaldi (1982) maintains that new nursing home investment in California, Connecticut, Massachusetts, and Minnesota has virtually ceased. If this is true, whether it is the result of strict certificate of need laws or a lack of profitability has yet to be determined.

TABLE XVII-9
Change in Nursing Home Bed Supply, 1973–1976

Increasing		Decreasing	No Change
Alabama	Missouri	Arizona	Maine
Alaska	Montana	California	New Jersey
Arkansas	Nebraska	District of Columbia	New Mexico
Colorado	Nevada	Florida	Ohio
Connecticut	New Hampshire	Iowa	Wisconsin
Delaware	New York	Massachusetts	Wyoming
Georgia	North Carolina	Minnesota	
Hawaii	North Dakota	Oklahoma	
Idaho	Rhode Island	Oregon	
Illinois	South Carolina	Pennsylvania	
Indiana	South Dakota	Utah	
Kansas	Tennessee	Washington	
Kentucky	Texas		
Louisiana	Vermont		
Maryland	Virginia		
Michigan	West Virginia		
Mississippi			

Source: U.S. Department of Health and Human Services, Under Secretary's Task Force on Long-Term Care, 1980, "Report of the Work Group on Nursing Home Bed Supply," August 12, 1980.

Conclusion and Policy Implications

This industrial organization analysis of the nursing home industry has revealed three fundamental aspects of the market: (1) the buyers (or recipients, in the case of those whose care is purchased by government) of the industry's services seem to have a weaker market position than the buyers of most goods and services within the U.S. economy, mainly because of age-related limited physical and mental capacities; (2) given that it paid for 57 percent of nursing home services in 1979, government would seem to possess considerable monopsonistic buying power; and (3) partially related to (1) above, most nursing homes in the industry possess a certain amount of market power in their ability to pick and choose their patient population. Due to public reimbursement mechanisms and certificate of need regulations, public-pay patients probably feel the effects of that market power more fully than do private-pay patients, because the former represent the residual claimants on available nursing home beds.

Scanlon (1980) has argued persuasively that the public patient excess demand issue has both efficiency and equity implications. Although the analytic distinction between demand and need is

616

TABLE XVII-10
Changes in Bed/Population Ratios, 1973–1976

Increasing	Decreasing		No Change
Alabama	Arizona	Nevada	Connecticut
Alaska	California	New Jersey	Georgia
Arkansas	Delaware	New Mexico	Hawaii
Colorado	District of Columbia	North Dakota	Idaho
Michigan	Florida	Ohio	Illinois
Nebraska	Iowa	Oklahoma	Indiana
South Dakota	Kansas	Oregon	Louisiana
Tennessee	Kentucky	Pennsylvania	Maryland
Texas	Maine	South Carolina	Mississippi
Vermont	Massachusetts	Utah	Missouri
Virginia	Minnesota	Washington	Montana
		Wyoming	New Hampshire
			New York
			North Carolina
			Rhode Island
			West Virginia
			Wisconsin

Source: U.S. Department of Health and Human Services, Under Secretary's Task Force on Long-Term Care, 1980, "Report of the Work Group on Nursing Home Bed Supply," August 12, 1980.

clear, the amount of resources that society wishes to devote to the care of the elderly is not. Under the present system, some vague concept of need for *nursing home* care is funded and presented to the forces of the nursing home market. And the market reacts with predictable results. Public patients queue up behind private-pay patients, the less disabled are preferred to the more disabled, and, under present public financing, access to a nursing home becomes partially a function of geographic location.

By its very nature, the first fundamental aspect of this market is basically beyond the control of any person or institution. To some extent, the situation could be ameliorated if government provided more information to those elderly capable of accepting it and acting upon it, or to their relatives and friends. Some would argue that government is not using its monopsonistic power effectively. Because the quality dimension of the output of the nursing home industry is so important,[34] government could use reimbursement practices

---

[34] Quality is "important" in the sense that very few citizens would knowingly vote for reimbursement rates which were so low that the level of care provided in nursing homes actually caused the condition of the residents to deteriorate markedly.

617

in combination with enforced regulation to secure some level of quality. Much of the literature on regulation analyzes and empirically demonstrates that it does not achieve its stated goals, but this result seems to stem from the fact that regulation often attempts to work at cross purposes with market forces. In the end, poorly designed regulations seem to influence behavior powerfully in many perverse directions. Reimbursement practices that bend the profit motive in a sought-after direction could offer incentives for the achievement of quality objectives. Probably the most significant reform needed in reimbursement practices is recognition of different levels of debility and dependence.[35] Otherwise, nursing home operators have a positive incentive to first accept only less demanding cases. A restructuring of the reimbursement system and elimination of certificate of need regulations would probably have more expensive long-run effects. Given proper incentives, quality would improve. The industry would become more profitable, and thus we would expect the entry of more firms into it. The final result would no doubt be that total expenditures on nursing homes would increase.

Many would argue that the existing situation is not optimal both from the perspective of society as a whole and from the perspective of the elderly (General Accounting Office, 1979). Publicly-financed programs for the long-term care of the elderly are heavily biased toward the subsidization of the medical model in nursing home care to the virtual exclusion of subsidies for other forms of long-term care. Estimates vary (Congressional Budget Office, 1977), but it is generally agreed that there are many elderly in nursing homes who need not be there if alternative financial incentives and living arrangements were available. It would not be difficult to design such a system of financial incentives that would call forth a supply response on the part of providers of alternative forms of care. The investment model discussed in this chapter provides the basic incentive variables for this design. However, it is also agreed that a broadly-based subsidy program for alternative forms of long-term care would monetize presently-provided informal and family care.

---

[35] In this same vein, Mead Over offers a proposal similar to the one that we made earlier: nursing homes would bid on a daily rate that they are willing to accept for each hard-to-place patient. Each patient could have a separate market-clearing price. The bid, if accepted, must constitute a binding contract to perform a certain minimum set of services, and inspectors would visit periodically. Bonuses could be paid if the patient's functions were improved compared to his/her initial condition. The patient would have the option of paying the difference between the lowest bid and that of a preferred home. No home would be required to accept any patient. Despite some scandals involving high winning bids, followed by insufficient care, most homes, once they bid on an individual, would have an incentive to maintain him/her alive and healthy to minimize their costs without changing their reimbursement levels. Some homes would specialize in difficult cases.

Even though substitution would take place,[36] the end result would be that nursing homes would not be emptied, and the other forms of long-term care would be used more extensively (Congressional Budget Office, 1977; General Accounting Office, 1979). Perhaps societal expenditures *per elderly person* would decrease (though even this is not clear); it is virtually certain that total societal expenditures on the elderly would increase, even if the elderly were to remain a stable proportion of the population (Grimaldi and Sullivan, 1981).

Given the predicted shift in the age and debility distribution of the population (See Chapter III), the percentage of society's resources devoted to long-term care could be expected to increase dramatically. Thoughtful persons have expressed concern about this eventuality straining the social fabric.

The third fundamental aspect of the nursing home market (and, it would seem, of any market where the debilitated marginal elderly consume), namely the market power of providers, can be altered to a degree. A seller will always have some measure of market power if consumers are uninformed. But in this market, the characteristics of the marginal consumer may be qualitatively different than those of marginal consumers in other markets because of age-related disabilities. That is why an argument can be made that government, as the surrogate buyer of services, should provide as much information as can be used by consumers, and effectively use its monopsony power to create a proper balance of forces.[37]

---

[36] Price and income elasticities of substitution between alternative forms of long-term care have not yet been reliably estimated empirically.

[37] The theoretical literature implies that *local* government (probably at the State level) is the proper locus of such activity. The classic discussion on this subject is Tiebout (1956). Related discussions may be found in Borcherding and Deacon (1972), Epple and Zelenitz (1981), and Oates (1981).

Appendix

Accountants use the term "book rate of return," and people in finance speak of "maximizing cash flow." In essence, the accounting and finance approaches are the same.[1] The real rate of return is determined by the expected value of the future flow of receipts and outlays and is independent of the historical cost of the investment. On the other hand, the book rate of return, or cash flow approach, is determined by accounting conventions, which rely to a large extent on historical cost and are independent of future expectations. The book rate of return differs from the economist's definition of real rate of return because accounting definitions of net income differ from economic definitions of income and because accounting measures of capital diverge from its market value.

The economic concept of income is defined as the change in wealth from one period to the next, that is, the net change in consumption opportunities available. The accounting definition of net income is a cash flow which may or may not reflect the underlying economic realities because of the way in which revenues and costs are expensed. For example, a machine might have a real economic life of 10 years, after which it will have been completely exhausted and have zero value. If the value of the machine deteriorated at a constant rate, it would lose one-tenth of its value each year. If accelerated depreciation were allowed for tax purposes, the accountant would write the machine off at a more rapid rate than one-tenth per year. In this example, economic net income would be greater in the early years of the life of the machine than accounting net income; in later years, the opposite would be true.

McCaffree *et al* (1978) believe that a "more serious problem with book rates of return" arises because assets are typically carried on the books at their historical cost rather than at their current market value. The market is continually revising its expectations (as exemplified by movements of prices on stock exchanges), and the historical value of an asset may bear little relation to its market value.

Given the potential differences in the real rate of return and the book rate of return, especially in periods of inflation, any inquiry into the investment decision on nursing home care has to raise the question as to *which* rate of return the investor uses in his or her investment calculations. The answer seems to be: "portions of each." In the long run, fundamental economic values are deter-

---

[1] As McCaffrey *et al* (1978) point out, the accounting and financial literature recognizes the conceptual superiority of the real rate of return approach, but claims that it has limited usefulness because the real rate of return cannot be easily observed.

mined by the market forces that prevail. On the other hand, institutional circumstances do change, and these changes alter the time stream of revenues and outlays. Using equations (3) and (5), it is easy to see that the real rate of return will be higher: (a) the larger the difference between R and $(C + D)$, especially if that difference is greater in the early years of an investment, rather than in the later years and (b) the smaller the marginal tax rate, and *vice-versa*. Equation (6) illustrates the trade-off among decision parameters.

$$Y_o = \sum_{t=1}^{n} \frac{[R_t - (C_t + D_t)] (1 - \tau)}{(1 + i)^t} + \frac{S (1 - \tau)}{(1 + i)^n} + \frac{L (1 - \tau)}{(1 + i)^n}$$
(6)

High rates of depreciation in the early years of an investment bring about lower tax liabilities; tax laws which allow accelerated forms of depreciation or even linear depreciation, when the economic life of an asset is not linear, create high book after-tax rates of return and encourage further investment in other projects. Equipment maintenance costs may be written off as operating expenses, but they can also be viewed as extending the economic life of the assets involved. Expectations of continuing high rates of inflation engender expectations about increases in the values of R and C but also bring about increases in the values of S and L. Differences in the relative rates of inflation in these variables must also enter the investment calculations.

Conceptually, there should be no difference between an investment decision for a nursing home, or any other form of long-term care, and that for a steel mill. In a private market economy, the R in the investment equation would be the result of a forecast of the height, shape, and elasticity of the demand curve for nursing home care, other forms of long-term care, or for steel ingots. In the short run, accounting conventions, influenced by tax, legal, and institutional realities, would determine the time stream of receipts and outlays.

References

American Nursing Home Administration, *Nursing Home Fact Book* (Washington: ANHA, 1971).

Bain, Joe S., *Industrial Organization*, (New York: Wiley & Sons, Inc., 1959)

Baldwin, Carliss Y., "Nursing Home Finance: Capital Incentives Under Medicaid," Background Paper, University Health Policy Consortium, Brandeis University, July 1980.

Bishop, Christine E., "Nursing Home Cost Studies and Reimbursement Issues," *Health Care Financing Review*, Spring 1980, pp. 47–63.

Borcherding, Thomas E. and Robert T. Deacon, "The Demand for the Services of Non-Federal Governments," *American Economic Review*, Vol. LXII, December 1972, pp. 891–901.

Brody, Elaine, "Institutional Settings: Nursing Homes and Other Congregate

Living Facilities," Lecture, University of Southern California, July 16, 1969.

Congressional Budget Office, *Long-Term Care for the Elderly and Disabled* (Washington: U.S. Government Printing Office, August 1977).

Congressional Budget Office, *Long-Term Care: Actuarial Cost Estimates* (Washington: U.S. Government Printing Office, August 1977).

Day, Suzanne R., *Survey of Nursing Homes and Retirement Homes in the State of Delaware*, (Delaware: Bureau of Aging, 1972).

Di Paolo, Vincent, "Nursing Home Survey," *Modern Health Care*, June 1979.

Epple, Dennis and Allan Zelenitz, "The Roles of Jurisdictional Competition and of Collective Choice Institutions in the Market for Local Public Goods," *American Economic Review*, Vol. 71, No. 2 May 1981, pp. 87–92.

Feder, Judith and William Scanlon, "Intentions and Consequences of Regulating the Nursing Home Bed Supply, *Milbank Memorial Fund Quarterly*, Vol. 58, Winter 1980.

Fisher, Irving, *The Theory of Interest*, (New York: MacMillan, 1930).

Fox, Peter D. and Steven B. Clauser, "Trends in Nursing Home Expenditures: Implications for Aging Policies," *Health Care Financing Review*, Vol. 2, No. 2, Fall 1980.

Fraundorf, Kenneth C., "Competition and Public Policy in the Nursing Home Industry," *Journal of Economic Issues*, Vol. XI, No. 3, September 1977, pp. 601–634.

Fraundorf, Kenneth C., "The Nursing Home Industry: A Reply," *Journal of Economic Issues*, Vol. XII, No. 4, December 1978, pp. 922–927.

Frech, H. E. III and Paul B. Ginsburg, "The Cost of Nursing Home Care in the United States: Government Financing, Ownership, and Efficiency," paper presented at the World Congress on Health Economics, Leiden, The Netherlands, September 1980, revised November 1980.

Friedman, Milton, *Essays in Positive Economics* (Chicago: University of Chicago Press, 1952).

General Accounting Office, *Entering a Nursing Home—Costly Implications for Medicaid and the Elderly*, (Washington: U.S. Government Printing Office, November 1979).

General Accounting Office, *Home Health—The Need for a National Policy to Better Provide for the Elderly* (Washington: U.S. Government Printing Office, December 1977).

Gottesman, Leonard E., "Nursing Home Performance as Related to Resident Traits, Ownership, Size, and Source of Payment," paper presented at the Annual Meeting of the American Public Health Association, Mental Health Section, November 15, 1972.

Grabowski, Henry G., *Drug Regulation and Innovation* (Washington: American Enterprise Institute, 1976).

Grimaldi, Paul L. and Toni J. Sullivan, *Broadening Federal Coverage of Noninstitutional Long-Term Care* (Washington: American Health Care Association, 1981).

Grimaldi, Paul L., *Medicaid Reimbursement of Nursing Home Care* (Washington: American Enterprise Institute, 1982).

Grossman, Michael, *The Demand for Health: A Theoretical and Empirical Investigation* (New York: National Bureau of Economic Research, 1972).

Henderson, James M. and Richard E. Quandt, *Microeconomic Theory*, (New York: McGraw Hill, 1971).

622

Kahn, Alfred E., *The Economics of Regulation: Principles and Institutions* (New York: John Wiley and Sons, Inc., 1970).

Kent, Donald P., "Aging—Fact or Fancy," *The Gerontologist*, Vol. 5, No. 2, June 1965.

Liu, Korbin and Jana Mossey, "The Role of Payment Source in Differentiating Nursing Home Residents, Services, and Payments," *Health Care Financing Review*, Summer 1980.

Lowenthal, Marjorie, *Lives in Distress* (New York: Basic Books, Inc., 1964).

Lutz, Friedrich and Vera Lutz, *The Theory of Investment of the Firm* (Princeton: Princeton University Press, 1951).

McCaffree, Kenneth, Suresh Malhotra, John M. Wills, and Michael Morrissey, *Profits, Growth and Reimbursement Systems in the Nursing Home Industry,* (Seattle: Batelle Human Affairs Research Centers, 1978, HCFA Contract No. 600–77–0069).

Mendleson, Mary A., *Tender Loving Greed* (New York: Alfred A. Knopf, 1974).

Merrill Lynch, Pierce, Fenner and Smith, Inc., *Institutional Report: Nursing Home Industry Review*, October 31, 1979.

Moreland Act Commission on Nursing Homes and Residential Facilities, *Reimbursement of Nursing Home Property Costs: Pruning the Money Tree* (Albany: State of New York, 1976).

Newhouse, Joseph P., "The Erosion of the Medical Marketplace," in Richard Scheffler, ed. *Research in Health Economics*, Vol. 2 (Westport: J. A. I. Press, 1981) and Rand Publication R–2141–1–HEW, August 1978.

New York State Department of Health, *The Resident Patient Profile* (Albany: State of New York, 1971).

Noll, Roger, "The Consequences of Public Utility Regulation of Hospitals," in Institute of Medicine, *Controls on Health Care* (Washington: National Academy of Sciences, 1975).

Pincus, Allen, "Toward A Developmental Viewing of Aging for Social Work," *Social Work* Vol. 12, No. 3, July 1967.

Ruchlin, Hirsch S., "A New Strategy for Regulating Long-Term Care Facilities," *Journal of Health Politics, Policy and Law*, Vol. 1, September 1977, pp. 190–211.

Oates, Wallace E., "On Local Finance and the Tiebout Model," *American Economic Review*, Vol. 70, No. 2, May 1981, pp. 93–98.

Salkever, David S. and Thomas W. Bice, *Hospital Certificate of Need Controls: Impact on Investment, Costs and Use*, (Washington: American Enterprise Institute, 1979).

Samuelson, Paul A., *Foundations of Economic Analysis* (Cambridge: Harvard University Press, 1947).

Scanlon, William J. and Judith Feder, "Regulation of Investment in Long-Term Care Facilities," Urban Institute Working Paper, 1218–9, January 1980.

Scanlon, William J., "A Theory of the Nursing Home Market," *Inquiry*, Vol. 17, Spring 1980, pp. 25–41.

Scott, John E. and David A. Whitaker, Jr., "The Economics of Nursing Home Development," *Appraisal Journal*, Vol. 43, July 1975.

Sloan, Frank A., and Bruce Steinwald, "Effects of Regulation on Hospital Costs and Input Use," *Journal of Law and Economics*, Vol. XXIII, April 1980, pp. 81–109.

Stigler, George J., "The Theory of Economic Regulation," *Bell Journal of*

Economics and Management Science, Vol. 2, Spring 1971, pp. 3–21.

Tiebout, Charles M., "A Pure Theory of Local Government Expenditures," *Journal of Political Economy*, Vol. 64, No. 5, October 1956, pp. 416–424.

Townsend, Claire, *Old Age: The Last Segregation* (New York: Grossman, 1971).

U.S. Department of Commerce, Bureau of the Census, *1976 Survey of Institutionalized Persons*, (Washington: U.S. Government Printing Office, 1978).

U.S. Department of Health, Education, and Welfare, National Center for Health Statistics, *The National Nursing Home Survey 1977: Summary for the United States*, Vital and Health Statistics, Series 13, Number 43 (Washington: U.S. Government Printing Office, 1979).

U.S. Department of Health and Human Services, Health Care Financing Administration, Office of Legislation and Policy, *Long-Term Care: Background and Future Directions* (Washington: HCFA 81–20047, 1981).

U.S. Department of Health and Human Services, Under Secretary's Task Force on Long-Term Care, 1980, "Report of the Work Group on Nursing Home Bed Supply," August 12, 1980.

U.S. Senate, Subcommittee on Long-Term Care, *Nursing Home Care in the United States: Failure in Public Policy* (Washington: U.S. Government Printing Office, 1976).

Vladeck, Bruce C., *Unloving Care: The Nursing Home Tragedy* (New York: Basic Books, 1980).

Washington State Department of Social and Health Services, *The Needs of the Elderly 1978, An Analysis of the Needs of Older Citizens in Washington State* (Olympia: Washington State DSHS, 1978).

624

CHAPTER XVIII

Provider Incentives Under Alternative Reimbursement Systems

by Philip G. Cotterill

Introduction

In many parts of the country there is excess demand for nursing home care, and the persons most in need of that care often have the most difflculty obtaining it. Current public programs contribute to the excess demand by subsidizing institutional care much more heavily than community services and by restricting expansion of the nursing home supply of beds. At the same time, public programs do little to ration the limited number of beds so that persons with the greatest care needs can obtain the services they require. All too often, efforts to constrain public nursing home expenditures reinforce nursing homes' tendencies to skimp on the care they provide. "Skimping" may mean denying access to heavy care patients or providing poor quality care.

While Medicaid reimbursement systems cannot be blamed for all of these problems, their role as contributors to both the problems and the potential solutions is increasingly being examined. Attention has focused on how reimbursement incentives affect public patients' access to care (especially those with heavy care needs), quality of care, and cost.

Medicaid Reimbursement Policies

Three key ideas have influenced nursing home reimbursement methods in recent years. The first is that rates should be related to costs to elicit an adequate supply of acceptable quality care. The second is that retrospective cost reimbursement of the type traditionally used to pay hospitals by both public and private third parties is excessively costly. The third is that there is a potential conflict between cost containment and improvements in quality and access.

Section 249(a) of the 1972 Social Security Amendments reflected each of these ideas. Section 249 supported the basic principle of cost-related reimbursement, without requiring that it take the specific form of retrospective cost-based reimbursement. It also gave States flexibility in the ways they might incorporate cost containment incen-

A portion of this chapter was presented at the meetings of the Eastern Economic Association in Philadelphia, Pennsylvania, April 9–11, 1981. The author would like to thank Christine Bishop, William Scanlon, and Robert Seidman for their comments.

tives and in the emphasis to be placed on cost containment *vis-a-vis* quality and access. However, "reasonable cost-related" reimbursement, as mandated by Section 249, proved difficult to implement precisely because the term is quite general. Section 249 did not satisfy those who wanted to use reimbursement policy to improve quality and access, and it annoyed others who viewed it as federal interference in States' decision-making.

Dissatisfaction with Section 249 led to its being replaced by Section 962 of the Omnibus Reconciliation Act of 1980 (P.L. 96–499). Section 962 increases the authority and flexibility of the States in using reimbursement policy to restrain nursing home expenditures but does not totally abandon the concept of cost-related rates. It states that rates should be "reasonable and adequate to meet the costs which must be incurred by efficiently and economically operated facilities."

Even without Section 249, the view that cost-related rates were needed to improve quality and access for public patients would probably have influenced Medicaid reimbursement systems. In response to recurring criticism that their traditional flat rate systems failed to pay the costs of acceptable quality care, many States began adopting one form or another of a cost-related system in the late 1960s and early 1970s. According to Weiner and Lehrer (1981), by 1973, just after the passage of Section 249, only 16 States had a form of flat rates that clearly did not conform to the amendment.

By 1978, the most common Medicaid reimbursement system set prospective rates based on the past costs of the individual facility (AHCA, 1978). These rates are usually subject to ceilings based on the costs of groups of facilities (often categorized by factors such as certification status, bed size, and geographical location). In 1982 only five States (Arkansas, California, Louisiana, Oklahoma, and Texas) set rates for individual facilities on the basis of the costs of groups of facilities. For example, California classifies facilities by type of certification (SNF–ICF), location and bed size. The State pays each facility a *per diem* rate for routine services equal to the median *per diem* allowable cost of the facilities in the class. These group-based rate systems are essentially "flat rate" systems, in that the individual facility cannot significantly affect the rate it will receive by altering its own costs.[1]

Flat rate systems have been generally favored for their cost containment incentives and criticized for poor quality and access incen-

---

[1] This statement is generally correct as long as the number of facilities in a group is large. The statement oversimplifies to the extent that facilities can affect their rate by changing groups (for example, in some cases, it may be advantageous for an ICF to incur the higher staffing costs required to become an SNF). Even when changes of this type are possible, they would not be frequent events for an individual home.

626

tives. The reverse is true of systems that base rates on individual facility costs ("cost-based" systems). Providers will only be willing to accept heavy care patients or provide quality care if they can recover the additional costs they must incur by doing so. The introduction of cost limits or ceilings into cost-based systems has added a decidedly flat rate element to those systems. Ceilings strengthen the cost containment potential of these systems and essentially convert a cost-based system to a flat rate system for facilities for whom the ceiling is binding.

A few States have tried to improve either access, quality, or both, by relating a facility's rate (or ceiling rate) directly to the characteristics of its patients (Illinois, West Virginia, and Ohio). Other States have attempted to account for differences in the cost of patients' care needs by refining the level-of-care classification. However, the most detailed plan to influence admission practices, length of stay, and quality is the experiment in nursing home incentive payments, sponsored by the National Center for Health Services Research, which is being conducted in San Diego (Weissert et al, 1980). All of these reimbursement systems, in one way or another, acknowledge differences in the cost of caring adequately for different types of patients. As a result, they attempt to incorporate the good features of Medicare-style, cost-based reimbursement without inheriting the bad features as well. In this way, they attempt to improve the trade-off between higher costs and improvements in quality and access.

To analyze the impact of reimbursement alternatives on providers' incentives, it is necessary to cut through the diversity of reimbursement methods and identify critical differences. The fact that aspects of cost-based and flat rate reimbursement are now found in the same reimbursement system does not lessen the importance of the cost-based and flat rate distinction for analyzing differences in incentives. To the extent that the modifications have attempted to strengthen the weaknesses of cost-based and flat rate systems, analysis of simplified "pure" examples of these systems should highlight their respective weaknesses.

Overview of the Chapter

This chapter analyzes providers' incentives under pure (or "stylized") cost-based and flat rate systems and then draws inferences for specific aspects of actual, more complex reimbursement systems. Unlike previous studies of nursing homes' incentives under alternative types of reimbursement (Pollak, 1977; Vladeck, 1980), the analysis is conducted in the context of an explicit model of nursing home behavior. The basic nursing home model presented in the section on analytical framework is a slightly simplified composite of the model used in most previous economic studies (Abt Associates, 1979; Bishop, 1980; Grana, 1978; Palmer and Vogel, 1980;

Scanlon, 1980). Unlike some of these studies, we examine only the incentives of for-profit nursing homes, and we assume in general that homes provide services to both private and public patients. Further, the reimbursement of capital costs is not explicitly addressed.

The purpose of this chapter is not to explain nursing home behavior, but to identify the economic incentives inherent in different reimbursement systems. Nursing homes may or may not behave as predicted. They may have non-economic objectives, and/or they may not be maximizers. However, for the purpose of understanding alternative reimbursement methods, the incentives of the profit-maximizing firm are a useful benchmark.

We describe the basic assumptions of the model and the stylized reimbursement systems and present a graphical solution to the model. However, the basic model provides only limited insight into the incentives we wish to examine. Therefore, in subsequent sections, we expand the model to permit more explicit analysis of these incentives.

Scanlon (1980) and others have analyzed access incentives, while assuming that all Medicaid patients are alike. Bishop (1980) has analyzed incentives to provide an intensity of services measure of quality that is the same for both private and public patients. While also limiting our analysis to intensity measures of quality, we add separate case-mix and quality variables for private and public patients. These variables enable us to show that in general, firms have different incentives in providing care to private and public patients under both cost-based and flat rate reimbursement.

Because of the strong potential impact of excess demand for nursing home care on facilities' willingness to accept heavy care patients, we compare providers' incentives under alternative assumptions about the impact of market supply and demand conditions on the individual facility. We first compare cost-based and flat rate reimbursement under the assumption that a facility can fill its beds with whatever type of patient it chooses. Second, we compare the two types of reimbursement under the assumption that, to fill its beds, a facility must accept patients with greater care needs.

As might be expected, we find that facilities have no incentive to select Medicaid patients requiring special care when market conditions yield plenty of patients with light care needs, and Medicaid reimbursement discourages acceptance of heavier care patients. Perhaps unexpectedly, we find that this result holds for *both* cost-based and flat rate reimbursement, as long as a facility serves both Medicaid and private patients. Further, this result is independent of the *level* of Medicaid rates.

When facilities are unable to fill their beds solely with light care patients, the level of Medicaid rates has a significant impact on access incentives. Even in this case, however, cost-based reimbursement does not necessarily have a definite advantage over flat rate reimbursement. Much depends upon whether the severity of the public or the private case-mix is increasing more rapidly at the margin.

Finally, we attempt to draw from our analysis some implications for improving access and quality incentives by tailoring reimbursement rates to the specific care needs of a facility's case-mix. While a system of fixed rate differentials linked to case-mix or quality requirements may marginally improve incentives, reform of nursing home reimbursement systems cannot be expected to offset totally the influence of excess demand in accommodating providers' preferences for light care patients.

In the section on cost containment incentives, we analyze reasons for the weakness of cost control under cost-based reimbursement. We show that the incentive to inflate profits by over-reporting costs is probably the chief source of weak cost containment incentives under cost-based reimbursement. The weakness of cost containment incentives under cost-based reimbursement is frequently attributed to an absence of efficiency incentives. Efficiency incentives may be stronger than commonly believed, as long as the firms attempt to maximize profits and are not totally financed by cost-based systems.[2] For the same type of firm, we also show that the incentives to seek efficiency gains through innovation are identical under both cost-based and flat rate reimbursement, as long as the "search" costs of innovation are allowable costs.

A wide variety of cost control measures have been incorporated into cost-related systems: general cost limits, specific cost center limits, limits on administrative salaries, restrictions on transactions with related parties, and "efficiency allowances" (sometimes called incentive payments). An efficiency allowance is either a proportion, or the entire amount, of any difference between actual per diem costs and the cost limit.

Of these measures, limits on administrative salaries and restrictions on transactions with related parties are most directly applicable in counteracting the incentive to over-report costs under cost-based reimbursement. The other types of cost limits are more commonly viewed as methods of screening and penalizing inefficient providers. Efficiency allowances are typically intended to provide

---

[2] William Scanlon has pointed out that this argument assumes that there is no difference between accounting costs and economic costs. Assuming that profit maximization is based on the latter, firms may be willing to incur additional accounting costs, even if those costs are not fully reimbursed, as long as economic costs are reduced. For example, a firm may be willing to pay higher wages under cost-based reimbursement if the net cost of the higher wages is more than offset by reduced costs in labor turnover.

incentives for efficient operation. While efficiency allowances could be used to discourage cost over-reporting, our analysis suggests that, except for the predominantly Medicaid facility, they are not required as an efficiency incentive.

How tightly limits are set determines whether their primary impact is to screen relatively inefficient (or heavy case-mix) providers or to be a *de facto* flat rate. A cost-based system with strict general cost limits and 100 percent efficiency allowances creates essentially the same incentives as a flat rate system, in which the rate equals the cost limit of the cost-based system.

Finally, in the conclusion, we state the implications of our analysis for nursing home reimbursement reform given the larger problems of financing and excess demand which confront the long-term care system. We discuss both the limitations and the potential of reimbursement reform.

Analytical Framework

This chapter analyzes the incentives of a profit maximizing nursing home which provides care to both private and public patients. The private market is assumed to be monopolistically competitive by virtue of homes' differentiation of their service mix and location. Hence private demand for patient days is assumed to be inversely related to the price private patients are charged. Other things equal, private patients are assumed to be willing to pay higher *per diem* rates for more intensive care and greater amenities.

The quantity of public patient days demanded depends upon the eligibility criteria for the public program. (These criteria are independent of the rate paid nursing homes for public patients.) The nursing home is assumed to supply as many public patient days of care at the public rate as it wishes. That is, nursing home beds are in short enough supply that the facility faces a perfectly elastic supply of public patients at the given public rate.

The firm's costs depend upon its total output of private and public patient days, the level of general amenities, and the intensity of services provided. Licensure and certification standards for different levels of care are not explicitly included in the cost function. Implicitly, they are assumed to be constant with respect to the variables included in the model.

The model is a single period model. As a result, several interesting issues are excluded from the analysis: (1) Since the facility's bed size is taken as given, we do not investigate the impact of the reimbursement system on investment in beds. (2) Property costs are reduced to a single category of fixed costs, which does not change over time. Hence dynamic effects of property cost reimbursement, such as incentives to "traffic" in homes, are not ad-

630

dressed. (3) The model does not account for the conversion of private patients to Medicaid when their private resources are exhausted.

We analyze two simple stylized public reimbursement systems. First, in the cost-based system, the public rate is equal to the firm's average total cost. All costs incurred are assumed to be allowable, and there are no limits imposed on either specific cost components or on total cost. Cost is assumed to include a "normal" profit. Since only a single period exists, there is no distinction between retrospective and prospective rates. (In the appendix, we argue that differences in incentives under retrospective and prospective cost-based systems are of secondary importance.)

In the flat rate system, the public rate is exogenously determined by the rate setting authority. The important difference from the cost-based case is that the public rate is assumed to be independent of the facility's *own* costs. The rate may be determined in a variety of ways. For example, it may be based on the costs of a group of facilities. However, we assume that the nursing home cannot alter its rate by changing its characteristics to obtain advantageous reimbursement.

Under the cost-based system, the facility can influence its public rate by altering its costs. For example, if the facility incurs a lower average cost by choosing to produce a larger total output, it will receive a lower public rate than if it produced a smaller output. However, if it incurs costs that raise average cost (as a result of providing higher quality care or accepting a more severe case-mix), the public rate will be higher than it would be otherwise. In the flat rate system, the public rate does not respond to the individual facility's decisions regarding factors such as output, quality of care, and case-mix. This distinction is the main source of differences in incentives between the two types of reimbursement.

The firm's decision-making problem involves determining optimal (or profit-maximizing) values of key variables under its control. In the basic model, which we present first, the only "choice variables" are total output and the public-private output mix. Later in the chapter, we expand the list of choice variables to include public and private quality and case-mix levels, as well as other variables. "Decision rules" are the conditions that define the optimal values of the choice variables. Our analysis of incentives consists of deriving and then comparing the decision rules for each choice variable under the alternative reimbursement methods.

Figure XVIII–1 illustrates the solution to the basic model for both our cost-based and flat rate reimbursement systems. As will be proved more rigorously later, the decision rule for total output under both reimbursement systems involves choosing total output so that

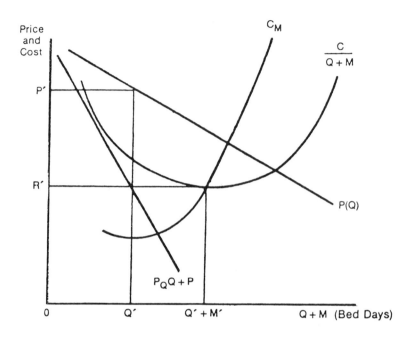

FIGURE XVIII-1
Profit Maximization Under
Cost-Based and Flat Rate Reimbursement

the revenue derived from another patient day is equal to the cost of an additional patient day. Given our assumption that it is profitable for the facility to produce both private and public patient days, and our assumptions about the private and public demand conditions, the decision rule is satisfied at output $Q' + M'$, where the public rate, R', equals marginal cost, $C_{M'}$.

The decision rule for allocating total output between private and public patient days is that the marginal profit earned on private and public patient days should be equal. In Figure XVIII–1, this rule requires choosing Q and M so that the private marginal revenue equals the public rate (at Q').

In Figure XVIII–1, we assume that the public rates are equal under cost-based and flat rate reimbursement. Under cost-based reimbursement, the rate is determined by (1) the decision rule for total output, which states that the rate should be equated to marginal cost and (2) the fact that our stylized cost-based reimbursement system pays a rate equal to average cost. For a U-shaped average cost curve, marginal cost and average cost will be equal at the minimum point of the average cost curve. Hence in Figure XVIII–1, R' is the cost-based rate. The flat rate is assumed to be equal to R'. The flat rate could be set either above or below R', and the same decision rules for total output and its allocation between private and public patient days would apply. Of course, the optimal values of total output and the public-private output mix would be different than when R equals R'.

Since the cost-based rate is endogenously determined by the average cost curve and the decision rules, it will be equal to R' unless the average cost curve shifts. Hence, while there are many possible flat rates, there is only one equilibrium cost-based rate for this facility for a given average cost curve.

While this discussion provides a basic understanding of the operation of the model and the reimbursement systems analyzed in the chapter, it provides very limited insights into the firm's incentives regarding access, quality, and cost containment. We will now expand the model to explore these issues.

Access and Quality Incentives

The limited empirical evidence indicates that nursing home access varies significantly for different types of patients. Using 1976 hospital discharge data from Massachusetts, Gruenberg and Willemain (1980) found evidence that nursing home placement took longer for Medicaid patients than for other patients, and particularly longer for Medicaid patients with special care needs. Other data of a more anecdotal nature support similar conclusions (U.S. Department of Health and Human Services, 1980).

633

Feder and Scanlon (1980) relate the placement problem to the existence of excess demand for nursing home beds. They state, "When nursing home beds are insufficient to satisfy demand, the people most in need of the service have the greatest difficulty finding it." Others, such as Gruenberg and Willemain, emphasize the role of the regulatory and reimbursement systems in determining homes' preferences for patients with light care needs. Analyses of alternative reimbursement systems have typically concluded that better access and quality incentives exist under cost-based than under flat rate reimbursement (Pollak, 1977; Vladeck, 1980).

None of the studies cited have systematically examined the interactions between bed supply and reimbursement methods in an explicit model of nursing home behavior. In the analysis that follows, we compare providers' access and quality incentives under alternative assumptions about the impact of market supply and demand conditions on the individual facility. We first compare cost-based and flat rate reimbursement under the assumption that a facility can fill its beds with whatever type of patient it chooses. In this case, output and case-mix are independent of one another. Second, we compare the two types of reimbursement under the assumption that, to fill its beds, a facility must accept patients with greater care needs. In this second case, case-mix levels and output are positively related.

To explicitly analyze facilities' incentives to accept patients with various levels of care needs, we add case-mix variables to the model. Private and public case-mix variables (S and T) are defined as the mean intensity of services required by the given caseload to meet a minimally acceptable standard of care. This standard of care is probably best thought of as one which is internal to the firm or is self-imposed. That is, it represents an intensity of care the firm feels compelled to provide if a given caseload is accepted. It could be interpreted as a legal standard, but we do not explicitly include non-compliance in the model. Hence it is simpler to regard the standard as firm specific.

S and T can be written as functions of a measure of patient characteristics: $S = S(Z)$, $T = T(Z)$. We assume that (1) each facility provides the same standard of care to public and private patients with the same characteristics ($S^i(Z)$, $= T^i(Z)$ for $i = 1, \ldots, n$, where n is the total number of facilities); (2) within each facility, patients with greater care needs (as measured by a higher value of Z) receive more intensive care (S_z^i, $T_z^i > 0$); and (3) across facilities, standards of care vary so that the same patient in one facility might receive a greater or lesser intensity of care if he or she were in another facility ($S^i(Z) \gtrless S^j(Z)$ and $T^i(Z) \gtrless T^j(Z)$ for i not equal to j).

Our single period model assumes that each facility staffs appropriately for the case-mix it selects and ignores adjustment problems associated with short-run changes in case-mix. Hence, assumptions (2) and (3) are consistent with the empirical result that, within a facility, the proportion of a facility's resources a patient receives increases to match greater care needs, but across facilities, no clear relationship exists between resource consumption and patient care needs (McCaffree et al, 1976).

Next we define private and public quality variables ($E - S$ and $F - T$), which measure the difference between the mean intensity of services actually provided and the minimum standard intensity of care. Taken together, the firm's choice of optimal case-mix levels measures the severity of the case-mix it is willing to accept, while the choice of optimal quality indicates whether or not the facility provides more than the minimum standard of care.

As in previous economic models of the nursing home, our quality variables are intensity measures. The implicit assumption is that more intensive care is better quality care. The model does not directly incorporate other concepts of quality, such as the extent to which services provided match independent professional judgment of care needs for the facility's patients. (See Shaughnessy and Kurowski (1980) for a discussion of this approach to quality.) However, we do introduce an independent standard of care needs in defining rate differentials as a means of improving quality incentives.

Finally, we include in the model one other quality variable. This variable (A) is analogous to Bishop's (1980) quality variable and is assumed to have the same value for both private and public patient days. We interpret this variable as reflecting the level of amenities that are shared in common by all of the facility's residents (such as the size and attractiveness of common dining, living, and recreation facilities).

Incorporating all these variables into the model, the firm's decision-making problem can be stated as follows:

$$\text{Maximize } \pi = PQ + RM - C \tag{1}$$

$$\text{Subject to: } P = P(Q, S, E - S, A) \tag{2}$$

where $P_Q \leq 0$, $P_S \geq 0$, $P_{E-S} \geq 0$, and $P_A \geq 0$.

$$C = C(Q, M, S, E - S, T, F - T, A) \tag{3}$$

$$C_i \geq 0 \text{ for all } i = Q, \ldots, A$$

$$C_M = C_Q \text{ for all } M = Q$$

$$C_S = C_T \text{ for all } S = T$$

$$C_{E-S} = C_{F-T} \text{ for all } (E-S) = (F-T)$$

Equation (1) states that total profit (π) is the sum of the revenues derived from private and public patient days ($PQ + RM$) minus total cost (C). The price charged private patients (P) is assumed to vary

635

inversely with the quantity of private patient days (Q) and directly with the private case-mix level (S), the private quality level ($E - S$), and the general amenities level (A).

The *per diem* price that an individual or his/her family is willing to pay is assumed to increase as the individual's care needs increase, because the cost of providing care in an alternative setting depends upon the individual's care needs. For example, a patient who requires a 24-hour private nurse at home would be willing to pay a higher nursing home rate than a patient who requires only limited home visits from a nurse. The more persons in the nursing home with greater care needs, the higher the private price the home can charge.

Similarly, if private patients place a positive value on receiving more care than the amount dictated by the facility's minimum standard, then the private price will rise as $E - S$ increases. As defined, $E-S$ cannot be negative because S is defined as the minimum standard of care that the home feels compelled to provide for a given caseload. Finally, if private patients value the general amenities offered by the home, the private price will be positively related to the amount of amenities offered.

Several assumptions are made about the cost function. First, marginal costs are assumed to be non-negative for all variables. Second, the home is assumed to treat equivalent patients in the same manner, regardless of whether they are public or private. Hence, the cost impact of an increase in Q, S, or $E - S$ is the same as that of an increase in M, T, or $F - T$ for equal values of the corresponding variables. This does not mean that the optimal values of the corresponding private and public variables will be equal.

Case 1: Case-Mix and Output are Independent

In Case 1, we assume that the facility can fill its beds with whatever types of patients it chooses, so that the private and public case-mix levels S and T are both choice variables. Under cost reimbursement, the first order conditions for profit maximization may be written as follows:

$$\pi_Q \quad = P_Q Q + P \qquad + R_Q M \quad - C_Q \qquad = 0 \quad (4)$$

$$\pi_M \quad = \qquad\qquad R + R_M M \quad - C_M \qquad = 0 \quad (5)$$

$$\pi_S \quad = (P_S - P_{E-S}) Q + R_S M \quad - (C_S - C_{E-S}) = 0 \quad (6)$$

$$\pi_{E-S} = \qquad P_{E-S} Q + R_{E-S} M \quad - C_{E-S} \qquad = 0 \quad (7)$$

$$\pi_T \quad = \qquad\qquad R_T M \quad - (C_T - C_{F-T}) = 0 \quad (8)$$

$$\pi_{F-T} = \qquad\qquad R_{F-T} M \quad - C_{F-T} \qquad = 0 \quad (9)$$

$$\pi_A \quad = P_A Q + \qquad R_A M \quad - C_A \qquad = 0 \quad (10)$$

Each of these equations reflects the basic principle of profit maximization that a choice variable should be increased up to the point at which the marginal revenue and the marginal cost are equal.

A significant asymmetry exists between the equations for the private variables (Q, S, and $E - S$) and those for the public variables (M, T, and $F - T$). Specifically, marginal revenue is derived from both private and public sources for the private variables, but only from public sources for the public variables. For example, the marginal revenue associated with a private patient day consists of that from private sources ($P_Q Q + P$) plus that from public sources ($R_Q M$). However, the marginal revenue of a public patient day ($R + R_M M$) is derived entirely from public sources. This asymmetry results because, in the cost-based reimbursement system, changes in total cost—incurred for either *public* or *private* patients—will in general alter the *public* rate. The presence in equations (4) through (10) of R_Q, R_M, R_S, R_{E-S}, R_T, R_{F-T}, and R_A reflects this fact.[3]

Under flat rate reimbursement, the public rate is independent of the individual facility's costs, so that R_Q, R_M, R_S, R_{E-S}, R_T, R_{F-T}, and R_A are all zero. Hence, the first order conditions for profit maximization under flat rate reimbursement are the following:

$$\pi_Q \quad = P_Q Q + P \qquad\qquad - C_Q \qquad\qquad = 0 \qquad (18)$$

$$\pi_M \quad = \qquad\qquad\qquad R \quad - C_M \qquad\qquad = 0 \qquad (19)$$

---

[3] When $R = \dfrac{C(Q, M, S, E - S, T, F - T, A)}{Q + M}$, the partial derivatives of R with respect to the arguments of the cost function can be written as follows:

$$R_Q = \frac{1}{Q + M}\left(C_Q - \frac{C}{Q + M}\right) \qquad (11)$$

$$R_M = \frac{1}{Q + M}\left(C_M - \frac{C}{Q + M}\right) \qquad (12)$$

$$R_S = \frac{C_S - C_{E-S}}{Q + M} \qquad (13)$$

$$R_{E-S} = \frac{C_{E-S}}{Q + M} \qquad (14)$$

$$R_T = \frac{C_T - C_{F-T}}{Q + M} \qquad (15)$$

$$R_{F-T} = \frac{C_{F-T}}{Q + M} \qquad (16)$$

$$R_A = \frac{C_A}{Q + M} \qquad (17)$$

637

$$\pi_S = (P_S - P_{E-S})Q \quad - (C_S - C_{E-S}) = 0 \qquad (20)$$

$$\pi_{E-S} = P_{E-S}Q \quad - C_{E-S} = 0 \qquad (21)$$

$$\pi_T = \quad - (C_T - C_{F-T}) = 0 \qquad (22)$$

$$\pi_{F-T} = \quad - C_{F-T} = 0 \qquad (23)$$

$$\pi_A = P_A Q \quad - C_A = 0 \qquad (24)$$

Under each type of reimbursement, the first order conditions enable us to determine the profit maximizing values of (1) total output, (2) the allocation of public and private patient days, (3) the private case-mix and quality levels, (4) the general amenities level, and (5) the public case-mix and quality levels.

Total Output

The results for total output presented in this section are the same as those illustrated graphically in Figure XVIII-1. Given our assumptions that (1) it is profitable for the facility to provide care to both private and public patients, and (2) the facility can provide as many public patient days as it wishes at the public rate, the first order conditions for public patient days (equations (5) and (19)) will determine total output. (At the output margin, the marginal revenue of a public patient day will exceed that of a private patient day. If this were not the case, the facility would provide only private patient days.) Substituting equation (12) for R_M in equation (5) and simplifying terms yields the following decision rule for the profit-maximizing total output under cost-based reimbursement:

$$\frac{Q}{Q+M}\left(R - C_M\right) = 0 \qquad (25)$$

Hence, cost-based reimbursement requires that total output be chosen so that the public rate equals marginal cost. Since R also equals average cost in our stylized cost-based reimbursement system, it follows that the optimal total output is the output at which average cost reaches its minimum.

In the flat rate case, equation (19) determines total output. As in the cost-based case, the firm should equate marginal cost and the public rate. However, since R is exogenous, total output depends upon the choice of the rate-setting authority. If R is equal to minimum average cost, total output would be the same as in the cost-based case.

Public-Private Allocation of Output

The results for the public-private output mix presented in this section are the same as those illustrated graphically in Figure XVIII-1. Under both cost-based and flat rate reimbursement, the profit-

638

maximizing allocation of total output between public and private patient days requires that private marginal revenue $(P_Q Q + P)$ be equated to the public rate (R):

$$P_Q Q + P = R \qquad (26)$$

This condition can be derived from equations (4) and (5) for the cost-based case and from equations (18) and (19) for the flat rate case. Hence, for equal public rates, cost-based and flat rate reimbursement yield the same profit-maximizing, public-private mix of patient days. A flat rate less than the cost-based rate will yield a lower public-private mix, and *vice-versa.*

Private Case-Mix and Quality

Cost-based reimbursement subsidizes a more severe private case-mix and a higher quality level than would be chosen under flat rate reimbursement. The subsidy effect is due to the presence of $R_S M$ and $R_{E-S} M$ in equations (6) and (7). The subsidy effect is absent under flat rate reimbursement (equations 20 and 21).

This comparison can be made in a more straightforward manner. Substituting equation (14) for R_{E-S} in equation (7) and simplifying terms yields the following decision rule for private quality under cost-based reimbursement:

$$P_{E-S} = \frac{C_{E-S}}{Q + M} \qquad (27)$$

Substituting equation (13) for R_S and equation (27) for P_{E-S} in equation (6) yields the following decision rule for private case-mix severity under cost-based reimbursement:

$$P_S = \frac{C_S}{Q + M} \qquad (28)$$

(Note that equation (28) assumes that equation (27) holds, that is, that quality is chosen optimally. Equations (27) and (28) also assume that the second derivatives of the P and C functions permit interior solutions to exist for positive values of S and $E - S$.)

Under flat rate reimbursement, the decision rule for private quality can be written:

$$P_{E-S} = \frac{C_{E-S}}{Q} \qquad (29)$$

Substituting equation (29) for P_{E-S} in equation (20) and rearranging terms yields the following condition for optimal private case-mix under flat rate reimbursement:

$$P_S = \frac{C_S}{Q} \qquad (30)$$

639

A comparison of equations (27) and (28) with equations (29) and (30) yields the following interpretation: Under cost-based reimbursement, the subsidy effect permits the facility to average the marginal costs of increased case-mix severity and higher quality over both private and *public* patient days. Under flat rate reimbursement, it only pays to increase private case-mix severity and quality to the point where private willingness to pay a higher rate (P_{E-S} and P_S) equals the marginal cost per private patient day (C_{E-S} and C_S).

However, under both reimbursement systems, facilities may be willing to provide a higher quality of private care than the minimum level associated with the optimal private case-mix severity. The key factor under both types of reimbursement is the private willingness and ability to pay for higher quality (P_{E-S}).

General Amenities

Formally, the decision rules for general amenities are the same as for private quality. Substituting equation (17) for R_A in equation (10) and simplifying yields the following expression:

$$P_A = \frac{C_A}{Q + M} \tag{31}$$

For flat rate reimbursement, rearranging equation (24) yields:

$$P_A = \frac{C_A}{Q} \tag{32}$$

Hence, applying exactly the same argument we used for private case-mix and quality, we see that cost-based reimbursement encourages a higher level of general amenities than does flat rate reimbursement.

However, while public patients receive no benefits from cost-based reimbursement's subsidization of a more severe private case-mix and higher private quality, they may benefit from a higher level of general amenities. As Bishop (1980) points out in a slightly different context, the benefits will not be evenly distributed among public patients. They will accrue to those public patients fortunate enough to gain access to homes where the private patients are willing (and able) to pay for general amenities. Of course, homes of this type will typically be unwilling to accept many public patients.

Public Case-Mix and Quality

Equation (9) implies that under cost-based reimbursement the level of public quality should be chosen so that the additional revenue derived from an increase in public quality equals the marginal cost of such an increase. However, substituting for R_{F-T} from equation (16), we can show that the marginal revenue associated with higher public quality ($R_{F-T}M$) is always less than the marginal cost of higher public quality, as long as the facility has some private patients $\left(\frac{M}{Q+M} \neq 1 \right)$:

640

$$R_{F-T}M = \frac{M}{Q+M}C_{F-T} \qquad (33)$$

Since the facility cannot cover its marginal cost of providing quality above the minimum standard, the profit-maximizing response is to provide only minimum standard care to public patients. That is, equation (9) can only be satisfied by setting C_{F-T} equal to zero, as long as $\frac{M}{Q+M} \neq 1$. In turn, C_{F-T} will be zero when F, the actual intensity of care provided, equals T, the minimum standard of care required by the public case-mix. Since F and T are measured in the same units, C_{F-T} is the segment of the C_T function for $F \geqslant T_0$, where T_0 is any given value of T. Hence, by definition, C_{F-T} is always zero for $F = T$.

The optimal public case-mix level can be determined from equation (8). Letting $C_{F-T} = 0$ and substituting equation (15) for R_T in equation (8), we can show that, just as in the case of public quality, the marginal revenue of an increase in T, ($R_T M$), will always be less than the marginal cost, C_T:

$$R_T M = \frac{M}{Q+M}C_T \qquad (34)$$

Hence, the profit-maximizing response is to minimize the public case-mix level. (Equation (8) can only be satisfied as an equality by setting $C_T = 0$ as long as $\frac{M}{Q+M} \neq 1$. Although it may not be possible to satisfy equation (8) as an equality, we interpret it as implying that the facility selects as light a public case-mix as possible.)

While cost-based reimbursement partially covers the marginal costs of higher public quality and case-mix levels, equations (22) and (23) show that flat rate reimbursement provides the facility no compensation for these marginal costs. As a result, the firm's incentives, as under cost-based reimbursement, are to minimize public quality and case-mix severity.

Comparison of the public case-mix and quality results under the two types of reimbursement yields an important insight: for a profit-maximizing firm, reimbursing only a portion of marginal cost has the same effect on incentives as paying none of the marginal cost. To induce the firm to accept a more severe public case-mix, or to provide more than minimal quality care, it is necessary to fully cover the accompanying marginal costs.

Case 2: Case-Mix Depends on Output

In contrast to Case 1, in Case 2 we assume that the facility cannot readily fill its beds with the patients of its choice. Instead, we assume that mean case-mix levels will be higher for larger outputs: [4]

$$S = S(Q) \qquad S_Q \geq 0$$
$$T = T(M) \qquad T_M \geq 0 \tag{35}$$

Because the model is static, the facility does not admit patients sequentially, but rather selects all its patients and patient days simultaneously. Thus the S and T functions represent ordered queues of potential patients (patient days) in ascending order with respect to care needs. Since the firm would always prefer patient days requiring less nursing care, rational ordering of the queue rules out the possibility that S_Q and T_M might be negative. In contrast to the previous case in which case-mix and output were independent, S and T are no longer choice variables for the firm. Instead, they are endogenous variables, the values of which are determined by the optimal values of Q and M. In other respects, the firm's decision-making problem is the same as in Case 1.

Under cost-based reimbursement, the first order conditions for profit maximization can be written:

$$\pi_Q = (P_Q + P_S S_Q - P_{E-S} S_Q) Q + P + R_Q M \\ - (C_Q + C_S S_Q - C_{E-S} S_Q) = 0 \tag{36}$$

$$\pi_M = R + R_M M - (C_M + C_T T_M - C_{F-T} T_M) = 0 \tag{37}$$

$$\pi_{E-S} = P_{E-S} Q + R_{E-S} M - C_{E-S} = 0 \tag{38}$$

$$\pi_{F-T} = R_{F-T} M - C_{F-T} = 0 \tag{39}$$

$$\pi_A = P_A Q + R_A M - C_A = 0 \tag{40}$$

Equations (38), (39), and (40) are the same as (7), (9), and (10). Hence, the decision rules for private and public quality and general amenities are the same in Case 2 as they were in Case 1. The first order conditions for Q and M (equations (36) and (37)) are more complicated than in Case 1, since now S depends on Q, and T depends on M.[5] However, they still have the same meaning: that Q and M should be chosen so that their respective marginal revenues equal their marginal costs.

---

[4] It would be more complete to write $S = S[Z(Q)]$ and $T = T[Z(M)]$. As in Case 1, we can subsume Z, the index of patient characteristics, without loss of content. Consistent with the assumptions made in Case 1, S and T in Case 2 are assumed to be equal for equal values of Z. However, it does not follow that S and T are equal when Q equals M, because Z may have different values when Q and M are equal.

Under flat rate reimbursement, R_Q and R_M are zero, as they were in Case 1. Hence, the first order conditions for profit maximization under flat rate reimbursement are the following:

$$\pi_Q = (P_Q + P_S S_Q - P_{E-S} S_Q)\, Q + P$$
$$\qquad - (C_Q + C_S S_Q - C_{E-S} S_Q) \qquad = 0 \quad (41)$$

$$\pi_M = R - (C_M + C_T T_M - C_{F-T} T_M) \qquad = 0 \quad (42)$$

$$\pi_{E-S} = P_{E-S} Q \qquad - C_{E-S} \qquad = 0 \quad (43)$$

$$\pi_{F-T} = \qquad - C_{F-T} \qquad = 0 \quad (44)$$

$$\pi_A = P_A Q \qquad - C_A \qquad = 0 \quad (45)$$

Equations (43), (44), and (45) are the same as (21), (23), and (24). As a result, the Case 1 analysis of the decision rules for private and public quality and general amenities is directly applicable to Case 2. For this reason, we will focus our attention on the determination of the profit-maximizing values of (a) total output and (b) the allocation of public and private patient days. The optimal private and public case-mix levels are determined by evaluating the S and T functions at the optimal values of Q and M.

Total Output

If we make the same assumptions that we did in Case 1, then the first order conditions for public patient days (equations (37) and (42)) will determine total output. Equation (37) can be simplified by substituting equation (37a) for R_M and combining terms. If we also use the result that optimal public quality requires that $C_{F-T} = 0$, then equation (37) can be written:

$$\frac{Q}{Q + M} \left[R - (C_M + C_T T_M) \right] = 0 \qquad (46)$$

Equation (46) implies that under cost-based reimbursement, total output should be chosen so that the public rate equals the marginal

[5] R_Q and R_M are interpreted the same way as in Case 1. However, they are defined slightly differently:

$$R_Q = \frac{1}{Q + M} \left[(C_Q + C_S S_Q - C_{E-S} S_Q) - \frac{C}{Q + M} \right] \qquad (36a)$$

$$R_M = \frac{1}{Q + M} \left[(C_M + C_T T_M - C_{F-T} T_M) - \frac{C}{Q + M} \right] \qquad (37a)$$

R_{E-S}, R_{F-T}, and R_A are the same as in Case 1. See equations (14), (16), and (17).

643

cost of a public patient day. In turn, since R equals average cost, the firm should produce at the output where average cost reaches its minimum point. The only difference between Cases 1 and 2 is that in Case 2, average and marginal costs rise as output rises, in part because case-mix levels rise.

Under flat rate reimbursement, C_{F-T} will also be zero, so equation (42) can be written:

$$R - (C_M + C_T T_M) = 0 \qquad (47)$$

Equation (47) implies that total output should be chosen so that the public rate equals the marginal cost of a public patient day. Consequently, the same decision rules apply under both types of reimbursement. As in Case 1, equal public rates will yield equal optimal total outputs under both types of reimbursement.

Public-Private Allocation of Output

In Case 2, the rules for allocating total output between private and public patient days reflect the same principle as in Case 1 (that the marginal profitability of a private and public day should be equated). However, the specific form of the decision rules differs from Case 1 as a result of the S and T functions. For cost-based reimbursement, the following condition is derived from equations (36) and (37):

$$(P_Q + P_S S_Q) Q + P = R + \frac{Q}{Q + M} \left[C_S (S_Q - T_M) \right] \qquad (48)$$

For flat rate reimbursement, the following condition is derived from equations (41) and (42):

$$(P_Q + P_S S_Q) Q + P = R + C_S (S_Q - T_M) \qquad (49)$$

In deriving equations (48) and (49), we have assumed that private and public quality are chosen optimally. That is, we have substituted equation (27) for P_{E-S} in equation (36) and equation (29) for P_{E-S} in equation (41). In addition, we have assumed that C_{F-T} is zero.

Unlike Case 1, equal public rates are not sufficient to yield the same profit-maximizing, public-private mix of patient days under cost-based and flat rate reimbursement. In Case 2, the optimal patient mix depends on both the relative severity of marginal case-mix $(S_Q - T_M)$ and the type of reimbursement. There are three possible relationships between private and public marginal case-mix severity: (1) When $(S_Q - T_M) > 0$, the mean intensity of care requirement is increasing more rapidly for the *private* than for the public patients in the neighborhood of the optimal solution; (2) when $(S_Q - T_M) < 0$, the *public* patients' care requirement is increasing

644

more rapidly at the margin than that of the private patients; (3) if $S_Q = T_M$, equations (48) and (49) reduce to the same decision rule that applied in Case 1. That is, output should be allocated between private and public patient days so that the public rate is equal to the private marginal revenue of a private patient day.

The relative severity of marginal case-mix has the following impact on the public-private mix of patient days: if $(S_Q - T_M) > 0$, the greater the difference, the larger the public share of total output. That is, the greater the amount by which the private marginal case-mix severity exceeds that of the public case-mix, the greater the extent to which the facility will substitute public for private output. Conversely, if $(S_Q - T_M) < 0$, the larger the absolute value of the difference, the smaller the public proportion of output, that is, the greater the amount by which the public marginal case-mix severity exceeds that of the private case-mix, the greater the extent to which the facility will substitute private for public output.

Assume that private marginal revenue—the left side of equations (48) and (49)—declines for greater Q. When $(S_Q - T_M) > 0$, a greater positive addition to the right side of equations (48) and (49) implies a greater optimal private marginal revenue and a smaller optimal value of Q. Conversely, when $(S_Q - T_M) < 0$, a greater value subtracted from the right side of equations (48) and (49) implies a lower optimal private marginal revenue and a larger optimal value of Q.

The type of reimbursement system also affects the optimal public-private output mix. For a given difference, $(S_Q - T_M) > 0$, a smaller proportion of public output will result under cost-based than under flat rate reimbursement. However, for a given difference, $(S_Q - T_M) < 0$, a greater proportion of public output will result under cost-based than under flat rate reimbursement. When the severity of the private case-mix is increasing faster than the severity of the public case-mix, cost-based reimbursement pays a part $\left(\dfrac{M}{Q + M} \right)$ of the difference in marginal cost attributable to the private patients, and vice-versa. This is reflected by the presence of $\dfrac{Q}{Q + M}$ in equation (48). Only $\dfrac{Q}{Q + M}$ of the marginal costs due to relative case-mix severity are not covered under cost-based reimbursement.

Two general conclusions emerge from this analysis of the public-private allocation of output. One is that we do not know enough about the probable shapes of the S and T functions to make explicit statements about their impact on the public-private mix. Note also that comparisons of case-mix levels are not helpful in evaluating the sign of $(S_Q - T_M)$. For example, $(S_Q - T_M)$ could be positive even if S were less than T. Second, neither reimbursement system unambiguously provides better access incentives for public or private patients. Cost-based reimbursement tends to cushion the negative effect on access caused by a relatively worse marginal case-mix. Hence, if $(S_Q - T_M) < 0$, cost-based reimbursement will be better for public patients than flat rate reimbursement. However, if $(S_Q - T_M) > 0$, the converse will be true.

Comparison of Cases 1 and 2

These analyses demonstrate that supply and demand conditions have a significant effect on the incentives of providers to accept public patients with special care needs. When market conditions permit providers to fill their beds with the patients of their choice (Case 1), neither of our stylized reimbursement systems offers providers any incentive to accept public patients with anything but the lightest care needs. Contrary to common opinion, cost-based reimbursement has no advantage over flat rate reimbursement.

Under both cost-based and flat rate reimbursement, raising public rates will expand access for public patients by (a) increasing total patient days (subject to the fixed beds constraint) and (b) increasing the proportion of public patient days. However, in Case 1, higher public rates will not increase access for public patients with heavier care needs.

The patient day method of apportioning costs to public patients under cost-based reimbursement does not provide any incentive for the individual facility to accept public patients who will raise the average severity of the public case-mix. This is because the cost apportionment method reimburses only a portion of the increased costs due to increased severity of the public case-mix. None of these costs are reimbursed under flat rate reimbursement, but the effect on incentives is the same as in the cost-based case.

Finally, patient day cost apportionment has a perverse effect from the point of view of the public program. Since the public rate depends on costs, whether they are incurred for public or private patients, cost-based reimbursement subsidizes a more severe private case-mix than is optimal under flat rate reimbursement.

In Case 2, where the output and case-mix levels are not independent of each other, the impact of the level of rates and the cost apportionment process on access incentives cannot be separated. In contrast to Case 1, higher public rates not only alter total output and the public-private allocation of total output, they also induce a facility to accept a more severe case-mix under both cost-based and flat rate reimbursement. A higher public rate enables the facility to fully cover the marginal costs of patient days requiring more intensive services.

In Case 2, patient day cost apportionment affects the profit-maximizing rule for allocating total output between public and

646

private patient days. Patient day cost apportionment cushions the negative impact on access for the type of patient whose mean case-mix is increasing more rapidly. Whether a more severe private case-mix is induced under cost-based than under flat rate reimbursement, as in Case 1, depends upon whether the severity of the private or public case-mix is increasing more rapidly at the margin. Neither type of reimbursement system unambiguously offers better access incentives. However, both cost-based and flat rate systems offer better access incentives than they did in Case 1.

Finally, some of the model's implications for quality incentives should be noted. In both Case 1 and Case 2, it is optimal for the facility to provide only the minimum level quality of care to public patients. This result differs from that for case-mix, where the optimal level of public case-mix rises when heavier care patients must be accepted to attract the optimal number of patients. The difference results from the fact that in neither Case 1 nor Case 2 is it necessary for the firm to raise quality to attract public patients ($F - T$ is not a function of M).

In general, a facility will have an economic incentive to provide a higher level of quality to provide patients than to public ones. (As long as $P_s > 0$, the optimal value of $E - S$ will exceed the optimal value of $F - T$ in both Case 1 and Case 2.) This result also suggests that some public patients or their families may be willing to (illegally) supplement the public rate to obtain higher quality care. We know of no empirical evidence to support either the hypothesis that quality levels differ between private and public patients within the same facility or that public patients supplement the public rate.

Both our case-mix and quality variables are more difficult to measure than are the actual intensity of services variables, E and F. Therefore, it is of empirical interest to summarize the predictions of the model for the private and public intensity variables. Recall that E and F depend on both the case-mix and quality decisions of the firm.

In Case 1, we would expect private intensity, E, to exceed public intensity, F, because both S and $E - S$ are expected to be greater than T and $F - T$. In addition, since cost-based reimbursement subsidizes a more severe private case-mix and higher quality than would occur under flat rates, the difference between E and F is expected to be greater under cost-based than under flat rate reimbursement.

In Case 2, we cannot predict the relationship between E and F a priori. Although private quality is expected to exceed public quality, we do not know which case-mix level will be greater. We can, however, predict that the difference (in absolute value) between E and F will be smaller under cost-based than under flat rate reimbursement. Since cost-based reimbursement tends to cushion the negative access effects of the case-mix that is relatively severe at the margin, the difference (in absolute value) between S and T will be smaller under cost-based than under flat rate reimbursement.

Improving Access and Quality Incentives
Through Reimbursement Reform

Our model suggests two approaches to improving access and quality through reimbursement reform, and, at the same time, indicates problems with their implementation.

First, Case 1 suggests that the way to improve access and quality incentives is to alter the patient day cost apportionment method under cost-based reimbursement so that the full marginal costs of public patients' care needs are reimbursed. In principle, this can be achieved by basing the public rate solely on public patients' costs. Assume the total cost function is separable so that R can be defined as the average total cost of a public patient day: $R = \dfrac{C\,(M, T, F - T)}{M}$ (We ignore the practical difficulties that might complicate efforts to isolate public costs.) Then substituting for R_T in equation (8), the first order condition for optimal T in Case 1, we obtain the following condition:

$$\frac{(C_T - C_{F-T})}{M} M - (C_T - C_{F-T}) = 0 \qquad (50)$$

Similarly, substituting for R_{F-T} in equation (9) yields the following condition for optimal public quality in Case 1:

$$\left(\frac{C_{F-T}}{M}\right) M - C_{F-T} = 0 \qquad (51)$$

Since equations (50) and (51) are satisfied for all values of T and $F - T$, the facility should, in principle, be neutral with respect to the case-mix and quality levels of public patients.[6] (The public subsidization of private case-mix and quality under cost-based reimbursement would also disappear.)

There is, of course, a flaw in this solution to the access problem.[7] Although a facility would not face the previous disincentive to accept heavy care public patients, neither would it have any incentive to control the costs of caring for these patients. Whatever the level

---

[6] In practice, there may be other reasons why facilities would continue to avoid heavy care patients. (See Bishop, Plough, and Willemain (1980), pp. 35–36.)

[7] The problem extends beyond determination of the optimal T and $F - T$ to the determination of total output (equation (5) for Case 1 and equation (37) for Case 2). Public output (and, in turn, total output) is indeterminate because total profit on public patient days is the same for all potential outputs.

of costs incurred, public rates adjust to fully cover those costs. This case illustrates the familiar tradeoff (commonly associated with cost-based reimbursement) between cost containment or efficiency incentives and access/quality incentives.

An alternative method of improving access and quality incentives is to modify flat rate reimbursement so that rates depend, at least in part, on the severity of the individual facility's public case-mix. For example, in Case 1, suppose equations (8) and (9) were adapted so that R_T and R_{F-T} represented fixed rate differentials linked to increases in T and $F - T$. In this case, the facility's optimal public case-mix severity and quality would be determined as follows:

$$R_T = \frac{C_T}{M} \tag{52}$$

$$R_{F-T} = \frac{C_{F-T}}{M} \tag{53}$$

With R_T as a fixed case-mix rate differential, the facility would have an incentive to increase T until the net marginal cost of increased case-mix severity per patient day equals R_T. For quality, there would also be an incentive to increase $F-T$ until the marginal cost of increased quality was equal to R_{F-T}. This solution is illustrated in Figure XVIII-2. We assume that the marginal costs $\frac{C_T}{M}$ and $\frac{C_{F-T}}{M}$ are initially less than the respective rate differentials R_T and R_{F-T} but that they increase as T and $F-T$ increase, so that interior solutions exist for positive values of T and $F-T$.

How would the rate-setting authority determine values for R_T and R_{F-T}? The policy goal of increasing access for heavy care patients does not imply a clear standard for determining R_T. Further, since T is defined in terms of a minimum care standard that may vary among facilities, the same R_T will affect access differently in different facilities. For simplicity, we just assume that R_T is determined to meet some desired access objective.

It is a little easier to specify guidelines for the determination of a quality rate differential, R_{F-T}. The critical questions are (1) how can the care standard (quality of care) that the State is willing to pay for be defined and (2) can the facility be induced to provide the acceptable quality level of care? Although our analysis can be applied in general, we limit our discussion to the case in which the facility's minimum standard of care is less than the State's acceptable level of quality. In this case, a positive rate differential, R_{F-T}, is required to induce an increase in the quality level.

Following the process approach to quality, we define the State's acceptable level of care in terms of the mean intensity of services (for example, nursing hours per day) for a specific group of patients.

649

FIGURE XVIII-2
Equilibrium Public Casemix and Quality
Levels for Given Fixed Rate Differentials

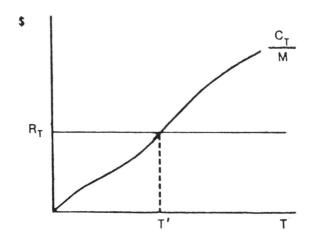

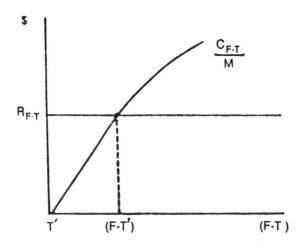

We assume that this quality standard, T, represents a consensus of professional judgment about the care needs of specific groups of patients. This approach to quality is described in Shaughnessy and Kurowski (1980, 1981) and has been incorporated into the Medicaid reimbursement system instituted in Ohio in July 1981.

The quality standard $\overline{T}$ can be used to determine the appropriate R_{F-T}. Our model implies that for every R_T, there exists an R_{F-T} such that the following condition holds:

$$T' + (F-T)' = \overline{T} \qquad (54)$$

That is, for every case-mix rate differential, there is a quality rate differential that will induce the facility to provide the State's acceptable quality of care to the group of patients selected by the facility.

Limitations

Although the fixed rate differential approach is preferable to full cost reimbursement that eliminates all cost containment incentives, it too faces numerous difficulties. Incorporation of case-mix and quality differentials into the reimbursement system involves, first, determination of appropriate measures of case-mix and quality and, second, determination of appropriate rate differentials for these measures. Case-mix severity must be measured in a manner that can be readily assessed and monitored. The case-mix measure should not be subject to easy manipulation by providers for their reimbursement advantage. Finally, linking rate differentials to suitable case-mix measures is not a simple process.

Walsh (1979) has described the problems of patient-related reimbursement based on the Illinois experience. He cites the administrative complexity that results from regular patient assessment. In Illinois, SNF patients are evaluated every 60 days, and ICF patients once every quarter. The administrative costs approach $4 million per year. Another administrative problem concerns the autonomy and authority conferred on caseworkers by the periodic patient evaluation process, which creates potential problems ranging from inconsistency and arbitrariness to corruption.

Finally, there is the problem of relating differences in patient conditions to differences in the cost of providing care. Particularly troublesome is the fact that if the reimbursement system pays more than it costs the facility to provide a service, such as feeding a bedridden patient, an incentive is created to keep as many patients bedridden as possible.

Various measures have been proposed as a basis for defining rate differentials, ranging from discrete categories (Ruchlin, Levey, and Muller, 1975) to continuous measures. One possible discrete approach is to adapt the diagnostic related group (DRG) concept to nursing homes to define sets of patient conditions (not necessarily

651

based on diagnosis) associated with differential resource utilization (Fries and Averill, 1980). The Illinois point count system (Walsh, 1979) is an example of a continuous measure.

Various ways of arriving at appropriate rate differentials have also been suggested. Both Walsh (1979) and Dean and Skinner (n.d.), have proposed regression analysis; Walsh also discusses engineering time and motion studies. There are problems with all of these methods, but it is not possible at present to specify a most feasible approach. Results from the NCHSR experiment (Weissert et al, 1980) should provide useful information on the feasibility of altering access/quality incentives with fixed rate differentials.

Willemain (1980) has used simulation techniques to analyze several different ways of differentiating rates according to differences in patient conditions. He shows that the benefits of greater refinement in categorizing patients (a potentially better match between patient "needs" and reimbursement) must be weighed against the costs associated with greater complexity. He particularly emphasizes the difficulties of accurately assessing patients' needs for service. For the set of environmental conditions he considers most realistic, Willemain finds that a case-mix adjustment based on only a sample of a facility's patients performs "best." ("Best" means the method yields the lowest mean "loss" where loss is a function of the difference between the simulated values of a patient's reimbursement rate and the value of the services he/she "needs.") The second best system was a two-level one similar to the SNF–ICF categories.

In addition to the complexity and operational difficulties of this approach, it does not alter the fundamental preference of providers for light care patients. At best, modifications of existing reimbursement methods can *marginally* improve access incentives for heavy care Medicaid patients. More basic changes in the availability and financing of long-term care services would be required to ensure priority nursing home access for those most in need of intensive nursing services. For example, it would be necessary to shift demand for nursing home care by light care patients to other forms of care.

Cost Containment Incentives

It is conventional wisdom that cost containment incentives are strong under flat rate reimbursement and weak under cost-based reimbursement. The weakness of cost containment incentives under cost-based reimbursement is frequently attributed to cost-based reimbursement's full coverage of costs so that facilities have no incentive to operate efficiently.

However, this problem only arises if the public rate is based solely on the costs of public patients. To illustrate the problem, note that for the totally public firm, $\pi = RM - C$ and $R = \dfrac{C}{M}$. Substituting for R in π, we see that π is zero for all values of M. That is, assuming that cost includes a normal profit, firms can do no better or worse than earn a normal profit whatever level of costs they incur or output they choose to produce. However, as long as the facility has both private and public patients, and the public rate is based on the average cost of care for both types of patients, this problem does not arise, at least in theory.

The problem does not emerge gradually as the share of public patient days increases because of the assumption that facilities *maximize* profit. Under other types of behavior, the incentive problem may appear under cost-based reimbursement before firms become totally publicly financed. It depends on how vigorously they pursue profits. There is no empirical evidence to indicate how high the public share of total output must be before this problem becomes serious. Abt Associates (1979) reported that, while over 60 percent of nursing home patients were publicly supported in 1974, over 54 percent of nursing homes had 80 percent or more publicly supported patients.

In this section, we investigate two other aspects of cost containment incentives. First, we compare the incentives under cost-based and flat rate reimbursement to pursue efficiency gains through innovation. That is, we investigate the incentive to undertake activities that lead to increased efficiency in the long run. Second, we examine the incentive to over-report costs under cost-based reimbursement. Our analysis suggests that over-reporting costs is potentially a more serious cause of weak cost containment incentives than is failure to operate efficiently. Finally, we evaluate the role of cost limits and efficiency allowances in strengthening cost containment incentives under cost-based reimbursement.

Efficiency Gains from Innovation

In the long run, cost containment also depends upon firms' incentives to become more efficient through innovation. We demonstrate that if two conditions are met, the incentives to "invest" in the search for cost-saving innovation are the same under cost-based and flat rate reimbursement. The two conditions are that (1) the investment or search costs must be included in the allowable costs for reimbursement, and (2) the facility must not be totally publicly financed. (This problem might typically be approached as an investment problem, but it can be analyzed using the single period, long-run model without serious loss of content.)

The analysis assumes that, given existing technology, facilities produce in a technically and economically efficient manner. That is, output is produced in the least cost manner.[8] However, we assume that it is possible to achieve levels of greater efficiency or lower cost by incurring additional costs that are assumed to lead to the discovery of cost-saving innovations.

To incorporate this analysis within the model, a shift variable (X) representing productivity is added to the total cost function:

$$C = C(Q, M, X(Y)), \text{ where } C_X < 0, X_Y > 0 \tag{55}$$

X depends on the level of effort (Y) devoted to the discovery of cost-saving innovations. An increase in innovative effort (Y) is assumed to increase productivity (X), which in turn lowers patient care costs (C). The cost of Y is denoted by the function $W(Y)$, where $W_Y > 0$. Total cost is now the sum of total patient care costs (C) and search costs (W). An increase in the search for cost-saving innovations affects costs in two ways: it raises investment or search costs (W) and it reduces production costs (C) by increasing the shift variable (X).

Incorporating innovation into the analysis of cost-based reimbursement yields the following profits function:

$$\pi = PQ + RM - C(Q, M, X(Y)) - W(Y) \tag{56}$$

Assume first that the search costs (W) are reimbursable, so that R can be written as follows:

$$R = \frac{C + W}{Q + M} \tag{57}$$

The profit-maximizing level of Y is obtained by differentiating equation (56) with respect to Y and setting the result equal to zero:

$$\frac{M}{Q + M}(C_X X_Y + W_Y) - (C_X X_Y + W_Y) = 0 \tag{58}$$

$C_X X_Y$ represents the marginal reduction in production costs due to innovation. (X_Y can be interpreted as the marginal productivity of the search activities, and C_X measures the (marginal) cost impact of innovation.) Since W_Y is the marginal search cost, $C_X X_Y + W_Y$ represents the net marginal cost saving of increased Y. Further, as long as the decrease in production cost ($C_X X_Y$) exceeds W_Y (in absolute value), $C_X X_Y + W_Y$ will be negative, and increased Y will result in a net cost saving.

Equation (58) shows the relationship between the change in profits and the net cost saving resulting from a change in Y. The first term shows that public reimbursement declines by a fraction $\dfrac{M}{Q + M}$ of the net cost saving. (For every dollar change in total costs, R

_____
[8] This assumption is a necessary condition for profit maximization.

changes by $\dfrac{1}{Q+M}$. The change in total costs is equal to $C_X X_Y + W_Y$. The change in total public reimbursement is the number of public days (M) multiplied by $\dfrac{1}{Q+M} \cdot (C_X X_Y + W_Y)$.) While the reduction in public reimbursement decreases profits, the net cost saving tends to increase them. Since the reduction in public reimbursement is only a fraction of the net cost saving, profits will rise as long as an increase in Y yields a cost saving.

It is useful to rewrite equation (58) as follows:

$$\left(\frac{M}{Q+M} - 1\right)(C_X X_Y + W_Y) = 0 \qquad (59)$$

Two results are apparent. First, as long as the facility is not totally public $\left(\dfrac{M}{Q+M} \neq 1\right)$, profit maximization implies that Y should be increased to the point that $C_X X_Y + W_Y = 0$, or until the net cost saving becomes zero.[9] Second, if $\dfrac{M}{Q+M} = 1$, equation (59) will be satisfied for all values of Y, and again we see that economic incentives do not exist for the totally public facility.

The optimal level of Y under flat rate reimbursement can be determined by differentiating equation (56) with respect to Y, under the assumption that R does not depend on Y:

$$- (C_X X_Y + W_Y) = 0 \qquad (60)$$

Equations (59) and (60) imply that the incentives to seek greater efficiency through innovation are the same under cost-based and flat rate reimbursement.

Disallowance of Search Costs

To show that these results depend upon the costs $W(Y)$ being included as allowable costs, we derive the optimal value of Y for the case when $W(Y)$ is disallowed. In this case, the public rate equals $\dfrac{C}{Q+M}$, and equation (56) is still the relevant profit function. The following condition determines the optimal value of Y:

---

[9] An interior solution may not exist either because W_Y is everywhere greater than $- C_X X_Y$, in which case, the optimal value of Y is zero, or because $- C_X X_Y$ is everywhere greater than W_Y in which case the optimal value of Y is its maximum feasible value. These corner solutions may be empirically relevant. However, from the perspective of the incentives created by the reimbursement system, they can be ignored because they depend on the actual C, X, and W functions and not on the nature of the reimbursement function.

$$\frac{1}{Q + M}\left(C_X X_Y M\right) - (C_X X_Y + W_Y) = 0 \qquad (61)$$

Public reimbursement declines by a greater amount when Y increases than when $W(Y)$ is included in allowable cost. (The marginal reduction is now $\frac{M}{Q + M} \cdot C_X X_Y$, rather than $\frac{M}{Q + M}(C_X X_Y + W_Y)$.) Hence, a larger marginal net cost saving $(C_X X_Y + W_Y)$ will be required to satisfy equation (61). That is, Y will not be increased to the point where the marginal net cost saving becomes zero, only to the point at which it is equal to $\frac{M}{Q + M} \cdot C_X X_Y$. Note also that the incentive to pursue greater efficiency weakens as the facility's public proportion of patient days increases.

Impact on Program Costs and Profits

As a final comment on incentives for long-run efficiency, we note the different impacts on public program costs and facility profits under cost-based and flat rate reimbursement. Under flat rate reimbursement, the facility pays the full costs of search (W) and retains, in the form of higher profits, the entire net cost saving $V = -\int_0^Y (C_X X_Y + W_Y)\, dY$. Public program costs ($RM$) are unchanged. Under cost-based reimbursement, the total search costs are shared between the facility, which pays $\frac{Q}{Q + M} \cdot W$ and the public program, which pays $\frac{M}{Q + M} \cdot W$. Similarly, the net cost saving is shared. The facility's profits are increased by $\frac{Q}{Q + M} \cdot V$, and public program costs are reduced by $\frac{M}{Q + M} \cdot V$.

Cost Over-Reporting

Under cost-based reimbursement there is an economic incentive to report greater costs than are actually incurred. The potential for boosting profit through excessive cost reporting is also contingent upon the owner's ability to capture the difference between reported and actual costs. Examples include paying inflated salaries and/or wages to oneself or one's family and, more generally, establishing "kick-back" arrangements with employees and suppliers.

The problem can be demonstrated analytically by writing the public rate (R) as a function of reported costs (C_R), which are the sum of actual costs (C_A) and a difference (D) that represents hidden profits:

$$R = R\,(C_A + D) = \frac{C_A + D}{Q + M} \qquad (62)$$

Substituting for C_R and C_A in the profits function yields

$$\pi = PQ + R\,(C_A + D)\,M - C_A \qquad (63)$$

Differentiating π with respect to D yields the following expression for the incentive to report costs in excess of actual costs:

$$\pi_D = R_D M = \frac{M}{Q + M} \qquad (64)$$

Equation (64) states that for every dollar that C_R exceeds C_A, profits increase by $\dfrac{M}{Q + M}$ dollars under the cost-based reimbursement system analyzed here. Hence, the return to over-reporting costs is higher the greater the proportion of patient days that are publicly financed. (This result contrasts with that of the previous section in which long-run efficiency incentives under cost-based reimbursement did not depend on the proportion of public patient days, short of the facility becoming totally public.)

It follows that cost-based reimbursement requires scrutiny of reported costs to control this potential abuse. The alternatives are cost audits and/or limits on those cost items which are particularly vulnerable to over-reporting. States commonly place limits on administrative salaries and attempt to restrict "related party" transactions.

Although the incentive to over-report costs is not as straightforward under flat rate reimbursement, it may not be totally absent if cost reports are used to determine group rates. In this case, the individual facility's incentive to report excessive costs depends on both its proportion of public patient days and the number of facilities in its group. For example, if the group rate were set as the mean cost per day of the facilities in the group, then $\pi_D = \dfrac{M}{Q + M} \cdot \dfrac{1}{n}$, where n is the number of facilities in the group.

Alternatively, if medians or percentiles are used to determine group rates, the number of facilities in a group will have no effect on the incentive to over-report costs. In this case however, facilities that expect to be at the critical percentile may have an incentive to over-report their costs. States typically use medians or percentiles, as opposed to means, in setting group rates or group cost limits.

Implications for Cost Containment Policy

We have discussed inefficiency and cost over-reporting as causes of poor cost control under cost-based reimbursement. Many States have adopted a variety of measures to deal with inefficiency: general cost limits, specific cost center limits, and efficiency allowances. Common measures aimed specifically at controlling cost-over-reporting include limits on administrative salaries and restrictions on related party transactions. Our analysis implies that, except where facilities are so heavily dependent on Medicaid that they behave as if they were totally financed by the program, cost over-reporting is likely to be the more important cause of excessive costs.

This analysis implies that measures to control cost over-reporting are likely to be important in containing costs, but that measures intended to control inefficiency are only required for facilities catering predominantly to Medicaid recipients. For example, specific cost center limits that attempt to establish efficiency standards for cost categories, such as nursing services, dietary costs, etc., may be unnecessary. Also, efficiency allowances may not be required to induce a facility to keep its costs below allowable limits. Although the analysis also implies that general cost limits may not be needed to screen inefficient providers, general limits are likely to be a convenient way of meeting budgetary constraints in many cases.

Of course, the dichotomy we have drawn between measures aimed at inefficiency and those aimed at over-reporting of costs is not a strict one. The measures that are intended to control inefficiency may also curb cost over-reporting.

Other types of interactions should be noted. For example, the size of the potential cost saving from the elimination of efficiency allowances depends on how tightly general cost limits are set. When the limits are binding for a large proportion of facilities, the benefits of eliminating efficiency allowances would be small. In addition, it should be noted that efficiency allowances may also discourage over-reporting of costs. Tradeoffs involving administrative costs should also be considered. A flat rate system that, in effect, pays 100 percent efficiency allowances but incurs lower administrative costs associated with audits, cost finding, and reporting, may be less expensive than a cost-based system without efficiency allowances.

Although the task would be complex, our model suggests a means of empirically testing the relative importance of inefficiency and over-reporting costs. The basis for the test is the model's prediction that the incentive to over-report costs increases as the Medicaid share of a facility's output increases. However, the inefficiency problem does not emerge until the facility becomes totally financed by public sources. It is important to investigate empirically how heavily financed by Medicaid a facility must be before it operates as if it were totally Medicaid.

The assumptions we have made about private demand for nursing home care are also critical to our analysis. Our conclusions regarding efficiency depend both on the presence of private patients in a facility and on a certain degree of competitiveness among facilities for private patients. In particular, it is important that facilities not be able to totally pass on higher costs to private patients in the form

658

of higher private rates. There is some empirical evidence to support this hypothesis. Both Bishop (1980) and Mennemeyer (1979) found private demand to be highly price elastic. However, further empirical analyses of private demand are needed, especially ones that consider the common conversion of private pay patients to public sources of funding.

Conclusion

This chapter has analyzed the pros and cons of cost-based and flat rate reimbursement. Past studies of providers' incentives under these alternative reimbursement systems have emphasized the trade-off between incentives for cost containment and those for access and quality. Although poor cost control is generally regarded as the chief liability of cost-based reimbursement, our analysis implies that when profit-maximizing facilities have some private pay patients, cost-based reimbursement also offers providers poor access and quality incentives. The problem is especially serious for heavy care public patients when excess demand for nursing home care permits facilities to readily fill their beds with light care patients.

In recent years, States have increasingly adopted cost-based systems which they have modified to provide greater cost containment incentives than do pure cost-based systems. These modifications typically have involved the addition of elements of flat rate reimbursement, such as cost limits. As a result, there has been a convergence of cost-based and flat-rate systems. For example, a cost-based system with strict general cost limits and 100 percent efficiency allowances provides basically the same set of incentives as a flat rate system with rates equal to the cost limits.

These changes might be expected to have worsened public patients' access to quality care. However, we have shown that, for the typical for-profit nursing home that serves both private and public patients, cost-based reimbursement offers weak access and quality incentives, even in the absence of cost containment pressures.

The disadvantages of cost-based reimbursement are particularly serious when the demand for nursing home care is so great that facilities can readily fill their beds with whatever severity of case-mix they choose. Under these circumstances, cost-based reimbursement subsidizes a more severe private case-mix and higher quality of care for *private* patients than does flat rate reimbursement. However, neither type of system gives providers any incentive to accept heavy care public patients or to provide more than minimal quality care for public patients.

A possible solution to these problems is to modify flat rate systems to incorporate rate adjustments that depend upon a facility's public case-mix and quality of care. However, systems of this type are complex and involve significant administrative costs. Furthermore, whether systems of this general type can improve access and quality, especially in the current environment of excess demand and budgetary problems, remains an open question. A critical issue is their ability to offset providers' preferences for light care patients.

Careful attention should be paid to the Medicaid reimbursement systems in Illinois, West Virginia, and Ohio, as well as the results from the NCHSR Incentive Payment Experiment in San Diego. These reimbursement systems can help define more clearly the potential and the limitations of reimbursement reform for improving access and quality.

Appendix

Retrospective Versus Prospective Reimbursement

Various advantages are frequently claimed for prospective over retrospective reimbursement, including stronger incentives for cost containment and efficiency, greater certainty of revenues, and lower bookkeeping and other administrative costs. There are real administrative differences between prospective and retrospective systems which may affect firms' behavior. However, we show in this Appendix that a prospective flat rate based on past costs of the individual facility yields essentially the same output decision as a retrospective cost-based rate. More generally, cost containment and efficiency incentives will not differ solely as a function of the prospective/retrospective difference. The chief difference between the two is that the prospective case may contain a short-run dynamic element not observed in the retrospective case.

The basic equivalency of the two cases can be shown by assuming that costs are constant in real terms over time so that the reimbursement function can be written (in real terms) as $R(C_{t-1}) = R(C_t)$. If the past and present cost curves are the same, retrospective and prospective reimbursement will yield the same result. Figure XVIII–A–1 illustrates the different dynamics between the two cases. Assume, arbitrarily, that initially the public rate is R_1. The firm will choose to produce where R_1 equals marginal cost, which yields a total output of $Q_1 + M_1$. This choice will, however, result in a lower rate next period, R_2; the equilibrium solution is at a rate R' which is equal to the minimum point on the average cost curve. R' also corresponds to the retrospective equilibrium. (It should be noted that unless costs are fraudulently reported, efforts by the firm to permanently raise its rate above R' will either not succeed or will be inconsistent with profit maximization.) This analysis demonstrates that in theory the distinction between retrospective and prospective payment does not alter the firm's basic incentives when rates are based on individual facility costs.

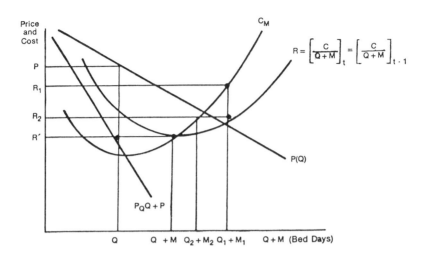

FIGURE XVIII A-1
Prospective Cost-Based Reimbursement

References

Abt Associates, Inc., *Reimbursement Strategies for Nursing Home Care: Developmental Cost Studies*, Cambridge: Abt, 1979, HCFA Contract No. 600–77–0068.

American Health Care Association, *How Medicaid Pays for Long-Term Care*, Wolfe and Company, Washington, D.C., 1978.

Bishop, Christine E., "Nursing Home Behavior Under Cost-Related Reimbursement," University Health Policy Consortium Paper DP–13, Brandeis University, August 1980.

Bishop, Christine, Alonzo Plough, and Thomas Willemain, "Nursing Home Levels of Care: Problems and Alternatives," *Health Care Financing Review*, Vol. 2, No. 2, Fall, 1980, pp. 33–45.

Deane, Robert T. and Douglas E. Skinner, "Development of a Formula Incentive Reimbursement System for Long Term Care," unpublished paper, Applied Management Sciences, Silver Spring, Maryland, no date.

Feder, J. and William Scanlon, "Intentions and Consequences of Regulating the Nursing Home Bed Supply," *Milbank Memorial Fund Quarterly*, Vol. 58, No. 1, Winter 1980, pp, 54–88.

Fries, Brant and Richard Averill, personal communication, March 1980.

Grana, John Murray, *The Impact of Reimbursement on the Nursing Home Industry in Massachusetts,* Unpublished Ph.D. dissertation, University of Massachusetts, Department of Economics, 1978.

Grimaldi, Paul, *Costs, Utilization, and Reimbursement of Nursing Home Care,* Washington: American Enterprise Institute, forthcoming, 1981.

Gruenberg, Leonard and Thomas R. Willemain, "Hospital Discharge Queues in Massachusetts," University Health Policy Consortium Paper DP–29, Brandeis University, November 1980.

McCaffree, Kenneth M., Sharon Winn, and Carl A. Bennett, *Cost Data Reporting Systems for Nursing Home Care*, Final Report, Grant No. HSO1115–O1A1, Battelle Human Affairs Research Center, Seattle, WA., October 1, 1976.

Mennemeyer, Stephen T., "The Elasticity of Demand for an Imperfectly Competitive Firm," *Economic Letters*, Vol. 2, No. 1, 1979, pp. 9–12.

Palmer, Hans C. and Ronald J. Vogel, "Towards An Analysis of Some Long-Term Care Providers' Behavior," Working Paper 18, Office of Research, Demonstrations, and Statistics, Health Care Financing Administration, November 1980.

Pollak, William, "Long-Term Care Facility Reimbursement," in *Altering Medicaid Provider Reimbursement Methods*, John Holahan *et al*, eds. Washington, D.C.: The Urban Institute, 1977, pp. 103–142.

Ruchlin, Hirsch S., Samuel Levey, and Charlotte Muller, "The Long-Term Care Marketplace: An Analysis of Deficiencies and Potential Reform by Means of Incentive Reimbursement, *Medical Care*, Vol. XIII, December 1975, pp. 979–991.

Scanlon, William J., "A Theory of the Nursing Home Market," *Inquiry*, Vol. XVII, Spring 1980, pp. 25–41.

Scanlon, William and Judith Feder, "Regulation of Investment in Long-Term Care Facilities," The Urban Institute, Working Paper 1218–9, January 1980.

Shaughnessy, Peter, Robert Schlenker, Barbara Harley, Nancy Shanks, Gerri

Tricarico, Vann Perry, and Bettina Kurowski, "Long-Term Care Reimbursement and Regulation: A Study of Cost, Case Mix and Quality," First Year Analysis Report, Center for Health Services Research, University of Colorado Health Sciences Center, February 1980, HCFA Grant No. 18–P–97145/8–01.

Shaughnessy, Peter and Bettina Kurowski, "Quality Assurance Through Reimbursement?" Working Paper 8, Center for Health Services Research, University of Colorado Health Sciences Center, December 1980.

U.S. Department of Health and Human Services, Office of the Inspector General, "Restricted Patient Admittance to Nursing Homes: An Assessment of Hospital Back Up," August 1980.

Walsh, Thomas J., "Patient-Related Reimbursement for Long-Term Care," in *Reform and Regulation in Long-Term Care,* Valerie LaPorte and Jeffrey Rubin, eds. New York: Praeger, 1979, pp. 153–167.

Weiner, Sanford L. and Susan Sanders Lehrer, "The Afterthought Industry: Developing Reimbursement Policy for Nursing Homes," *Milbank Memorial Fund Quarterly*, Vol. 60, No. 1, Winter 1981.

Weissert, William G., William J. Scanlon, Thomas T. H. Wan, and Douglas E. Skinner, "Encouraging Appropriate Care for the Chronically Ill: Design of the NCHSR Experiment in Nursing Home Incentive Payments," paper presented at the Annual Meeting of the American Public Health Association, October 19–23, 1980, Detroit, Michigan.

Willemain, Thomas R., "Nursing Home Levels of Care: Reimbursement of Resident-Specific Costs," *Health Care Financing Review*, Vol. 2, No. 2, Winter 1981, pp. 47–52.

Vladeck, Bruce C., *Unloving Care: The Nursing Home Tragedy.* New York: Basic Books, 1980.

CHAPTER XIX

Studies of Nursing Home Costs

by Hans C. Palmer with the assistance of Philip G. Cotterill

The Study of Costs

Any productive facility incurs costs in providing the output which it sells or gives away, and nursing homes are no exception. Much economic literature has focused on theoretical specifications of the relationship between volume of output and level of costs—average, marginal, total—for a given product. Alternatively, some of these analyses have sought to identify a link between costs and the characteristics of a given product or the manner of its production, holding the volume of product constant. These approaches, among others, emphasize that the cost of production, usually cost per unit or average cost, is determined by a number of aspects of the production process: volume of output, nature of inputs, combination of inputs, characteristics of the provider, scale of operation, and so on.

For nursing homes and other medical facilities, unlike many other types of producers, concern with cost considerations has often been stimulated by the need to link costs to reimbursement, usually provided from public sources. The growth of Medicare, Medicaid, and other forms of public, third-party payment as well as, to a lesser extent, the growth of private health insurance, has forced concern with cost as a proper basis for those reimbursements. The approach is similar to that used with agricultural parity payments and public utility "fair rate of return" rate-setting. The need to provide an appropriate basis for reimbursement to nursing homes and hospitals has yielded a rich supply of cost studies, many of which have been analyzed and compared by Christine Bishop, whose work guided much of the section on cost analyses. (See Figure XIX–1 for a list of studies analyzed by Bishop.) In what follows, we will use Bishop's analysis as a road map to identify key elements in nursing home costs, not only from the reimbursement perspective but, more importantly, to understand the nursing home as a productive entity (Bishop, 1980).

Among the first cost-determining factors listed by Bishop are those associated with facility characteristics, that is, scale of operations, provider type (non-profit versus profit), and location and regional differences in input costs. Secondly, she suggests consideration of the nature of the product and the manner of payment:

We wish to thank Christine Bishop for her very helpful suggestions.

665

FIGURE XIX-1
Nursing Home Cost Studies

Study, Dependent Variable	Data Description			R^2 [1]
	Number of Facilities	Location	Date	
Average Total Cost				
Ruchlin and Levy (1972)	638	Mass.	1965–1969	.61
Mennemeyer (1979)	405 to 516	New York	1975, 1976	.51–.66
Bishop (1980)	417	Mass.	1976	.70
Average Operating Cost				
Christianson (1977)	30	Montana	1974	.51
Reis and Christianson (1977)	50	Montana	1974	.51
Walsh (1979)	136	Illinois	—	.57
Jensen and Birnbaum (1979)	1127	National	1973	.58
Lee and Birnbaum (1979)	479 to 504	New York	1974–1976	.65–.77
Bishop (1979)	438 to 468	Mass.	1973–1975	.66–.72
Jensen (1979)	78 to 86	Indiana	1973–1975	.47–.63
Lee et al (1979)	1127	National	1973	—
Private Price				
Deane and Skinner (1978)	4000 private pay patients	National	1973	.60

[1] Proportion of variation explained by the regression
Source: Bishop, Christine E., "Nursing Home Cost Studies and Reimbursement Issues," *Health Care Financing Review*, Vol. 1, Spring 1980, p. 49

certified level of care (SNF versus ICF), the nature and volume of services offered and actually provided, patient characteristics, patient turnover, and source of payment (public versus private). Other factors, such as occupancy and patient turnover rates, were also found to be important.

In this chapter we will consider, first, the body of nursing home cost studies based on single equation cost functions. We will discuss many of the facility, patient, and reimbursement characteristics which are important cost determinants in the nursing home. Because of some methodological and theoretical difficulties associated with single-equation models, we review various multi-equation models which incorporate interactions among regulation, private demand conditions, and cost. We then turn to a consideration of new approaches to the relationship between patient mix and cost, including production function analyses, methods of improving patient grouping, and manipulations of the case-mix/quality/cost interactions.[1] The chapter concludes with a section on research needs.

Single Equation Approaches

The research considered in this section employed single equation cost models using regression analysis, a technique through which the influences of a number of actors can be simultaneously estimated. For cost analysis, the dependent variable (that which is determined or influenced by output level, input use, etc.) is usually cost per unit, or average cost, of output. In nursing homes, the unit of output is conventionally the bed or patient day of care, rather than the case or episode as used in some hospital studies. Birnbaum et al and McCaffree et al used other variables as well.

In some instances, average operating (or variable) cost has been preferred to total costs, including capital costs. This choice reflects the belief that fixed costs do not vary greatly once a given nursing home has been established and that such costs are not linked to the other variables reflecting scale and product mix. Presumably, the latter are determined by ". . . historical construction costs, age of the facility, method of financing, and ownership type, as well as by the type and number of patient days provided (Bishop, 1980)." Omission of capital is also justified on the grounds that the amount and value of an enterprise's capital are difficult to measure, often reflecting accounting and tax conventions rather than any objective measures. Moreover, there is scant possibility of substituting capital

---

[1] Among the works considered at length will be a recent study by Howard Birnbaum, Christine Bishop, Gail Jensen, A. James Lee, and Douglass Wilson, cited as Birnbaum et al. We will also consider recent studies by McCaffree et al (1975), Meiners (1978), and Frech and Ginsburg (1980).

Birnbaum et al imaginatively used so-called structural and reduced form analyses of the nursing home industry and of nursing home provider behavior which usefully augment the more conventional, cross-sectional static analysis implicit in the techniques of most other research. Meiners used additive and multiplicative models, the latter estimated in a log-linear form as the "best" for the cost-size relationship. His data set was taken from the 1973–74 National Nursing Home Survey (NCHS).

Frech and Ginsburg employed translog and log-linear analyses of the influences of output, input costs, ownership, and reimbursement system variables on total operating expenses. They standardized patient conditions, services provided, and services available among homes. Their objective was to examine the effects of these variable on costs and on efficiency in the context of a property rights model. Another study concerned with reimbursement effects is Morrisey (1979).

for labor in most nursing care. Furthermore, it can be argued that since variable costs (especially labor costs) are such a large element in total nursing home costs, and since the short run for such facilities is actually very long because of the nature of their clientele, variable costs are more relevant and behavior-determining in any event. Additionally, the existing reimbursement systems emphasize operating costs and, indeed, translate capital charges into operating costs because of specific allowances for depreciation, etc. For these and other reasons, questions about capital charges merit special analyses to be considered elsewhere.

Although we would conventionally assume that operations will continue in the short run as long as variable costs are covered, and despite the seeming reasonableness of some of these capital cost arguments, all cost must be covered in the long run, at least for proprietary facilities, if the productive entity is to remain viable. For non-profit or government-operated facilities, the same requirement might hold, although usually the government or charity agrees, at least implicitly, to cover shortfalls arising from operations as long as these shortfalls remain within budgetary limits. Even in these latter cases, however, costs of operation genrally are supposed to bear some stable relationship to budget allocation levels and to "reasonable" charges for operations, as defined either by the political process or some group of trustees.

Facility Characteristics

Scale Effects

Consistent with conventional biases about mass production and the efficacy of large scale production, much analysis of the effect of scale of output on nursing home costs has assumed scale-related declines in average costs followed by increases in costs due to communications difficulties, etc.[2] This combination presumably yields a conventional U-shaped cost curve.

Actually, the empirical evidence on scale impacts on costs is equivocal. As Bishop notes, some researchers (for example, Deane and Skinner, 1978) found that average cost (or price) increases, rather than decreases, with scale (bed size). New York State's Moreland Commission found similar results for that State for 1976, whereas the Social Security Administration found no systematic relationship between bed size and costs (Deane and Skinner, 1978). Age of facility may also have some role to play, since newer nursing homes tend to

---

[2] Scale is measured either in number of beds or the average daily census (that is, the quotient of yearly patient days divided by 365). Empirically, there appears to be little difference in these two measures. (See Birnbaum *et al*, I, p. 36.)

be both larger and more expensive than older ones. For example, Ruchlin and Levy found a negative impact of scale (that is, scale economies) once they had controlled for age; Mennemeyer, however, found a positive impact even when controlling for age. While no studies have found overwhelming evidence of sizeable scale economies, both Birnbaum *et al* and Mark Meiners have found statistically significant scale influences (Bishop, 1980; Meiners, 1978, Ruchlin and Levy, 1972; Walsh, 1979).

Birnbaum *et al,* using national data from 1972 to 1976 and data of a five-State sample from the same period, identified some mild economies of scale, especially in facilities with less than 40 beds (1979). Cost decreases steeply as census rises from near zero to 20 patients per day, the decrease amounting to 20¢ per unit increase in average daily census up to the 20-patient level. Between 21 and 40 patient days, decline in costs is considerably more modest. Surprisingly, beyond 40 patients the average cost curve becomes virtually flat. New York and Massachusetts figures again show a flat relationship between cost and scale. Massachusetts seems to indicate that cost declines below a size of 80 beds are very gentle: 2.7¢ per bed. Above that scale, however, the relationship is not statistically significant. What is striking about the New York data is the inconsistency across size groupings from year to year. For example, in·1974 facilities with more than 300 beds had average costs almost $4.89 per patient day higher than those of smaller units. In 1976, the class of facilities 200 to 300 beds was $2.23 less costly. Birnbaum *et al* attribute these vagaries to a "dynamic regulatory environment in New York state," (1979).

Meiners, using bed size, found that nursing home production is initially subject to economies of scale and eventually to decreasing returns to scale (that is, there is a U-shaped cost curve.) His results for both characteristics of the average cost curve are significant at the 99 percent level of confidence. He found optimum facility size to be 330 beds, all else equal (Meiners, 1978). Very importantly, however, he found that, at the level of the mean bed size for his sample (121 beds), a 10 percent increase in the number of beds would reduce costs by only 0.78 percent. In other words, in that size region the average cost curve is almost flat. Meiners argues that given the external costs imposed on patients and families by moves between facilities, it is not surprising that such modest economies of scale do not suggest great cost and price reductions and thus do not dictate larger nursing facilities on technical grounds. The average size of the nursing home remains small. Overall, one might conclude on the basis of the Bishop survey and the Birnbaum *et al* and Meiners analyses that the effects of scale economies are small. Regulatory authorities, therefore, may not be able to achieve much in the way of program cost reductions through reimbursement rate shifts designed to change (enlarge) facility bed size or average daily census.

Occupancy Factors

In considering the effects of scale, one must remember that two factors are actually at work: capacity of the facility and degree of utilization or occupancy rate. For both of these elements, one can again hypothesize a region of declining costs followed by one of increasing costs. Viewed in this manner, the conventional hypothesis about scale of operations breaks into two sub-hypotheses: (1) average costs first decline and then increase with bed size (holding *occupancy rate* constant) and (2) average costs first decrease and then increase with occupancy rate (holding *bed size* constant). The simultaneous effects of these two influences can be examined using multiple regression analysis, assuming that scale (size) and occupancy are not intercorrelated.

Unlike the scale factor, the occupancy factor in the national Birnbaum study did not appear to significantly influence costs across any grouping of facility sizes, although costs fell gently as occupancy rates increased. On an individual State basis, occupancy rates in New York were not statistically significant, although costs in 1974–75 did appear to fall gently up to 90 percent of capacity and, for 1976, over all ranges of output. The outcomes were not statistically significant, however. In Massachusetts, where occupancy rate penalties apply for rates under 90 percent, costs fell significantly up to that figure. Beyond 95 percent, however, costs appeared to rise, suggesting some real constraints as capacity limits are approached. Overall, this study concluded that State regulatory environments were more important than underlying "real" factors of scale or occupancy rates. Nationally Birnbaum *et al* could only conclude that scale and occupancy rates appear unimportant except in very small facilities.

It should be noted that firm conclusions about the scale aspects of nursing home data are based mainly on Birnbaum's analysis of a fairly small number of States and on a small number of State-specific studies (for example, Ruchlin and Levy, 1972; Walsh, 1979). Clearly, one needs to analyze a sample even larger than that provided by the National Nursing Home Survey to develop firm conclusions about supposedly typical nursing home behavior.

By contrast with some of the ambiguous occupancy results in the Birnbaum study, those in the Deane and Skinner, Walsh and Meiners research were statistically significant and relatively large. (See Figure XIX–2). Meiners also shows that, with a combined linear and quadratic measure, a 1 percent increase in the occupancy rate will reduce average costs by almost 2.7 percent. He also suggests

670

FIGURE XIX-2
Effect of Scale

Independent Variables

Study, Dependent Variable	Beds	Occupancy Rate	Total Patient Days or ADC
Average Total Cost			
Ruchlin and Levy	Insignificant	Negative: $.06 per percentage point	—
Mennemeyer	Positive	Negative	—
Bishop (1980)	—	Inverse of occupancy rate positive: + $13.232, implying a negative effect of about − $.20 to − $.13 per percentage point for occupancy rates between 80 and 100 percent	Insignificant
Average Operating Cost			
Ries and Christianson	Quadratic form significant: costs fall over range toward minimum at 122 beds	Insignificant	—
Walsh	Negative: − $.0002 per bed	Negative: − $.0957 per percentage point	—

(Continued)

671

FIGURE XIX-2 (Continued)

Study, Dependent Variable	Beds	Occupancy Rate	Total Patient Days or ADC
Jensen and Birnbaum	—	—	Negative, then insignificant: cost falls by $.20 per unit ADC for range 1–20, flat thereafter
Lee and Birnbaum	Negative or insignificant	Negative to 90%, then insignificant	—
Bishop (1979)	Negative	Negative then positive: −$.12 to −$.24 per percentage point for 0–90% range; increasing over some ranges above 95%	—
Lee et al	Positive: +$.007 per bed	Negative: −$.02 per percentage point	—
Private Price			
Deane and Skinner	Positive: +$1.52 for facilities with 60 + beds	Positive: +$.52 for facilities with 93% + occupancy	

Source: Bishop, Christine E., "Nursing Home Cost Studies and Reimbursement Issues," *Health Care Financing Review*, Vol. 1, Spring 1980, p. 51

that economies to increased capacity utilization are available throughout the entire range of feasible operations (1978).

Disagreement among the various studies about scale and occupancy rate requires further investigation, not only from the analytical perspective but also in view of policy considerations. Many States establish reimbursement rates based on classification of facilities by size. Many of them also impose penalties on facilities not meeting minimum occupancy rates. Although these regulations often reflect the desire to force facilities to accept public patients, they may have some unsuspected cost implications which must be addressed. Of course, any analysis of this type must proceed from an understanding of differences among States with respect to input prices, a given State's unique nursing home history, and the impact of past regulatory policies. The Medicare/Medicaid balance, as well as the role of private pay patients, also should not be overlooked.

Non-Profit and For-Profit Providers

In contrast with the equivocal results shown for scale of operations, the analyses for provider type consistently indicate that government and non-profit homes are more costly than for-profit, proprietary facilities. As shown in studies analyzed by Bishop, as well as in some other research, non-profit homes range from about $1.75 to almost $12 per day more costly than profit-oriented homes, while government homes are anywhere from $2.50 to over $7 more expensive than their proprietary counterparts (Bishop, 1980). Similar wide divergences are reported in the Birnbaum study (1979). Meiners found that average costs in proprietary homes are about 7.5 percent lower than in voluntary, non-profit homes (1978). He suggests that proprietary homes may be similarly advantaged compared with government facilities. Such disparities might arise from profit-oriented, cost-minimizing actions by proprietors, from possibly "lighter" case loads in the proprietary homes, and from the impact of regulation.

Frech and Ginsberg (1980) also found that non-profit and government homes were more costly to operate than were for-profit institutions. Greatest differences were found in States with flat rate reimbursement systems, indicating an interaction among ownership type and reimbursement practices. In addition, they found that private non-profit homes were more costly than for-profits, but the differences were statistically significant only in the flat rate States. Government homes were the most costly, 34 percent more than for-profits in non-flat rate States and 51 percent more in the flat rate States. Frech and Ginsberg found such differences to be unrealistically large, but they believed that some underlying behavioral differences were being revealed.

673

It is tempting to argue that these ownership-reimbursement cost differences reflect efficiency differences, but at least two other sets of factors may contribute to the cost variations. First, the data may not pick up real differences in patient needs and quality of care among the various ownership categories. One may speculate, for example, that government homes may be filled with highly dependent, high cost patients. Second, non-profit and government homes may practice what Martin Feldstein calls philanthropic wage policy, that is, they pay their staffs more than market rates for various non-economic reasons.

While more aggressive cost minimization may characterize proprietary homes, more research is needed on this issue. One might well surmise that output maximization by non-profits could explain their higher average costs, but investigations to test such hypotheses have yet to be undertaken. As discussed subsequently, there is little evidence to support the proposition that proprietary nursing homes "skim" the long-term care population for light cases and lower costs. On the other hand, as noted in Frech and Ginsburg, regulation may explain a significant amount of observed profit versus non-profit cost differentials, though the exact mechanism of these effects remains unknown.

Free-Standing Facilities

Another common classification relates to a nursing home's being free-standing or incorporated within another facility. Usually, such other facility is a hospital, although many homes are linked to retirement centers. The Health Care Financing Administration (HCFA) has recently analyzed cost differences between free-standing and other nursing homes (Cotterill, 1980). Data from the 1977 Medicare cost reports for skilled nursing facilities (SNFs) suggest that hospital-based units experience over 60 percent higher average costs than do free-standing institutions. In metropolitan areas, the differences may be on the order of 85 percent, while in rural areas they may be over 50 percent. (These results are preliminary, and a number of methodological questions remain unanswered.) Similarly, Shaughnessy et al found in Colorado that hospital-based nursing homes were $10 more costly (average cost) per patient day than were free-standing homes (1980).

Chain Ownership

It is often assumed that members of nursing home chains will enjoy lower costs because of presumed economies of scale in management, buying supplies, and obtaining finance. Neither Birnbaum et al nor Meiners, however, found chain membership to be of much importance nationally. Regionally, the former found chain membership to exact a significant downward influence on

674

costs. If these findings hold up, they will resolve one of the most inflammatory elements in current nursing debates. In any event, this question should be further analyzed, especially in view of the somewhat surprising national findings (Birnbaum et al, 1979; Meiners, 1978).

Other facility characteristics have often been cited as influencing costs, for example, changes in numbers of beds, percent of services provided under external contracts, in-house training programs, and average number of beds per room. Somewhat surprisingly, Birnbaum et al found the first two to be of no significance, while Meiners found that the latter two exerted no significant influences. Because these findings run counter to intuition, however, additional research is in order.

Location

By contrast, location and related input price differentials do appear significantly related to cost differences. Most of the explanation derives from wage rate differences in various parts of the country. Alternatively, some studies have indicated cost variations based on rural versus urban sites or on population size. From reports on the studies cited by Bishop, it appears that location in the nation (northeast, south, central, west or in specific HHS planning regions) were statistically significant in explaining cost differences. For Boston, the rural-urban split was significant, although in the Birnbaum data, the rural-urban and population density variables were not. Again, in that analysis county retail trade wages and facility nurse, or licensed practical nurse (LPN), wages were positively and significantly related to costs (Bishop, 1980; Birnbaum et al, 1979).

Meiners found the same hierarchy of locational costs as did Birnbaum et al: the Northeast is 36 percent more costly on average than is the West and 22 percent more costly than the South and North Central regions, in both of which average costs were similar (1978). He also found that wages of LPNs were significant determinants of average costs; a 10 percent increase in average wages accounted for 2.2 percent increase in average costs.

Nature of Nursing Home Product

Level of Care

Not surprisingly, certified level of care is found to increase costs significantly in the studies considered, including that of Meiners. Certification classification was based on Federal level of care distinctions (SNF versus ICF) or on eligibility for Medicare reimbursement, which usually is more stringent than certification for Medicaid. Additionally, some studies incorporated characteristics jointly identified with SNFs and intermediate care facilities (ICFs).

675

As the Birnbaum study points out, however, it is important to recognize distinctions among State patterns of certification when considering these effects. First, States set certification standards subject only to imprecise Federal guidelines. Second, as in the case of size groupings and identification of provider characteristics, States use certification (SNF versus ICF, etc.) as the basis for rate-setting for reimbursement purposes, but only within very broad limits. This link to the reimbursement process may create a condition in which the grouping procedure, employed for rate-setting purposes, may perpetuate the differences which the grouping initially reflected. If rates for SNFs and ICFs are initially set on the basis of average operating costs, there is no reason to expect that cost differences between types of facilities will change, since both facility owners and regulators know that the reimbursement system will pick up any changes in costs, including those associated with the original classification schema (Birnbaum et al, 1979).

Also, although one might expect rate-related certification to reflect differences in patient characteristics, the imprecision of the placement process with respect to patient requirement casts some doubt on any legitimate link between certification and costs, at least those presumably appropriate to meeting needs of specific groups of patients. In short, certification may not be a valid guide to matching expenditure per patient with the level of dependency of that patient. Therefore, level of care cost differences may reveal more about the impact of regulations and reimbursement schedules than about the impact of patient need.

Undoubtedly, State-specific reimbursement patterns of the type cited by Birnbaum et al are reflected in Meiners' finding that only Medicare certification appears to exert any statistically significant influence on costs. He determined that Medicare certification accounts for costs 5 percent higher than those for Medicaid certified SNFs and 15 percent higher than for Medicaid certified ICFs. He was, however, unable to identify any statistically significant difference between the latter two groups. He ascribes this lack to relatively high negative correlations among the Medicaid, SNF, and ICF variables (1978).

In considering both an average of national data and data for specific States, Birnbaum et al (1979) established that the SNF-ICF cost differences were large and significant, though much greater in New York ($9–$11) than in Massachusetts ($4–$6) and Indiana ($1–$3). National SNF-ICF differences of over $2, while significant, were considered to excessively reflect the impact of individual State regulatory practice for them to have any applicability across the nation. Two other interesting findings, however, emerge from their study of SNF-ICF certification cost differences. One is that in New

York, data suggest some efficiencies in operating a mixed SNF/ICF facility from which both parts benefit. In Massachusetts, on the other hand, the joint facilies were more expensive. The second is that, again in Massachusetts, the method of setting rates in combined type facilities by assigning a joint weighted (by bed proportions) SNF-ICF rate to all Medicaid patients, whether SNF or ICF, reduced any stimuli to cost reduction if ". . . facilities concentrated on public patients at the ICF level and private patients at the SNF level."

An interesting set of findings from Meiners' analysis is related to characterization of the home. In comparison with so-called nursing homes (presumably some form of SNF), ICFs had average costs lower by 10 percent, while those characterized as ". . . providing some other type of residential health care" were about 26 percent lower. (Meiners, 1978). Convalescent or rest homes had costs not appreciably different from those of nursing homes. Among those more costly, on average, were extended care units of hospitals (17 percent more) and nursing care units of retirement centers (23 percent more). It should be noted, however, that these results do not hold up in statistical significance when a linear functional form is used for the cost equation. Also, level of care (SNF/ICF) was not compared.

Services Provided per Patient

It seems reasonable to assume, on intuitive grounds at least, that volume of services provided per patient should be positively related to average operating costs. After all, more services per patient means more staff time used, which in turn implies a larger wage bill, more fringes, and more usage of complementary factors of production. Actually, on both methodological and empirical grounds, it appears that the service intensity issue cannot be separated from patient characteristics (especially patient disability), and from the quality of care to which the facility aspires. These possible interactions between inputs and outputs must be kept in mind when reading the balance of this sub-section.

As Bishop's survey shows, most cost studies do find a link between service provision and costs, yet careful methodological analysis will show that some of this relationship may be spurious unless the nature of services is identified and some attempt is made to tie volume of services to the type and amount of service appropriate to patient condition.

First, it is necessary to distinguish between the availability of service and the dosage or actual amount offered and/or provided. Second, one must recognize the distinction between services associated with routine caring and special services, for example, rehabilitation, physical therapy, psychiatric care, etc., needed to minister

677

to specific conditions. Third, one must acknowledge that what passes for higher quality (in the form of more nursing or therapist hours, for example) may actually be evidence of inefficiency. In the absence of any specifications about the amount and type of service associated with a given quality of care for any given condition, it is impossible to distinguish between high quality and waste. Pursuant to these reservations, Birnbaum *et al* (1979) found that services *offered* were more important for cost levels than were services *provided*. It appears, from their analysis, that homes gear up for a given quality of provision for this case-mix and that this level of intention tells more about costs than what is actually used.

The effects of services offered show quite clearly both in the Birnbaum volumes and in the Meiners analysis. In the former, the offer of occupational therapy added $0.86 to average daily operating costs, while the offer of physical therapy added $0.91 (Birnbaum *et al*, 1979). Other offers of services (for example, recreational therapy, rehabilitation therapy, education, etc.) were not statistically significant.

In a similar vein, Meiners (1978) found that the number of therapies offered was a highly significant and large influence on costs, for example, the addition of one type of service added 4.5 percent to average costs. He also found that the presence of a physician as supervisor of clinical services could add as much as 16 percent to average daily cost. Another measure of attempted quality of care, an index of quality of staff coverage of nursing shifts, likewise positively influenced costs. A one unit increase in this index value pushed average costs up by 2.2 percent. Overall, this factor could change costs by as much as 11 percent in light of the all shift combinations involved. In terms of services *used,* the Birnbaum study found that providing one or more specific services (physical, occupational, speech, hearing, or recreational therapy, professional counseling) to a patient added $.08 a day to costs. Since each patient in the Birnbaum survey received an average of 4.1 services a month, the cost of the services added $.33 per patient day to costs.

Patient Condition

Patient condition, like volume of services provided, intuitively appears linked to operating costs, and many studies of nursing home costs have included measures of patients' ability to perform activities of daily living (ADL) and/or their medical diagnoses in analytical cost functions. Essentially the argument has been that different types of patients require different types of care, may need different nursing home products, and account for different levels of costs. The fundamental proposition is that a "basic" patient requires basic services and that more difficult cases require add-ons, augmenting costs. This approach, which in some formulations has been carried to very

678

sophisticated lengths, must, however, confront two questions: (1) Can we really measure patient status and (2) What is the quality of care (however measured) in terms of the given patient population? In effect, the product of the care facility may not vary with the types of patient served, since the volume and type of care provided may be inappropriate to the patients' problems and to the outcomes which may be sought for them (Bishop, 1980; McCaffree et al, 1975).

In addition, it must be recognized that including patient status in an econometric cost function implies a linkage between some status index and the cost of care. The problem with this approach is that most status indexes are ordinal in nature, and the differences among levels of condition do not necessarily imply equivalent differences among care requirements. For example, a patient with a five rating on a given ADL disability scale may require twice as much care as one with a rating of three or even four. This difficulty arises because most indexes attempt to measure the number of problems and to attach some numerical values reflecting number count rather than severity. Even in the case of indexes identifying patients as dependent or independent or partially dependent, the care implications of those characterizations are unspecified, unless some theoretical and empirical care coefficients have been defined through time and motion studies or similar operations research techniques. This latter may be a formidable task, given the numbers of conditions and potential numbers of patients.

To evade some of the technical and methodological problems discussed earlier, the econometric cost function might group patients by general types of condition. This technique could ease the accounting problems and alleviate the ordinality difficulty, but only at a loss of predictive power as to prognoses of individual patients and outcomes of regimes of care which, even among grouped patients, will have selected individual effects. Cost links to patient descriptions would still remain spurious. Alternatively, it may be possible to include proportions of patients with certain characteristics as independent variables in the cost equations, but the results may be hard to interpret. For one thing, patients tend to present clusters of conditions, diagnoses, and dependencies which would introduce multicollinearity into the equations and the statistical manipulation of the data. Multicollinearity cannot be evaded by including only certain "significant" patient descriptors in the equations, since we do not yet know which clusters of conditions, diagnoses, and dependencies are thus represented. Again, the links among conditions, care, costs, and outcomes might be spurious, diluting the predictive value of such exercises. As noted by Bishop, using patient grouping variables presents a data problem, since much available information on patients is based on samples taken from facilities. The samples may be unbiased, but the variance of the estimates based on the samples depends on the size of the parent populations in each of the facilities and on the proportions of patients sampled. As a result, any actual effects of patient conditions may be hidden in the biasing toward zero of the relevant coefficients because of large variances in the statistics obtained from the samples (Bishop, 1980).[3]

The Interaction Between Quality, Case-Mix, and Cost

A more fundamental problem is whether the health or dependency status of an individual directly affects the nature and amount of service provided, an issue raised earlier. Assuming that one might accurately assess patients or clients, and accepting the proposition that sicker or more dependent people will receive more care than the less sick, the question remains—will those with a given level of dependency or illness receive the same type and amount of care in any home in which they may find themselves? Much anecdotal evidence suggests that they will not. To be sure, some of the perceived differences may reflect differences in efficiency of resource use, at least as far as meeting the needs of a given dependent person is concerned. One home, for example, may provide twice as many bed baths daily as another, yet there may be no difference between the two with respect to patient well-being. On the other hand, differences in provision may reflect the decision to offer the same quality of care to all patients. The analytical problem then becomes one of identifying the predetermined level of quality of care before attempting to examine the impact of patient condition on costs. The analysts must thus control for quality in linking condition to cost. The argument can be illustrated by Figures XIX–1 and XIX–2.

These diagrams indicate that, given the level of quality chosen (as shown by the rays in Figure XIX–1 or the curves in Figure XIX–2), the volume of inputs, and thus the cost of care, will depend on the difficulty or dependency status of the patient(s). Consequently, any characteristics-cost analysis based on a sample of institutions will inevitably reflect the mix of quality decisions for those institutions. As a result, it will be impossible to accurately discern the relationship between case-mix and cost without a prior sort for facility quality. Unfortunately, there are complicated methodological problems associated with defining, let alone measuring, facility or care quality, and few studies have dealt with the qualitative issue in other than input terms. This is an inappropriate technique since quality is a characteristic of consequences, and we have no way of linking

---

[3] Bishop also notes that the 1973 and 1977 *National Nursing Home Surveys* of the National Center for Health Statistics are especially prone to this weakness, because, at most, 10 patients from a facility's population were sampled on a given day during a year.

680

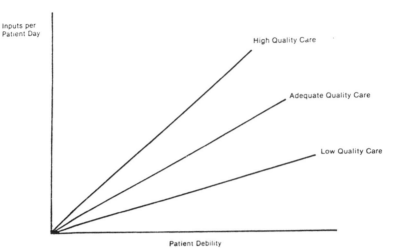

FIGURE XIX-3
Patient Debility and Inputs
per Patient Day

Inputs per
Patient Day

High Quality Care

Adequate Quality Care

Low Quality Care

Patient Debility

Source: Bishop, Christine E. "Nursing Home Cost Studies and Reimbursement Issues"
Health Care Financing Review, Vol. 1, Spring 1980, p. 57

FIGURE XIX-4
Patient Dependency and Quality of Care

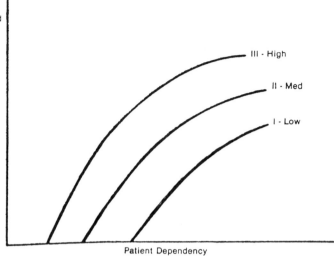

Quality
of
Care
(Sources and
Costs per
Patient
Day)

III - High

II - Med

I - Low

Patient Dependency

Source: Adapted from Birnbaum *et al.*, *Reimbursement Strategies for Nursing Home Care*, (Cambridge, Mass.: Abt, 1979, v. II).

682

consequence merely to levels of input use. Because of these limitations, we must conclude that studies showing high cost provision in some facilities, as compared to other facilities, may as well be showing waste as showing better care (Bishop, 1980).

Two studies do attempt, in a simple manner, to address the cost-characteristics questions, while controlling for quality. The Birnbaum analysis of New York data indicates that, on the basis of judgments about which facilities needed improvement and those which met predetermined standards of service and provision (and thus controlling for facilities' quality), "heavy" cases cost more. Indeed, their quality-adjusted New York analysis showed that ADL status was a significant determinant of costs, whereas, in their unadjusted national analysis, it was not. Among their other New York findings were those that showed average cost increasing 4.5¢ per day with every percentage point increase in those who required assistance with eating (1979).

Walsh also found that, on the basis of a quality-adjusted econometric analysis of the Illinois point-count system of patient assessment and reimbursement, average costs increased with severity of patient condition (directly reflected in number of disability points assigned to patients), and with the number of skilled nursing days, a ". . . complementary index of the severity of patients needs" (1979).

Walsh's study further shows that both county and voluntary homes are more expensive than proprietary facilities, and that costs are inversely proportional to proportion of Medicaid patients. A skilled care patient added $2.73 per day, while each additional point for disability increased costs by an amount dependent on the actual point score. To care for a 25-point patient cost $5.20 more per day than to care for one with a five point score, an important inducement to accept low-need patients in a flat-rate system. In the Walsh analysis, the qualitative dimension of a home was determined by long-term care professionals and included considerations of amount and preparation of food, quality of medical care, quality of housekeeping, and compliance with housing standards. A point score was given for quality, and this score was then entered into the regression equation, thereby allowing separate analysis of the impact of patient characteristics.

Neither the Birnbaum New York analysis nor Walsh's technique provide an unbiased and totally methodologically pure approach. Both rely heavily on subjective assessments of quality, while the Illinois point count system may misconstrue the actual relative costs of providing services for certain categories of patients, for example, is occasional oxygen really more expensive than a diet prescribed by a doctor? Nonetheless, both show the feasibility of a quality-adjusted, patient characteristics approach and should lead to a more aggressive research program to define the dimensions of quality and thus more accurately link resource use to outcomes. The implications for reimbursement, as well as for determination of the effectiveness of resource use, would be highly significant (Walsh, 1979).

Admission Rate

Patient turnover or admissions rate is another source of cost variation which appears related to patient characteristics. One might, for example, argue that this variable would distinguish post-stroke patients or rehabilitation candidates from patients needing long-term custodial care. Actually, the turnover indicator may also reflect discharge policies of the facility and/or the source of patient funding, that is, the using up of a given type of third party coverage for nursing care services. Whatever the combination of variables masked by the turnover rate, most studies show high positive cost effects associated with high turnover. Accounting reasons for this relationship may range from high administrative costs to patient type and condition.

The empirically derived influence of the admission rate in the studies surveyed by Bishop was very high. The addition to annual total cost per additional admission ranged from $385 to $1,720. The addition to annual average operating cost ranged between $262 and $1,050. In their national sample analysis, Birnbaum et al found that costs per admission were $419. That same analysis showed that an additional admission added about $0.017 per day to average operating costs. Similarly, Meiners found that one additional unit added to the annual admission rate accounted for 0.04 percent of added cost. Both results were statistically significant (Bishop, 1980; Birnbaum et al, 1979; Meiners, 1978).

Private Versus Public Pay

A number of analyses have shown that source of payment seems related to average costs, although this factor appears to work in a somewhat contradictory fashion. One could argue that a commitment to the private market, as shown by high percent private pay, should result in higher costs, since a key element in success in the private market is the provision of amenities (for example, more nursing hours), which cost more money. On the other hand, it can be argued that success in the private market might stem from offering lower cost (though not necessarily lower quality) care, since private buyers of care will have to pay out of their own pockets and so will shop for the best value.

Given the plausibility of both of these arguments, it is not surprising that empirical results show both types of outcomes, even within the same study. For example, Birnbaum et al and Bishop in Massachusetts, and Walsh in Illinois, found that per diem costs were

684

lower in public pay homes, while Birnbaum *et al* and Mennemeyer found the reverse in New York. The Birnbaum national analysis found the private pay to be a positive but statistically insignificant influence on costs, a finding which Bishop finds not surprising, since the national data average out the regulatory and third-party payer effects across the various States (Bishop, 1980; Birnbaum *et al*, 1979).

Actually, the seeming inconsistency both among arguments and evidence may be resolvable if the effects of providers' commitments and regulations are incorporated into the discussion. To do so, of course, involves the realization that the empirically identified effects of various factors, such as payment source, reflect the interaction of a number of other forces such as those in the services-quality-patient characteristics intersection. In the sources of payment case, one might well argue that a given provider makes a commitment to the private market and, thus, to the provision of more nursing services, implying higher average costs. Another provider may be more committed to the public market and thus to a lower nursing input per patient. The first provider, having to attract private pay patients, may have to be highly efficient in order to be price competitive with similar providers. The public pay-oriented homes, however, may not have to be as efficient, since their costs may be reimbursable, as under Medicaid, and since they may not have to compete for patients. Consequently, if one can control for nursing intensity (in effect holding it constant), the private pay, market-oriented homes can be more efficient for a given type of service. If the comparison is not made in these terms, the contrast is between two dissimilar types of provision and may be invalid.

According to Birnbaum *et al*, the New York and Massachusetts evidence would seem to bear out the latter argument. In New York, the public reimbursement rates have been high relative to the private market rates, and homes are more likely to be committed to the public market. The average home may not have to be as aggressive in price competition or as cost-efficient with their amenities-rich private offering, since they can cover their higher (private) costs through the public rate and since they do not have to compete so aggressively for patients. To attract private pay patients in the essentially public pay New York environment, the mainly private-oriented facility would have to be price competitive and cost-efficient. In Massachusetts, however, the incentive to go after private pay patients is greater, nursing services and other offered amenities may be more lavish, and average costs are higher in the privately oriented facilities, the reverse of New York. In both cases, then, it would seem that, assuming a constant level of amenities in both types of facilities and the same reimbursement and regulatory

685

environment, the private pay-oriented homes would find themselves having to be more efficient and less costly on an average cost basis (Bishop, 1980; Birnbaum et al, 1979).

The interplay among costs and the regulatory, reimbursement, and market environment are also shown in the Medicare (as distinct from Medicaid) reimbursement question. The Birnbaum study, for example, shows that filling a Medicare-certified bed with a Medicare-certified patient is more costly than filling a standard Medicaid bed with a public patient. In Massachusetts in 1975, the impact of a one percentage point increase in Medicare patients in Medicare beds was a highly significant 34¢ per day addition to average operating costs. Similar outcomes were obtained for New York, although the national data show a much more modest effect. These results indicate that studies should be undertaken to assess the cost implications of differing public pay certification among the various States, especially as they relate to the Medicaid-Medicare-private pay patient mix.

The State Regulatory Environment and Costs

Specific State or "internal" regulations also help to determine costs. For example, Birnbaum et al found that prospective reimbursement was associated with higher costs than were retrospective systems. Possible technical explanations for this somewhat surprising result may lie in their particular specification of equations. Also, the need to set higher rates to induce facility proprietors to accept reimbursement systems with high downside risks, as well as the possibility that prospective rates may be used in high cost States to contain future cost increases, may underlie these findings. In any event, as Birnbaum and his associates point out (1979), their results parallel those of Sloan and Steinwald on hospital cost prospective reimbursement schemes.

Birnbaum et al also found that other internal regulations, such as the presence and enforcement of life safety codes and so-called "absolute" staff requirements (the need for a nurse or dietician in every facility, regardless of size) and low occupancy penalties exerted statistically significant, positive effects on costs. Certificate of need programs, pre-admission patient assessment requirements, and uniform charts of accounts did not. By contrast, flat rate reimbursement systems, rate limit systems, and administrator salary limits produced insignificant negative effects on costs. It should be noted that they found similar results in both their static and structural analyses based on the behavioral analysis of providers.

Similarly, Meiners found that flat rate, or other cost control type, reimbursement systems exerted statistically significant downward influences on (average) costs, that is, they were about 12 percent lower than for homes with any other system. His study also appears to demonstrate that more liberal types of cost reimbursement systems, as well as those featuring cost reimbursement subject to limits, tend to raise average costs though the coefficients are not statistically significant. His conclusions are hedged, however, by the finding that, with a changed functional form (that is, a linear version) for the cost equation, the most liberal cost reimbursement systems do appear to significantly increase average costs (Meiners, 1978).

It should also be noted that Meiners combined prospective reimbursement and flat rate reimbursement as the most stringent reimbursement types. He also used terms showing proportion of patients in each home paid for under each reimbursement type, rather than State dummy variables as Birnbaum used in the national study.

Frech and Ginsburg also discerned important reimbursement influences on costs. Specifically, they found that pure cost reimbursement systems without ceilings had the highest costs, 21 percent more than flat rate systems. On the other hand, cost reimbursement systems with ceilings were much less costly than those without ceilings and, in fact, were not much more costly than flat rate systems. Ceilings appear to be binding constraints on individual home costs. Overall, Frech and Ginsburg also found that all types of prospective reimbursement systems together yielded costs between pure cost reimbursement and flat rate systems. Somewhat surprisingly, however, prospective systems without ceilings and those with reimbursement based on nursing home group characteristics produced costs much like those in flat rate systems. By contrast, prospective reimbursement systems with ceilings behaved like pure cost reimbursement systems. These last results, which run counter to what we might expect, may partially be explained by the relatively recent development of some reimbursement systems in 1972 (the year of the survey data) and by changes in the systems prior to the survey. Such findings indicate, however, that further research is needed on these types of interaction (Frech and Ginsburg, 1980).

Achievements and Limits of
Nursing Home Cost Function Analyses

It is clear that the range of variables and influences treated by cost function analysis is very wide. As Bishop notes, cost function research has identified systematic links between nursing home costs and certain key variables. Among the latter are occupancy rate, ownership and provider type, location, and certified level of care. Costs may also be influenced by patient mix and by services offered, although the connections are not as consistent.

On the other hand, a number of problems characterize cost studies of the type reviewed here. Again as cited by Bishop, the data are faulty in measuring product descriptors and quality of care. More fundamentally, the interactions among quality, case-mix, and service intensity present some special problems of definition and measurement. As Bishop says, future studies may have to measure new variables which are better suited to their purposes.

We must also recognize that measured costs and product variation reflect a very complex environment involving (among other factors) reimbursement policies, State-specific quality and certification standards, and private demand conditions. If this complexity is not mirrored in models of cost, the models will not faithfully reflect factors influencing nursing home costs. Also, their usefulness in the policymaking process will be very limited, since they may mislead policymakers into believing that the links between costs and certain variables are simpler than they actually are.

Other Approaches to Costs and Outputs

Because of the recognized limits to cost function analyses, other approaches to the question of costs and of regulatory impact have been suggested to assess the behavior of nursing homes as economic entities and subjects of regulation. Among these alternatives are a more "structural" examination of costs and the interactions among a number of other factors characteristic of nursing home behavior. Additionally, one might directly consider the nature of the production process for nursing home outputs (however defined) via the production function.

The Birnbaum group has recognized that single equation cost models emphasize average costs to the exclusion of other aspects of nursing home provider behavior, especially in a regulated environment. In analyzing these firms and this industry, we are clearly concerned with aspects other than costs, since we are dealing with a multi-dimensional output, the ingredients of which include bed days of care as well as quality of care. In this light, a focus solely on cost might lead an analyst or regulator to opt for regimes of care which are unacceptably low with respect to the objectives of a long-term caring institution or a caring system. Furthermore, given the possible types of interaction in the system, a single equation model could be misleading. For example, reimbursement may be related to service intensity as well as to costs. A single equation cost model would, therefore, identify only the direct effects of the reimbursement variable without correctly specifying its indirect effects through the service intensity variable.

These considerations led Birnbaum *et al* to formulate so-called structural and reduced form equations employing systems of simultaneous equations related to nursing home behavior. These allow the analysis of a number of interactions among various factors and a number of outcomes. In particular, they seek to incorporate inter-

688

actions among regulation, private demand conditions, and cost. Among relevant factors are average daily operating costs, service intensity as measured by nursing hours per patient day, intensity of rehabilitation services (measured by an index of such services), occupancy rate, public-private patient mix, and the private pay price or rate, a proxy for the competitiveness of private pay patients for available space. Multiple regression analysis of costs and simultaneous analyses of the other endogenous variables allow recognition of a number of relationships, for example, service intensity pushes costs up, yet simultaneously increases the occupancy rate and the percent of private pay patients, both of which can be shown to drive costs down. Similarly, prospective reimbursement usually leads to higher service intensity and higher costs, but it also may lead to a higher private rate and a smaller number of private pay patients, thus increasing access for public patients. Conversely, retrospective or flat rate reimbursement may reduce costs but will also curtail service intensity and the share of public patients. To capture these interactions, as well as the behavioral consequences of various reimbursement, regulatory, and certification provisions, Birnbaum *et al* devised simultaneous equation models in which the outcomes listed earlier were shown to be functions of each other as well as of the regulatory/reimbursement/certification climate.[4] Note that models reflect behaviors of individual nursing homes rather than behavior across market areas or defined catchment areas.

The results of the application of this model to the 1973–74 National Nursing Home Survey data generally reinforced the findings from the single equation model, although there were some startling differences which we will discuss. More importantly, the model shows the interrelations among the endogenous variables concerned with provider behavior and the impact of regulation, etc. Average costs, for example, are clearly influenced by newly introduced elements in the expected direction. Nursing intensity, omitted in the single equation model because of its intercorrelation with other variables, adds significantly to average costs, while occupancy rate reduces them. So also, private pay patient share accompanies lower cost levels. These latter findings appear connected with the impact of increased nursing service on keeping beds filled and on the desirability of the home to private pay patients.

Average Costs in the Structural Framework

All of the listed endogenous variables were found significant in influencing average costs. Nursing intensity, for example, showed

---

[4] See Birnbaum *et al* (1979), I, pp. 125–130 for a discussion of the structural approach. Results of the structural analysis are found in Volume II, pp. T-8–12 though T-8–42. The following discussion is based on the Volume II analysis of these results.

689

that for every 10 percent increase in that service, there would be a 4.6 percent increase in costs. Occupancy as a proxy for demand exerted a significantly negative influence on costs, as did percent private patients. Rehabilitation services were also positively related to costs. Bed size, a proxy for scale, is strongly and positively linked to costs. By contrast, the admissions rate (turnover) is not as influential as in the single-equation cost models, and the ICF variable is completely insignificant. These results, as well as those for occupancy and percent private patients, may reflect the inclusion of intensity of nursing services, a variable omitted from the single-equation cost models. In the case of ICF/SNF certification variable, the ICF factor may have included a lower amount of nursing services already. The effect was, however, masked in the single-equation cost analysis.

Reimbursement shows some strong and interesting influences. Retrospective reimbursement is, again, cost suppressing, more so than prospective reimbursement, reducing costs by $1.74 per day. Surprisingly, flat rate reimbursement is much less influential ($-50¢$ per day), and the coefficient is not statistically significant. Limits on administrative salaries, uniform charts of accounts, certificate of need programs, and minimum staffing requirements are all significant, but low occupancy penalties and regional wage levels are not.

Structural Analysis of Service Intensity

The role of service intensity was covered by two equations in the Birnbaum model. In effect, the intensity of services was denoted by nursing intensity and rehabilitative service level. There also seems to be an inverse relationship between the two types of service, that is, the more nursing service provided, the less rehabilitation would be available. (This result was only statistically significant in connection with rehabilitation, however.)

Among the exogenous variables (those affecting nursing homes from the outside), bed size (a proxy for the effects of scale) was not significant, although the influence seemed positive. On the other hand, frequency of admissions, a measure of turnover, was positively and significantly associated with rehabilitation services offered. Similarly, SNF certification was positively and significantly linked to intensity of nursing service. Number of bedridden patients was neither positively nor significantly tied with either measure of service intensity. These equations also show that reimbursement methods affect "quality" as shown by service intensity. Retrospective payment reduces nursing services by 0.2 hours per day in comparison with prospective reimbursement; rehabilitation services seem similarly influenced. Flat rate payment appears to have much the same effect as retrospective reimbursement. The choice of a flat rate or retrospective system can cut costs, but only at the expense of quality,

690

a result that may be undesirable. Flat rate systems also eliminate many rehabilitative services which appear to be the first to
go when providers are faced with fixed reimbursement limits.
Occupancy penalties, which might have reduced resources available
to nursing homes and thereby reduced services, were instead found
to be associated with greater intensity of nursing services. Possibly
nursing home operators increased nursing service intensity to keep
beds filled and penalties down.

Occupancy and Access

Occupancy rate, the percentage of beds filled, was used as proxy
for demand for nursing home services. It is influenced directly by
turnover and nursing intensity and indirectly by reimbursement
systems which may cut nursing intensity. Rehabilitation services
also were associated with occupancy rate (thus demand), though
not to a significant degree. Certificates of need, designed to prevent
an over-supply of beds and facilities, also raise occupancy rates by
perhaps 2.5 percentage points, possibly lowering costs as well. This
result may only be attained, however, by reducing access for public
patients. Again, proprietary, for-profit homes experience higher
occupancy rates, although it is difficult to determine whether this
is because of client preference or because of more aggressive cost
minimizing (and bed-filling) behavior by private proprietors.

On the negative influence side we find bed/population ratio in the
market area and private pay price, that is, there is an expected
negative relationship between private price and private quantity
demanded. Along the same lines, occupancy is negatively associated (though not significantly) with private price, perhaps because
private pay patients require faster access and no waiting in line.
Again, three-bed versus two-bed rooms exert a negative influence.
Apparently, the difference between SNF and ICF certification was of
little influence, indicating that any low occupancy penalties should
be uniformly applied across facilities regardless of level of care
classification. Low occupancy rate penalties themselves appeared
to have little effect on occupancy rates.

Private Price Factors

The supply-price interaction was sought with an inverse supply
function which showed price as a function of quantity provided, of
other constraints on its behavior, and of internal factors, for example,
nursing intensity, occupancy rate, etc. From the analysis, it appears
that private price is a function of occupancy rate and both types of
service intensity, nursing and rehabilitation. In fact, the relationship
is so strong and so much larger than that found in the average cost
equations that Birnbaum and his associates suggest the private pay
patients were being charged more than the marginal cost of pro-

691

ducing these services. Private rate is also strongly influenced by reimbursement formulae. Specifically, retrospective reimbursement strongly pushes up private prices as the policy-makers attempt to control public rates. The implication is that cost controls aimed at public pay patients are increasing the costs which private pay patients must bear. The same is less true of flat rate and allowable cost limit types of reimbursement. Controlling average public costs may be raising average private costs, a dubious policy outcome at best.

Results for private versus non-profit ownership are much the same as the effects of cost-cutting reimbursement formulae. For-profit ownership seems associated with higher private prices, indicating that private patients in those facilities are more heavily subsidizing public patients than is true in non-profit facilities. Either full costs are not being reimbursed for public patients, or excess profits are being made on private pay. Percentage of rooms with one bed is directly related to private prices. Coefficients for levels of disability, percentage of bedridden patients, and percentage of those needing aid with getting out of a bed or chair, were all significant but negative. Possibly public patients tend to be more debilitated than private patients and private patients shy away from facilities with more disabled patients. The study data do not permit a comparison of private and public patient characteristics.

The relation between the share of beds occupied by public and by private patients was examined to gain a more direct view of access for public patients. This equation appears to show that cost-reducing reimbursement actions by public authorities will put public patients at disadvantage. Of course, this result will have the same effect as direct cost-cutting via limitations on costs, so that there are double-barreled consequences from these policies. The outcome of public policy is also shown dramatically by the influence of retrospective reimbursement, which significantly reduced access for public patients. By contrast, low occupancy penalties increased access for public patients, that is, forcing facilities to fill beds may make them more receptive to public patients. Favoring the access, or at least utilization, by private patients were the degree of nursing intensity and the amount of rehabilitative service. These factors appear to attract private patients. ICF certification, non-profit status, and fewer beds per room are associated with private patients. Turnover is inversely related, indicating that private patients have longer average stays.

Reduced-Form Equations

In the reduced-form version of the Birnbaum multi-equation model, all endogenous variables (internal to the individual nursing home) are omitted as explanatory variables. This gives the impact of the exogenous variables, including reimbursement formulae, ICF/SNF certification, State-mandated occupancy penalties, etc. on the endogenous variables including average operating costs. Thus we can link cost-related reimbursement formulae not only directly to average operating costs, but also indirectly through their effects on other endogenous variables which, in their turn, affect average operating costs.

As suggested earlier, Birnbaum *et al* found that reimbursement types and rates have a complex relationship with nursing intensity and amount of rehabilitation service which are reflected in average costs. The reduced form of these analyses differs importantly from the structural version. On the surface, a retrospective type of system reduces average daily costs by $2.31 in comparison with a prospective system; a flat rate cuts them by $0.87. So also, a limit on cost-related reimbursement (a form of modified flat rate) brings costs down by $1.50 per day. Cost limits also seem to directly reduce access for public patients. Conversely, adoption of uniform accounting procedures by State governments as the basis for reimbursement costs appears to increase operating costs (by $2.41 per day) and the private rate (by $1.85 per day). Certificate of need and minimum staff requirements increased average costs and the private rate or price. This result may reflect a more positive stance toward public care, and thus higher regulatory cost impacts, in those States which have adopted such practices. This possibility emphasizes the fact that a regulatory posture and a stance toward public provision may be more influential in cost determination than some of the so-called more objective determinants of costs. Of course, we must recognize that the "progressive" States may be the most industrialized and/or unionized and thus higher priced from the standpoint of input cost.

Other than reimbursement formulae, facility characteristics and patient descriptors were important exogenous factors affecting costs and the other variables of interest. ICF certification, for example, led to $2.01 per day lower average costs than did SNF classification. It also led to 0.45 fewer nursing hours per day and lower rehabilitation intensity. Occupancy rates were also lower in ICFs than in SNFs by 2.2 percentage points, as were private rates (minus $2.50 per day) and percent of private patients (minus 7.4 percentage points). Admitting frequency (turnover) also raised costs and private rates, although the latter not so much as the former, presumably because of the smaller amount of paperwork required. Turnover was linked to service intensity, suggesting that short-stay patients are more concerned with rehabilitation. Occupancy rates also were lower with higher admissions, as might be expected given the necessity of

693

moving patients in and out of beds with a high volume of admissions and discharges.

Profit-oriented homes have lower costs ($1.50 less than non-profits per day), but their private rates are higher (plus $1.53 per day). This suggests that private facilities may either be making extraordinary profits on private patients or that private patients are subsidizing public patients, as was suggested in the positive relation between private pay rates and cost containment measures. Given much of the furor over the alleged behavior of proprietary facilities in seeking only private patients, it is perhaps surprising that in the Birnbaum et al study, such facilities contain a smaller proportion of private pay patients than do non-profits. Fewer patients per room also raises costs, as does the percentage of services purchased externally on contract.

Patient Characteristics

Among the aspects of nursing home operation attracting much attention has been patient condition and/or characteristics. Included in these attributes have been diagnosis, age, sex, and disability level, as measured by a Katz scale or some similar instrument. Interestingly, the Birnbaum et al reduced form analysis appears to show that age is relevant to average operating costs only for percent private pay in a facility. Private patients appears to be somewhat older than public, possibly because patients and their families will only spend their own money if the client is very ill and needs much attention. Female patients appear to cost more and were charged higher private rates.

A corollary of these private pay findings is that the relative youth of public pay patients may be symptomatic of relative over-utilization. Such a concept is imprecise, however, unless one defines it in terms of alternatives and examines the stimuli to institutionalization. Although the Birnbaum analysis did not consider the socioeconomic condition of patients, it is possible that low income or lack of social supports may force recourse to a nursing home for some elderly and their families for whom home care is not affordable.[5]

In the Birnbaum et al research, higher level of patient debility implied higher average costs as well as greater nursing intensity, more rehabilitation service, and higher private pay rates. Partial debility, however, appeared to influence increasing costs more than full disability, a finding which parallels those of Skinner and Yett, (1970). Evidently, highly debilitated patients require little care other than routine maintenance, usually being confined completely to bed. Mildly debilitated patients, on the other hand, also require little

---

[5] See Vladeck (1980) for a discussion of these factors.

care, often being able to manage much of their own care. However, moderately debilitated patients, usually private pay, are more active than the former and more in need of help than the latter, so they require more services on average. Severer medical diagnoses, as distinct from debility or disability, also boosted costs but reduced rehabilitative intensity, probably a reflection of the need for greater nursing services on one hand and the improbability of successful rehabilitation on the other.

By way of summary, it appears that the Birnbaum structural and reduced form models provide more insight into the behavior of providers with respect to cost, quality, and access to service than do the straight single equation models. In addition, these approaches offer more information on the impact of public reimbursement, rate-setting, and regulatory and certification policies. Among the more important implications of the structural approach are the following:

- The price elasticity of demand for an individual nursing home for pay provision is greater than one. This has been suspected for some time and incorporated in much previous modeling of nursing home behavior, but the analysis provides perhaps the most convincing proof.
- A corollary of the above is that by not requiring copayments or other devices to raise costs to public patients, we may be encouraging overutilization of institutions with adverse effects not only on the total social costs of providing long-term care but also on the development of cost-effective and satisfying alternatives.
- Cost control policies clearly restrict access for publicly supported patients.
- Cost control policies also restrict the volume of nursing services provided, possibly reducing the quality of care below desired levels.
- The lack of strong links between patient characteristics and average operating costs suggests that more debilitated patients may not be getting intense enough nursing or rehabilitative services. If so, more research must be undertaken on patient-centered or patient group-centered reimbursement procedures.
- Certificates of need increase occupancy rates.
- Low occupancy penalties have little effect on occupancy rates but may increase public patient access to care.
- Cost containment programs increase the difference between private and public pay rates. This implies either high profits from private pay and/or subsidization of public pay patients by private pay patients.

Although the Birnbaum *et al* analysis appears to provide these valuable insights, more research along these lines is needed, especially if new data bases are provided or discovered. Certainly their noteworthy conclusions warrant further investigation.

Are Patient Characteristics Appropriate?

Conventional cost function analysis usually does not include user descriptions or characteristics among the independent variables associated with cost determination. In short, costs are usually cast as functions of output, technology, and input prices. In cost analysis of health services, however, patient characteristics are often included because of the difficulty of identifying and quantifying output(s). Specifically, patient attributes or "case-mix" are often introduced as independent variables to control for the inadequacy of the patient day as a measure of the scope and intensity of services which compose health care outputs. In part for this reason, and also because it is important to know whether patients of varying disability levels receive different "bundles" of nursing care, nursing home cost analyses have followed the tradition of including patient characteristics in the cost function.

A number of problems are associated with this approach. First, there is the question of specification as to which characteristics are relevant. Second, other output descriptors or surrogates may interact with case-mix, for example, services offered, services provided, quality. These other descriptors may be as difficult as output to identify and specify; moreover, their analytical and causal interaction with case-mix may be harder to specify than the nature of the output itself. In addition, it is unclear which parts of possible output mix or set of descriptors influence which aspects of output, *per se.*

Because of these limitations on conventional cost function analysis and the difficulties associated with incorporating patient characteristics and other descriptors, it seems appropriate to consider other ways of analyzing cost. Among the possible approaches are production function analyses, analyses based on better patient groupings, and direct analyses of case-mix, quality, and cost interaction.

A Direct Case-Mix—Cost-Production Analysis

A 1975 study by the Battelle Institute in Seattle for the National Center for Health Services Research does attempt a direct calculation of the production and delivery of services to various categories of nursing home patients. This study used canonical correlation to model and calculate, simultaneously, a production function for care and the allocation of care in 140 nursing homes to sets of patients as defined by the Washington State reimbursement formula as of 1971 (McCaffree et al, 1975). Canonical correlation was chosen because conventional cost and production analyses run into complications from output variation, substitution among inputs, and the multiproduct nature of nursing homes (in that they provide care simultaneously to patients with differentially severe conditions).

Battelle's fundamental assumption about the nature of the nursing home is that it is an enterprise which produces, jointly, a series of outputs (that is, care to several levels of patients), although it experiences only one production function. In the Battelle model, a home will generate standard care units (SCUs) which will then be "packaged" in different amounts and provided to differing groups of patients. These groups will differ both in severity of condition and source of payment, whether private or public. It should be noted that the SCU is never defined, remaining an abstraction, although it is postulated to be composed of room, board, and labor services. The activity of interest is, first, the production of SCUs and, then, their allocation among categories of patients to maximize the profits of the firm.

Under the 1971 Washington State rules, there were five home groupings: extended care facilities (ECFs; essentially Medicare-eligible), three additional lower classes (I-III; some Medicare/Medicaid, some Medicaid only), and boarding homes. Patients could be private or public pay. Private and public patients were mixed in the same homes. Homes were classed by the types of patients they could serve, so that some could cater to all levels of care needs while others could take only less demanding patients. On the bases of patient characteristics and reimbursement eligibilities, there were essentially four groups for analysis: Group I (accepting all classes of Medicaid patients; 36 percent could take Medicare as well), Group II (taking less severe cases), Group III (essentially an ICF group), and the ECF or Medicare level homes serving only Medicare patients.

For the most part, the analysis supported conventional beliefs. In the Group I facilities, all private pay categories of patients received more service than did their public pay counterparts. The same was generally true for the ICF level of care homes.

The most surprising output allocation outcomes were those showing that private level 3 (lower care) patients received more services than the private level 2 (higher care) group, perhaps an artifact of the numbers in the sample. More surprising were the results of the production function analysis which showed that the dieticians in the Group I homes extended no appreciable effect on output and that nurses aides were more productive than licensed practical nurses (LPNs). The former may have been due to the fixed cost nature of dietician services, the latter to the barriers to entry to the LPN profession. Yet more startling was the finding that neither RNs nor LPNs exerted much influence on the production function among ICF-level homes. This result may stem from the existence of such

697

staff on scene as a matter of regulation or habit among such homes, which are often owned or managed by RNs or LPNs.

The canonical correlation analysis was also applied to facility characteristics to identify influences on production conditions and allocations. This effort showed no influences derived from level of Medicare certification among Group I firms but did reveal important consequences of profit versus non-profit orientation. For-profit entities were shown to produce more service for each patient class and also to use inputs more productively than the entire set of analyzed firms, profit and non-profit, in Group I. Facility bed size also did not influence production but did appear to affect the distribution of care among classes of using units, though not in a systematic manner. Overall, the facility size (and presumably scale) impacts were uncertain.

The analysis also purported to illuminate the relative pricing questions within and between care classes. Among firms providing only ICF-level services, the price per SCU seems to have been the same. Among Group I firms, however, each patient set within the public and private pay sectors paid the same amount per SCU, but the private paid more per SCU than did the public. So also, wages equaled marginal factor costs among Group I firms but not among ICF-type firms. The former behaved as profit maximizers; the latter did not. It is possible that the factor cost findings may reflect the higher standards required of SNF-level firms, whereas the failure of ICFs to maximize profit may reveal the larger number of public pay patients found there.

Dealing directly with production and allocation of the product with the canonical correlation technique rather than attempting to generate cost functions allows the analyst to consider the case-mix/output linkage without having to use case-mix as a surrogate for output. The inability to deal with output definition and measurement is also avoided, since no unique output is sought. Rather, the amounts of care delivered to each care group can be presumed to reflect corresponding multiples of the SCU without having to identify or quantify that abstract bundle.

McCaffree et al also assert that their analysis makes some definite statements about profitability and presumed subsidization by private patients. Specifically, they claim that patients who are exclusively Medicare (ECF) receive more care than the heaviest category of public pay (group 1) patients not in ECFs. Not surprisingly, light care patients receive fewer SCUs than heavy care cases, which are, however, more profitable, as are private (versus public) patients. Light care groups (public and private) are also shown to sometimes generate losses in Group I homes. The combination of greater profitability from heavy care and possible losses from light care may

698

provide a set of motivations for proprietors to keep or place patients in heavy care situations, as has sometimes been claimed by nursing home reformers. (This is at variance with another common assertion that proprietors skim the patient loads for only light care cases. Such action may occur only if the reimbursement rate is the same for both types of cases. The McCaffree analysis specifically excludes that possibility.) Overall, the analysis purports to show that firms maximize profits by providing services to loss-generating as well as profit-making patients and that the typical firm made positive profits on its operations. Losses on light care patients were less than losses on empty beds. It would seem that this empirical model comes to many of the same conclusions about allocating output as did the geometric expositions developed earlier in Chapter XVI.

The canonical correlation technique also allows the analyst to determine the effects of changes in staffing requirements and, potentially, of changes in other regulations and certification standards. For example, an increase in the requirement for registered nursing hours may raise standards of service for all classes of patients, public and private. However, if we use the amount of care provided public class No. 2 (moderate care need) as a *numeraire,* it can be shown that the private pay groups will all benefit more from such regulations than will any of the public pay groups. In effect, the care groups will share in the additional care, not equally, but in proportion to the amount of care each was receiving before the change in regulations. This result should not surprise us, nor should its policy implications, since proprietors will tend to allocate additional service (and costs) to those customers who pay higher prices and who are responsible for more profit. Also, private pay patients are subject to price rises, at least under certain circumstances, whereas public pay may not be because of reimbursement limits.

This lengthy discussion of the results of the application of the canonical correlation technique may appear overextended; yet it can be justified because of the interesting results and imaginative use of a new methodology in a way that may permit us to evade some of the output definition problems discussed earlier.

The McCaffree *et al* analysis is not without its shortcomings. Birnbaum *et al* note that the assumption of the provision of different qualities of care to patients with the same needs in the same facility depending on source of payment (public versus private) is somewhat artificial and is to be contrasted with their own assumption of uniformity of care within care groups regardless of payment source. So also, the definition of bed-related services, food, and housekeeping activity as fixed inputs in the Washington State study is unusual. Additionally, the McCaffree group allows for no capital/labor substitutions, nor do the researchers consider the possibility that the provision of more care to all levels of patients, regardless of payer, might generate higher private prices and more profits. While these and other criticisms may be valid, and while the McCaffree research may be preliminary, the point remains that a new production function approach to an otherwise awkward analytical problem can produce some interesting results. Clearly, similar research efforts should be encouraged.

Other Approaches to Patient Grouping

The analytical discussion up to this point has focused sharply on the intersection of patient characteristics, implied levels of care and types of services required to address those characteristics, and amount of service which a facility provides in actually caring for patients. Of concern also are the costs of the service "packages" and the impact of regulation on the total amount of care supplied and the nature of the care offering. For the analysis immediately preceding this section, these concerns can be reclassified as those of output identification and quantification and of the supply of care under various pricing systems and at differing levels of prices. Thus, in attempting to define provider behavior and define supply in a functional manner, the analyst is necessarily concerned with the cost implications as well as the output definitions associated with differing patient characteristics.

Diagnosis-Related Groups

One approach to the cost/characteristics linkage might be a type of analysis somewhat similar to the diagnosis-related groups (DRG) devised at Yale University (Fetter et al, 1980). This analytical technique explicitly determines the use of resources for specified medical conditions in an acute care setting. By assessing a large number of patients and their conditions, the Yale researchers claim the ability to predetermine resource requirements for various groups of patients, given the patient's medical and personal characteristics. The DRG system has three basic attributes: 1) a manageable number of patient classifications, 2) a medically meaningful care process reflecting most commonly accepted current practices, and 3) a statistically stable pattern of resource use among the group of patients treated by the facility(ies) in question. In effect, the DRG approach determines the time, skill level, equipment, and drugs necessary to deal with a given condition. These needs can then be assigned costs which can be assessed and predicted for each DRG. These predictions presumably allow providers (mainly hospitals), care planners, health planners, and utilization monitors (usually utilization review teams and/or Professional Standards Review Organizations [PSROs]) to predict resource use and costs and to assess care programs, at

700

least with respect to modal and conventional behaviors among health care professionals. The DRG has been tested and evaluated and is being used in New Jersey as a basis for diagnosis-specific reimbursement rates.

Although the DRG concept is appealing for application to the long-term care field, in which much controversy exists regarding both assessment and the determination of appropriate resource use, some fundamental analytical and methodological issues must be resolved in advance. First, the DRG concept reflects "best" current practice. It relies on modal patterns and leaves the decisions about best practice for serving specified groups of patients (the DRGs) in the hands of practitioners. Where best practice may be still a matter of philosophical as well as technical differences, the resource implications may be unclear. Certainly, the systemic nature of most long-term problems and of the conventional means of addressing them render DRG-type, direct condition-cost linkages of dubious value. So also, the concept of DRGs is grounded in the notion that identifiable groups of patients with specified conditions require definite bundles of care. Such certainty about condition-care package links does not exist in long-term care, since many patients experience multiple conditions which interact to preclude single treatments or outcomes. Also, many important indicators of need for long-term care are social (the availability of family supports) or functional (the ability to cope or to carry on the activities of daily living).

The interactive nature of long-term care requirements, as well as the extra-medical dimension of long-term care need, reveal themselves in the nursing soci support, housing, transportation, and income maintenance facets of best practice in the field. These complex patterns often mean that best practice reflects existing institutional arrangements (for example, recourse to a nursing home, which is a "home," service facility, and nursing center, as well as a hospital). By contrast, acute care usually does not involve such a complicated set of relationships. Similarly, acute procedures appear to have identifiable outcomes in most instances, whereas long-term care may result only in stability of functional condition and/or in death. Long-term care relates more to quality of life in most cases than it does to cure or some other single-valued outcome. The maintenance of health status implies that much long-term care is custodial or at best, rehabilitative, yielding changes that are very hard to measure.

Studies of Patient Condition and Service Needs

The intuitive and analytical appeal of attempting to relate patient conditions to services needs is reflected in a number of studies.

Four recent research efforts attempted to address these issues directly. Different questions motivated the individual research programs, and different analytical approaches were involved.

In 1979, Walsh published an analysis of the 10-year old Illinois point count system of determining the basis for cost-related reimbursement. Since the 1960s, Illinois has used a three-part formula comprising a base (or flat) rate paid for all patients regardless of need, a payment to adjust for needed services above the minimum level, and a special activity payment to facilities with rehabilitation nursing and social rehabilitation programs. The special need payments are determined with a point count system of patient evaluation, implemented by caseworkers from the Illinois Department of Public Aid. Walsh questioned whether the system has special problems for patient-related reimbursement in general and whether experience with the point count system has been favorable. These questions resulted from a series of problems with the system: the assessment instrument was viewed by many as too simple and undiscriminating, yet a complicated tool was too difficult to use; the system was complex and costly to administer; patients had to be re-evaluated too often; different evaluators differed in their assessments of the same patients, often to a considerable degree (15 percent among the various State regions); and the system was open to bribery from facility operators because of the potential gains from evaluating patients as highly disabled. (A one point change for each patient in a 100 bed facility could gain the owner $6,000 to $7,000 annually and cost the system as much as $3 million per year.) Most importantly, point count reimbursement was not empirically related to the cost of providing care. The relationship is (was) only approximate and may have led to perverse incentive effects. For example, if the actual cost of feeding a patient in bed is $2.00 per day and the State pays $2.50, operators will strive to keep many patients bedridden who might otherwise be ambulatory. Additionally, Federal mandates to develop cost-related reimbursement systems may lead to expensive time-and-motion studies if the point count system is to provide the basis for reimbursement. On the other hand, tying a patient assessment procedure to the reimbursement system has a greater advantage because it allows payments for a wide range of patients to be tailored to the care they actually need. Walsh argues that if objections to the point count system mandate its removal, some other system involving patient characteristics must be developed.

Having established that the point count system revealed the existence of patient differences related to care, Walsh then determined whether those differences imply cost differences. He proposed two lines of analysis: a statistical approach based on multivariate techniques and an engineering, or time-and-motion, study based on

702

measured care requirements on a per-patient basis. Working with a conventional profit-maximizing model, Walsh defines the nursing home revenue function to include quantity and amenity items as well as the Medicaid reimbursement rate and the proportion of Medicaid and private patients. The cost function constraining the maximizing of revenues and profits includes items for labor and capital devoted both to expanding quantity and amenities (the latter needed to attract private patients). The first order, profit-maximizing conditions are quite predictable in equating wage and interest rates with marginal revenues from uses of additional units of labor and capital for both private and public patients. These conditions also require equating marginal costs of amenities with marginal revenues from private patients brought about by changes in amenity level. Finally, they demand equating marginal revenues from using a unit of labor or capital to increase quantity with MR from using labor or capital to increase amenities. Facilities should choose a public-private mix so that the marginal revenue from private patients equals the Medicaid rate.

In estimating cost functions, it was assumed that the elasticity of substitution between capital and labor in nursing homes was near zero and that regional input price differences could be handled with an area-wide index. Amenities and quality were measured by an index of nursing home quality based on historical supervisory agency ratings, the proportion of public patients in a facility, and whether ownership was county, private, or voluntary. The nature of care was represented by average point count and by the proportion of patients receiving skilled level care. Managerial efficiency was represented by facility size, capacity utilization, and the presence of an owner on the scene. The cost function was for a series of products generated jointly but independently. (This assumption is similar to that in the McCaffree *et al* study discussed earlier.) The basic product was a day of ICF care meeting minimum standards, to which resources to produce skilled care, amenities, etc. were added. The cost function was generated by regression analysis. This analysis showed that patients' conditions as measured by point scores and levels of care were important for computing cost of providing care. A patient receiving skilled care added $2.73 to costs, and each additional point awarded to a patient increased costs by an amount dependent on the size of the point score. Public or voluntary facilities were significantly more expensive than private. The influence of quality was minor though significant. Capacity was not significant, but occupancy rate was.

Overall, Walsh concluded that patient condition did influence costs and that a satisfactory reimbursement formula could be devised

703

reflecting point count and skilled care in individual terms and all other factors in a constant term. That is,

$$\text{reimbursement} = K + a_1 \text{(point-count)} + a_2 \text{(skilled care)}$$
$$= 10.08 + .54 \text{ (number of points)} - .008$$
$$\text{(number of points)}^2 + 3.02 \text{ (skilled care binary)}$$

Although the statistical approach appears to offer much flexibility both to cost analysis and to framing a reimbursement formula, it may be more desirable to link specific patient conditions and the costs of care. Accordingly, Walsh proposed what he called an "engineering approach" based on time-and-motion studies of actual care situations. First, he identified the nature of long-term care needs and then linked them to their frequency in the population. He combined these needs with the number of personnel required to meet such needs and with the time input from each personnel type. Data generated in three facilities by time-and-motion studies allowed calculation of the following relationship:

staff time for condition i = number of staff times (frequency of service per month) times (duration of care) times group factor, that is, the proportion of staff time required to serve one member of a group with a given need.

He determined costs of providing service by constructing a weighted index of staff wages and multiplying that index by the calculated number of hours of staff time required. Overall cost also included a factor for non-labor costs.

The engineering approach has some appeal in terms of direct linkages of costs with conditions, but it displays some weaknesses. The level of expenditure predicted ran about 15 percent ahead of costs as reported by facilities, and the pattern of expenditures among facilities differed from that predicted by the formula. Possible underestimation of economies of scale, as well as the small number of facilities generating the time-and-motion data, may have been responsible for these anomalies.

Overall, Walsh shows that patient condition can be linked to care patterns and costs. He attempts to include quality provided as a cost influence in his statistical approach but does not explicitly do so in the engineering analysis in which he is directly comparing specific patient condition with costs. In 1977, McCaffree et al reported on another study explicitly linking patient condition and cost of care. This study developed a set of cost-finding tools and instruments and identified the relation between costs and the conditions of patients in nursing homes. Overall, the study's object was to test

704

the feasibility of collecting self-reported data on costs and adjusting costs for differences in the characteristics and conditions of patients. The study proceeded in four phases, of which the second generated data on patient characteristics and costs in a sample of selected nursing homes. The fourth extended the analysis to a sample of 50 nursing homes nationwide. Phases I and III involved development of cost data collection instruments and the education of nursing home operators and administrators in their use.

Phase II formally involved the 1974 collection of data on actual contact hours of various categories of nursing service staff for 1,615 patients in 12 facilities across five States. Data were gathered on the patients' medical, social, mental, and financial conditions, as well as on their dates of admissions, age, and sex, 192 descriptors in all. Additionally, all direct nursing service personnel reported on all direct contact activities over a specific 48 hour period. From these data, time weights (percentages of average contact time or PACTs) were calculated, the weights reflecting the proportional amount of total nursing contact time devoted to caring for patients with certain types of conditions. In the words of the report (p. xvii), ". . . the relationship between resident/patient characteristics and conditions and the distribution of direct care time is *relative* to, or expressed as a percentage of the average contact time per resident/ patient day in each facility." In common with the McCaffree *et al* canonical correlation study (using the SCU) and the Walsh study (using point count), this study sought to provide a common denominator of service (the average amount of contact time) and to express the percentage attribution of that time with respect to specific patient characteristics. The time weights provided the mechanism by which nursing costs would be adjusted across facilities with different mixes of patients and characteristics.

The facilities sampled demonstrated wide variations in time available per patient for different employee categories and for volunteers. For example, the facility with the most nursing time had 2.34 times as much as did the one with least. Homes also varied by amount and proportion of nursing contact time available to patients, ranging from .81 hours to 1.96 hours per day and from 36 percent to 57 percent of total tim In addition, among different staff categories there were large vai   ns in the amount of contact time per patient day and in the prop. .on of available time actually used in patient contact . These differences were even more marked for personnel providing specialized services of various types. Perhaps most interesting from the standpoint of analyzing patient condition-cost linkages is the finding that facilities displayed great variations in absolute amounts of contact time for patients having the same conditions across facilities. In general, more nursing contact time available implied more contact time with "heavy care" patients. Overall, 46 percent of variation in the aide/orderly contact time could be explained by selected, cost-related patient characteristics, but only 14 percent of the variation in nursing time could be so explained, perhaps because nurses are likely to encounter random demands on their time. For individual facilities, the amount of variance explained ranged from 16 percent to 71 percent for aide/orderly time, and from 1 percent to 32 percent for licensed nursing time. Use of non-nursing time was not explained. Bishop *et al* (1980, p. 37) conclude that the consistency of the proportional distribution of characteristic-related use of personnel time within and across facilities and the much smaller consistency of absolute time allocations across facilities suggest that ". . . an absolute standard of need for care, given patient characteristics, is not widely applied."

Analysis of the influence of different patient characteristics indicated that 11 of the 192 explained most of the variation in the use of aide/orderly time, and 12 explained most of the variation in the use of licensed nursing time. On the other hand, most of the characteristics did not explain much use of time or did not do so in a consistent manner. Senility, somewhat surprisingly, did not explain much, usually being associated with other characteristics with more explanatory power. For use of licensed nursing time, the most powerful explainer was the number of medicines required. Patients taking over 10 medications required .105 percent of average contact time. For aides/orderlies, the most important explanatory variable was functional capacity as measured by ADL function, which on average explained 80 percent of the variation in time use. The results on ADL capability are not surprising in light of other studies' findings. Although intermediate care (ICF level) patients received only about 60 percent as much of the aide/orderly time as skilled level patients, and 70 percent as much skilled nursing time, the source of payment (Medicare or Medicaid versus private) was not an important explanatory variable. Apparently, private pay patients were not receiving more care, given their level of care, than were publicly supported patients.

McCaffree and his associates concluded that it was technically feasible to develop a characteristic-related basis for more informed decision-making in allocating nursing home resources. Also, nursing costs across facilities could be compared after adjusting for cost-related characteristics and conditions. An equitable basis for reimbursing facilities with different mixes of patients was thus conceivable. On the other hand, this study did not explicitly consider the quality variable, other than by using sample homes which were supposedly "effective and efficient." The quality issue surfaces in connection with the variations in absolute amounts of contact hours across facilities. In this study, the clear implication is that the absolute amounts of care associated with given characteristics in individual facilities are strongly influenced by the total amount of contact time available, but no basis for that total is analytically proposed.

Although the research indicates the prevalent amounts of time used with respect to particular patient characteristics, it cannot indicate the absolute amount of care which should be received by patients with specific conditions. Indeed, facility differences in use of absolute time indicate on the one hand that standards vary and, on the other, that the data will not internally indicate which standard is preferred. In addition, variations in proportions of available time used for patient contact do not indicate any preferred proportion. Rather, they suggest that facility administrators differ in how they use employee time in training or patient charting and/or with respect to choices of employees with varying levels of competence. Standards for all these matters can only be produced by further work on the effects of services on care provided and on patient outcomes.

With respect to reimbursement, McCaffree *et al* point out that the results provide a set of relative weights and are therefore useful in allocating existing levels of reimbursement among services and among groups of patients. They cannot, however, be used to set the actual reimbursement rate, nor can they be used to determine or compare absolute costs of care for individual patients.

In 1979, McCaffree and another group of associates reported on a follow-up to the 1974 data. Although the earlier study's results indicated that, on average, a good deal of the variation in use of nursing staff time could be explained by patient characteristics on an individual facility basis, the sampled facilities had not been judged typical of the nursing home industry. In addition, another data base was needed to validate the results and coefficients linking characteristics to patterns of time use. Because of the encouraging results of the earlier study and because of its problems, another study was undertaken of 16 randomly-selected, dual-certified (SNF and ICF) nursing homes in Ohio, Vermont, and Washington (State). The researchers hypothesized that the average relative weights (ARWs or PACTs divided by 100 to get whole numbers) would explain a smaller proportion of the variation in contact time among patients with diverse characteristics in typical homes than in superior or efficient homes. Also, it was argued that the explanation of the variation in contact time would be improved by controlling for size, ownership or control, location, or staffing level. The hypotheses were tested by using data from the two samples (1974 and 1977) through estimating the following equation:

$$CT_{ij} = a + B (ARW)_{ij}(ACT_j)$$

707

in which CT_{ij} was the observed contact time in minutes per day for resident i in facility j; ACT_j was the observed contact time in minutes per day in facility j; ARW_{ij} was the average relative weight for resident i in facility j. The $ARW_{ij} = a' + U_1X_{1ij} + \ldots U_nX_{nij}$ where X_{kij} reflects the presence (absence) of characteristic k for resident i in facility j. The U's are the weights derived for the impact of specific individual characteristics on the time use of licensed nurses and aides/orderlies.

When facility, location, and staffing intensity (that is, the amount of licensed nurse contact) were added to the equation to help predict use of aide/orderly time, the overall results were not affected in any significant manner. Only the proprietary variable and the staffing variables were individually statistically significant (with negative coefficients). Reasons for the influence of the proprietary variable were not developed, but the substitutability of licensed nurses for aides/orderlies was clearly shown in the negative influence of staffing level. When bed size was entered as a continuous, not grouped, variable, the influence was small, yet significant for aides/orderlies. For licensed nursing staff, none of the facility characteristics appeared to be significant. "Patient characteristics, when weighted by the ARW's, remained the primary explanatory variables . . ."

Overall, the study concluded that the characteristics identified in the 1974 study and weighted according to the 1974 ARWs explained the variations in contact time of aides/orderlies and licensed nurses as well or better with the 1977 data. Furthermore, the 1974 weights could not be improved on as predictors. Using the 1974 ARWs, the cost-related characteristics explained over half the variation in the contact time of aides/orderlies and nearly 22 percent of the variation in the contact time of nurses. McCaffree et al also concluded that the principles underlying the allocation of contact time among different categories of patients remain applicable across both typical and exceptionally efficient facilities. By contrast, facility characteristics appeared to have had little influence on variations in use of labor time, with the exception of licensed nursing staff level on aides/orderlies.

In common with many other studies, and as shown in the Bruun analysis which will be discussed shortly, patient characteristics reflecting (in)abilities to carry on the activities of daily living (ADL) accounted for most of the variation in contact time of employees among residents. In considering the application of the research results to nursing home administration and reimbursement questions, however, the researchers concluded that the ARW technique (as in the 1974 study) was useful only for determining relative influences across facilities and for setting relative levels of cost-related reim-

708

bursement among different categories of patients. The question of absolute levels of service and of absolute reimbursement rates still requires judgments and choices about desired standards of care. To be sure, if a standard of care, say in terms of desired nursing hours per day, could be agreed upon or revealed by some research, then absolute allocations of time could be made and specific reimbursement levels set. For example, if the staffing standard is established at two hours per day per patient for aide/orderly time, ARWs combined with patient characteristics would imply that ICF patients would get 90 minutes per day of aide/orderly time and 30 minutes of licensed nurse time. Skilled nursing care patients would receive 150 minutes of aide/orderly time and 35 minutes of skilled nursing. With a $3.50 aide/orderly hourly wage rate and a licensed nurse rate of $7.00 per hour, the ICF patients would cost $8.75 for nursing and the SNF patient, $12.89. SNF and ICF reimbursement rates could then be established to reflect these differences. However, to repeat an earlier point, the standard must be set by administrators, policymakers, and/or analysts on the basis of research linking outcomes to care modes. Relative analyses of this type cannot produce such judgments.

A 1980 doctoral dissertation by Bruun was motivated by the need to plan nursing requirements to care for the dependent population in the nation's nursing homes over the remainder of the 20th century. Bruun tried to link patient characteristics to time requirements for various types of nurses (RNs, LPNs, nurses' aides) within an operations research framework. He examined data for 110 patients in 11 facilities in Maryland to determine nursing needs of a set of conditions measured by the Collaborative Patient Assessment Instrument (CPAI). This instrument picks up demographic, functional, specific impairment, general medical, and specific medical conditions. Using procedures and standards from the Health Services in Long-Term Care Study (HSLTC), Bruun linked various CPAI categories to decisions about appropriate assessment, appropriate placement, staffing requirements, and quality assurance. In light of these considerations he selected nursing homes which were well-staffed, had an RN on duty 40 hours a week, were not new at providing skilled care, and had 24 or more beds and an annual occupancy rate of at least 90 percent. Having analyzed patients in the 11 sample facilities, Bruun then tried to match CPAI characteristics with those shown by the 1973–74 National Nursing Home Survey. He used the CPAI Maryland data to sort patients into three categories (self-care, partial care, and total care) which were later shown to match patients sorted on Katz's six-level ADL functional scale. That is, there was consistency between Katz's scores (low score indicating low dependency, etc.) and a sort based on CPAI.

709

The Maryland analysis allowed Bruun to determine the hours of nursing services required to care for sets of patients sorted into the three care sets either using CPAI or Katz's methods. He found that Class I patients (independent in all areas) required an average of over 20 minutes per day of direct care. Class II (dependent in one to three areas) patients required about 76 minutes per day, and Class III patients required over 140 minutes per day. The class method of sorting allowed Bruun to discriminate between low and high using groups, rather than just using averages. In addition, his method permitted much closer monitoring of changes in patients' conditions, and presumably of patients nursing care needs over time. A series of cross-tabulations on the data showed that neither level of care (SNF, ICF) nor age were significantly related to care need. On the other hand, males needed more care than females, and blacks needed more care than whites.

Following his application of the method to the Maryland sample and his development of measures of care requirement from that data, Bruun validated the procedure on a data set of 192 patients from 14 nursing homes in Denver, Colorado. He found that the classification system applied in this way produced results similar to those from the Maryland data set. Bruun then classified the patient sample data from the 1973–74 National Nursing Home Survey (NNHS). He sorted these patients into the three categories based on the patient characteristics shown in the NNHS. From this sort, he was able to determine the number of patients nationwide who would need specific amounts of nursing care. He then projected these requirements outward to estimates of the nursing home population for the last years of the 20th century. Based on his estimates of the full-time equivalents of nursing staff required to care for the various levels of dependency (Classes I, II, III) in the nation's nursing homes, Bruun estimated a shortage of about 14,000 RNs in the nation's nursing homes in both 1974 and 1977. LPNs were present in the needed numbers in 1974, but were over 9,300 in surplus in 1977. Most interestingly, nurses' aides were significantly in surplus in both years, over 7,400 in 1974 and 34,300 in 1977. If Bruun is correct, not only was there a substitution of LPNs and aides for RNs in both years, but also the quality of nursing care in the nursing homes may have been much less than required by current standards and level of dependency. On the other hand, it may well be that aides and LPNs can be substituted for RNs without a significant erosion of quality of care. Further research is clearly needed to establish the linkages between amounts of care, types of care providers, and quality, particularly as measured by outcomes. By the year 2000, Bruun estimates that the shortfalls in RNs would be considerably aggravated if the 1977 shortfall is not redressed in the interval. In

710

absolute terms, given an expected nursing home population of two million (the estimate Bruun uses), the total required number of nurses of all types (including aides) would be almost 860,000, versus about 580,000 in 1977.

Bruun's type of research is clearly useful to analysts and planners of labor force requirements in long-term care and to those responsible for training adequate numbers of personnel to meet long-term care needs. Since he also was able to develop salary cost estimates by level of dependency (that is, Class I cost $2.94 per day in 1977; Class II, $8.85; and Class III, $15.73), Bruun was able to provide some benchmarks as to possible future expenditures, presuming, of course, that nursing patterns do not change. This is a very strong assumption, particularly in an environment of strong pressures for cost containment.

Bruun's approach to the linkages among patient characteristics, care needs, and costs is imaginative in its use of the CPAI to sort patients into cost and care categories, in its recognition of the comparability of sorts made on the basis of the three-category and Katz scales, and in its placing the research effort in the context of the Health Services in Long Term Care process. Since some of that type of analysis had already been undertaken by others, as Bruun himself acknowledged, it appears that an important contribution of his research lies in using the NNHS data with a three-class scheme for sorting patients nationwide into a few, statistically distinct, care categories with highly different care and cost implications. This process does not, however explicitly consider quality and standards, especially with respect to outcomes.

Kenneth McCaffree, in his review of the literature for the 1979 study, offers some important reflections on the interaction of time-and-motion study analysis and the more "statistical" approach taken by his group. He notes that numerous studies (task analyses) of the use of staff time in both hospitals and nursing homes have been done. Task analysis studies, however, tend to be employee-centered rather than patient-centered; the latter look at how much time was spent with patients having certain characteristics rather than looking at what service was provided. Task analysis also suffers from being unable to measure the interrelationship among tasks, while statistical distribution of time as influenced by resident characteristics allows the analyst to fold in both economies of scale and the interaction among tasks. For example, an aide may provide some service to a group of patients simultaneously, or a nurse might give several services to a given patient at about the same time. Task analysis would either have to consider each task, one at a time, or bundle large blocks of tasks into unwieldy analytical groupings. Although the Illinois point count system does attempt to link service to need,

711

McCaffree notes that even that method did not (at least before Walsh's work) establish the actual relationship of cost to various levels of care. Furthermore, in that system patient needs are determined subjectively by professional caseworkers in charge of initial assignments and re-evaluations. The McCaffree design relies instead on the actual amounts and patterns of time use as revealed in the actions of care providers.

Other approaches relating case-mix and cost have been tried by various analysts of hospitals who mainly used cost functions of the types discussed earlier. Other than the work of Skinner and Yett, not much had been done to relate patient characteristics to costs in nursing homes, the main output being a series of indexes linking ADL ability to costs of care. More recently, Deane, Skinner, *et al* have tried to build a debility index into a reimbursement system in which Medicaid rates for two States were predicted on the basis of facility location, input prices, and a debility index. A similar attempt to implement such a program in the State of Washington has so far not produced any useful results.

This discussion of studies tying patient characteristics, care requirements, and cost can close by repeating two points developed earlier:

(1) Standards of care are matters of administrative and political judgment and depend on resource availability and the care which society is willing to provide. Analysts have yet to provide empirical or theoretical bases for standards of long-term care.

(2) The ability of patients to carry on activities of daily living appears to be the best available predictor of nursing home care needs and costs, at least as of 1981. This finding, coming out of many studies and reinforced by Bruun's analysis, suggests that both medical diagnoses and heavy medical requirements may not be of particular value in considering long-term care, including nursing home, costs, and probably should be of secondary importance in developing rational bases for cost-related reimbursement systems. The finding also suggests, as other research has demonstrated, that ADL scales, perhaps of the Katz type, may be the most cost-effective sorters of patients for care needs and the most efficient bases for establishing cost-related reimbursement systems.

University of Colorado Cost, Case-Mix, and Quality Analysis

Linkages within nursing homes among case-mix, quality, and cost which use a method similar to the DRG are currently being sought by the Center for Health Services Research at the University of Colorado (Shaughnessy *et al,* 1980). In its experimental research, the Colorado group has sought to identify case-mix and devise means of classifying long-term care patients by nature and severity of condition. For each class, standards of care quality have been defined, and each resident's care, as well as each facility's (nursing) provision of care, has been assigned quality indicators. The cost consequences (mostly average variable cost) of case-mix and quality have been established in a preliminary manner, as have the implications of facility characteristics. The group has also assessed the implications of proportion of Medicaid patients, age of patients, bed size, and a number of other subcategories of the main groupings of patients. Facility characteristics were essentially those of size, nature of control (profit versus non-profit), certification level (SNF versus ICF, etc.) hospital linkage, proportion of Medicaid patients, and so on.

Case-mix variables were composed of 16 medical diagnostic groups, 21 (initially 27) long-term care problems identified by the Colorado Center, eight activities of daily living (ADL), and three other sets of ADL indexes, grades, and scores (for example, Skinner and Yett, Katz). Four major problem groupings were constructed from the individual problems in the medical, long-term care, and ADL sets. These four groups are nursing care-dependent, medical care-dependent, communicative skill-dependent (for example, impaired vision or hearing), and psychosocial service-dependent. A fifth group, relating to the effects of dehydration and malnutrition, was later added. The four groups were amended by indirect case-mix measures: percent of Medicaid residents in SNF-certified facilities, age distribution of residents, and ratio of admissions of licensed beds. (See Figure XIX–5.)

For each of the individual conditions in the four groups, as well as for the groups themselves, quality of care was defined in relation to a previously established, professionally specified quantity of each service necessary to treat the condition. Quality of service was then determined essentially by comparing the amount and type of service provided to treat actual patient conditions with the previously established norms for amounts and types of services. The Center's professional nursing staff then assigned quality "grades" to individual patients. Facilities were similarly graded and also rated on the basis of facility-wide provision of services for conditions affecting only sub-groups of their patients (for example, certain skin conditions, appearance of residents, need for specialized therapies).

The combinations of case-mix and quality standards in the Colorado research function like DRGs, in that they provide information on the resource use (service) implications of conditions of nursing home residents. This resource-use specification has clear implications for costs. By comparing standards of resource use with actual levels of provision, researchers can not only determine quality but can also tie quality to costs.

713

FIGURE XIX-5
Problem Groups Which Define Similar Sets of Service Modalities,
Based Upon the Set of 21 Frequently-Occurring Problems
In Long-Term Care

Problem Group A: Nursing Care-Dependent Problems
    Primary skin condition
    Dehydration
    Constipation
    Incontinence of bowels etc.
    Incontinence of urine
    Neurologic and/or orthopedic immobility
Problem Group B: Medical Care-Dependent Problems
    Secondary skin condition
    Dependent edema
    Malnutrition
    Hypertension
    Shortness of breath
Problem Group C: Communicative Skill-Dependent Problems
    Impaired vision
    Impaired hearing
    Speech disorder
    Loneliness/isolation
Problem Group D: Psychosocial Service-Dependent Problems
    Confusion
    Depression
    Anxiety
    Apathy
    Disruptive or disturbing behavior
    Discharge planning

Source: Shaughnessy, Peter *et al., Long-Term Care Reimbursement and Regulations: A Study of Cost, Casemix and Quality,* University of Colorado, Center for Health Services Research, 1980

Eight cost categories, each built up from cost centers, were identified. (See Figure XIX–6.) Most attention, however, was focused on average operating costs (AOC) and on nursing care (nurses and nurses aides) costs. Preliminary results from the Colorado cost analyses appear to show that case-mix variables account for significant percentages of the variance in daily operating per patient costs and of the variance in daily nursing and nurses aide costs (Shaughnessy et al, 1980). Initial results as summarized below lead the Colorado researchers to feel that they can explicitly bring case-mix and process quality into the regulatory process. More directly, since Medicaid and non-Medicaid patients in a given facility appear to display similar characteristics, it may be possible to devise Medicaid reimbursement formulae on the basis of the case-mix characteristics of all patients in a given facility. Research is needed, however, to test the hypothesis that Medicaid and other patients of the same case-mix receive comparable quality of care. The reimbursement rate-setting, quality assessment, and cost-finding tasks may also be simplified by the finding that only a small subset of the quality measures account for most of the variation in quality; hence the reimbursement-cost-quality relationship may be fairly straightforward for analytical and research purposes.

The following detailed findings on case-mix from the first year of the Colorado investigation are of the most interest:

- There were distinct and unrelated aspects of case-mix. For example, medical and psychosocial problems, in general, were not related to measures of functional disability. One of the most important groupings of variables shows need for nursing and personal care services. These seem related to ADL problems. Implications for the design of long-term care policy are profound if this finding holds up. Specifically, it suggests that nursing home policy, alternatives policy, and long-term care policy in general should be gearing up for more custodial and less medically-oriented provision. This would reflect much current opinion and intuition among analysts in the field.

- If case-mix clusterings hold up as in the preliminary analysis, it might be useful to define a measure of case-mix based on such groupings in a manner analogous to the DRGs discussed earlier. The Colorado group makes this reference quite explicitly.

- Different groups of long-term care problems appear to cluster in certain facilities. For example, circulatory and musculoskeletal problems are highly correlated. Mental retardation does not appear with non-organic psychiatric conditions.

- Case-mix clusters are often associated with specific types of facilities; for example, by contrast with patients in free-standing

715

FIGURE XIX-6
Cost Categories and Component Cost Centers

Cost Category	Component Cost Centers
Administrative and General Services	Administrative and General Travel and Entertainment Insurance, other than Property Medical Records
Room and Board Services	Dietary Food Laundry and Linen Housekeeping Plant Operation and 　Maintenance
Nursing and Aide Services	RNs LPNs Other (Aides and Orderlies)
Therapy Services	Occupational Therapy Physical Therapy Recreational Therapy Speech Therapy
Other Ancillary Services	Pharmacy Medical Supplies Laboratory X-Ray Physician Care Respiratory Care Social Services Medical Director Utilization Review Dental Care
Personal Services	Beauty and Barber Shop Personal Purchases for Patients
Property	Depreciation Amortization Real Estate Taxes Rent Interest Property Insurance Other Property Expenses
Other Expenses	Income Taxes Other Non-Health Care Non- 　Property Expenses

Source: Shaughnessy, Peter et al., Long-Term Care Reimbursement and Regulation: A Study of Cost, Casemix and Quality, University of Colorado, Center for Health Services Research, 1980.

716

facilities, patients in hospital-based facilities tend to have more problems, be older and more ADL dependent, and have more musculoskeletal problems.

- Percentage of beds certified for skilled care is positively associated with functional dependence but not with other case-mix variables.
- Percentage of Medicaid patients is negatively associated with increased debility, ADL weaknesses, and presence of multiple dependencies.

Most of the quality analyses were stated in terms of process quality rather than outcome quality. The necessity for a linkage between the two was, of course, recognized by the Colorado group. Among the more important quality conclusions, again admittedly tentative, were the following:

- Quality of care varied among individual long-term care clients in the sample. This finding was singled out as a subject for future research.
- Residents in skilled level situations experience higher quality than intermediate level residents for four of the six nursing-related problems and one of three medical care-related problems. Their quality scores were lower, however, in three of the four communication skill problem areas and three of the five sociopsychological areas.
- In general, average quality falls as age, numbers of problems, and functional disability increase. This finding demands more research.
- Average facility quality scores were higher in for-profit than in non-profit facilities. Psycho-social care tends to be better in larger and for-profit facilities than in non-profit and smaller facilities. Other facility characteristics appear unrelated to process quality.
- The interaction among process quality, outcome quality, case-mix, facility attributes, and cost must be further analyzed.

As stated, the initial cost analyses focused heavily on average total and operating costs per resident day and on the nursing and nurses aides costs. Free-standing facilities are about $10 per day less expensive than hospital-based facilities. This accords with other findings but should be researched further.

- Nursing and nursing aide costs are the largest components of operating cost per patient day, accounting for 44 percent. Room and board accounted for 35 percent, administrative costs for 17 percent, and special therapies and ancillary activities for 4 percent.

717

- Property costs accounted for 13 percent of total costs. The range was very wide, however, from 4 percent to 22 percent of total costs. In general, they account for 15 percent of average operating costs.
- For-profit facilities tended to have lower operating costs than did the non-profits. The same was true for facilities having larger proportions of Medicaid residents. Other facility characteristics were not related to total cost, average operating cost, and room and board costs.
- Nursing and aide costs were not related to facility control but rather to level of care (SNF versus ICF), possibly because of certification staffing requirements.
- About 20 percent of the homes could not meet facility operating costs in 1978. Revenues for the remaining 80 percent exceeded costs. For 20 percent of the facilities studied, Medicaid reimbursement rates were below costs, but 32 percent had rates 10 or more percentage points above costs. The average facility receives two-thirds of revenues from Medicaid reimbursement.
- Future research should analyze the costs of treating patients with different types of problems, at different quality levels, and under different sources of payment. The analysis of the quality/cost effects of services should be part of the same effort.
- Regional wage-price differences should be examined with respect to influences on costs.
- The relationship between Medicaid reimbursement and cost, quality, and case-mix needs further analysis.

Clearly, many of the factors analyzed in the Colorado study interact in complex ways. These relationships are often too convoluted to be revealed by other than multivariate techniques. Accordingly, the data were specifically examined for interrelationships. Findings were as follows:

- Case-mix, quality, and facility characteristics account for a substantial proportion of the variance in costs, between 68 percent and 75 percent in operating and nursing and aide costs per day.
- Functional disabilities (ADL) account for 38 percent of the variance in operating cost per day and 50 percent of that in nursing cost per day.
- Combining information on functional dependency (ADL) with that on groups of long-term care problems provides better indicators of the relationship between case-mix and cost than does either of those measures alone.
- Cost measures are more strongly related to nursing and medical care quality scores than to those for other problem groupings.

718

There appears to be an interaction between these two types of quality, that is, as quality increases for both problem groups, the actual cost of high quality care may diminish because of economies of scale.

- If case-mix and quality are taken into account, facility characteristics (other than non-profit versus for-profit) do not influence costs. Non-profits have higher operating costs per day, but nursing and aide costs appear not to be significantly linked to facility control.
- Certification level was not a significant influence on costs because it had, presumably, been picked up in the staffing and case-mix variables.
- Operating cost per day is negatively influenced by proportion of Medicaid residents. Nursing and aide costs are not. The interaction among Medicaid share and cost, case-mix, and quality should be further examined to determine if Medicaid patients in need of high quality (cost) care cannot get access to such care.
- The impact of for-profit versus non-profit control on cost, case-mix, and quality operating together needs further study.
- Similarly, the relationship among certification level, percentage of skilled care residents, staffing ratios, and more direct measures of case-mix and quality (process and outcome) are needed.

Although the Colorado procedures apparently allow the simultaneous analysis of case-mix, quality, and cost for an examination of their interrelationships, some difficulties remain. First, the analysis thus far is based on one year's work and relates only to nursing homes in Colorado. Second, as with the DRGs, the standards of quality of care are determined by practitioners, mainly in the nursing and health fields. Consequently, the approach may be excessively medical for groups of vulnerables whose difficulties may be more social, psycho-social, income-related, or housing-related. Means of diluting the institutional bias toward the nursing home have to be found if the Colorado methods are to assist with a broad range of long-term problems and if they are to be applicable to alternative sites of care. The use of the Katz, Landes, and Kahn methods of assessment by Colorado for ADL and long-term care "problems" are encouraging in this regard.

References

Birnbaum, Howard, Christine Bishop, Gail Jensen, A. James Lee, and Douglas Wilson, *Reimbursement Strategies for Nursing Home Care: Developmental Cost Studies,* 2 volumes, prepared for the Health Care Financing Administration under DHEW Contract No. 600–77–0068. (Cambridge, Mass.: Abt, 1979).

Bishop, Christine, "Nursing Home Cost Studies and Reimbursement Issues," *Health Care Financing Review,* Spring 1980, pp. 47–64.

Bishop, Christine E., Alonzo L. Plough, and Thomas W. Willemain, "Nursing Home Levels of Care: Problems and Alternatives," *Health Care Financing Review,* Fall 1980, pp. 33–45.

Bruun, Robert L., "A Patient Classification Methodology for Estimating Nursing Resource Requirements in Long Term Care Facilities," Ph.D. dissertation, Johns Hopkins University, Baltimore, Maryland, 1980.

Cotterill, Philip G., "Casemix and Cost: A Study of the Difference Between the Routine Per Diem Operating Costs of Hospital-Based and Free-Standing SNFs," Report, DRS, OR, ORDS, HCFA, April 1980

Deane, Robert T. and Douglas E. Skinner, "Development of a Formula Incentive Reimbursement System for Long-Term Care," Applied Management Sciences, Inc. under DHEW Contract No. 100–76–0029, April 20, 1978.

Fetter, Robert B., Youngsoo Shin, Jean L. Freeman, Richard F. Averill, and John D. Thompson, "Case Mix by Diagnosis-Related Groups," *Medical Care,* February 1980 (Supplement).

Frech, H. E. III and Paul Ginsburg, "The Cost of Nursing Home Care in the United States: Government Financing, Ownership, and Efficiency," paper presented at the World Congress on Health Economics, Leiden, The Netherlands, September 1980 (revised version, November 1980; mimeo).

LaPorte, Valerie and Jeffrey Rubin, eds., *Reform and Regulation in Long-Term Care.* (New York: Praeger, 1979.)

McCaffree, Kenneth M., Jean Baker, and Edward B. Perrin, "Long-Time Case Mix, Employee Time and Costs," prepared for National Center for Health Services Research, DHEW, Final Report on Contract No. HRA–230–76–0285 (Seattle: Battelle Human Affairs Research Centers, February 28, 1979).

McCaffree, Kenneth M., Lawrence Muller, and R. P. Johnson, "An Economic Analysis of the Production Process in Washington State Nursing Homes," prepared for the National Center for Health Services Research, DHEW, Report on Grant No. HS 01582 (Seattle: Battelle Human Affairs Research Centers, December 31, 1975).

McCaffree, Kenneth M., Sharon Winn, and Carl A. Bennett, "Final Report of Cost Data Reporting System for Nursing Home Care," prepared for American Association of Homes for the Aging and American Health Care Association under Grant No. HS 01114–01A1 and HS 01115–01A1 from Division of Long Term Care, National Center for Health Services Research, DHEW (Seattle: Battelle Human Affairs Research Centers, October 1, 1976; revised March 1977).

Meiners, Mark R., "Nursing Home Costs: A Statistical Cost Function Analysis Using National Survey Data," unpublished Ph.D. dissertation, Georgetown University, December, 1978.

Morrisey, Michael A., "The Effects of Reimbursement on Nursing Home Services," paper presented at the 54th Annual Conference of the Western Economic Association, June 17–21, 1979 (mimeo).

Ruchlin, Hirsch S. and Samuel Levey, "Nursing Home Cost Analysis: A Case Study," *Inquiry,* Fall, 1972, pp. 3–15.

Shaughnessy, Peter, Robert Schlenker, Barbara Harley, Nancy H. Shanks, Gerri Tricario, Vann Perry, Bettina Kurowski, and Arlene Woodson, *Long-Term Care Reimbursement and Regulation: A Study of Cost, Casemix*

720

and Quality, Working Paper No. 4, University of Colorado, Center for Health Services Research, 1980. (Report prepared pursuant to HCFA Grant No. 18–P–97145/8–01.)

Skinner, Douglas E. and Donald E. Yett, "Estimation of Cost Functions for Health Services: "The Nursing Home Case," paper presented to the Southern Economic Association, November 1970 (mimeo).

Vladeck, Bruce, *Unloving Care: The Nursing Home Tragedy.* New York: Basic Books, 1980.

Walsh, Thomas J., "Patient-Related Reimbursement for Long-Term Care," in LaPorte, Valerie and Jeffrey Rubin, eds., *Reform and Regulation in Long-Term Care* (New York: Praeger, 1979, pp. 153–167).

721

CHAPTER XX

The Labor Supply Question

by Jeffrey H. Horen

As Chapter I describes, the increasing number of elderly people could present a significant economic burden for the working population, and may do so in the forseeable future. The long-term care sector of the health care industry is expanding to meet this growing demand. The resource most critical to this expansion is manpower because long-term care is a labor intensive industry.[1]

This chapter examines aspects of the labor supply question in long-term care from a microeconomic perspective, viewing labor as an input to the production of long-term care. Classical microeconomic models of an industry depend on certain restrictive assumptions regarding the motives of firms and consumers, production technology, information flow, and freedom of entry. Under assumptions of perfect competition, any input will be supplied in the quantity that is optimal to the society. If there are exogenous changes in the system that change the optimal amount of the input, such as increased demand for the final product, then the models imply that the industry will adjust to use the input at the new optimal level.

Health care planners and administrators generally perceive that there is a shortage of labor in the long-term care industry, that is, the quantity of labor falls below what they perceive to be the optimal level. Therefore, the labor economics models, based on demand and supply equilibrium—making a "shortage" impossible—are at variance with the perceptions of the labor market of many health planners in long-term care. In this chapter we shall examine the reasons for the general perception of shortages.

In the first section we consider the need for manpower as seen by health care planners. The following section explores "shortage" and offers three alternative definitions of this concept. Next we propose some microeconomic models to explain the shortage by the three definitions in the supply of labor for long-term care. In the final section, we accordingly revise our view of the labor supply question and then discuss the feasibility of possible solutions.

---

[1] For example, according to the 1977 National Nursing Home Survey (National Center for Health Statistics, 1979), labor costs constituted 60 percent of all nursing home costs.

Manpower Needs as Seen by Planners

Many recent studies of long-term care examine current manpower availability and estimate requirements.[2]

Nursing personnel and service personnel compose the major category of personnel in nursing homes, and within this category, nurses' aides constitute the largest segment. As Table XX–1 shows, 89 percent of nursing home personnel were in nursing or service, including 65.6 percent who were nurses' aides. This percentage of service workers is the highest of all sectors in the health care industry.

In 1977, the Bureau of Labor Statistics compiled projections of the 1985 demand for selected occupations in long-term care. These projections are frequently cited in other manpower studies. They are based on a detailed method of estimation, briefly outlined below.

- The size and demographic composition of the labor force for the target year are projected from census data.
- Using assumptions of unemployment and output per demographic group, these labor force projections are translated into a projected 1985 level of the real gross national product (GNP).
- A macroeconomic model is used to distribute the potential growth in real GNP among consumer expenditures and other major demand components and then into subcategories. For example, seven of the 82 subcategories of consumer expenditures are for medical care.
- The estimates of demand by product or service are then allocated to industries using an input-output table developed for the U.S. economy by the Department of Commerce.
- Estimates of production by industry are translated into employment requirements using figures on average weekly hours worked and worker productivity that are estimated from past data and assessment of future trends.
- Projections of industry employment requirements are translated into occupational requirements using an industry-occupational matrix for 200 industries and 425 occupations.

According to the resulting projections, nursing home employment requirements will grow 73 percent between 1976 and 1985, reaching 1,431,000 persons in 1985. The projected annual rate of increase

---

[2] For example, in the legislative branch of the Federal government, studies have been done by the U.S. Senate Special Committee on Aging 1975) and the Congressional Budget Office (1977). In the Executive branch, the Department of Commerce has surveyed manpower requirements through the Bureau of the Census (1978). The Department of Health and Human Services has done related studies, through the Administration on Aging (1980), the Federal Council on the Aging (1981), the National Center for Health Statistics (1979), and the Bureau of Manpower Education (1980).

TABLE XX-1
Occupational Categories of Nursing Home Employees: 1977

Category	Number	Percent
Total	647,700	100.0
Administrative, Medical, and Therapeutic	70,600	10.9
Registered Nurse	66,900	10.3
Licensed Practical Nurse	85,100	13.1
Nurses Aide	424,900	65.6
(Total Nurses)	*(576,900)*	*(89.1)*

Source: U.S. Department of Health, Education, and Welfare, National Center for Health Statistics, *The National Nursing Home Survey: 1977 Summary for the United States.*

from 1976 to 1985 is 6.3 percent, compared with 4 percent for all the health industries combined. As a result, the proportion of employment in the total health industry that is in nursing homes is projected to rise from 14 percent in 1976 to 17 percent in 1985.[3]

Table XX–2 shows data from the Bureau of Labor Statistics on nursing home industry employment by occupational group. Requirements for professional and technical workers are expected to reach 157,000 by 1985; 101,000 for these are registered nurses. The number of health service workers is expected to reach 690,000, of whom 538,000 are nursing aides, orderlies, and attendants. This is the largest single category of workers, representing almost 38 percent of nursing home employment.

An unpublished dissertation based on an input-output model contains another set of projections (Bruun, 1980). Bruun classifies nursing home patients into groups defined by the level of care required and then uses regression analysis to estimate the amount of nursing care from each type of personnel (for example, RN, LPN, orderly) needed for a unit in each group. He then applies these estimates to the patient data collected from the National Nursing Home Survey and population projections to estimate the number of personnel needed now and in the future.

The resulting projections are summarized in Table XX–3. The figures for 1990 are comparable to those from the Bureau of Labor Statistics. As in Table XX–2, the greatest requirements are for orderlies and RNs.

[3] These figures are derived from unpublished data from the Bureau of Labor Statistics and are listed in "Human Resource Issues in the Field of Aging: The Nursing Home Industry (Revised)," *AoA Occasional Papers in Gerontology*, No. 1.

725

TABLE XX-2
Nursing Home Industry Employment
by Occupational Group, 1976 and Projected 1985

Occupational Group	1976	1985
Total, all Occupations	828,000	1,431,000
Professional, Technical, Kindred	111,000	157,000
Medical Workers, Except Technical	90,000	121,000
Health Technologists and Technicians	2,000	3,000
Managers, officials, proprietors	49,000	73,000
Sales workers	1,000	2,000
Clerical workers	40,000	82,000
Craft and kindred workers	9,000	17,000
Operatives	22,000	52,000
Service workers	591,000	1,037,000
Cleaning Service Workers	68,000	138,000
Food Service Workers	96,000	172,000
Health Service Workers	404,000	690,000
Personal Service Workers	21,000	33,000
Laborers, except Farm	6,000	11,000

Note: Because of rounding, individual items may not equal total.
Source: Bureau of Labor Statistics.

Turning to the projected need for physicians, the Graduate Medical Education National Advisory Committee (GMENAC) issued a report in 1980 on the projected supply of physicians to 1990. The estimates were based on a methodology adapted from the delphic method, using panels of representatives from each specialty field. The report caused heated debate in the health care community over the central finding that the U.S. will have an oversupply of 70,000 physicians and a surplus in 15 of 27 specialty groups by 1990.

None of the specialty groups that the study defined, however, were equivalent to geriatric medicine or long-term care. Thus, even if GMENAC's conclusions about an oversupply of physicians are valid, they do not directly relate to long-term care. Furthermore, the exclusion of geriatrics as a specialty is indicative of the relative inattention given to this field of medicine in the past.

A recent study by the Rand Corporation does project needs for geriatric physicians (Kane, 1980). The report estimates that the U.S. will need between 7,000 and 10,300 geriatricians by 1990, as compared to the 629 physicians in 1977 who reported geriatrics as one of their specialties.

TABLE XX-3
Projection of Nursing Personnel Requirements
from 1980 to 2000

	Actual	Projected			
	1977	1980	1985	1990	2000
Nursing Personnel Requirements (Full-time equivalents)					
RN	66,900	86,803	96,248	105,997	127,167
LPN	85,100	81,053	89,873	98,976	118,843
Aide/Orderly	424,900	417,862	463,327	540,258	612,680
Total	576,900	585,718	649,448	745,231	858,690

Note: The projection assumes that the ratio of institutional population to the total population by age is constant at the 1977 ratio and that the distribution of nursing home residents among classes is constant.
Source: Brunn, 1980

Although manpower requirements are difficult to estimate, these reports, along with those of many other writers in the health care field, are nearly unanimous in the opinion that manpower in long-term care falls short of current requirements (as they perceive them) and that in the future these requirements will grow.[4] In the following sections we shall re-examine these stated "needs" in the context of labor economic analysis.

The Meaning of "Shortage"

The previous section discussed aspects of long-term care (LTC) manpower as seen by various health care planners. The concensus of the studies was that shortages of manpower exist for the important categories of personnel, and that these shortages will continue for many years.

An analysis of a shortage requires a definition of "shortage" because the meaning is not clear. In this section we introduce three definitions that have been suggested by economists. In the next section we shall discuss some models of shortages that may be relevant to LTC manpower in terms of these definitions.

The remainder of this chapter presumes that the reader is familiar with the fundamentals of economic markets for consumer goods, that is, supply and demand analysis. For review, the interested reader can refer to any standard economics text.

Consider a competitive market for a labor input such as LTC nursing. Figure XX–1 illustrates the market supply curve SS′ and

---

[4] See, for example, Heilman (1981) and Sandroff (1980).

FIGURE XX-1

Types of Shortage

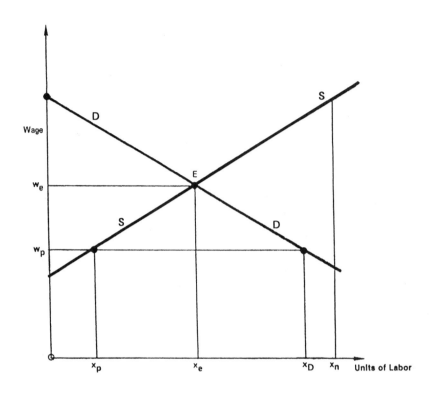

demand curve DD' The demand curve is derived from the individual firms' value of marginal product (*VMP*) curves and the supply curve is externally given. The curves intersect at the equilibrium point E. The equilibrium wage is w_e and the quantity of labor employed is x_e.

If the wage rate is below the equilibrium wage rate then a *market shortage* can occur. Suppose that the prevailing rate is w_p in Figure XX–1. Then the quantity demanded at this wage, x_D, exceeds the quantity supplied, x_p. Here the market shortage is $x_D - x_p$. This is the number of job vacancies that should occur for the wage w_p.

If the market is in equilibrium then there is no shortage in the market sense. At wage w_e, the number of people willing to work equals the number of openings, both x_e.

Another concept of shortage is used by planners. The *planning shortage* may be stated as the difference between the number "needed" for an industry and the number available or currently employed. Suppose that x_n is the number of LTC nurses that the planner states is needed. Then the shortage in the planning sense is $x_n - x_e$. Note that at wage w_p there is also a planning shortage of $x_n - x_p$.

A third concept of shortage is its economic definition. An *economic shortage* of an input exists if the marginal benefit to society exceeds the marginal cost of obtaining the input at the present quantity. If we consider the demand curve in Figure XX–1 as the marginal benefit curve of society (aggregated from the *VMP* curves of the individual firms) and the supply curve as the marginal expenditure curve of society, then there is a shortage in this third sense at x_p. Here the marginal benefit (demand price) exceeds the marginal cost (supply price). Therefore the last unit of x adds more benefit than it costs, meaning that the total surplus (benefit minus cost) could be increased by increasing the quantity of x. In fact, there is an economic shortage for any x to the left of x_e because the net benefit to society can be improved by increasing x. (Similarly, if x is greater than x_e then there is an *economic surplus* of x because the last unit of x has a higher cost than benefit. Thus, reducing x increases the net benefit.) Therefore x_e is the optimal quantity of x in the economic sense. The economic shortage for wage w_p is $x_e - x_p$.

We see then, that the existence and the amount of a shortage depends on how we define this term. In a competitive market, a shortage in the market sense or in the economic sense will not exist if the market is in equilibrium. But a planning shortage may exist if the stated need is large enough.

Current "needs" for an input such as labor are sometimes estimated by aggregating the estimated needs of firms in an industry. This method assumes the validity of a typical firm's stated needs. Future needs for LTC labor can also sometimes be pro-

729

jected by multiplying the current ratio of workers to patients by the estimated future patient population. This method assumes that the input is currently being used in the right quantities. Economists like to point out that a "need" has no clear meaning in the economic sense.

If needs were equated with wants, then our needs for any resource or product would be essentially unlimited. By this reasoning there should be shortages in every industry. For example there should be a "shortage" of Rolls Royces, since many people who would want a Rolls Royce do not have one. However, there is a definite perception of a "shortage" of manpower in LTC, and in the health industry in general, that is *not* stated elsewhere. This feeling is expressed by planners, administrators, and government studies (Sandroff, 1980).

Why then is a shortage seen as more critical in this industry? Using Figure XX–1, we suggest two reasons. First, if the market is not in equilibrium there may be a market shortage. Second, the perceived "need" x_n may exceed the equilibrium quantity x_e in LTC manpower more so than in other industries, even though the market is in equilibrium.

A relatively large $x_n - x_e$ may also occur from an inter-temporal change in market conditions. To illustrate, consider a "shortage" in another industry. In 1980, peanut crop failures caused a 45 percent reduction in the supply of peanuts. The market price increased from $.35/lb. in 1979 to $1.40/lb. in 1980. At this latter price the quantity supplied supposedly equaled the quantity demanded. Presumably there was no market shortage. Yet people spoke of a "peanut shortage." Why? There were fewer peanuts available in 1980 than at the previous year's prices. Alternatively, the number currently sold was smaller than last year.

In either case, the "need" stemmed from the difference in quantity that was previously available. Since market conditions changed in this particular industry to reduce the available quantity, a "shortage" arose. Therefore, the shortage can arise from a *change* in market conditions. (If peanuts had always cost $1.40 per pound and sold in the same quantities, then there would not have been a perceived shortage in 1980).

The following section discusses shortages, as we have defined them, that are caused by a change in market conditions.

Microeconomic Models of Labor Shortages

Two similar economic models were formulated to explain perceived shortages in the market for engineers in the 1950s. Both were applied by Donald Yett (1975) to the shortage of nurses (not necessarily in LTC). Both models are based on a change in market conditions and can be applied to any input market where the

730

demand is expanding faster than the supply. In this section we shall briefly describe both models and then use them to explain the perceived shortage of LTC manpower.

The first model, by David M. Blank and George J. Stigler (1957), defines a shortage as the market shortage that would exist at the wage rate that the firms are "used to." Figure XX–2 illustrates this concept for a simplified two-period version of the model. Suppose that the market for input x is at a competitive equilibrium in period 1 with demand $D_1 D'_1$ and supply $S_1 S'_1$. The wage is w_1 and quantity of input is X_1. Suppose that, due to increased demand for nursing home care, the input demand curve shifts in the next period to $D_2 D'_2$, but the supply curve shifts only to $S_2 S'_2$. Thus the supply of the input is increasing, but not as fast as the demand. The new equilibrium wage, w_2, is higher than w_1. If the market reaches equilibrium, then there is no market shortage or economic shortage. But Blank and Stigler assert that firms may perceive a shortage in period 2 because they would want more of x than is available at the period 1 wage of w_1. The perceived shortage is $x_{22} - x_{21}$ in Figure XX–2.

Suppose that the demand for long-term care labor, induced by the growing demand for nursing home care, increases faster than the supply. Then, according to this model, if nursing home operators do not expect wages to increase upward, they may perceive a labor shortage.

The second model, by Kenneth J. Arrow and William M. Capron (1959), is similar to the Blank-Stigler model. If demand increases faster than supply, Arrow and Capron assert that a market shortage can result if wages are slow to reach market equilibrium.

The Arrow-Capron model requires the following assumptions:

- Market demand and supply curves are linear, exogeneously determined.
- The demand curve is moving to the right over time relatively faster than the supply curve.
- The current wage is not the instantaneous market equilibrium wage but lags somewhere below this wage. However, the wage increases over time at a rate of speed that is proportional to the excess of demand over supply at the current wage.

Thus, Arrow and Capron hypothesize that the actual wage may be slow to adjust to the market equilibrium. This delay creates a shortage.

To illustrate, Figure XX–3 shows the same pairs of supply and demand curves as Figure XX–2.[5] Again, let the market be at

---

[5] Arrow and Capron actually assume a stationary supply curve and a moving demand curve, but this case can easily be generalized to that of a supply curve that moves more slowly than the demand curve.

FIGURE XX-2

Blank-Stigler Model of Input Shortage

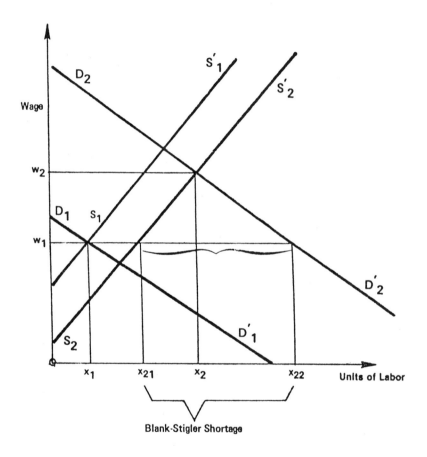

Blank-Stigler Shortage

FIGURE XX-3

Arrow-Capron Model of Input Shortage

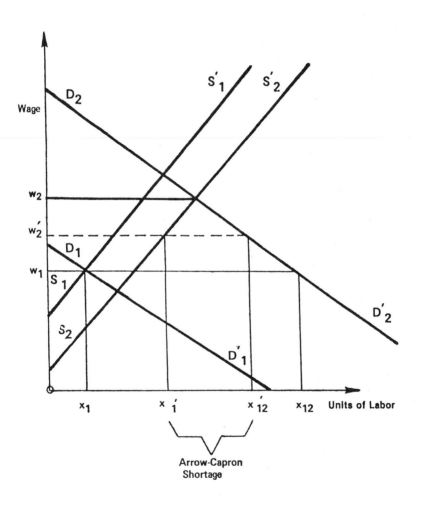

equilibrium in period 1 with wage w_1. If demand and supply shift in period 2 as before, then at wage w_1 there is a market shortage of $x_{12} - x_1$. Rather than moving instantaneously to the new equilibrium, suppose that the prevailing wage is slow to adjust, and in period 2 rises to w'_2, less than w_2. Then there is an actual market shortage of $x'_{12} - x'_1$. At this point, the speed at which the wage increases, which Arrow and Capron call the "reaction speed," is proportional to the shortage $x'_{12} - x'_1$.

The appendix to this chapter contains the formulation of the model and analysis. The results show that the market wage increases over time. The amount of the shortage also *increases* over time, approaching an upper limit. Therefore if such a formulation serves as a valid model of the nursing home industry, we should not expect the market shortage to vanish as long as demand continues to increase.

We see that the simplied forms of the two models differ only in where the "real" wage moves. Blank and Stigler assume that w reaches equilibrium immediately and define the shortages as perceived. Arrow and Capron assume that w lags behind the equilibrium and define the shortage as the actual market shortage. Both, however, rely on the major assumption of demand increasing faster than supply. We suggest that either market model (and definition of shortage) is appropriate for explaining current "shortages" of LTC manpower.

The most important assumption of both models is dynamically increasing demand for the input. As indicated throughout this book, demand for nursing home care has increased for many reasons, such as growth in Medicaid payments, health insurance, and tax incentives. This increased demand for the product has been passed on to increased demand for manpower (the input) in the manner discussed in the previous section.

On the supply side, the manpower supply has expanded relatively slowly in health care, particularly for nursing homes. Expanding employment opportunities for women in non-health care fields and improved wages and working conditions for nurses in hospitals have made nursing homes a less desirable location for nurses. This change lowers the supply curve for LTC nurses because fewer nurses are willing to work for a given wage. Increased welfare benefits raise the opportunity costs of jobs of attending to the needs of the elderly and make them less desirable in comparison. Here again, the increased welfare benefits move back the supply curve for nurses' aids. Therefore demand increases faster than supply, and we can expect the perceived shortage of the Blank-Stigler model.

In addition, wages may be slow to adjust upward. Arrow and Capron suggest that this slow adjustment can result from:

> ... the time it takes the firm to recognize the existence of a shortage at the current salary level, the time it takes to decide upon the need for higher salaries and the number of vacancies at such salaries, and either the time it takes employees to recognize the salary alternatives available and to act upon this information or the time it takes the firm to equalize salaries without outside offers.

All of these factors may be true for nursing homes as well as for other firms.

In addition, however, many nursing homes are reimbursed either by cost or at a flat rate, as discussed in Chapter XVIII. If a nursing home is reimbursed at cost, then the wage that a nursing home offers in year 2 may be based on reimbursement for costs (and prevailing wage rate) in year 1, causing a lag in adjustment.

If a nursing home is reimbursed at a flat rate, the operator may be more reluctant to raise wages unless the reimbursement rate is raised. A recent empirical study of nursing home wages (Borjas, Frech, and Ginsburg, 1981) concludes that flat-rate reimbursement tends to hold down wage rates of nursing home staff. Therefore, the structure of nursing home reimbursement may be an added hindrance to the adjustment of wages, one that is not found in other industries.

For both the Blank-Stigler and Arrow-Capron models, we assume that demand for LTC labor increases relatively faster than supply. If either model is valid, we may turn to the supply side and ask why, in the long run, the rising wage does not induce a greater increase in supply. We suggest that the movement of labor into long-term care is less than into other industries. As Vladek (1980) and many others point out, attending the elderly is considered an unpleasant job. Accordingly, the annual turnover rate for nursing home orderlies is estimated to be 50 percent. (See Vladek, 1980.) The degree of mobility of labor into LTC is, however, an empirical question.

Imperfect competition in the input market from the buyers' side is another reason for an economic shortage of an input that is also a perceived shortage. G. C. Archibald (1954) used this scenario to explain hiring behavior in the market for skilled craftsmen.

Figure XX–4 illustrates the market for a monopsony. The demand curve of a single firm for labor is given by dd' and the market supply curve faced by the firm is given by SS'. The curve EE' depicts the firm's marginal expenditure, defined as the additional cost in total wages to the firm in hiring one additional unit of the input x. The

FIGURE XX-4

Input Demand for a Monopsonistic Firm

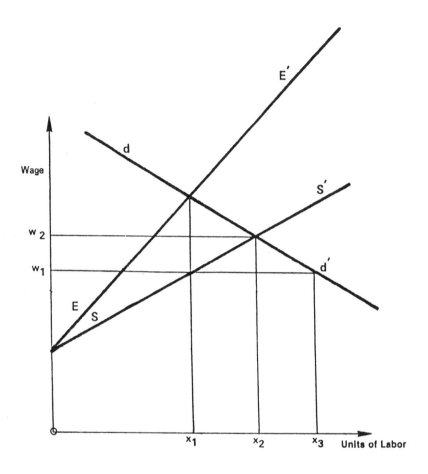

curve EE' lies above the supply curve SS' because, for a given x, the cost of hiring one more unit is the unit wage for x (given by SS') *plus* the increase in wage that must be paid to the units before x.

If dd' was a competitive market demand curve, then the competitive equilibrium would be the intersection of dd' and SS' in Figure XX–4, at wage w_2 and input quantity x_2. However, a profit-maximizing monopsonist will hire the quantity of x where the curve dd' (which is also the marginal revenue curve) intersects the marginal expenditure curve EE'.

In Figure XX–4, this is at wage w_1 and quantity x_1. The monopsonistic wage w_1 is below the competitive market wage of w_2 and the input quantity x_1 is less than the competitive equilibrium quantity x_2. Therefore there is an economic shortage of $x_2 - x_1$. Furthermore, the monopsonist would be willing to hire more labor X if it were available at wage w_1 up to $x = x_3$, where the dd' curve falls to w_1. The input buyer has $x_3 - x_1$ vacancies at the current wages w_1. Therefore we have a perceived shortage. The analysis can be extended to oligopsonies (markets with few buyers) with similar results.

The markets for low-skilled labor in nursing homes are probably competitive. However, a market for hospital nurses within a geographical area is frequently modeled as oligopsonistic. To the degree that there may be few nursing homes within geographic areas, the market for nurses in general may show some degree of imperfect competition. Therefore, some market shortages may be caused by imperfect competition. The degree of competition for nurses for nursing homes, however, is an empirical question.

Our discussion of shortages emphasizes that we must re-evaluate the concept of a "need" for LTC labor. Meeting any need entails a cost. The cost is the resources that are used to meet other "needs." In the final section we discuss ways of reducing the perceived shortage of LTC labor while remaining aware of these costs.

Summary and Conclusions

We have shown that the "shortage" in LTC manpower can result from rapidly increasing demand for the product, and the institutional factors that hinder rapid adjustment by the market. If the Arrow-Capron model is valid then the slow adjustment creates both a market shortage and an economic shortage of labor. One recommendation is to facilitate adjustment by the market. For example, one can disseminate information on position openings and salaries or change the reimbursement mechanisms. But here we are assuming that market equilibrium is the ideal state. This assumption is true only if the market demand curve for labor represents the real marginal benefit to society and the supply curve, the true marginal cost.

Statements in other chapters lead us to question this first premise. Some demand may be artificially induced by government reimbursement, health insurance, and tax laws. That is, the price offered on the demand curve for a certain quantity of nursing home services does not represent the real benefit to the consumer. This distortion in demand for the final product is then passed on to the demand for labor input.

Therefore, facilitating adjustment of the input market so that the quantity of labor supplied equals the quantity demanded may not lead to the most desirable outcome. If the demand for inputs is artificially high then the induced supply may in turn be too high.

A better general solution to the "shortages" of labor, then, may be to reduce the demand for the final product, nursing home care. Many studies have indicated this, asserting that patients in nursing homes would be more appropriately cared for in other settings. For example, the Congressional Budget Office (1977) concludes that:

> . . . a number of persons in Skilled Nursing Facilities and Intermediate Care Facilities either do not need the presumably high level or degree of care provided or could be maintained at home if adequate home care services were available.

The study goes on to suggest, among other possible plans, liberalized Medicare and Medicaid coverage of home health services. A fiscally conservative approach might be, alternatively, to lower the Medicaid and other present incentives for nursing home care. Either suggestion would make nursing home care relatively less desirable and lower the demand for it. Therefore the question of shortages of supply of labor in long-term care may be better addressed by focusing our attention on the causes of increasing demand.

The previous section also suggested that shortages may be caused by imperfect competition in the input market. Any solution to this condition would involve radical changes in the structure of the market. For example, we could take steps to increase the mobility of nurses or encourage more and smaller nursing homes, thereby losing some advantages of scale. It is doubtful that the benefit of more competition would justify such extreme measures.

As the section on labor economics mentioned, if the price of one input increases, it is economical to substitute other inputs for it. We ask if this is feasible with respect to labor in nursing homes. Since labor is relatively scarce, can other resources be substituted for it? Or can less skilled labor, such as nurses' aides, be substituted for more skilled labor, such as RNs?

Nursing homes, unfortunately, are a labor–intensive industry. We cannot see how other resources can be economically substituted for labor. (Graphically speaking, the isoquants between labor and non-labor would be very steep.) Furthermore, with regard to substitution of less skilled labor for more skilled labor, it appears that this has been done already. As Table XX–1 showed, nurses' aides greatly outnumber RNs and LPNs. Thus, nursing homes already seem to have revised their input mixes in response to market forces.

As this chapter shows, specific policy recommendations for the "shortage" of labor in the long-term care industry require the answer to certain empirical questions. Below we reiterate some of these questions:

- Is the demand for long-term care increasing? Does this induce an increase in the demand for long-term care labor?
- Do the reimbursement mechanisms or any other factors cause slower adjustment of wages to market conditions in the nursing home industry than in other industries?
- What is the degree of competition among nursing homes in the markets for labor?
- How mobile is labor transferring into the long-term care sector?

Subject to our limited answers to these questions, we believe that the best way to address the problem of labor shortage in nursing homes is to focus our attention on the demand for nursing home care. To solve the problem, we may need to direct more resources into alternative modes of care, as other chapters assert. In any event, we must face the fact that any long-range solution to this problem will entail a sizeable and permanent cost.

Appendix

This appendix contains a mathematical formulation of the Arrow-Capron model of a labor shortage. The analysis is identical to that in Arrow and Capron (1959), except that their assumption that supply is stationary and demand is dynamically increasing is generalized here to that of demand dynamically increasing relatively faster than supply.

Let w be the current wage, D, demand, S, supply, and t, the time. The market movement over time is formulated as:

$$D = -aw + c + et, \tag{1}$$

$$S = bw + d + ft, \tag{2}$$

$$\frac{dw}{dt} = k (D - S) \tag{3}$$

$$\text{and } e > f \tag{4}$$

where a, b, c, d, e, f, and k are positive constants.

FIGURE XX-A-1
Illustration of Arrow-Capron Shortage

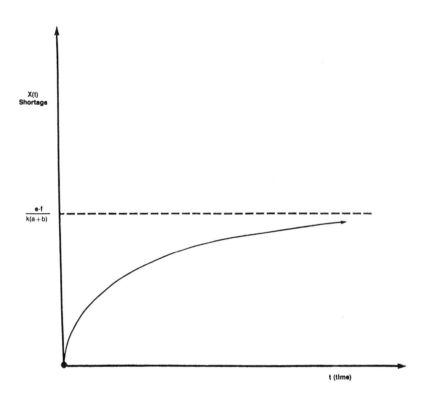

Equations (1) and (2) are assumptions that the supply and demand curves are linear in w and increasing linearly in time. Equation (3) expresses the assumption that the wage rises in proportion to the current shortage. The constant k determines the "reaction speed," or the rate at which w rises. Equation (4) means that demand increases faster than supply.

Let X represent the shortage, that is, $X = D - S$.

From (1) and (2),

$$X = -(a + b)w + (c - d) + (e - f)t \qquad (5)$$

Differentiating (5) with respect to time t,

$$dX/dt = -(a + b)(dw/dt) + e - f \qquad (6)$$

Now (3) can be rewritten using $X = D - S$,

$$\frac{dw}{dt} = kX \qquad (7)$$

Substituting (7) for dw/dt into (6),

$$dX/dt = -(a + b)kX + e - f \qquad (8)$$

Assume that at the beginning there is no shortage. Then,

$$X = 0 \text{ at } t = 0 \qquad (9)$$

Equations (8) and (9) specify a differential equation with the unique solution

$$X = \frac{-(e - f)}{k(a + b)} \exp[-(a + b)kt] + \frac{e - f}{(a + b)k} \qquad (10)$$

where exp is the exponential function. Differentiating (10) we see that,

$$\frac{dX}{dt} = (e - f) \exp[-(a + b)kt] > 0 \qquad (11)$$

and we also see from (10) that

$$\lim_{t \to \infty} X(t) = (e - f) / k(a + b) \qquad (12)$$

Therefore the shortage X is increasing over time and approaches a limit, as is shown in Figure XX–A–1. Thus Arrow and Capron's model implies a permanent and increasing market shortage.

References

Archibald, G. C., "The Factor Gap and the Level of Wages," *Economic Record*, Vol. 30, 1954, pp. 187–99.

Arrow, Kenneth J. and William M. Capron, "Dynamic Shortages and Price Rises: The Engineer-Scientist Case," *Quarterly Journal of Economics*, Vol. 73, 1959, pp. 292–308.

Blank, David M. and George J. Stigler, *The Demand and Supply of Scientific Personnel*, New York: National Bureau of Economic Research, Inc., 1957.

Borjas, G. J., H. E. Frech III, and P.B. Ginsburg, "Property Rights and Wages: The Case of Nursing Homes," Unpublished Paper, University of California, Santa Barbara, May 1981.

Bruun, Robert L., *"A Patient Classification Methodology for Estimating Nursing Resource Requirements in Long Term Care Facilities*, Unpublished Dissertation, Johns Hopkins University, 1980.

Heilman, Joan R., "Nursing—Can We Solve the Crisis?," *Parade*, March 15, 1981, pp. 21–24.

Kane, Robert L., David H. Solomon, John C. Beck, Emmet Keeler, and Rosalie A. Kane, *Geriatrics in the United States: Manpower Projections and Training Considerations* (Rand Corp. Report R–2543–HJK), Santa Monica, Ca.: The Rand Corporation, May 1980.

Kane, Robert L., David H. Solomon, John C. Beck, Emmet Keeler, and Rosalie A. Kane, "The Future Need for Geriatric Manpower in the United States," *The New England Journal of Medicine*, Vol. 302, June 12, 1980, pp. 1327–1332.

Sandroff, Ronni, "The Shortages," *RN*, November 1980, p. 55.

Smith, Phil M., *Influence of Wage Rates on Nurse Mobility*, Chicago: Graduate Program in Hospital Administration, University of Chicago, 1962.

U.S. Congress, Senate, Special Committee on Aging, *Nursing Home Care in the United States: Failure in Public Policy* (No. 1–4, 94th Congress, 1st Session). Washington, D.C.: Government Printing Office, April 1975.

U.S. Congress, Congressional Budget Office, *Long-Term Care for the Elderly and Disabled,* Washington, D.C.: Government Printing Office, 1977.

U.S. Department of Commerce, Bureau of the Census, *1976 Survey of Institutionalized Persons*, Washington, D.C.: Government Printing Office, 1978.

U.S. Department of Health, Education, and Welfare, Administration on Aging, *Human Resources in the Field of Aging: The Nursing Home Industry (Revised)*, (AoA Occasional Papers in Gerontology, No. 1), Washington, D.C.: Government Printing Office, 1980.

U.S. Department of Health, Education and Welfare, Bureau of Manpower Education, *Quantitative Measurement of Nursing Services* (Nursing Home Research Study), Washington, D.C.: Government Printing Office, 1980.

U.S. Department of Health, Education, and Welfare, National Center for Health Statistics, *The National Nursing Home Survey: 1977 Summary for the United States*, Washington, D.C.: Government Printing Office, 1979.

U.S. Department of Health and Human Services, Federal Council on Aging, *The Need for Long-Term Care*, Washington, D.C.: Government Printing Office, 1981.

U.S. Department of Health and Human Services, Public Health Service, *Report of the Graduate Medical Education National Advisory Committee to the Secretary* (DHHS Publication No. (HRA) 81–657) 1980.

Vladek, Bruce C., *Unloving Care: The Nursing Home Tragedy*, New York: Basic Books, 1980.

742

Index

Page numbers in *italics* indicate illustrations and tables.

743

744

745

748

749

754

Outpatient psychiatric care, Medicare coverage for, possible changes in, to encourage appropriate services, 493-494

Output, determinants of, in nursing home industry, 594

Outreach services of voluntary nursing homes, 533, *534*

Patient(s), nursing home
characteristics of
in nursing home cost studies, 694-696
nursing time requirements and, 709-711
condition of
cost of care and, 704-709
in nursing home cost studies, 701-712
grouping of, in nursing home cost studies, 700-701
service needs of, in nursing home cost studies, 701-712

Patient management components, long-term care system agencies providing, *59*

Payments to voluntary nursing home industry, sources and amount of, 526, *527-528*

Peer review, voluntary, in quality assurance, 117-118, 122-124

Pennsylvania
national long-term care demonstration in, 206-208
study of, on domiciliary care facilities, 446-453

Personal care facility(ies) in voluntary nursing homes, 531-532

Personal care services in Medicaid program, 154-157

Personnel staffing, integer programing approach to, 69-72

Pharmacy services, skilled nursing, capitated reimbursement for, HCFA demonstration projects on, 241-243

Physically impaired, sheltered housing program for, AMS study on, 294-295

Physician as gatekeeper, 29-30

Physician nursing home visitation, Medicaid, 204-206

Planning shortage of labor, 729

Point count system for cost-related reimbursement, 702-704

Policy goals for long-term care, 15-16

Policy issues of Health Care Financing Administration, 170

Population
effect of, on long-term care expenditures, estimation strategies for, 95-99
elderly. *See* Elderly population

Poorhouses in nursing home history, 507

Price, determinants of, in nursing home industry, 594

Price factors, private, in nursing home cost studies, 691-692

Private payment plus Medicaid coverage, nursing home demand and, 545-550

Process measures in quality measurement, 106-112

Product differentiation of nursing home services, geographical structure of market and, 592-593

Professional Standards Review Organizations, nursing homes and, 518

Product efficiency in nursing home industry, 615

Professionals
as managers, 30
as providers, 30-31

Profitability nursing home industry, 607-615

Programing, linear, 77-78

Prospective reimbursement versus retrospective, 661, *662*

Provider incentives
  Medicaid reimbursement policies
    and, 625-627
  under alternative reimbursement
    systems, 625-662
    for access, 633-653
    access improvement and,
      648-651
    analytical framework for,
      630-633
    with case-mix dependent on
      output, 641-643
    public-private allocation of
      output in, 644-646
    total output in, 643-644
    with case-mix and output
      independent, 636-641
    amenities in, 640
    private case-mix and quality
      in, 639-640
    public case-mix and quality
      in, 640-641
    public-private allocation of
      output in, 638-639
    total output in, 638
    comparison of cases 1 and 2 in,
      646-648
    for cost containment,
      652-659
    for quality, 633-652
Psychiatric care
  inpatient, Medicare coverage for,
    possible changes in, to
    encourage appropriate services,
    494-495
  limited financing for, 492
  outpatient, Medicare coverage for,
    possible changes in, to
    encourage appropriate services,
    493-494
Psychiatric day care, Medicare
  coverage for, possible changes
  in, to encourage appropriate
  services, 496
Psychological impact of family
  caregiving, 321

Psychosis with cerebral
  arteriosclerosis, 489
Public policy and lack of system, 9,
  12-13
Public provisions for long-term care,
  15-16

Quality
  measurement of, 103-128. *See
  also* Quality assurance
    introduction to, 103-104
    outcome measures in, refining,
      112-115
    studies using process and
      outcome measures in, 108-112
    studies using structure and
      process measures in,
      106-108
  of nursing home services
    incentives for, under alternative
      reimbursement systems,
      635-636
    problem of, 604-607
Quality assurance, 115-125. *See
  also* Quality, measurement of
    certification in, 117
    programs for, 118-122
    licensure in, 116
    programs for, 118-122
    medical care review in, mandatory,
      117
    programs for, 122-124
  for nursing homes, HCFA
    demonstration project on,
      247-252
    in New York State, 247-249
    in Wisconsin, 249-252
    peer review in, voluntary, 117-118,
      124-125

Reduced-form equations, in nursing
  home cost studies, 692-694
Region III study of domiciliary care
  facilities, 442-444
Rehabilitation Act of 1973 on public
  transportation, 472

758

Contributors

Wiley S. Alliston is presently a Ph.D. candidate in economics at the University of Texas. While working on this project, he was an intern in HCFA's Division of Economic Analysis.

Philip G. Cotterill received his Ph.D. in economics from Northwestern University. He is currently an economist in the Division of Economic Analysis, HCFA.

Dolores A. Cutler received her M.F.A. from the University of California, Los Angeles. She is currently a private consultant. While working on this project, she was a social science research analyst in HCFA's Division of Long-Term Care Experimentation.

Nancy T. Greenspan received her M.A. in economics from the University of North Carolina. She is chief of the Economic and Long-Range Studies Branch, Division of Economic Analysis, HCFA.

Marni J. Hall received her Ph.D. in sociology from Boston University. She is presently a sociologist in HCFA's Division of Economic Analysis.

Linda V. Hamm received her M.S.W. from the University of Maryland. She is currently Director, Division of Long-Term Care Experimentation, HCFA.

Jeffrey H. Horen received his Ph.D. in operations research from Yale University. He is a faculty member at the University of Iowa. When he was working on this project, he was a Brookings Institution Economic Policy Fellow in the Division of Economic Analysis, HCFA.

Thomas M. Kickham received his Ph.D. in economics from the University of Pittsburgh. He is currently Chief, Long-Term Care Coverage Branch, Division of Long-Term Care Experimentation, HCFA.

Bettina D. Kurowski received her D.P.A. from the University of Colorado. She is presently Director, Graduate Program in Health Administration, University of Colorado.

Korbin Liu received his Sc.D. in population sciences from Harvard University. He is currently a demographer in the Division of Economic Analysis, HCFA.

Susan Lloyd received her M.P.H. from U.C.L.A. She was an intern in the Division of Economic Analysis and is now engaged in a health and economic development project on the Ivory Coast.

763

Kenneth G. Manton received his Ph.D. in sociology from Duke University. He is currently Assistant Medical Research Professor, Duke University.

Hans C. Palmer received his Ph.D. in economics from the University of California, Berkeley. He is the Stedman-Sumner Professor of Economics at Pomona College. During the first eight months of this project, he worked in the Division of Economic Analysis on an Intergovernmental Personnel Act loan to HCFA.

Judith A. Sangl received her M.P.A. and M.P.H. from the University of Pittsburgh. For two years she was a Presidential Management Intern in the Division of Economic Analysis, HCFA. She is currently a social science research analyst there.

Peter W. Shaughnessy received his Ph.D. in mathematics from Catholic University. He is currently Director, Center for Health Services Research, University of Colorado.

Steven G. Thomas received his M.A.P.P.S. from Duke University. He was an intern in HCFA's Division of Economic Analysis and is now a budget analyst with the City of New York.

Ronald J. Vogel received his Ph.D. in economics from the University of Wisconsin. During the course of this project, he was Director, Division of Economic Analysis, HCFA. He is presently a faculty member at the University of Arizona.

Saul Waldman received his B.A. from Brooklyn College. He was a social science research analyst in the Division of Economic Analysis, HCFA, and is now retired.

764